Clinical Approach to
Pediatric Neurology

For Postgraduate Students & Practicing Pediatricians

Clinical Approach to Pediatric Neurology

For Postgraduate Students & Practicing Pediatricians

SECOND EDITION

Jaya Shankar Kaushik
MD DNB DM
Additional Professor and Head
Department of Pediatrics
All India Institute of Medical Sciences
Guwahati, Assam, India

Piyush Gupta
MD FAMS FRCPCH
Professor
Department of Pediatrics
University College of Medical Sciences and
Guru Teg Bahadur Hospital
New Delhi, India

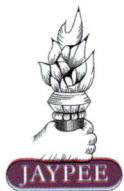

JAYPEE BROTHERS MEDICAL PUBLISHERS
The Health Sciences Publisher
New Delhi | London

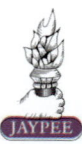 **Jaypee Brothers Medical Publishers (P) Ltd**

Headquarters
Jaypee Brothers Medical Publishers (P) Ltd
EMCA House, 23/23-B
Ansari Road, Daryaganj
New Delhi 110 002, India
Landline: +91-11-23272143, +91-11-23272703
+91-11-23282021, +91-11-23245672
Email: jaypee@jaypeebrothers.com

Corporate Office
Jaypee Brothers Medical Publishers (P) Ltd
4838/24, Ansari Road, Daryaganj
New Delhi 110 002, India
Phone: +91-11-43574357
Fax: +91-11-43574314
Email: jaypee@jaypeebrothers.com

Overseas Office
JP Medical Ltd.
83, Victoria Street, London
SW1H 0HW (UK)
Phone: +44 20 3170 8910
Fax: +44 (0)20 3008 6180
Email: info@jpmedpub.com

Website: www.jaypeebrothers.com
Website: www.jaypeedigital.com

© 2024, Jaypee Brothers Medical Publishers

The views and opinions expressed in this book are solely those of the original contributor(s)/author(s) and do not necessarily represent those of editor(s) or publisher of the book.

All rights reserved. No part of this publication may be reproduced, stored or transmitted in any form or by any means, electronic, mechanical, photocopying, recording or otherwise, without the prior permission in writing of the publishers.

All brand names and product names used in this book are trade names, service marks, trademarks or registered trademarks of their respective owners. The publisher is not associated with any product or vendor mentioned in this book.

Medical knowledge and practice change constantly. This book is designed to provide accurate, authoritative information about the subject matter in question. However, readers are advised to check the most current information available on procedures included and check information from the manufacturer of each product to be administered, to verify the recommended dose, formula, method and duration of administration, adverse effects and contraindications. It is the responsibility of the practitioner to take all appropriate safety precautions. Neither the publisher nor the author(s)/editor(s) assume any liability for any injury and/or damage to persons or property arising from or related to use of material in this book.

This book is sold on the understanding that the publisher is not engaged in providing professional medical services. If such advice or services are required, the services of a competent medical professional should be sought.

Every effort has been made where necessary to contact holders of copyright to obtain permission to reproduce copyright material. If any have been inadvertently overlooked, the publisher will be pleased to make the necessary arrangements at the first opportunity.

Inquiries for bulk sales may be solicited at: jaypee@jaypeebrothers.com

Clinical Approach to Pediatric Neurology for Postgraduate Students & Practicing Pediatricians

First Edition: 2021
Second Edition: **2024**

ISBN: 978-93-5696-760-1

Printed in India at Sterling Graphics Pvt. Ltd.

Dedicated to

Blessings of Late Smt G Vijayalakshmi (mother) for Jaya Shankar Kaushik; and also, to our students and our patients who remain our best teachers.

Preface to the Second Edition

We are delighted to present this second edition of *Clinical Approach to Pediatric Neurology for Postgraduate Students & Practicing Pediatricians.* The first edition has been received very well by the readers, including students and teachers. Pediatricians often use the book as the first reference before presenting a neurological case. Based on feedback from residents, we have included several new chapters. We hope this edition helps postgraduate students and practicing pediatricians approach clinical cases in pediatric neurology.

This edition comes up with a detailed chapter on Neurological Examination. It covers all components of neurological examination in a simple language. The chapter on developmental history and examination is a new addition in this edition, considering its importance in exam case presentation and day-to-day practice. Approach to a Child with Macrocephaly and Microcephaly, Vision Loss, and Hearing Loss are new chapters that make this edition more appealing. Cerebral palsy is the most common case presentation in the examinations, so a chapter on the Approach to a Child with Cerebral Palsy has been added to this edition. The chapter on Case of Paraplegia has been expanded with a more detailed discussion. All other chapters have been updated based on recent developments in pediatric neurology.

We sincerely thank our residents who have provided valuable feedback on the first edition, which helped us revise and update it. We have tailored the contents to make it resident-friendly with appealing flowcharts and tables. We sincerely hope this second edition becomes integral to pediatric training programs nationwide. We shall be happy to receive feedback and further suggestions for improvement to *jayashankarkaushik@gmail.com*. Please also let us know if there are any unintentional errors in the book

We thank M/s Jaypee Brothers Medical Publishers (P) Ltd, New Delhi, India for its meticulous sketches, typesetting, and expeditious publication. Jaya Shankar Kaushik is thankful for the blessings and support of Professor Ashok Puranik, Executive Director, All India Institute of Medical Sciences, Guwahati, Assam, India who has encouraged and supported all academic endeavors. Jaya Shankar Kaushik also wanted to thank all his family members, especially Dr Kausalya, who gave him ample time to revise the book. We also wish to thank Dr Murchana, Dr Bipul, Dr Shantasree, Dr Shabnam, Dr Sreejana, and Dr Abhishek for their help with proofreading. We also immensely thank Ms Anju Kumari (PA to Piyush Gupta) for her help.

Jaya Shankar Kaushik
Piyush Gupta

Preface to the First Edition

Pediatric neurology has evolved tremendously over the last decade. A substantial proportion of outpatient and inpatient admissions to pediatric services have neurological etiology. Right from the undergraduation days, nervous system often freaks out the students to *"neurophobia".* When it comes to dealing with delicate children, it is even more complicated. There is a great need for pediatricians and residents to understand the basic approach to diagnosis of childhood neurological problems. Children with neurological problems do not present with a diagnosis; they present with symptoms and signs. We felt that existing textbooks do not help approach a clinical case and logically conclude with the differential diagnoses. Apart from understanding the clinical approach, students need guidance on presenting a neurological case and understanding the necessary investigations and outline preliminary management. This book is an attempt to gather the most practice relevant aspects of pediatric neurology in a comprehensive and simplified manner.

The book has four sections. The first section covers clinical neuroanatomy, neuroimaging, electrophysiology, and other essential investigations in pediatric neurology. The second section focuses on how to approach a child with a specific neurological problem. Chapters on clinical approach highlight the points to be covered in history and examination. The text is replete with clinical pearls of wisdom to reach a clinical diagnosis and plan relevant investigations. The third section is the core of the book called "Residents' Corner," to help the residents to present a neurological case, thus imploring them to think in a logical sequence. Practical key boxes provide the templates that can help the residents on how to present important aspects of relevant neurological history or examination in a particular case. The book ends with quick notes on management issues of common neurological ailments encountered in day-to-day practice, relevant to both residents and practitioners. We have used figures, flowcharts, tables, anecdotes, and mnemonics liberally making it reader-friendly and enhancing retention.

Considering rapid progress in the field of pediatric neurology, controversies and difference of opinion are bound to exist in the clinical approach to various conditions. This is the first edition, and we will be happy to rectify any unintentional and unknown errors in the book. Please let us know your thoughts, critical comments, and suggestions to *jayashankarkaushik@gmail.com*

Jaya Shankar Kaushik
Piyush Gupta

Contents

SECTION 1: Neurological Evaluation

1. Clinical Neuroanatomy 3
2. Developmental History, Examination, and Analysis 41
3. Examination of Central Nervous System 54
4. Making a Clinical Neurological Diagnosis 104
5. Neuroimaging 118
6. Neurophysiologic Evaluation 139
7. Cerebrospinal Fluid and Tissue Diagnosis 166
8. Genetic Evaluation in Neurological Diseases 177
9. Neural Control of Urinary Bladder 188

SECTION 2: Neurological Approach to Diagnosis

10. Seizures, Epilepsy, and Other Paroxysmal Disorders 195
11. Approach to a Child with Altered Sensorium and Coma 212
12. Approach to Global Developmental Delay and Intellectual Disability 233
13. Approach to a Child with Cerebral Palsy 246
14. Approach to a Child with Developmental Regression 254
15. Approach to Neuromuscular Weakness 272
16. Spectrum Disorder and Attention-deficit Hyperactivity Disorder 289
17. Approach to Diagnosis of Movement Disorders 302
18. Approach to Diagnosis of Ataxia 316
19. Approach to Diagnosis of Headache 331
20. Approach to a Child with Macrocephaly and Microcephaly 343
21. Approach to Neural Tube Defects 353
22. Approach to a Child with Vision Loss 357
23. Approach to a Child with Hearing Loss 361

SECTION 3: Residents' Corner: Exam-oriented Cases

24. A Case of Cerebral Palsy 367
25. A Case of Tubercular Meningitis 381
26. A Case of Acute Hemiplegia 392
27. A Case of Paraplegia 402
28. A Case of Acute Flaccid Paralysis/Guillain–Barré Syndrome 414
29. A Case of Floppy Infant 424
30. A Case of Muscular Dystrophy 433
31. A Case of Neurodegenerative Disorder 443
32. A Case of Hydrocephalus 452

SECTION 4: Common Therapeutic Dilemmas

33. Antiseizure Medications 465
34. Management of Acute Seizure and Status Epilepticus 476
35. Treatment of Infections of Nervous System 485
36. Management of Raised Intracranial Pressure 498
37. Medical Management of Acute Vascular Stroke 504
38. Management of Developmental Disorders 520
39. Treatment of Neuropathies and Myopathies 531

Index *543*

SECTION 1
Neurological Evaluation

1. Clinical Neuroanatomy
2. Developmental History, Examination, and Analysis
3. Approach to a Child with Cerebral Palsy
4. Making a Clinical Neurological Diagnosis
5. Neuroimaging
6. Neurophysiologic Evaluation
7. Cerebrospinal Fluid and Tissue Diagnosis
8. Genetic Evaluation in Neurological Diseases
9. Neural Control of Urinary Bladder

CHAPTER 1: Clinical Neuroanatomy

GENERAL ORGANIZATION OF NERVOUS SYSTEM

The nervous system is broadly divided into central nervous system (CNS), peripheral nervous system (PNS), and autonomic nervous system **(Fig. 1)**. CNS includes brain and spinal cord, whereas PNS includes all neural structures outside CNS including 12 pairs of cranial nerves (CNs), 31 pairs of spinal nerves, and their ganglia. Autonomic nervous system consists of sympathetic and parasympathetic nervous systems.

There are two types of cells in nervous system—neurons and neuroglial cells.

Neurons

Neurons are the excitable cells, which have a cell body, dendrites, and axon **(Fig. 2)**. Dendrites receive the signal from another neuron and send it to the cell body. Axon passes the signal from the cell body to other neurons.

- *Cell body:* A collection of cell bodies in CNS is called a nucleus (e.g., CN nucleus

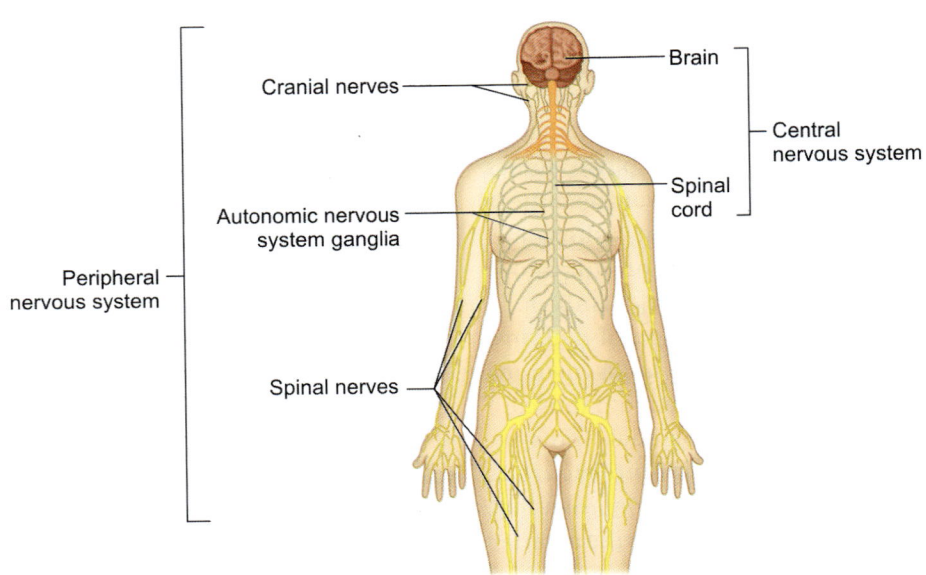

Fig. 1: Organization of nervous system.

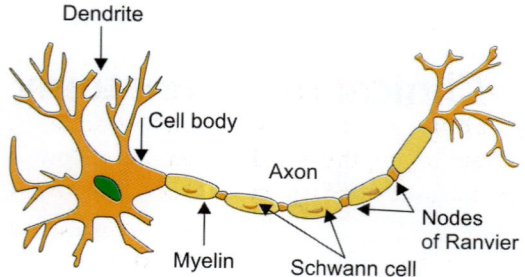

Fig. 2: Structure of neuron.

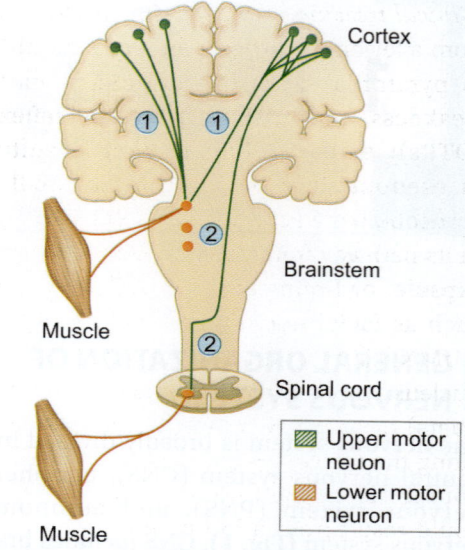

Fig. 3: Upper motor neuron in green [corticobulbar tract (1) and corticospinal tract (2)] and lower motor neuron (red).

in brainstem). Ganglion is the collection of nerve cell bodies in PNS (e.g., dorsal root ganglia and trigeminal ganglia).

- *Axons:* Axon of a neuron is called *nerve fiber*. A bundle of nerve fibers in CNS is called a *tract* (e.g., corticospinal tract and corticobulbar tract) whereas a collection of nerve fibers in PNS is called a *nerve* (e.g., median nerve and radial nerve).

Neurons are the functional unit of nervous system and cannot regenerate (except in parts of hippocampus and olfactory bulb). When neurons fire, an action potential is generated, which traverses the axon to reach dendrite of the next neuron through a junction called *synapse*. A synapse consists of a presynaptic terminal and a postsynaptic terminal. The chemical neurotransmitters like acetylcholine and adrenaline carry the impulse across the two terminals. The neurotransmitters may be excitatory (noradrenaline, adrenaline, glutamate, and aspartate) or inhibitory [glycine and γ-aminobutyric acid (GABA)].

Depending on the function of neurons, they are classified as *motor neurons* (neurons that stimulate skeletal and smooth muscle), *sensory neurons* (neurons that transmit sensation to CNS), and *interneurons* (connecting neurons). Motor neurons that transmit signals from the brain to the anterior horn cell or from the brain till the CN nuclei are called *upper motor neurons (UMNs)*.

Motor neurons located in spinal cord that transmit signals from the spinal cord to muscle or those that transmit from CN nuclei to muscles of head and neck are called *lower motor neurons (LMNs)* **(Fig. 3)**. A lesion in the motor neuron is accordingly categorized as a UMN lesion or an LMN lesion.

Upper motor neurons have their cell bodies in the motor area of the cerebral cortex. Their axons descend through the internal capsule and brainstem to end at spinal cord (corticospinal tract) or end at CN nuclei in the brainstem (corticobulbar tract). A lesion of corticospinal tract or corticobulbar tract is called a UMN lesion. LMNs have their cell bodies at the spinal cord (called anterior horn cell) or at the brainstem (in case of CN nuclei). The anterior horn cells of the spinal cord supply the skeletal muscles of the limbs and trunk. CN nuclei at the brainstem supply skeletal and smooth muscles of head and neck. A lesion anywhere along this pathway is called LMN lesion.

Clinical relevance: UMN lesion could result from a lesion in corticospinal tract [resulting in pyramidal signs like spasticity, motor weakness, and brisk deep tendon reflexes (DTRs)] or corticobulbar tract (resulting in pseudobulbar palsy). Corticospinal or corticobulbar tract can be affected anywhere in its pathway from cerebral cortex, internal capsule, or brainstem. Similarly, CN palsy such as facial nerve palsy can result from a UMN lesion (if the lesion is above the CN nucleus, similar to the lesion of corticobulbar fibers) or an LMN lesion (lesion anywhere along the nerve, e.g., along the facial nerve course as in Bell's palsy). LMN lesion could result from a lesion anywhere in the pathway of LMN—anterior horn cell (e.g., poliomyelitis), nerve (e.g., Guillain–Barré syndrome), neuromuscular junction (e.g., myasthenia), or muscle (e.g., viral myositis).

Neuroglial Cells

Glia means "glue" in Latin. It was believed that neuroglial cells only provide physical support to neurons, but their functions are far wider. Neuroglial cells include astrocytes, oligodendrocytes, microglia, and ependymal cells. Nerve cells (cell body) embedded in neuroglia comprise gray matter, whereas nerve fibers or axons embedded in neuroglial cells comprise white matter.

- *Astrocytes* form a supporting framework for nerve cells and nerve fibers.
- *Oligodendrocytes* are responsible for formation of myelin sheath of nerve fibers of CNS. Schwann cells form the myelin sheath of peripheral nerves.
- *Microglial cells* are specialized reticuloendothelial cells in CNS.
- *Ependymal cells* line the cavities of the brain and assist in circulation of cerebrospinal fluid (CSF).

Clinical relevance: Mild injuries result in neurons to undergo swelling, with displacement of nucleus and Nissl granules. Neurons tend to recover from this state. In severe injury, there is degeneration followed by phagocytosis by microglial cells. Microglia migrates to and proliferates at the site of injury in inflammatory and degenerative diseases of CNS. There is fibrous proliferation of neuroglial cells resulting in gliosis. This proliferation does not compensate for neuronal loss; rather, it leads to volume loss. In contrast, on surgical excision, there is no residual traumatized nervous tissue and thus there is minimal or no gliosis.

■ PERIPHERAL NERVOUS SYSTEM

Peripheral nerves are bundles of nerve fibers enveloped by Schwann cells, which form its myelin sheath. A nerve fiber can be myelinated or nonmyelinated. Myelin sheath is segmented at a regular interval called nodes of Ranvier (**Fig. 2**). It enhances the conduction of impulses across the nerve.

There are three types of peripheral nerve fibers—type-A fibers (myelinated large diameter fibers), type-B fibers (medium diameter and myelinated fibers), and type-C fibers (small diameter and nonmyelinated fibers). Majority of PNS (motor and sensory) has type-A fibers, which have the highest conduction velocity. Type-A fibers serve to carry proprioception (Aα), touch/pressure (Aβ), motor signals to muscle spindle (Aγ), and pain/cold/touch sensation (Aδ). Type-B fibers are preganglionic sympathetic neurons. Type-C fibers are located in dorsal root carrying pain/temperature and postganglionic sympathetic system. Certain types of peripheral nerves are susceptible to pressure damage (type A), hypoxic injury (type B), and local anesthesia (type C).

BOX 1: Names of 12 cranial nerves.

1. *I CN:* Olfactory nerve
2. *II CN:* Optic nerve
3. *III CN:* Oculomotor nerve
4. *IV CN:* Trochlear nerve
5. *V CN:* Trigeminal nerve
6. *VI CN:* Abducens nerve
7. *VII CN:* Facial nerve
8. *VIII CN:* Vestibulocochlear nerve
9. *IX CN:* Glossopharyngeal nerve
10. *X CN:* Vagus nerve
11. *XI CN:* Spinal accessory nerve
12. *XII CN:* Hypoglossal nerve

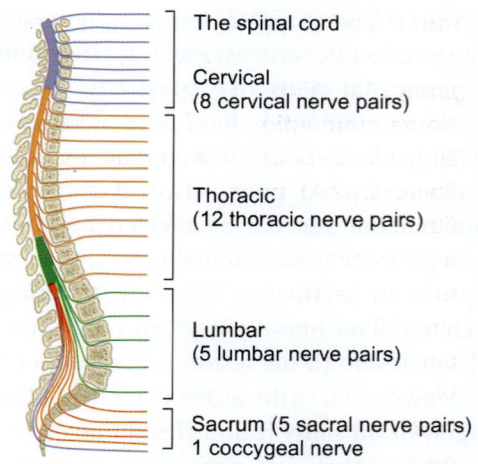

Fig. 4: Segments of spinal cord.

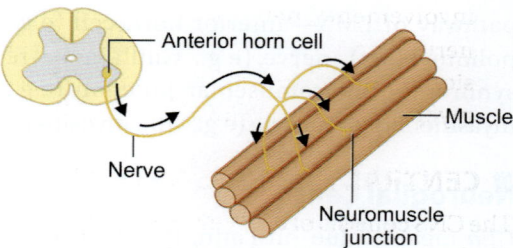

Fig. 5: Components of motor unit.

The PNS consists of 12 pairs of CNs **(Box 1)** and 31 pairs of spinal nerves. Among the 12 CNs, olfactory nerve (I), optic nerve (II), and vestibulocochlear nerve (VIII) are pure sensory nerves; oculomotor (III), trochlear nerve (IV), abducens nerve (VI), accessory nerve (XI), and glossopharyngeal nerve (XII) are pure motor CNs; and rest are mixed. Among the spinal nerves, 8 arise from cervical, 12 from thoracic, 5 from lumbar, 5 from sacral, and 1 from coccygeal segment of spinal cord **(Fig. 4)**.

Most spinal nerves are mixed nerves that have both motor and sensory fibers. A spinal nerve arises from the spinal cord by union of an anterior motor efferent and a posterior sensory afferent. *Sensory ganglion* (collection of cell bodies) is located on the posterior or dorsal sensory afferent nerve. The motor efferent arises from anterior horn cell in the spinal cord and supplies motor impulses to the muscle. A *motor unit* is composed of anterior horn cell, peripheral nerve, neuromuscular junction, and the muscle fibers supplied by it **(Fig. 5)**.

Clinical relevance:
- Injury to peripheral nerve can involve both axon and myelin (neurotmesis), only axon (axonotmesis), or could spare both (neuropraxia—transient nerve compression). Neuropraxia has better chances of recovery than axonotmesis and neurotmesis.
- If only one peripheral nerve is affected, it is called *mononeuropathy*. If more than one noncontiguous nerve are involved, it is called *mononeuritis multiplex*. When multiple peripheral nerves are affected, it is called *polyneuropathy*. Majority of systemic diseases result in polyneuropathy or mononeuritis multiplex.
- Guillain–Barré syndrome is a polyneuropathy. If it damages the myelin, it is called *demyelinating polyneuropathy* [acute inflammatory demyelinating polyneuropathy (AIDP)]. If it damages axons as well, it is called *axonal polyneuropathy* [acute

motor axonal polyneuropathy (AMAN) or *acute motor-sensory axonal polyneuropathy* (AMSAN)].
- Nerve conduction study can study only large diameter and fast conducting nerve fibers (type A). Injury to type B and type C fibers may result in clinical symptoms of neuropathy, but nerve conduction study may be normal. Hence, patients with small fiber neuropathy can have normal nerve conduction study.
- Weakness that results from lesion in the motor unit is called neuromuscular weakness. Neuromuscular diseases can be classified depending on the site of lesion as neuronopathies (anterior horn cell involvement), neuropathies (peripheral nerve disease), neuromuscular transmission disorder (myasthenic syndromes), or myopathies (muscle involvement).

■ CENTRAL NERVOUS SYSTEM

The CNS consists of the brain and spinal cord. The brain consists of cerebrum, diencephalon, brainstem, and cerebellum. Cerebrum consists of two cerebral hemispheres and basal ganglia. Diencephalon consists of thalamus, hypothalamus, metathalamus, epithalamus, and subthalamus. Brainstem consists of midbrain, pons, and medulla **(Fig. 6)**.

The brain and spinal cord have gray matter where cell bodies of neurons are located, and their axons constitute the white matter. Gray matter is peripherally located, and white matter is centrally located in the brain, and the reverse in the spinal cord. Both brain and spinal cord are covered by meninges and are suspended in CSF. Meninges consist of dura mater, arachnoid mater, and pia mater (outermost layer to innermost layer). The inner two layers (pia mater and arachnoid mater) are called leptomeninges. The space between the two is called the subarachnoid space that contains CSF. In meningitis, there is leptomeningeal enhancement that is evident on contrast neuroimaging. Dura mater is also called pachymeninges.

Spinal Cord

Spinal cord is located inside the vertebral column, occupying its upper two-third. The cord is shorter than vertebral column and ends at L1 vertebral level. It continues caudally from the medulla and ends in a conical structure called *conus medullaris*.

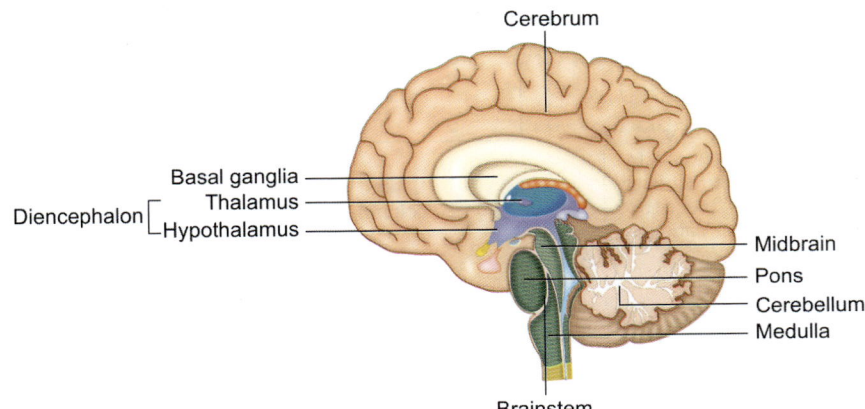

Fig. 6: Components of central nervous system (excluding spinal cord).

The conus medullaris continues as a thin filament called *filum terminale*. The spinal cord is segmented into 31 spinal segments; from each segment, a pair of spinal nerves arises on both the sides. Spinal segment always arises above the corresponding vertebral body level. Below the level of L1 spinal segment, the spinal nerve roots descend vertically to form a tuft, called *cauda equina* (**Fig. 7**) due to its similarity to a horse tail.

Cross section of spinal cord is composed of inner core of gray matter with surrounding white matter. Gray matter projects into anterior, posterior, and lateral horn. White matter has dorsal, lateral, and ventral funiculus (**Fig. 8**). Anterior and posterior spinal nerve roots pass from spinal cord to the level of vertebral foramina where they unite to form a *spinal nerve*. The level of spinal nerve and vertebral levels are depicted in **Table 1**. Each spinal nerve is a mixed nerve, consisting of motor and sensory fibers. Once they exit vertebral foramina, they divide into *anterior and posterior ramus*. Posterior ramus supplies the muscles of the back and anterior ramus continues anteriorly to supply the appendicular muscles. Ascending (toward brain) and descending (from brain) tracts of spinal cord are summarized in **Table 2 and Figure 9**. The spinal cord is supplied by anterior spinal artery (ASA) and a pair of posterior spinal artery.

Spinothalamic tract carrying sensation to sensory cortex via thalamus includes anterior and lateral spinothalamic tract. Anterior spinothalamic tract carries light touch and pressure; it crosses over to contralateral side after ascending for one to two segments.

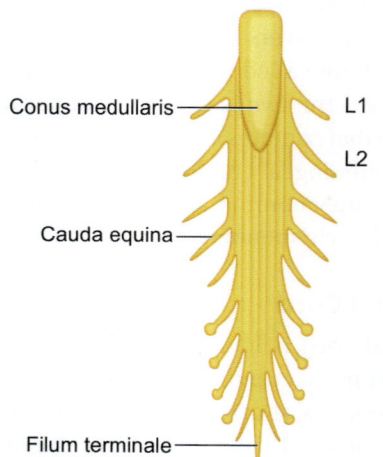

Fig. 7: Spinal cord structure showing conus medullaris, cauda equina, and filum terminale.

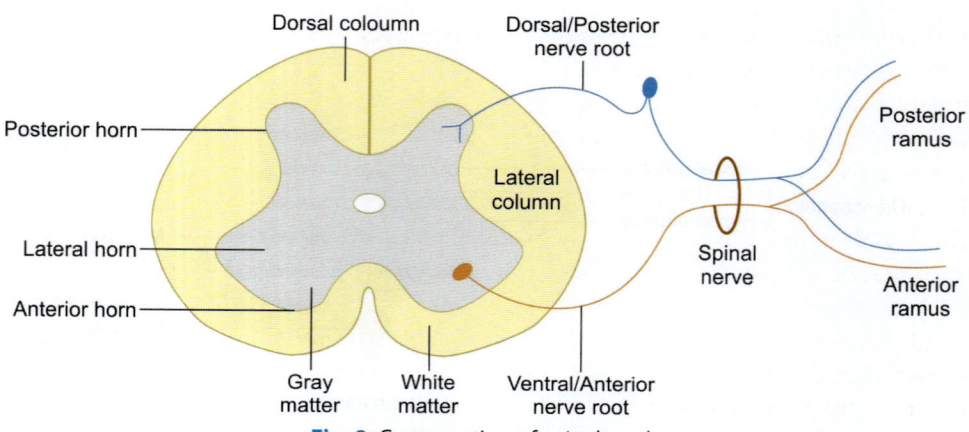

Fig. 8: Cross-section of spinal cord.

CHAPTER 1: Clinical Neuroanatomy

TABLE 1: Corresponding spinal nerve with vertebral level.

Vertebral level	Spinal segment
Upper cervical	Same
Lower cervical	Add 1
Thoracic (1–6)	Add 2
Thoracic (7–9)	Add 3
10th thoracic	L1–2 cord segment
11th thoracic	L3–L4
12th thoracic	L5
1st lumbar	Sacral and coccygeal segments

TABLE 2: Ascending and descending tracts of spinal cord.

Ascending fibers	Descending fibers
Fasciculus gracilis	Lateral and anterior corticospinal tract
Fasciculus cutaneous	Rubrospinal tract
Spinocerebellar tract (anterior and posterior)	Reticulospinal tract
Spinothalamic and spinoreticular tract	Vestibulospinal tract
Spino-olivary tract	Tectospinal tract

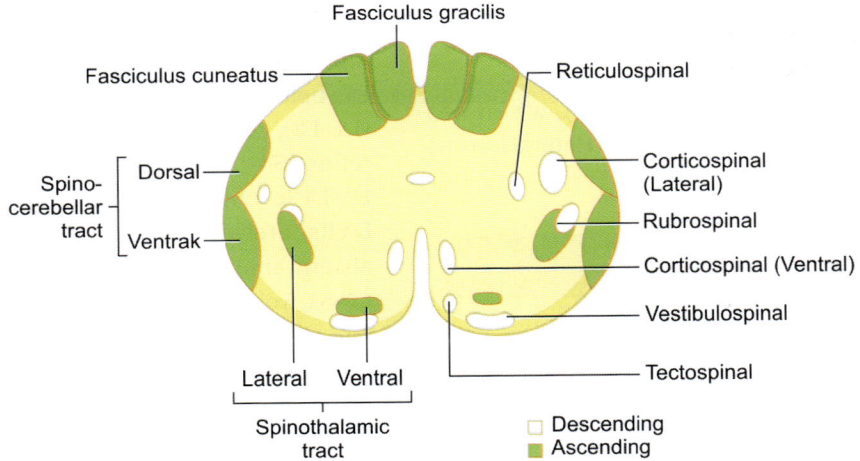

Fig. 9: Ascending and descending tracts of spinal cord.

Lateral spinothalamic tract carrying pain and temperature crosses over immediately to contralateral side. If there is loss of light touch sensation at L2–L3 dermatome on the right side, it is possible that the lesion in spinal cord could be at the level of L1–L2 (left side).

The dorsal column carrying discriminative touch, vibration sensation, and proprioception ascends at the same level and on the same side till medulla and then crosses over at the medullary level.

The corticospinal tract controls skilled motor activity. The lateral corticospinal tract descends and crosses over at the level of medulla to supply the contralateral side of the body. In contrast, the anterior corticospinal tract descends uncrossed till the level of spinal cord, where it crosses to supply the contralateral side. Hence, corticospinal tracts will always control the movement of the opposite side of the body. Reticulospinal tract has cortical control of voluntary motor function. Rubrospinal tract facilitates flexors and inhibits the extensors. In contrast, vestibulospinal tracts facilitate the extensors and inhibit the flexors for balance control.

Clinical relevance:
- Spinal cord ends at L1–L2. Hence, spinal cord is shorter than vertebral column. **Table 1** helps us to determine the site of vertebral level that corresponds to the given spinal cord level. Hence, if there is a lesion clinically compatible with L1–L2 spinal level, then the corresponding vertebra would be T10.
- *Sensory dermatome helps in localization:* A rough guide to key landmarks is given in **Table 3**. T10 corresponds to umbilicus—L1: groin; L2: upper medial thigh; L3: lateral lower thigh; L4: medial upper leg; L5: lateral lower leg; S1: foot; S4–S5: perianal area **(Fig. 10)**. Hence, if there is a loss of sensation in the leg with preserved sensations at the thigh region, we know the lesion has to be below L4 (lateral lower thigh is supplied by L4 which is intact), either L5–S1 or below.
- Root value of DTR is useful to determine the site of lesion. Commonly elicited DTRs (with root values) are knee jerk (L2–L4), ankle jerk (L5–S1), biceps (C5–C6), brachioradialis (C5–C6), and triceps (C7–C8). DTRs are usually lost at the level of the lesion and are exaggerated below that level.
- Similarly, superficial reflexes are useful in localization, as they are absent or hypoactive below the site of lesion and are preserved above it. Root value of superficial reflexes include abdominal reflex [T6–T10 (above umbilicus); T10–L1 (below umbilicus)], cremasteric reflex (L1–L2), plantar reflex (L5–S1), and anal reflex (S4–S5). For example, a lesion at L2–L4 level would result in loss of knee DTRs, preserved abdominal reflex, and absent anal reflex. Similarly, a lesion at L5–S1 would result in loss of ankle DTRs and mute or absent plantar reflex.
- Any lesion at the spinal cord level will result in LMN signs (loss of DTR, flaccid weakness, and fasciculation) at that level and UMN signs (spasticity and brisk DTR) below that level. Hence, a lesion at L5–S1 would result in loss of ankle reflex (L5–S1 root value). L2, L3, and L4 will result in loss of knee reflex (L2–L4 root value) and brisk ankle reflex.
- Muscle power testing is useful to determine the severity of weakness (plegia vs. paresis). Overall, one can remember that majority of leg and foot muscles are supplied by L4–L5–S1. Hip flexors L1–L2; thigh adductors: L2–L3; knee extensors: L3–L4; ankle dorsiflexors: L4–L5; ankle plantar flexion: S1–S2; hip extensor; and abductors: L5–S1.

TABLE 3: Rough guide to determine the sensory dermatome.

Spinal cord level	Spinal dermatome
C5	Clavicle
C5, C6, and C7	Lateral aspect of upper limb
C8 and T1	Medial aspect of upper limb
T4	Nipple
T10	Umbilicus
T12	Inguinal area
L1	Lateral-to-medial aspect of upper thigh (put your hand in your pant pocket, i.e., L1 area)
L2	Medial aspect of lower thigh (think as if your hand drops medially if your pant pocket was torn)
L3	Lateral aspect of upper leg
L4	Medial aspect of lower leg
L5–S1	Foot
S2–4	Perineum

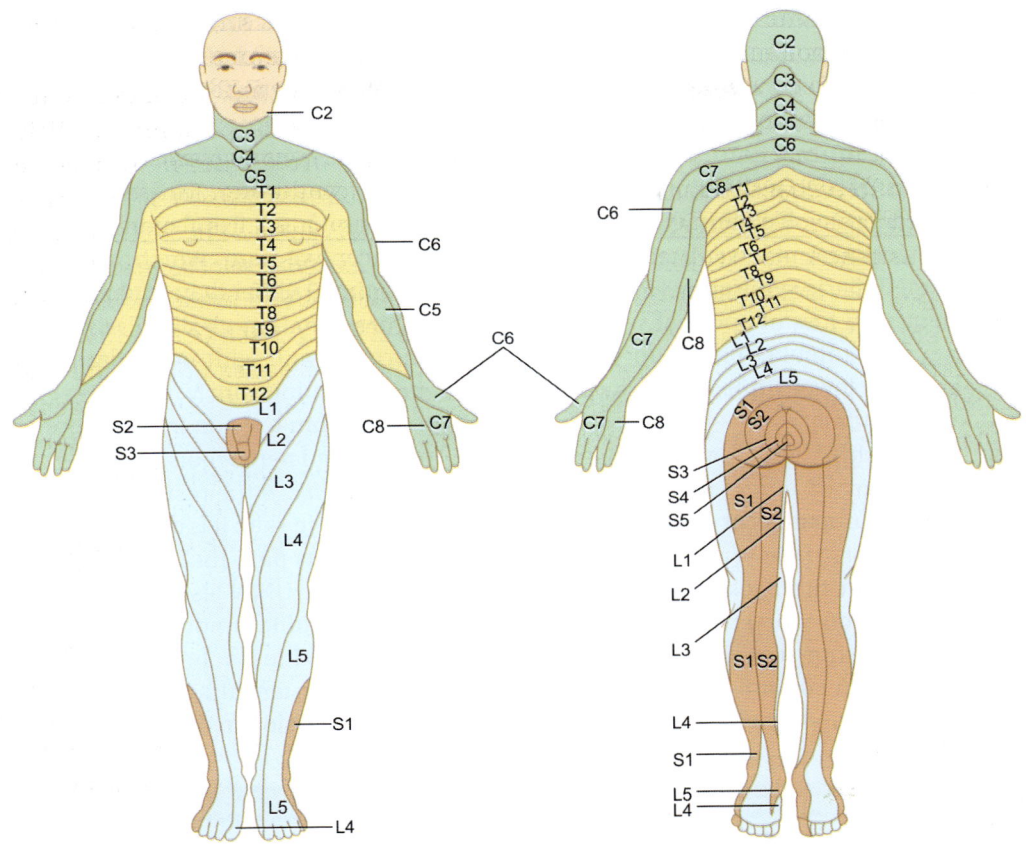

Fig. 10: Sensory dermatomal levels.

- If there is a hemisection of spinal cord at one spinal level, there will be spastic paralysis on the same side below that spinal level (descending motor tracts of spinal cord supply on the same side), loss of joint position sensation and vibration on the same side below that spinal segment (posterior or dorsal columns ascend on the same side), and loss of pain and temperature on the contralateral side (lateral spinothalamic tract lesion cross to the opposite side). This clinical syndrome of hemisection is called Brown–Sequard syndrome.
- If the patient has loss of pain and temperature sensation (lesion of lateral spinothalamic tract) but preserved sensation of vibration and joint position (posterior columns are spared), then the lesion is affecting the center of spinal cord and sparing the dorsal aspect. This dissociated sensory loss is characteristic of conditions like syringomyelia.
- If the patient has isolated loss of joint position and vibration sensation and starts swaying with closed eyes (Romberg sign), then it indicates posterior column involvement as in vitamin B_{12} deficiency. Proprioception, vestibular function, and vision are required. In dorsal column lesion, proprioception is impaired, which results in swaying while standing

- that becomes evident once the vision is blocked by asking the patient to close his eyes.
- Loss of perianal sensation is observed in cauda equina/conus medullaris syndrome. In such a situation, if there is early bladder involvement with minimal muscle weakness of lower limb, it favors conus medullaris syndrome. However, if a patient with loss of perianal sensation has severe radicular pain and spastic weakness of lower limb, it favors cauda equina syndrome.
- Pain in a child with paraparesis can provide a lot of clues. Pain could be radicular, neuropathic, or nociceptive.
  - *Radicular pain* (radiculopathy) starts from the back, radiates down the leg, and worsens with Valsalva or leg raising test. This is typically observed in compressive myelopathy secondary to vertebral involvement resulting in stretching of nerve radicals. Such radicular pain is also observed in vertebral disk prolapse with resultant compression or polyradiculoneuropathy (Guillain–Barré syndrome). This needs to be differentiated from neuropathic or nociceptive pain, which indicates a peripheral rather than cord pathology.
  - *Neuropathic pain* is distal, severe, and burning pain with no radiation and no worsening with Valsalva/crying. It results from a lesion in the peripheral nerves and nerve roots.
  - *Nociceptive pain* results from pain receptors in skin; it is dull aching, near continuous pain that is relieved with analgesics. UMN lesions never result in neuropathic or nociceptive pain.

Table 4 provides a few clinical case scenarios to understand these basic principles of localization of lesion in the spinal cord.

TABLE 4: Localization of lesion based on clinical case vignettes.

Case scenario (clinical findings)	Possible anatomical site of localization
Right lower limb weakness, tingling and numbness, radicular pain (right), areflexia, and mute plantars on right side	Nerve root (radiculopathy) or plexopathy (lumbar plexus) on right side
Isolated right foot drop, atrophy of right foot muscles, especially extensor digitorum brevis (EDB), absent ankle reflex, preserved knee jerk, and mute plantar (right)	Right common peroneal nerve injury (peripheral nerve involvement)
Flaccid paraparesis, areflexia, mute plantars (bilateral), and presence of fasciculations	Anterior horn cell involvement (e.g., poliomyelitis)
Spastic paraparesis, brisk DTRs, and extensor plantars	Spinal cord involvement (e.g., transverse myelitis)
Paraparesis with positive Romberg sign	Posterior column involvement (e.g., vitamin B_{12} deficiency)
Weakness (proximal hip girdle predominant) with hyporeflexia and muscle pain	Myopathy (inflammatory) (e.g., viral myositis)
Proximal hip girdle weakness with associated ptosis and diurnal variation of weakness	Neuromuscular weakness (e.g., myasthenia gravis)

(DTRs: deep tendon reflexes)

Brainstem

Brainstem consists of three main structures—midbrain, pons, and medulla. It hosts all the CN nuclei and other vital autonomic functions. Brainstem regulates vital cardiac and respiratory functions.

- Midbrain is known to play a role in the vision [Edinger–Westphal nucleus (EWN)]. It also hosts the reticular activating system that controls sleep and wakefulness. The site for temperature regulation is also governed by the midbrain.
- Pons communicates signals from cerebellum to brain. It hosts vital respiratory centers as well as a center for bladder control (pontine micturition center).
- Medulla is the most crucial part hosting vital cardiac, respiratory, emetic, and vasomotor centers.

Cranial nerve nuclei and their fibers are classified into afferent fibers and efferent fibers. Types of fiber and functions of CN nuclei are enumerated in **Table 5**. There are 12 pairs of CN, 10 of which arise from brainstem **(Table 6)**. First CN (olfactory nerve) arises from olfactory mucosa and reaches the brain through cribriform plate; second CN (optic nerve) arises from the optic disc to end at optic chiasma. CN nuclei are in midbrain (III and IV CNs), pons (V, VI, VII, and VIII CNs), and medulla (IX, X, XI, and XII CNs). Each pair of CN nuclei in the brainstem supplies ipsilateral muscles of head and neck.

Blood supply of midbrain is posterior cerebral artery, pons is supplied by basilar artery (midline) and anterior inferior cerebellar artery (AICA) (lateral), and medulla is supplied by ASA (midline part of medulla) and posterior inferior cerebellar artery (PICA) (lateral medulla) **(Fig. 11)**.

Clinical relevance: Brainstem can be broadly divided into midline and lateral sides. The structures that are in midline include CN III, IV, VI, and XII. Midline tracts also include medial longitudinal fasciculus (MLF), motor tract (corticospinal tract), and medial lemniscus (contralateral vibration and proprioception) (all start with letter M are midline). Hence, a midline lesion of the pons on the right side would affect right sixth CN nucleus (impaired abduction of right eye), right MLF (impaired adduction of left eye), and right corticospinal tract (left hemiparesis). This may occur secondary to the top of basilar artery syndrome where the

Fiber type	Function
General somatic efferent	Innervates skeletal muscle
General visceral efferent	Innervates smooth muscles of viscera, extraocular muscles, heart, and salivary gland
Special visceral efferent	Innervates skeletal and cardiac muscle derived from brachial arches
General somatic afferent	Conducts impulses from skin and skeletal muscle spindles
Special somatic afferent	Conducts impulses from retina, auditory apparatus, and vestibular apparatus
General visceral afferent	Conducts impulses from viscera and blood vessels
Special visceral afferent	Conducts impulses from taste and olfactory mucosa

TABLE 5: Types of cranial nerve fiber and its functions.

TABLE 6: Cranial nerve fiber and its function.

Cranial nerve	Fiber type
Olfactory	Special sensory
Optic nerve	Special sensory
Oculomotor nerve	• *Somatic motor:* All extraocular muscle except LR and SO • *Visceral motor:* Sphincter pupil
Trochlear nerve	*Somatic motor:* Superior oblique
Trigeminal nerve	• *Somatic sensory:* Face • *Visceral motor:* Masticators, tensor tympani, and tensor palati (branchial arch derivatives)
Abducens	*Somatic motor:* Lateral rectus
Facial nerve	• *Somatic sensory:* Posterior ear canal • *Special sensory:* Taste (anterior two third) • *Somatic motor:* Facial muscles • *Visceral motor:* Salivary gland and lacrimal gland
Vestibulocochlear	*Special sensory:* Auditory
Glossopharyngeal	• *Somatic sensory:* Posterior one third tongue • *Visceral sensory:* Carotid body • *Special sensory:* Posterior one third tongue • *Somatic motor:* Stylopharyngeus • *Visceral motor:* Parotid gland
Vagus	• *Visceral sensory:* Carotid bulb • *Special sensory:* Taste over epiglottis • *Somatic motor:* Soft palate, pharynx, and larynx • *Visceral motor:* Causing bronchoconstriction and peristalsis
Spinal accessory	*Somatic motor:* Trapezius and sternocleidomastoid
Hypoglossal	*Somatic motor:* Tongue

(LR: lateral rectus; SO: superior oblique)

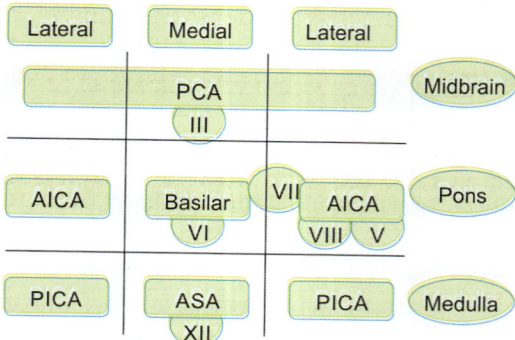

Fig. 11: Blood supply of brainstem. (AICA: anterior inferior cerebellar artery; ASA: anterior spinal artery; PCA: posterior cerebral artery; PICA: posterior inferior cerebellar artery)

basilar artery that supplies the midline part of pons is affected.

Structures that are present laterally include CN V, VII, IX, and XI. Lateral columns include sympathetic tract and spinothalamic tract (both start with letter S are *inside*). Hence, a right lateral pontine infarct would affect right VIIth CN nucleus (right facial palsy), right spinothalamic tract (loss of pain and temperature sensation on the left side), and right fifth CN nucleus (loss of facial sensation on the right side).

Clinical features of various brainstem syndromes are summarized in **Table 7**.

TABLE 7: Brainstem syndromes.

Level	Structure involved	Clinical finding
Midbrain (medial) (Benedict syndrome)	• CN III • Medial lemniscus • Red nucleus	• Oculomotor palsy • C/L loss of posterior sensation • Tremor/ataxia
Midbrain (peduncle) Weber syndrome	• CN III • Corticospinal • Corticobulbar	• Oculomotor palsy • C/L hemiparesis • Pseudobulbar palsy (spastic dysarthria)
Pons (medial)	• Corticospinal • VI CN • VII CN • MLF, VI CN	• C/L hemiparesis • I/L VI CN palsy • I/L VII CN palsy • Lateral gaze restriction
Pons (lateral)	• Vestibular nucleus • Spinothalamic tract • V CN • VII CN • Sympathetic	• Vertigo/ataxia • C/L pain and temperature loss • I/L loss of facial sensation • I/L VII CN palsy • Horner syndrome
Medulla (medial)	• Corticospinal • Medial lemniscus • XII CN	• C/L hemiparesis • C/L loss of posterior column sign • XII CN palsy
Medulla (lateral)	• Vestibular nucleus • Spinothalamic tract • V CN • Sympathetic tract	• Vertigo/ataxia • I/L pain and temperature loss • C/L loss of facial sensation • Horner syndrome

(C/L: contralateral; CN: cranial nerve; I/L: ipsilateral; MLF: medial longitudinal fasciculus)

Cerebellum

Cerebellum is connected to brainstem by superior, middle, and inferior cerebellar peduncle. Inputs to cerebellum reach via middle and inferior cerebellar peduncle. Efferents from cerebellum leave via superior cerebellar peduncle. Cerebellum is composed of vermis in the midline, two cerebellar hemispheres, and a flocculonodular lobe **(Fig. 12)**. Vermis controls the truncal stability and proximal limb movement, whereas cerebellar hemispheres control the distal limb movement. Cerebellum modifies motor command of corticospinal pathway to make the movement smooth, adaptive, and accurate. Main functions of cerebellum include maintenance of posture and balance, coordination of voluntary movement, and motor learning (learning new motor movements with trial and error).

Anatomically, cerebellum has two parts—cerebellar cortex (neurons) and cerebellar deep nucleus (output). There are three deep nuclei of cerebellum:

1. Fastigial nucleus
2. Interpositus nucleus (emboliform and globose nucleus)
3. Dentate nucleus (projects to contralateral red nucleus and ventrolateral thalamus)

Clinical relevance:
- Midline cerebellar dysfunction leads to truncal ataxia.
- Cerebellar hemispheric lesions lead to limb ataxia, dysmetria, dysdiadochokinesia, intentional tremors, dysarthria, and hypotonia.

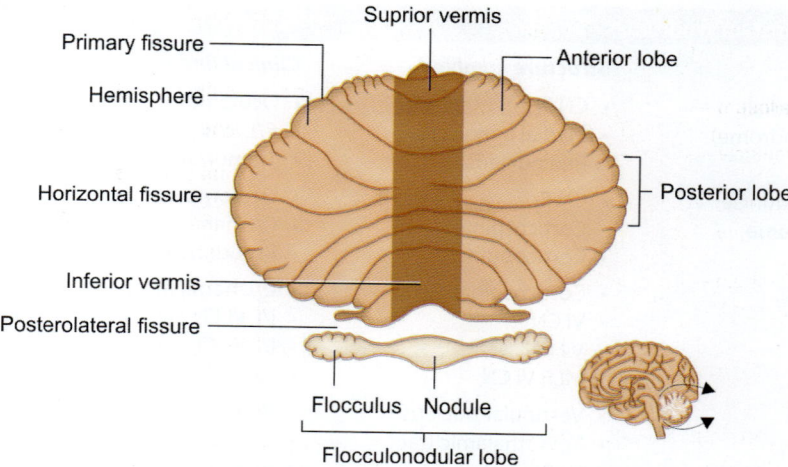

Fig. 12: Anatomy of cerebellum.

- Involvement of flocculonodular lobe results in nystagmus and ocular movement disorders.

Diencephalon

Diencephalon is the structure between brainstem and cerebrum. It consists of thalamus, metathalamus, epithalamus, subthalamus, and hypothalamus. Thalamus acts as a sensory relay station for all sensations of the body except the olfactory system. All sensations such as pain, touch, and temperature from the limbs ascend the spinal cord to be relayed to parietal cortex through thalamus. Similarly, auditory sensations from medial geniculate nucleus relay through thalamus to auditory cortex. Thalamus also regulates consciousness and emotional content.

Clinical relevance: Thalamic syndromes are characterized by variable clinical presentations including loss of sensation in the limbs, ocular motility deficits, visual processing defects, memory problems, alteration of sensorium, or auditory problems. Thalamic lesions in children result in movement disorders including dystonia, myoclonus, athetoid movements, or tremors. Hence, there is a wide variation in neurological manifestations of thalamic lesion depending on the thalamic nucleus that is affected.

Basal Ganglia

Basal ganglia are a set of gray matter nuclei, which consist of caudate, putamen, globus pallidus, subthalamic nucleus, substantia nigra (SN), and ventral tegmentum **(Fig. 13)**. Corpus striatum is a term used to denote head of caudate plus putamen. Lentiform nucleus consists of putamen and globus pallidus. Functions of basal ganglia are complex. They constitute an extrapyramidal system that controls movement. In addition, basal ganglia have a role in emotion, memory, and cognitive functions. Dysfunction of basal ganglia results in movement disorders. The basal ganglia circuit is complex, and it is difficult to clinically localize different types of movement disorders.

The basic concept in regulation is that reduced inhibition will increase output and

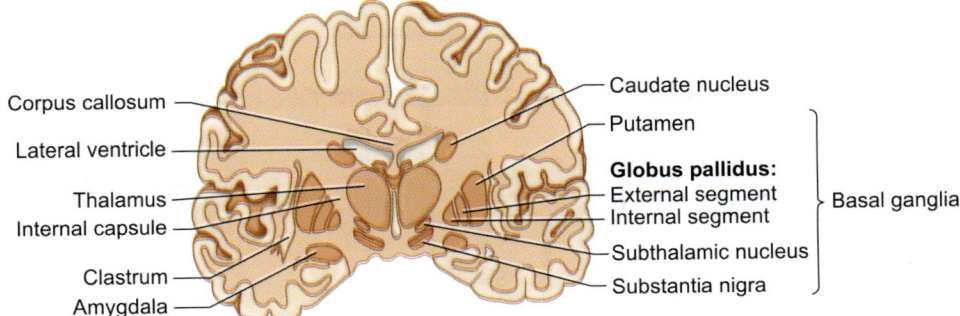

Fig. 13: Anatomy of basal ganglia.

increased inhibition will decrease the output. There is a direct and an indirect pathway (**Fig. 14**). Direct pathway stimulates muscle movement and indirect pathway inhibits the muscle movement. Globus pallidus internus is the main output of basal ganglia that is inhibitory to thalamus and thus to the cortex. When a patient wants to move a limb, the cortex stimulates the putamen, which in turn inhibits globus pallidus interna (GPi), thus reducing the inhibition of GPi on thalamus. This in turn excites the cortex to perform the movement. This pathway where putamen directly inhibits GPi is called direct pathway. The inhibitory neurotransmitters are GABA and dopamine, and excitatory neurotransmitters are glutamate and dopamine. Basal ganglia pathology results in increased inhibition of GPi, thus decreasing its inhibition on thalamus, resulting in increased movements. This forms the basis for hyperkinetic movement disorders in children.

At rest, cortex activates putamen, which in turn increases inhibition on globus pallidus externa (GPe) that releases inhibition on GPi. This makes GPi more active which will inhibit thalamus, thus leading to lesser excitation to motor cortex. This pathway of inhibition of GPi through GPe is called indirect pathway,

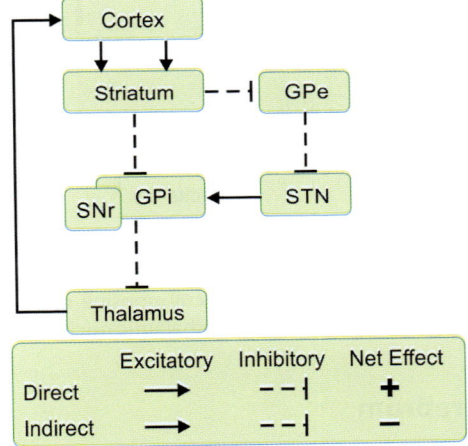

Fig. 14: Basal ganglia motor circuit. (GPe: globus pallidus externa; GPi: globus pallidus interna; SNr: substantia nigra pars reticulata; STN: subthalamic nucleus)

which inhibits muscle movement. SN is like a hand brake of car that needs to be released when a car starts moving. SN receives cortical input that we are starting movement, which stimulates direct pathway and inhibits indirect pathway at rest. Subthalamic nucleus is excitatory to GPi. Degeneration of the dopaminergic nigrostriatal pathway might lead to increased inhibition of movement even when the movements are desired. This leads to a hypokinetic movement disorder with Parkinsonian features (**Fig. 15**).

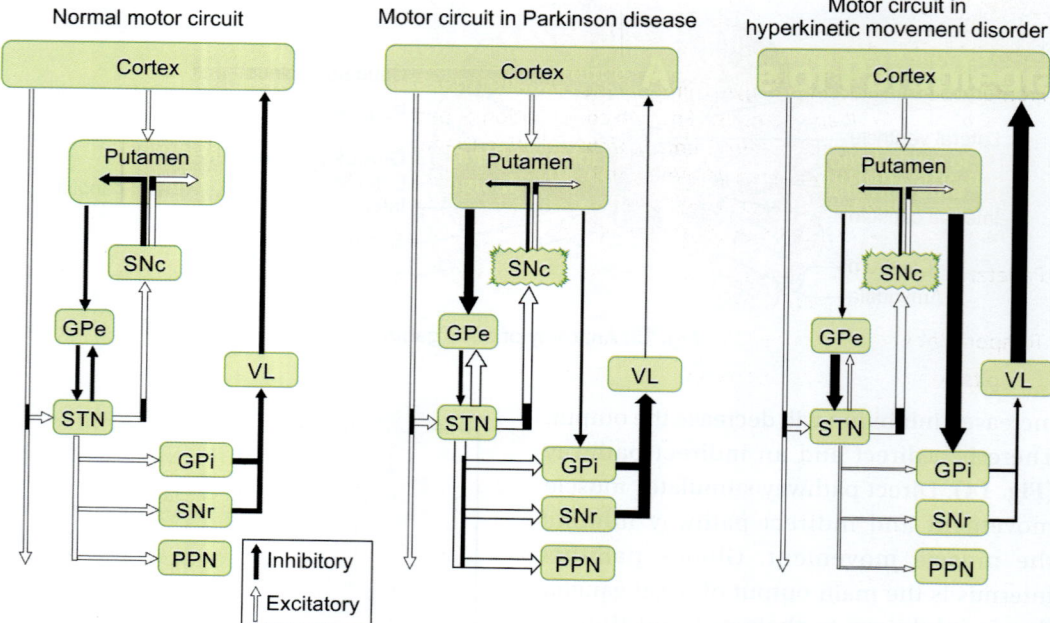

Fig. 15: Abnormalities in basal ganglia motor circuits (dark lines indicate inhibition, light lines indicate excitation, thickness of the line depicts the strength of output). (GPe: globus pallidus externa; GPi: globus pallidus interna; PPN: pedunculopontine nucleus; SNc: substantia nigra pars compacta; SNr: substantia nigra pars reticulata; STN: subthalamic nucleus; VL: ventrolateral nucleus of thalamus)

Cerebrum

Cerebrum consists of two cerebral hemispheres connected by corpus callosum. Cerebral cortex (gray matter) runs into folds called *gyri* and fissures in-between are called *sulci*. Based on the large sulci, cerebral cortex is divided into four lobes—frontal, temporal, parietal, and occipital. Based on the area represented in the lobe, there are various functions of these four lobes of the brain **(Table 8)**. Frontal lobe is largely responsible for cognitive function, expressive language, and voluntary movement. Parietal lobe processes all sensory inputs like pain, temperature, pressure, and touch. Occipital lobe is responsible for processing the visual signals and temporal lobe processes the auditory signals and memory.

Consciousness

Consciousness refers to the state of awareness of self and the environment. It has two dimensions—*wakefulness* and *awareness*. Wakefulness or arousal is mediated by the ascending reticular activating system, a diffuse network of neurons originating in the tegmentum of the pons and midbrain and projecting to diencephalic and cortical structures. Awareness is dependent on the integrity of the cerebral cortex and its subcortical connections **(Fig. 16)**.

Clinical relevance: Consciousness is altered in lesions of reticular activating pathway in the brainstem above the mid pons level or thalamic or extensive cortical lesion. **Flowchart 1** summarizes the stages of altered sensorium into conscious, minimally

TABLE 8: Main function of four lobes of the brain.

Lobes of brain	Function
Frontal lobe	• *Precentral gyrus:* Primary motor cortex • *Premotor cortex:* Smooth coordination of motor • *Supplementary motor cortex:* Initiating the movement • *Frontal eye field:* Horizontal conjugate movement of eyes • Broca motor speech area (left); lesion results in nonfluent aphasia • *Prefrontal cortex:* Intellectual functioning, emotions, personality, and disinhibition
Parietal lobe	*Postcentral gyrus:* Perceives somatosensory events (touch, temperature, body position, and pain)
Temporal lobe	*Wernicke area:* Understand spoken language (comprehension); lesion results in fluent aphasia
Occipital lobe	Visual reception and interpretation

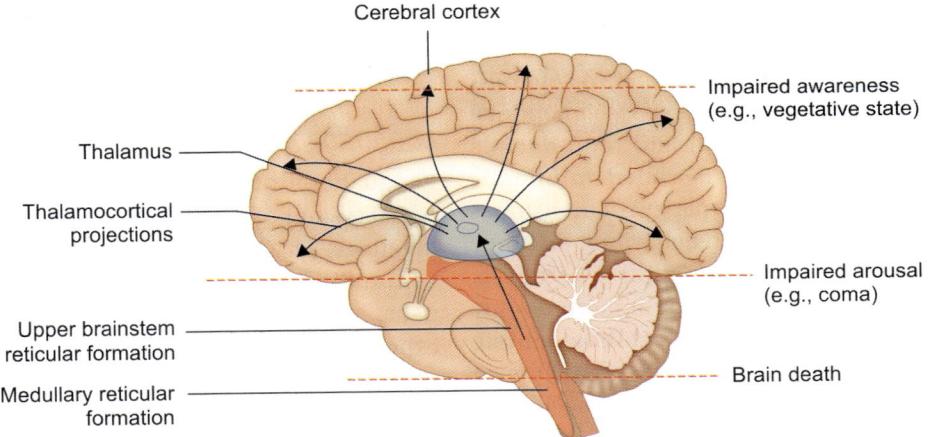

Fig. 16: Pathway for consciousness in brain.

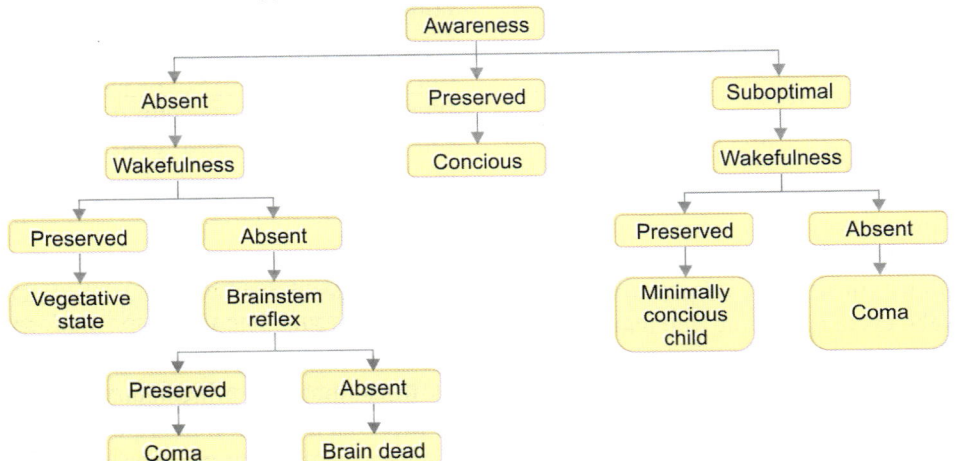

Flowchart 1: Approach to clinical diagnosis of stage of altered sensorium.

conscious state, vegetative state, and coma. Impaired consciousness implies a significant impairment in the awareness of self and of the environment, with variable degrees of wakefulness. Descriptive terms such as *somnolence, stupor, obtundation*, and *lethargy* used to denote different levels of consciousness are best avoided, given the lack of uniformity in the way these states are defined in the literature.

States of altered consciousness can be categorized into one of the following:
- *Conscious:* If the patient has preserved awareness and wakefulness (arousal), then the patient is conscious.
- *Minimally conscious state:* If wakefulness is preserved but awareness is suboptimal with few meaningful and reproducible response, then it is called minimally conscious state. The patient demonstrates minimal but definite behavioral evidence of self or environmental awareness. Patients in this state are able to do any or all of the following—follow simple commands, gesturally or verbally give yes–no responses (regardless of accuracy), verbalize intelligibly, or perform movements or affective behaviors in contingent relation to environmental stimuli (and not due to reflexive activity).
- *Vegetative state:* If wakefulness is preserved but awareness is completely absent, then it is called vegetative state. If the same vegetative state persists for >30 days, it is called persistent vegetative state. It results from extensive cortical damage with preserved brainstem and reticular activating system. The patient might show signs of preserved sleep–wake cycle and some behavioral arousal (like yawning and sneezing). States like akinetic mutism, coma vigil, and abulia are also often used to describe this state. These terms are best avoided.
- *Coma:* If both wakefulness and awareness are impaired but brainstem reflexes (such as Doll's eye response and corneal reflex) are preserved, then this state is called coma. A comatose patient has no meaningful eye opening.
- *Brain death:* Absence of awareness, wakefulness, and brainstem reflexes suggests brain death.
- *Locked-in syndrome:* If wakefulness and awareness are preserved but the patient is unable to communicate or move owing to ventral pontine lesion, this state is called locked-in syndrome. The movement or speech is locked leading to a mute and quadriplegic patient.

Language

Language is defined as use of a conventional system of symbols (spoken word, sign language, written words, and pictures) for communication. It has two main components—receptive (listening and reading) and expressive (speaking and writing). *Receptive component* is perceived by Wernicke area in the superior temporal gyrus, whereas *expressive motor component of speech* is governed by Broca area located anteriorly in inferior frontal gyrus **(Fig. 17)**. Wernicke area is connected to Broca area through arcuate fasciculus, which governs the repetition in the language. If the repetition is preserved, receptive aphasia is called *transcortical sensory aphasia* and expressive aphasia is called *transcortical motor aphasia*. **Flowchart 2** summarizes the types of aphasia based on comprehension and repetition.

Clinical relevance:
- Dysfunction of language is called aphasia. Aphasia occurs when there is a lesion in the dominant hemisphere.
- Lesions in the anterior part of language area result in *expressive aphasia*, where

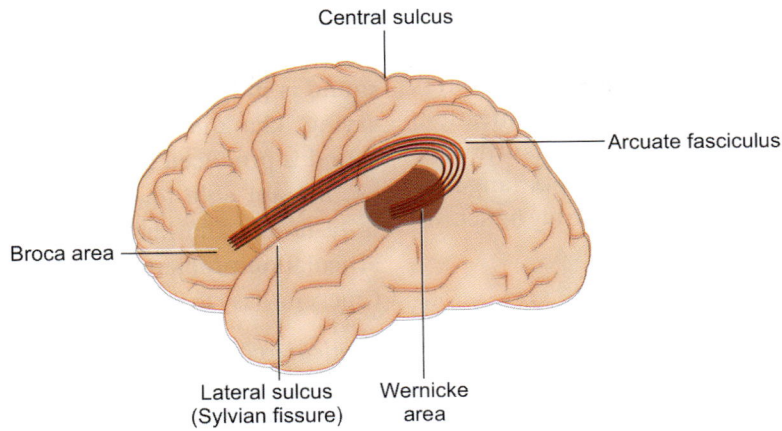

Fig. 17: Broad areas for language in cerebral cortex.

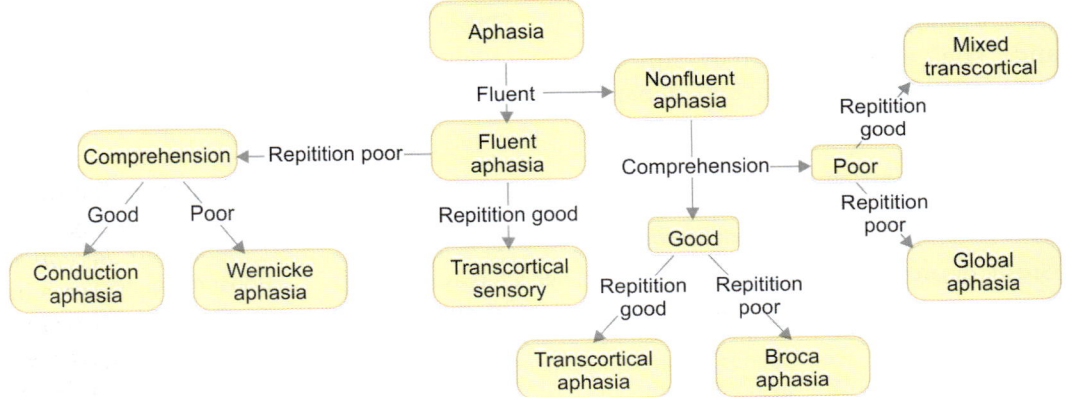

Flowchart 2: Clinical approach to characterizing the type of aphasia.

the child omits words, especially nouns, and has nonfluent speech. Most children with nonfluent aphasia often have associated right hemiparesis considering the proximity of motor cortex to Broca area and left hemisphere being the dominant hemisphere.
- In contrast, lesions in the posterior part of language area (stroke involving parieto-occipital cortex) result in *receptive aphasia* where the speech will be fluent but will have a lot of word substitutions and neologistic words making the speech incomprehensible.
- In dense middle cerebral artery (MCA) stroke of left side, all functions of language including comprehension, fluency, and repetition are affected resulting in *global aphasia*.
- Isolated lesion of angular gyrus results in *nominal aphasia* (inability to name an object).

For instance, if you are looking for an object in a dark room, you start your search, you might end up getting the right thing (or the right word), you might get something that was different from what you were searching for (neologistic words), or you might not get anything. This is what happens to an aphasic patient when commanded to respond. Hence, aphasia is inability to under-stand or express words for the purpose of communication, even though the primary sensorimotor pathways to receive and express language and the mental status are relatively intact.

Speech

Speech is defined as expressive production of sound that includes articulation, fluency, with voice and resonance quality. Defects of articulation are called dysarthria. Sound in the speech is produced by lips (labial), tongue (lingual), and soft palate (guttural). Syllables like "pa" are produced by lips (labial sounds), "ta" are produced by tongue (lingual sounds), and "kha" are produced by soft palate (guttural sounds). Try saying "papapapa"; you can see that sound is produced by lips. Try saying "ta-ta-ta-ta" you can feel that this sound is produced by tongue. Similarly, try saying "kha-kha-kha" you can feel that this sound is produced from the depth of throat. So, if I am able to clearly say "pa-pa-pa-ta-ta-ta-kha-kha-kha", I know I do not any articulation problems (pa-ta-kha in Hindi is Crackers; easy to remember).

Clinical relevance: Articulation of speech is governed by cerebellum, pyramidal, and extrapyramidal pathways. Dysarthria results from disturbance in the muscular control over the speech mechanism. It could be cerebellar, spastic, or extrapyramidal dysarthria **(Table 9)**. Dysarthria is different from dysphonia, which refers to abnormalities of voice secondary to local laryngeal abnormality.

TABLE 9: Types of dysarthria.

Type of dysarthria	Speech description	Condition
Spastic dysarthria	Child speaks with strained effort as if trying to speak from the depth of his/her stomach. Child is hardly able to open the mouth, and the speech sounds is slurred and strained. This speech is associated with brisk DTR, pseudobulbar signs	Upper motor neuron lesion (spastic cerebral palsy) or acquired bilateral upper motor neuron lesion
Extrapyramidal dysarthria	• Monotonous speech without any rhythm and prosody. • All words look jumbled with lack of clarity. Majority of these children will have dyskinesia, dystonia, or choreoathetoid movement	Dyskinetic cerebral palsy, Wilson disease, and other neurological disorders with extrapyramidal involvement
Cerebellar or ataxic dysarthria	The child speaks slowly or deliberately as if scanning a line of poetry. The speech sounds slurred as if drunk. Sometimes, each syllable is given equal emphasis. For example, artillery pronounced as ar-til-ler-y. Patient will have associated cerebellar signs	Acquired cerebellar pathology
Bulbar dysarthria	Nasal speech along with weak gag reflex and drooling of saliva are indicators of bulbar dysarthria. Most of these children are hypotonic with areflexia	Guillain–Barré syndrome, 9th and 10th cranial nerve palsy

(DTR: deep tendon reflex)

Homunculus

The term homunculus in Latin means representation of a small human being.

If one draws a miniature human being in the precentral gyrus (motor cortex) according to the part of the body that is represented by the area, it is called motor homunculus and if the same is drawn over the postcentral gyrus (sensory cortex), it is called sensory homunculus. Cortical representation is largest for face, hands, and thumb owing to their dense innervations. Foot and leg are represented in the medial portion of cerebral cortex whereas, hand, thumb, and face are represented in lateral cerebral cortex **(Fig. 18)**.

Brain has two hemispheres (right and left). It is well known that right side controls the movements and sensations of the left side of the body and vice versa. Although the functions of both sides of brain are similar, hemisphere that controls language is referred to as dominant hemisphere. In the dominant hemisphere, there is also integration of language with intellect and emotions.

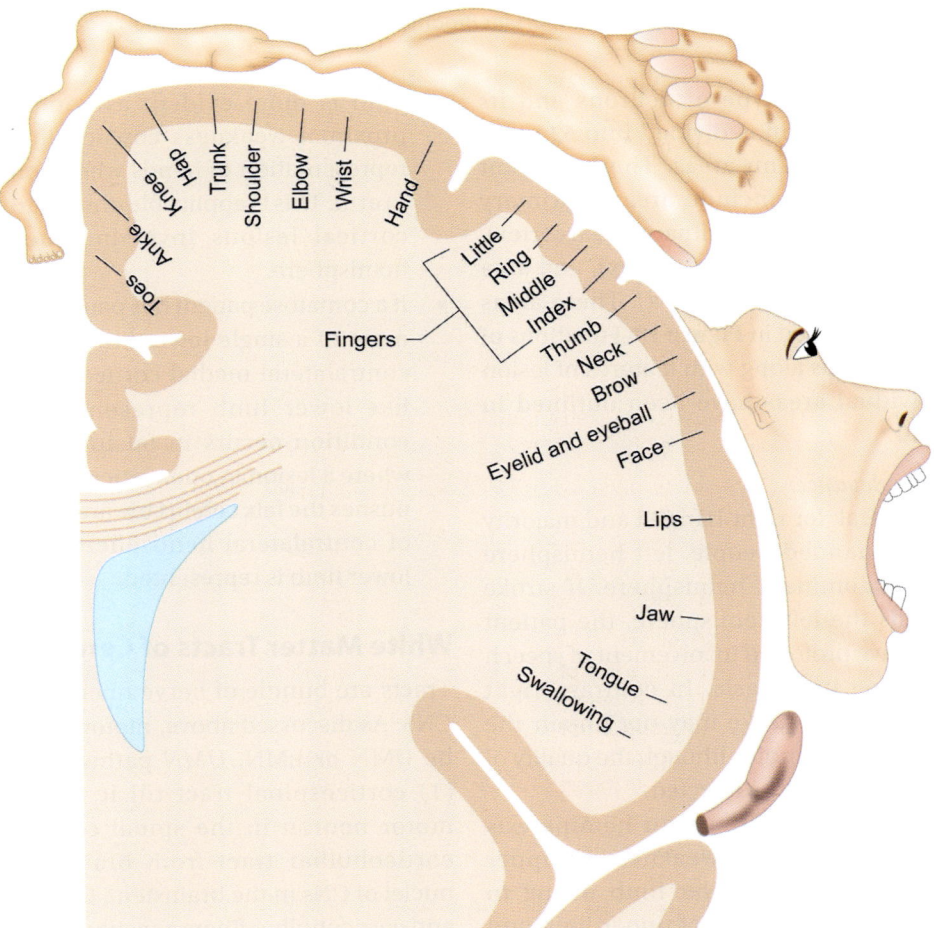

Fig. 18: Representation of body parts in cerebral cortex (motor homunculus).

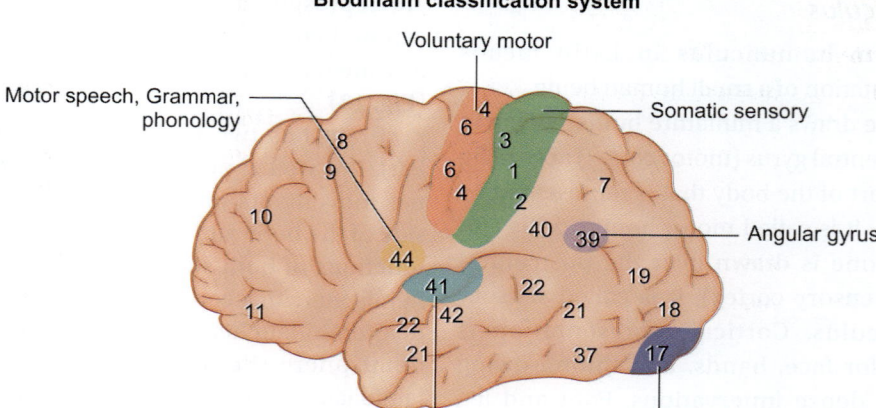

Fig. 19: Cortical mapping of important Brodmann areas of human cerebral cortex.

Based on the type of neurons and its organization, brain is divided into 52 areas called as Brodmann areas. The important Brodmann areas include area 4 (primary motor cortex), area 17 (primary visual cortex), area 22 (primary auditory cortex), and area 44 (Broca motor speech area). These areas have been mapped in **Figure 19**. Functions of important areas along with features of lesion in individual areas have been outlined in **Table 10**.

Clinical relevance:
- In general, for right-handed and majority of left-handed people, left hemisphere is the dominant hemisphere. If stroke affects the left hemisphere, the patient will have profound involvement of speech resulting in aphasia. In contrast, right hemispheric stroke may not impair the speech profoundly although the quality of the speech may be affected.
- Majority of children with hemiparesis have predominant weakness of upper limb more than lower limb owing to larger representation of upper limb and face. Similarly, distal weakness of upper limb is more evident as compared to proximal weakness considering larger representation of hands when compared to arm. This is applicable only in extensive cortical lesions involving the entire hemisphere.
- If a comatose patient has paucity of movement of a single lower limb, it indicates contralateral medial cortical lesion that has lower limb representation. This condition occurs in falcine herniation where a lesion in one cortical hemisphere pushes the falx cerebri toward medial side of contralateral hemisphere where the lower limb is represented.

White Matter Tracts of Cerebrum

Tracts are bundle of nerve fibers present in CNS. As discussed above, motor neuron can be UMN or LMN. *UMN* pathway includes (1) corticospinal tract till it reaches the motor neuron in the spinal cord and (2) corticobulbar tract from brain to motor nuclei of CNs in the brainstem. Corticospinal and corticobulbar fibers constitute pyramidal tracts. Voluntary motor function of the body

TABLE 10: Brodmann area of brain and localization in cortical lesion.

Lobe of brain	Area of brain	Function
Frontal	Area 4 (primary motor cortex)	Lesions result in paralysis in contralateral side of the body
	Area 6 (supplementary motor cortex)	Lesions affect sensory guidance of movement and control of proximal and trunk muscles of body
	Area 44/45 (Broca speech area)	Lesion results in motor aphasia
	Area 8 (frontal eye field)	Supranuclear control of horizontal conjugate movement
	Areas 9 and 10 (dorsolateral prefrontal cortex)	Controls executive functions
	Area 11 (orbitofrontal area)	Lesions result in personality changes and disinhibition
Parietal	Area 3, 1, and 2 (primary somesthetic area)	Lesions result in loss of contralateral touch, pressure, and proprioception
	Areas 5 and 7 (somatosensory association area)	Lesion results in ideomotor apraxia and astereognosis
	Area 39 (angular gyrus)	Lesions result in alexia and agraphia
Temporal	Areas 41 and 42 (auditory area)	Loss of awareness of sound in bilateral lesion
	Areas 20, 21, 22, and 38 (auditory association area)	
	Area 22 (Wernicke area)	Lesions result in receptive aphasia
Occipital	Area 17 (primary visual cortex)	Bilateral lesion result in cortical blindness
	Areas 18 and 19 (secondary visual cortex)	Visual agnosia (difficulty in recognizing and identifying objects)

and face are controlled by pyramidal tract and extrapyramidal tracts. These tracts are described below:

- *Corticospinal tract:* Pathway starts from cortex, travels through subcortical structures, internal capsule, midbrain, pons, and then crosses at medulla to reach motor neuron along contralateral spinal cord. Most of corticospinal fibers cross to form the lateral corticospinal tract; few remain uncrossed and enter the spinal cord as anterior corticospinal tract **(Fig. 20)**. These pathways directly control the voluntary movement.
- *Corticobulbar tract:* Pathway from the cerebral cortex to ipsilateral and contralateral brainstem motor nucleus is called corticobulbar tracts. CN nuclei usually have bilateral innervation, except for a part of seventh CN that supplies lower half of the face, which has only contralateral innervation.

Extrapyramidal tracts consist of rubrospinal tracts, tectospinal tracts, reticulospinal tracts, and vestibulospinal tracts. Extrapyramidal pathway is involved in initiation of voluntary movement and selective control of agonist and antagonist group of muscles. Hence, pyramidal tract is the main performer and extrapyramidal tracts are modulators of voluntary motor activity.

Clinical relevance:
- UMN and LMN involvement can be differentiated clinically. UMN syndrome has spasticity, brisk DTRs, and extensor plantar response. In contrast, LMN syndrome is characterized by weakness, flaccidity, atrophy of muscles with decreased or normal DTRs. **Table 11** summarizes the clinical differentiation between UMN and LMN lesions.
- Injury to pyramidal tract will result in spastic paralysis (weakness, spasticity, and brisk DTRs) and injury to extrapyramidal pathway would result in movement disorders like chorea, athetosis, ballismus, and dystonia.

Upper motor neuron lesion often results in spastic hemiparesis. In a child with spastic hemiparesis, the lesion could be anywhere from the cortex, subcortical structures, internal capsule, or at the level of brainstem. Following points need to be considered while localizing the UMN type of lesion:
- *Cortical involvement:* Presence of seizure, altered awareness, and coexistent motor and sensory deficit (as motor and sensory cortices are nearby) suggest cortical involvement. Involvement of frontal eye field (in frontal region of same side) will result in eye deviation to same side (eyes deviate toward destructive lesion). Hence, if there is a block in superior division of left MCA, it will involve left motor cortex, sensory cortex, inferior frontal gyrus (that lodges Broca area of speech),

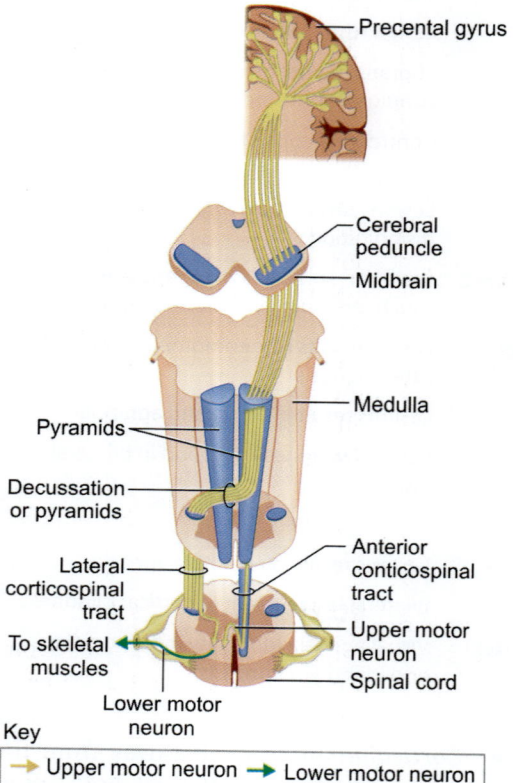

Fig. 20: Course of corticospinal tract.

TABLE 11: Differences between upper motor neuron (UMN) and lower motor neuron (LMN) lesion.

Finding	UMN lesion	LMN lesion
Weakness	Spastic weakness	Flaccid weakness
Deep tendon reflex	Brisk	Sluggish or absent
Atrophy	May or may not be present	Present
Babinski reflex	Extensor response	Flexor response
Fasciculations/fibrillation	Absent	Fasciculation present in anterior horn cell involvement; fibrillation in muscle involvement

and frontal eye field. This will result in right hemiparesis, hemisensory loss on right side, Broca aphasia, and eyes being deviated to left side.
- *Internal capsule:* Internal capsule has five parts—anterior limb, genu, posterior limb, sublentiform (carries auditory fibers), and retrolentiform (carries visual fibers) **(Fig. 21)**. Sensory fibers from thalamus to cortex called thalamic radiations traverse through both anterior and posterior limb of internal capsule. Genu of internal capsule has corticobulbar tract and posterior limb has corticospinal tract **(Fig. 21)**. Internal capsule is supplied by lenticulostriate branch of MCA (superiorly) and recurrent artery of Huebner, a branch of anterior cerebral artery (ACA) (inferiorly in the anterior limb and genu) and anterior choroidal artery, a branch of internal carotid artery (inferiorly in posterior limb). A lesion in internal capsule will result in one or more of the following—hemiplegia (corticospinal tract involvement), hemisensory loss (thalamic radiation involvement), and CN palsy (corticobulbar fibers). Since the fibers for arm, trunk, and legs are closely packed, it results in dense hemiplegia involving both arms and legs equally. This is in contrast to cortical lesion where upper limb (which has a larger representation in the cortex) is involved more compared to lower limb. A lenticulostriate artery stroke on the right side can result in left-sided dense hemiplegia with right UMN type of facial palsy. The sensory tracts of posterior limb are often supplied by anterior choroidal artery and hence may be spared completely in lenticulostriate artery stroke. Involvement of lenticulostriate artery is common in adults with chronic hypertension or diabetes mellitus.
- *Brainstem:* Most of brainstem syndromes are crossed. This is obvious as CNs descend along same side whereas corticospinal tract will decussate at the level of medulla to supply opposite side of the body. Depending on CN involvement, lesion can be localized to midbrain (III or IV CN), pons (V, VI, VII, or VIII CN) or medulla (IX, X, XI, or XII CN).

■ BLOOD SUPPLY OF BRAIN

Arterial supply consists of anterior circulation (internal carotid artery) and posterior circulation (vertebral artery). Internal carotid artery divides into ACA and MCA. MCA divides into superior and inferior divisions. Anterior communicating artery connects right and left ACA. Two vertebral arteries join at the level of pons to form basilar artery that subsequently divides into two posterior cerebral arteries. Posterior communicating artery connects posterior cerebral artery with MCA and is a branch of internal carotid artery.

Circle of Willis is formed by terminal portion of internal carotid artery, proximal portion of ACA, anterior communicating artery, posterior communicating artery, and

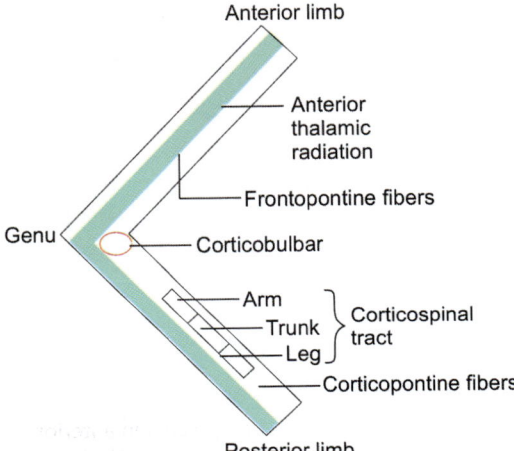

Fig. 21: Fibers across the internal capsule.

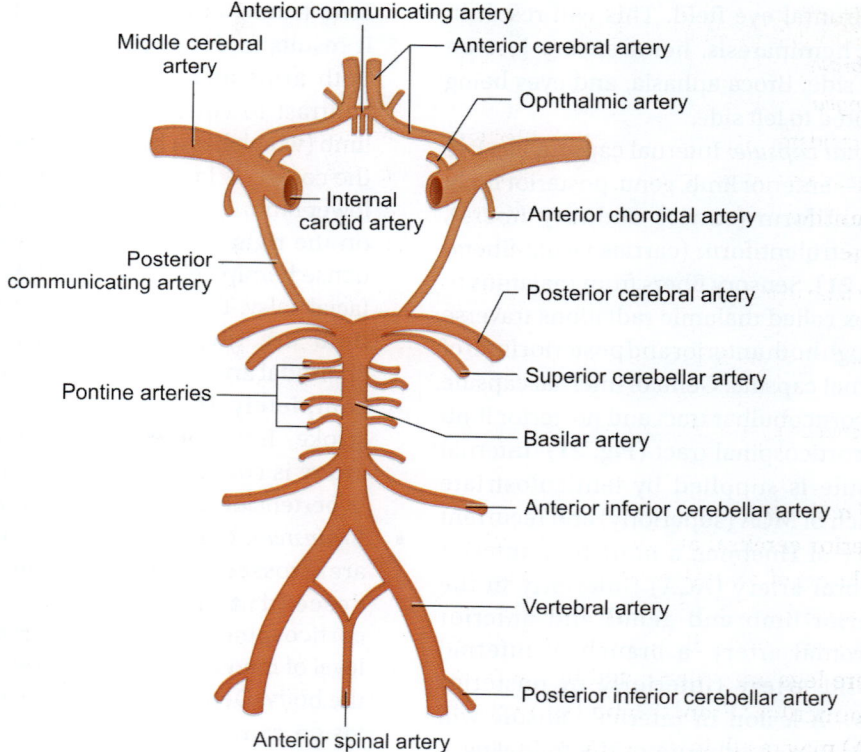

Fig. 22: Circle of Willis.

proximal portion of posterior cerebral artery (**Fig. 22**). Vertebral artery has two branches—ASA and PICA. Branches from the basilar artery include superior cerebellar artery and AICA.

Anterior cerebral artery supplies anteromedial portion of brain, MCA supplies the lateral surface of brain, and posterior cerebral artery supplies both medial and lateral surface of posterior portion of brain (**Fig. 23**). ACA through its medial lenticulostriate artery supplies medial basal ganglia, corpus callosum, and genu of internal capsule. **Table 12** summarizes the blood supply of various basal ganglia structures.

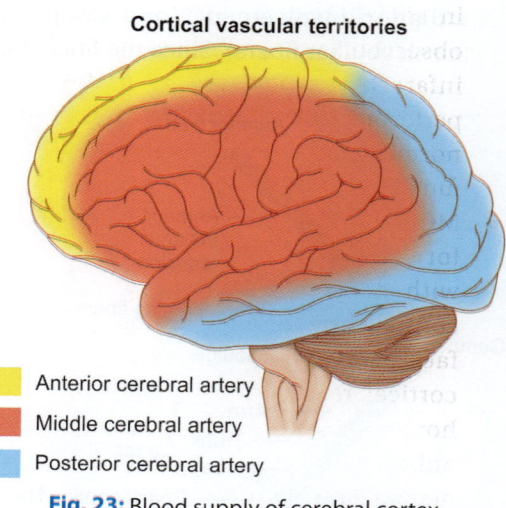

Fig. 23: Blood supply of cerebral cortex.

TABLE 12: Blood supply of basal ganglia.

Area of brain	Blood supply
Basal ganglia	
Head of caudate	Recurrent branch of ACA
Rest of caudate and putamen	Penetrating branches of MCA
Globus pallidus	Anterior choroidal artery
Thalamus	Posterior cerebral artery and posterior communicating artery
Anterior limb of internal capsule and genu	• Lenticulostriate branch of MCA • Recurrent branch of ACA
Posterior limb of internal capsule	• Lenticulostriate branch of MCA • Anterior choroidal branch of ICA

(ACA: anterior cerebral artery; MCA: middle cerebral artery)

Clinical relevance:
- Anterior cerebral artery infarct results in weakness of contralateral lower extremity, gait apraxia, and urinary incontinence, as ACA supplies medial portion of the brain where legs are represented in the motor homunculus. Frontal lobe (supplied by ACA) may result in gait apraxia. Similarly, cortical control of bladder is governed by frontal lobe. Urinary incontinence in socially inappropriate situations is observed in frontal lobe lesion (ACA infarct). (Apraxia means inability to perform a learned skilled action despite normal motor, sensory, and cerebellar functions.)
- MCA supplies sensorimotor cortex except for lower extremity. Hence, a patient with dense MCA stroke would have contralateral motor weakness (affecting face and upper limb considering its cortical representation), sensory loss, homonymous hemianopia, along with aphasia (dominant hemisphere), and hemineglect (nondominant hemispheric lesion).
- Posterior cerebral artery supplies thalamus and temporo-occipital cortex. Most common presentation is visual field defect (homonymous hemianopia) with cortical lesion (area 17). Brainstem lesion would often result in alteration of sensorium (reticular activating system in brainstem is responsible for wakefulness) and multiple CN palsies (CNs emerge at the level of brainstem). More examples are provided in **Chapter 37**.

Venous Drainage of Brain

Venous drainage of the brain can be divided into superficial venous system and deep venous system. Superficial venous system consists of superior cerebral veins, middle (superficial), and inferior cerebral veins. The two important veins in superficial venous system are superior anastomotic vein of Trolard (connects superior sagittal sinus to superficial middle cerebral vein) and inferior anastomotic vein of Labbe (connects superficial middle cerebral vein to transverse sinus). Superficial venous system especially superior sagittal sinus drains the entire cortex. Lateral sinus including transverse sinus and sigmoid sinus drains cerebellum, brainstem, and posterior regions of cortex. Inferior sagittal sinus drains into straight sinus that joins the confluence of sinuses along with superior sagittal sinus and a pair of transverse sinuses. Transverse sinus continues on each side to form sigmoid sinus that ultimately drains into internal jugular vein.

Thalamostriate vein and choroidal vein join to form internal cerebral vein, which joins basal vein of Rosenthal to form great cerebral vein. The great cerebral vein (vein of Galen) drains into straight sinus **(Fig. 24)**. Deep venous system drains cerebellum, brainstem, and posterior regions of cortex. Deep white matter and basal ganglia are also drained by the deep venous system.

Clinical relevance:
- In contrast to arterial stroke, venous strokes do not have any clinical localization considering extensive collaterals between various venous channels. Among the superficial and deep venous system, superior sagittal sinus is the most common site of thrombosis in children.
- Since venous collaterals are well formed, majority of patients with venous thromboses have insidious onset of symptoms in contrast to sudden onset of focal deficit in arterial stroke.
- Children with venous stroke often present with features of raised intracranial pressure (headache, vomiting, irritability, or alteration of sensorium) and seizures. Motor deficits are more common in arterial stroke in comparison to venous stroke.
- Since capillaries and veins are fragile, venous stroke often have hemorrhage. Hence, in the presence of intraparenchymal hemorrhagic infarct, one must always consider venous thrombosis, especially when there are predisposing risk factors like diarrheal dehydration, severe anemia, postoperative period, or any underlying cyanotic congenital heart disease.
- Venous sinus thrombosis is best picked up in magnetic resonance venography, which may demonstrate nonvisualization of the sinus, flow defect, and presence of collaterals.

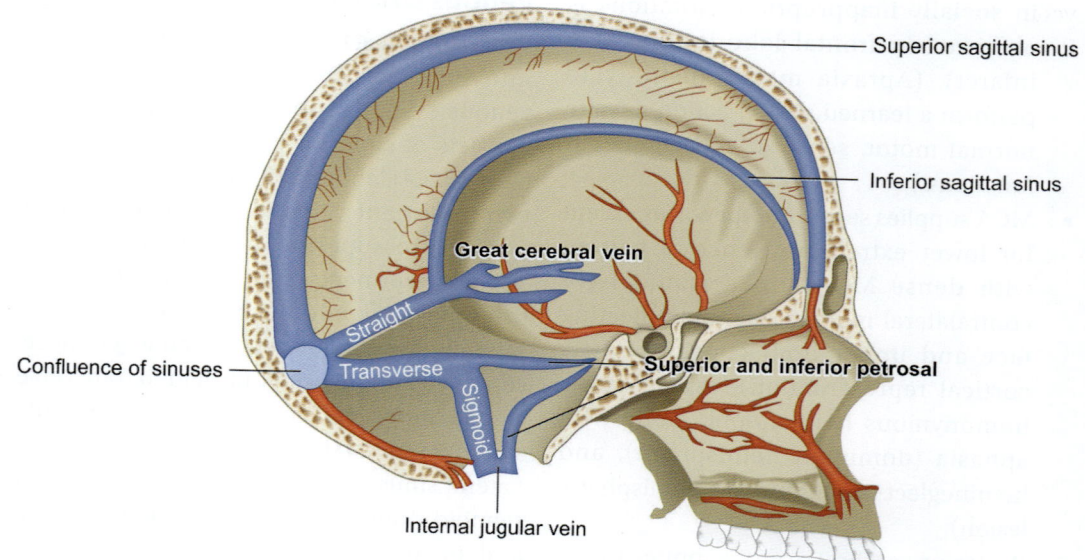

Fig. 24: Venous drainage of brain.

CEREBROSPINAL FLUID

Cerebrospinal fluid is formed by choroid plexus located in walls of lateral ventricle. CSF flows from lateral ventricle to third ventricle through foramen of Monro. It then passes through aqueduct of Sylvius to the fourth ventricle, and via foramen of Luschka and foramen of Magendie and ultimately drains into the basal cisterns and subarachnoid space **(Fig. 25)**. CSF from subarachnoid space flows over the surface of brain parenchyma to be finally drained into venous circulation (superior sagittal sinus). Arachnoid granulations are considered as the main site for CSF reabsorption. CSF is produced at the rate of approximately 500 mL/day. CSF has lower protein, glucose, and potassium than plasma but higher chloride. It acts as a cushion to brain and spinal cord.

Clinical relevance: Enlargement of ventricles (ventriculomegaly) can result from accumulation of CSF resulting in hydrocephalus. Hydrocephalus can be *communicating* or *noncommunicating*. If lateral ventricle, third ventricle, and fourth ventricle are all dilated, it would be considered as communicating hydrocephalus. However, if only lateral and/or third ventricle are dilated, and fourth ventricle is normal, it would be considered as noncommunicating hydrocephalus.

MENINGES

Meninges consist of pia mater, arachnoid mater, and dura mater (P-A-D). Pia mater is a vascular structure closely adherent to the surface of brain. Dura mater lies against the bone with thick connective tissue and contains the venous sinuses. There are two layers of dura mater—periosteal layer attached to skull bone and the meningeal layer. The space between these two layers has venous sinuses. The space between the periosteal layer of dura mater and skull is called extradural space. The space between dura mater and arachnoid mater is called subdural space. CSF lies in the subarachnoid space between arachnoid mater and pia mater. Pia mater is very closely stuck to the brain. Falx cerebri is dura mater that dips in-between the cerebral hemisphere. Dura mater that separates cerebellum from the overlying cerebral surface is called tentorium cerebelli **(Fig. 26)**.

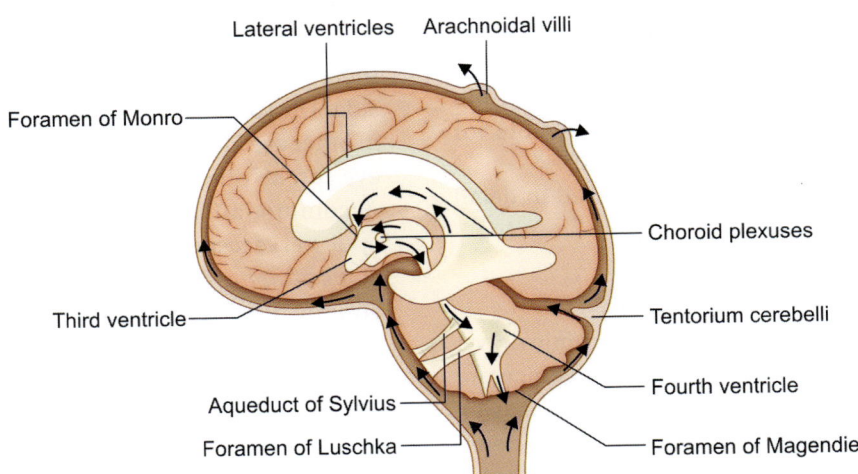

Fig. 25: Flow of cerebrospinal fluid.

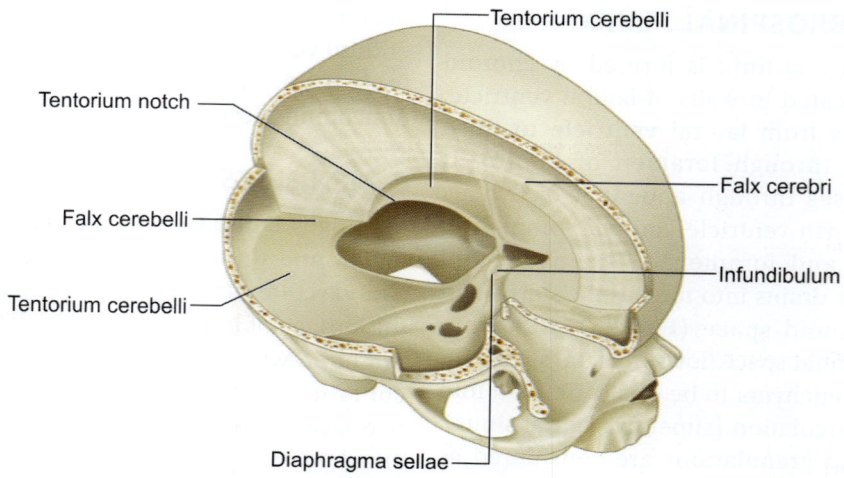

Fig. 26: Dural folds.

SPECIAL SENSES AND THEIR NEURAL PATHWAY

Special senses include smell, vision, sound or hearing, balance, and taste. The olfactory system transmits the sense of smell from olfactory epithelium to olfactory cortex through olfactory nerve (first CN).

Auditory pathway starts from cochlea, cochlear nerve, cochlear nucleus, trapezoid body, lateral lemniscus, inferior colliculus, medial geniculate body, and auditory radiation, and it ends at the auditory cortex. The vestibular nucleus in brainstem receives signals from vestibular receptors in labyrinth (utricle and saccule). It is responsible for maintenance of balance and posture.

The visual pathway is discussed in detail below.

Visual Pathway

Visual pathway consists of retina, optic nerve, optic chiasma, optic tract, lateral geniculate body, optic radiations, and visual cortex **(Fig. 27)**. The optic nerve is a sensory nerve that is covered by meninges rather than neurilemma. Hence, the optic nerve does not regenerate when cut. It lies in close relation to the sphenoid sinus, which accounts for retrobulbar neuritis among children with sphenoid sinus infection. Optic chiasma lies over the pituitary (sella turcica) leading to a visual field defect in lesions of pituitary like adenoma. Lesions along the optic pathway can be determined by testing field of vision.

Clinical relevance:
- *Optic nerve lesion:* Lesions of optic nerve result in ipsilateral blindness with loss of direct as well as consensual light reflex (observed in unaffected eye) on the same side. Direct light reflex will be preserved in other eye and consensual reflex of other eye can be observed in the affected side. Accommodation reflex is preserved in optic nerve lesion.
- *Optic atrophy:* There are two types of optic atrophy. Primary optic atrophy results in chalky white optic disc with well-defined margins. Secondary optic atrophy results as a sequelae of previous papilledema, which is seen as blurred disc margins with peripapillary sheathing and tortuous veins.

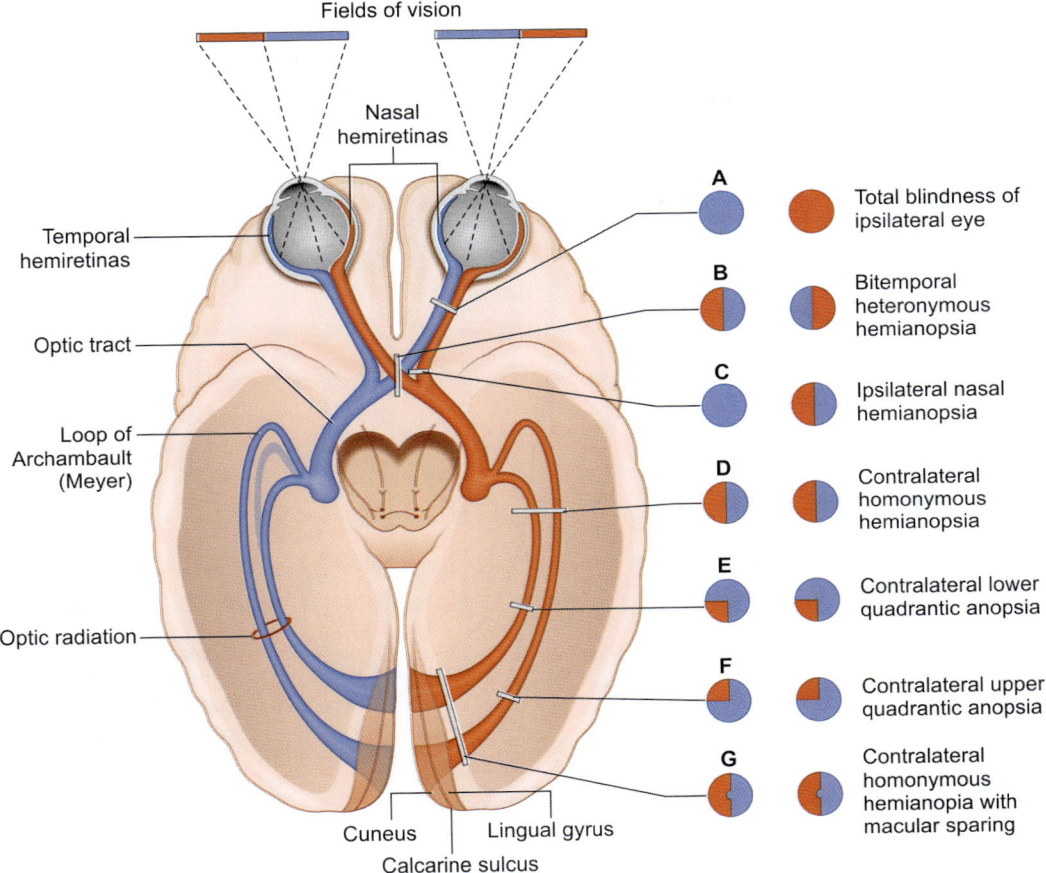

Fig. 27: Visual pathway along with visual field defects resulting from lesion in optic nerve (A), optic chiasma (B and C), and optic radiations (D to F) and occipital cortex (G).

- *Lesion at optic chiasma* (tumors of pituitary gland, suprasellar aneurysm) results in bitemporal hemianopia. Lateral chiasmal lesion (distention of third ventricle) is characterized by binasal hemianopia.
- *Optic tract lesion* results in homonymous hemianopia, whereas lesions in occipital lobe cortical lesion results in homonymous hemianopia with macular sparing.
- *Parietal lobe lesion* results in inferior quadrantanopia hemianopia, whereas temporal lobe lesion results in upper quadrantanopic hemianopia.

Ocular Reflexes

Light Reflex

Light reflex is mediated via fibers from optic tract to pretectal nucleus to EWN located in the midbrain. Fibers from optic tract enter brachium of superior colliculus instead of lateral geniculate body **(Fig. 28A)**. Fibers from EWN enter ciliary ganglion and supply the ciliary muscles causing pupillary constriction. The pathway for light reflex does not pass through occipital cortex. Hence, children with cortical blindness will have vision loss with preserved pupil light reflex.

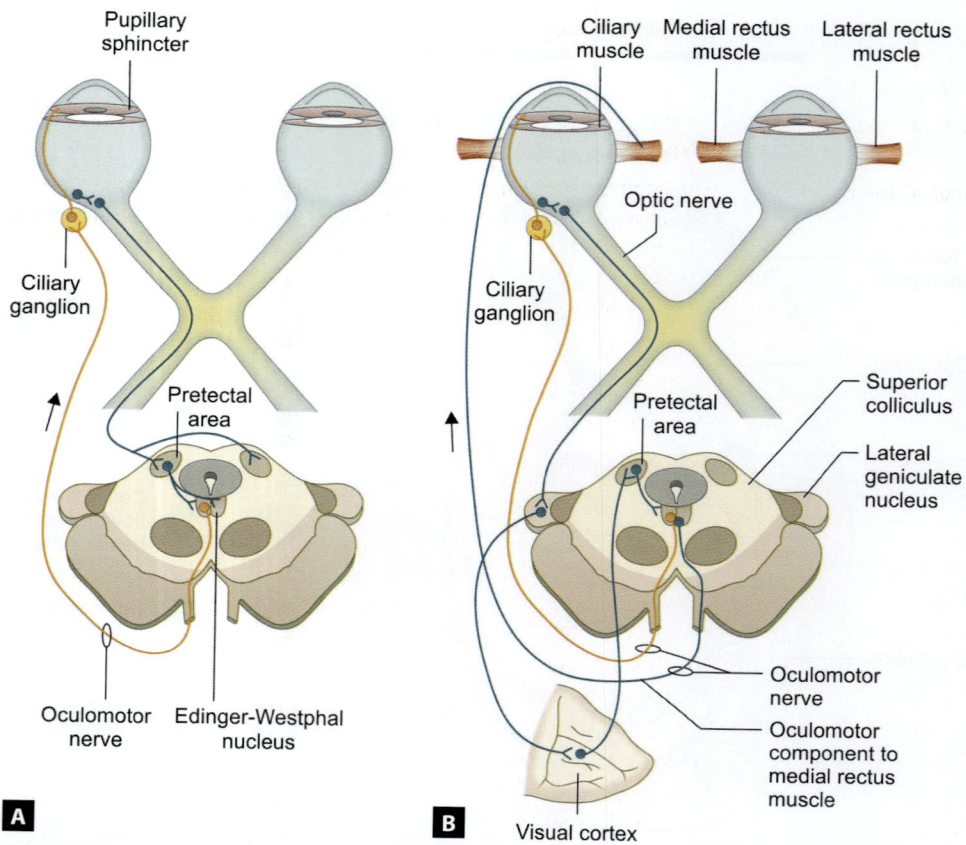

Figs. 28A and B: Pupillary light reflex pathway (A) and accommodation reflex pathway (B).

Accommodation Reflex

Accommodation reflex is mediated via occipital cortex.

Fibers from optic tract reach lateral geniculate nucleus, which in turn relays signals to occipital visual cortex. Signals from visual cortex reach pretectal area to ultimately relay to EWN (ciliary muscles cause pupillary constriction and thickening of lens) and prefrontal cortex (convergence through frontal eye field and area 8 [not shown in figure]) **(Fig. 28B)**. Accommodation involving convergence and pupillary constriction to focus on a nearby object requires intact visual cortex.

Abnormalities in Pupil

Normally, pupils are normally equal in size, round, centered in iris, and react to direct and consensual light reflex. There are various abnormalities of pupil **(Table 13)**.

Ocular Motility

Extraocular Muscle Innervation

Monocular eye movements are called ductions (abduction and adduction). Binocular conjugate eye movements are called version (right or left sided version). Disconjugate eye movements are called vergences. Convergence is movement of both

TABLE 13: Common abnormalities of pupil.

Pupillary abnormality	Description
Unilateral fixed dilated pupil	Third nerve palsy (in a comatose patient, it could indicate uncal lobe herniation)
Marcus–Gunn pupil	Relative afferent pupillary defect (RAPD) is observed in optic nerve pathology: Dilation of pupil when the light is swung from unaffected eye to affected eye
Holmes–Adie pupil	Unilateral dilated pupil that constricts sluggishly and slowly to light (tonic pupil)
Horner syndrome	Unilateral constricted pupil (miosis), associated with anhidrosis, ptosis, and enophthalmos
Argyll–Robertson pupil	Bilateral small pupil that does not constrict on light but constricts on accommodation (mnemonic: accommodation reflex present: ARP: Argyll Robertson pupil)

eyes nasally and divergence is movement of both eyes temporally.

We know that the 4th nerve supplies superior oblique [SO supplied by 4, can be remembered as SO_4 (sulfate)] and 6th nerve supplies lateral rectus (LR6). The rest of extraocular muscles, levator palpebrae superioris (LPS), and sphincter papillae are supplied by 3rd CN. Hence, complete third CN palsy will result in:
- Bilateral or unilateral ptosis (LPS involvement)
- Pupils are dilated and nonreactive to light and accommodation
- Eye movements are restricted to lateral gaze; eyes are turned out and down

Ptosis may result from 3rd CN palsy or weakness of tarsal muscles (due to sympathetic involvement) but in the latter, the lid can be raised voluntarily. The most common cause of unilateral complete ptosis is 3rd CN palsy. The most common cause of unilateral partial ptosis is Horner's syndrome and bilateral mild ptosis is myasthenia gravis and other neuromuscular causes. Ptosis can be congenital or acquired. In congenital ptosis, LPS is fibrosed, leading to lid lag on downgaze.

Squint or Strabismus

Deviation of eye, which is otherwise not appreciable but manifests on cover–uncover test, is considered *latent squint (phoria)*. When the deviation is obvious on primary gaze, it is called *tropia*: eyes deviated laterally (exotropia), eyes deviated medially (esotropia), eyes deviated upward (hypertropia), and eyes deviated downward (hypotropia).

When normal eye is fixing, the deviation that occurs in the affected eye is called primary deviation. On covering the normal eye, when the affected eye starts fixing, the movement of normal eye under the cover is called secondary deviation. When secondary deviation is more than primary deviation, it is called paralytic squint.

Broadly, there are two main types of strabismus—concomitant squint and paralytic squint. When the misaligned eye maintains its abnormal position in all directions of gaze, it is called concomitant squint. Hence, in right eye exotropia, in primary position, the right eye is deviated out and it remains deviated out when moved right, left, upward, or downward whereas if there is paralytic squint in right eye (right exotropia), in primary gaze, eyes are deviated to right. When a patient is asked to look right, his eyes will move to right; when asked to look left, his eyes will not move; when asked to move up, his eyes will move up and out; and when asked to look down, it will move down and out. Hence, in paralytic squint, deviation is more evident in one gaze when compared to other gaze, whereas in concomitant squint, deviation is same in all gaze.

Clinical relevance:
- Paralytic squint, as the name suggests, results from CN palsy (3rd, 4th, or 6th CN), whereas concomitant squint usually has no definitive etiology.
- Face turn, head tilt, and chin lift will be seen in paralytic squint.
- Similarly, diplopia or double vision will be a complaint in paralytic squint and not in concomitant squint.

Ophthalmoplegia

Ophthalmoplegia refers to the inability to move eye muscles. When paralysis involves pupillary and ciliary muscles, it is called internal ophthalmoplegia. When paralysis involves extraocular muscles alone, it is called external ophthalmoplegia.

Supranuclear Control of Eye Movement

Supranuclear control of eye movements is summarized in **Table 14**. Pathways involved in the supranuclear control of saccadic movements are depicted in **Figure 29**. Left-sided cortex stimulates right parapontine reticular formation (PPRF), which in turn stimulates right-sided 6th CN (moving the right eye to look right) and through MLF also stimulates the left 3rd CN (moving the left eye to look at right). Hence, normally, the left cortex will cause conjugate deviation of eyes

TABLE 14: Supranuclear control of eye movement.

Eye movement	Localization
Saccadic eye movement	Frontal lobe
Pursuit eye movement	Parieto-occipital lobe
Horizontal eye movement	Pons
Vertical eye movement	Midbrain reticular formation

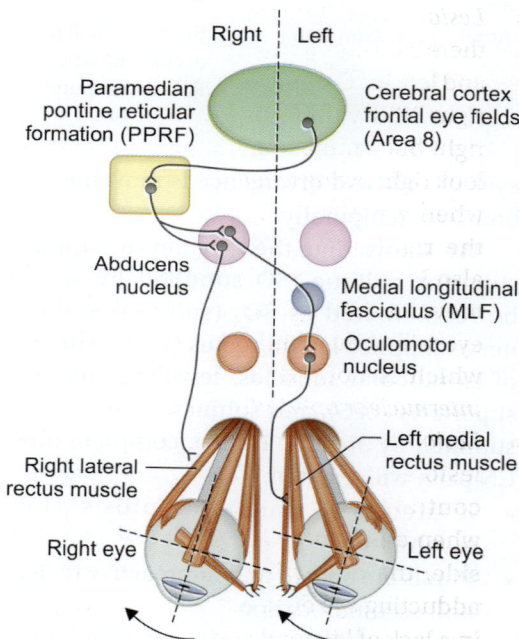

Fig. 29: Pathways involved in supranuclear control of eye movement.

toward the right. Types of lesions that can occur in this pathway include the following:
- *Lesion at right 6th CN:* Right eye cannot look toward the right but can look in all other directions and the left eye can look in all directions. The only restriction is abduction of right eye. This indicates isolated right 6th CN palsy.
- *Lesion in right PPRF:* We know that right PPRF is responsible for stimulating the

right 6th nerve and through MLF it will stimulate the left 3rd nerve. If there is a right PPRF lesion, right 6th nerve and left 3rd nerve will not be stimulated. Hence, there will be a right-sided gaze palsy (neither right eye nor left eye can look toward right). But the right cortex continues to stimulate left PPRF forcing the eyes to look toward left. Hence, the eyes are tonically deviated to the opposite side with PPRF lesion.
- *Lesion at left MLF:* With left MLF lesion, there is disconnection between right PPRF and left 3rd CN nucleus. When stimulated, right PPRF will command right eye to look right but cannot command the left eye to look right owing to left MLF lesion. Hence, when a patient is asked to look toward the right side, right eye abducts (and also has nystagmus) and left eye has no movement. When asked toward left, left eye will abduct and right eye will adduct, which is normal. This lesion is called *internuclear ophthalmoplegia (INO)*.
- *Lesion involves both MLF:* Bilateral MLF lesion will disconnect both PPRF to contralateral 3rd CN nucleus. Hence, when a patient is asked to look at either side, the abducting eye moves but the adducting eye does not move. This results in a lack of bilateral adduction.
- *Lesion involves right PPRF and both MLF:* If there is a lesion in right PPRF, there will be right gaze palsy. In addition, if there is a bilateral MLF lesion as well, there will be no adduction in both the eyes. This results in no adduction in both eyes and no abduction in right eye. Hence, only the left eye can abduct; the rest of three movements (abduction of right eye and adduction of right and left eyes) are not possible (so, three out of four movements are restricted: 1½). This is called *one and half syndrome*.
- *Lesion at cortex:* Left-sided destructive lesion will result in no signal to right PPRF. The right cortex will stimulate left PPRF to look at left. Hence, a destructive cortical lesion will result in eye deviated to the same side. In contrast, an irritative cortical lesion will hyperstimulate contralateral PPRF. Hence, the eye looks toward the destructive cortical lesion and looks away from the irritative cortical lesion.

Common Abnormal Eye Movement

The common abnormal eye movements include opsoclonus, ocular dysmetria, ocular flutter, ocular bobbing, and ocular myoclonus **(Table 15)**.

TABLE 15: Types of abnormal eye movements.

Eye movement	Description	Localization
Opsoclonus	Random, chaotic eye movement in all directions	Can be seen in opsoclonus–myoclonus ataxia syndrome, neuroblastoma
Ocular dysmetria	Overshoot of eyes on rapid fixation	Cerebellar dysfunction
Ocular flutter	Horizontal oscillatory movement with forward gaze	Cerebellar dysfunction, hydrocephalus
Ocular bobbing	Downward jerking from primary gaze	Pontine lesion
Ocular myoclonus	Pendular oscillation of eye synchronous with eye muscle movement	Red nucleus and inferior olivary nucleus

Limbic System

The limbic system in brain is responsible for emotional behavior, memory formation, olfaction, and control of food habits. It is composed mainly of hypothalamus, hippocampus, amygdala, limbic cortex (cingulated gyrus and parahippocampal gyrus), olfactory bulb, and septal area **(Fig. 30)**. Spatial memory is governed by parahippocampal gyrus, whereas long-term memory is governed by hippocampus. Amygdala controls aggression, anxiety, emotional memory, and social cognition. Hence, a lesion in amygdala would result in docile behavior, hypersexuality, and compulsive attentiveness (Kluver–Bucy syndrome). Cingulate gyrus controls autonomic function regarding heart rate and blood pressure.

Papez postulated that a circuit linking consciousness, thought, and emotion involves hippocampal formation, cingulated gyrus, mammillary body (hypothalamus), and anterior nucleus of thalamus (Papez circuit) **(Flowchart 3)**. The structures involved in memory are summarized in **Table 16**.

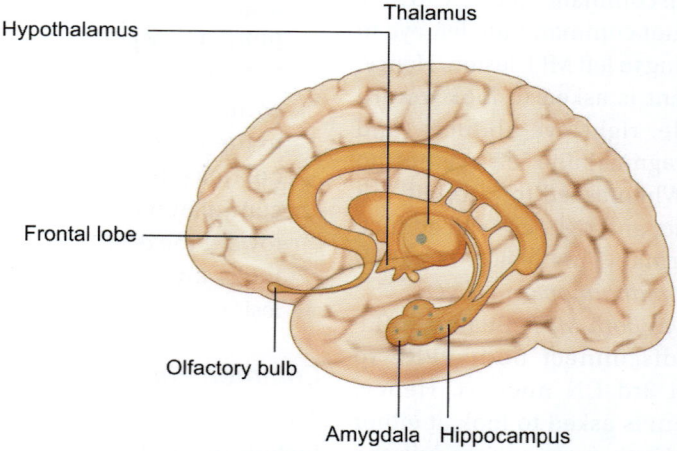

Fig. 30: Anatomy of limbic system.

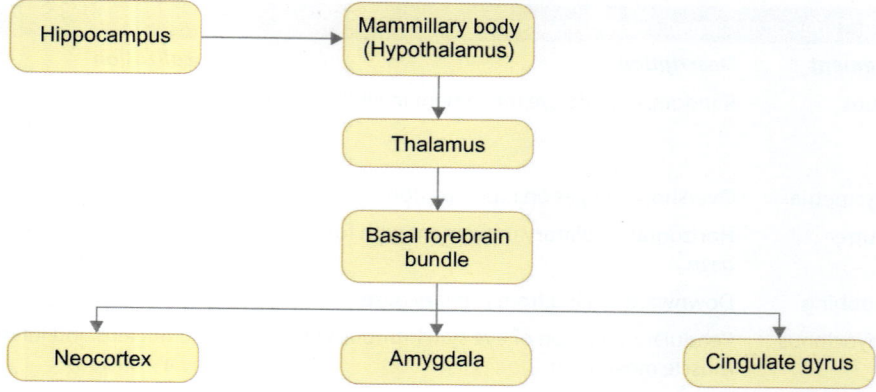

Flowchart 3: Papez circuit showing the link among hypothalamus, anterior thalamus, cingulated cortex, and hippocampus.

TABLE 16: Areas of the brain that control the memory.

Memory	Area of brain that controls
Short-term to long-term memory	Hippocampus and medial temporal lobe
Recent memory/acquiring new memory	Hippocampus
Past memory	Cerebral cortex
Emotions to memory or fear memory	Amygdala
Working memory and higher order processing of memory	Prefrontal cortex
Storing of long-term memory and episodic memory	Frontal cortex

■ AUTONOMIC NERVOUS SYSTEM

Autonomic nervous system consists of sympathetic and parasympathetic nervous systems. Sympathetic nervous system has thoracolumbar origin (T1 to L3–L4) and parasympathetic nervous system has craniosacral origin [CN 3, 7, 9, and 10 and sacral (S2–S4)]. Autonomic nervous system has noradrenergic neurons and cholinergic neurons. In autonomic nervous system, motor neurons are categorized into preganglionic neurons (cell bodies lie in the brain and spinal cord) and postganglionic neurons (cell bodies lie outside the CNS). Cholinergic neurons include all preganglionic autonomic, postganglionic parasympathetic, neuromuscular junction, and few postganglionic sympathetic (sweat gland, skeletal muscle, and blood vessel). Adrenergic neurons include postganglionic sympathetic neurons, adrenal medulla, and hypothalamus.

Activation of sympathetic nervous system (fright and flight reaction) results in dilated pupil, tachycardia, hypertension, constriction of skin blood vessel, bronchial dilatation, inhibition of salivary secretion, urinary sphincter contraction, and detrusor relaxation. In contrast, parasympathetic stimulation results in constricted pupil, bradycardia, bronchial constriction, and increased salivary secretion.

Hypothalamus

Hypothalamus (*below the thalamus*) consists of various nuclei that synthesize and secrete neurohormones through pituitary. It consists of suprachiasmatic nuclei (controls sleep–wake cycle and circadian rhythm), paraventricular nucleus [secrete releasing hormone for thyroid stimulating hormone (TSH) and adrenocorticotropic hormone (ACTH)], preoptic nucleus [secrete gonadotropin-releasing hormone (GnRH)], arcuate nucleus (secrete releasing hormone for prolactin), and periventricular nucleus (secrete growth hormone).

Fibers from supraoptic nucleus (secrete oxytocin) and paraventricular nucleus (secrete vasopressin) connect with posterior pituitary, and the hormones are released at the end of nerve terminal in posterior pituitary. Hypothalamus controls sleep, circadian rhythm, temperature regulation, thirst, and hunger. It also controls the autonomic nervous system.

KEY MESSAGES

- Upper motor neuron (UMN) weakness will have spasticity, brisk deep tendon reflexes (DTRs), and extensor plantar response; lower motor neuron (LMN) weakness may have flaccidity, diminished or absent DTRs with flexor or mute plantar response.
- The presence of seizures, aphasia (cortical lesion), and dense hemiplegia (internal capsule lesion) could point to UMN involvement.
- Pyramidal tract lesion would result in spastic weakness, whereas extrapyramidal tract lesion would result in dyskinesia or movement disorders.
- *In the LMN weakness:* Presence of tongue fasciculations points to anterior horn cell involvement; distal atrophy with diminished or absent DTRs points to neuropathy; ptosis and weakness of extraocular muscles point to neuromuscular pathology; proximal muscle weakness is seen in myopathy.
- *Few symptoms and signs have specific localizing value in neurology:* Dystonia/ choreoathetosis (basal ganglia), ataxia (posterior column, vestibular pathway, or cerebellar), and bladder retention (spinal cord pathology).

Developmental History, Examination, and Analysis

CHAPTER 2

INTRODUCTION

Development of a child is a continuous sequential process and is intimately related to maturation of nervous system. There is loss of primitive reflexes for acquiring purposeful desired voluntary movement. For example, till asymmetric tonic neck reflex (ATNR) persists, infant is unable to roll from back to front or bring hands in the midline to reach for objects. Similarly, once the child achieves the desired motor milestones, the righting reflexes help them develop stability. The advanced postural reflexes that are protective like parachute reflex and propping reflex often are not developed in children with cerebral palsy.

ASSESSMENT OF PRIMITIVE REFLEXES

Moro's Reflex

Hold the infant in your hand and forearm with infant's head rested on your palm hold the infant at 45° to ground. Slightly drop your palm for the infant's head to come back to fall on your dropped palm. This will result in extension of infant's both arms with opening of hands. It appears at 28 weeks and persists till 3–6 months **(Fig. 1)**.

Asymmetric Tonic Neck Reflex

While the infant is supine with head in midline, turn the head to one side. The ipsilateral limb [upper limb/lower limb

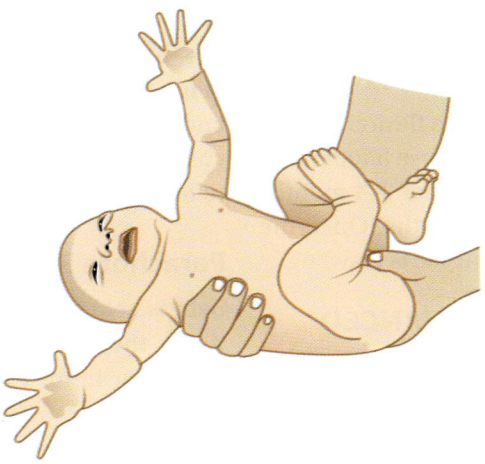

Fig. 1: Moro reflex.

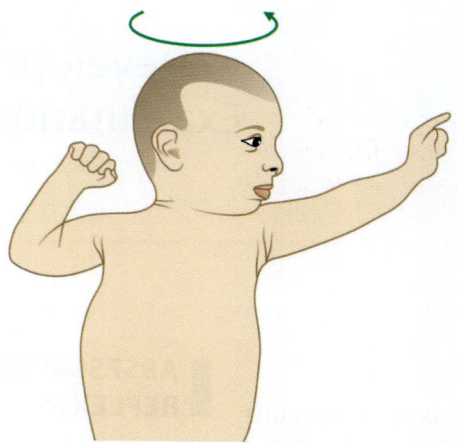

Fig. 2: Asymmetric tonic neck reflex.

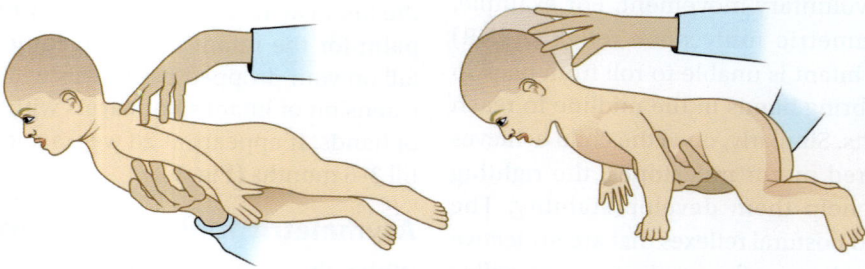

Fig. 3: Landau reflex.

(UL/LL)] extends and contralateral UL/LL flexes. It appears at 1 month and disappears by 3–4 months **(Fig. 2)**.

Symmetric Tonic Neck Reflex

Flexion of infant head leads to flexion of arms and extension of legs and reverse happens on extension of head. It appears at 3–4 months and disappears by 9–10 months. Once the reflex disappears, the infant starts crawling.

ASSESSMENT OF ADVANCED POSTURAL REFLEXES

Landau Reflex

When the baby is ventrally suspended in the prone position in the air, there is an extension of the neck with arching of the back and extension of upper and lower limb. When the head is flexed in this position, the upper limb and lower limb flexes **(Fig. 3)**. This reflex appears at 3 months and disappears at 12 months. It represents a combination of labyrinthine reflex and visual reflex.

Parachute Reflex

Baby is held in ventral suspension face down. When the head is suddenly lowered, both the upper limbs extend as if to prevent the face getting injured **(Fig. 4)**. It appears at 6–9 months and persists through life. It is a protective reflex.

Propping Reflex

Like parachute reflex, when the infant is titled suddenly to one side, the same-sided arms extend to prevent falling. This reflex appears at 5–7 months and allows pivoting/sitting (**Fig. 5**).

Delayed disappearance of primitive reflexes or persistence of primitive reflexes with non-development of advanced postural reflexes is observed in children with cerebral palsy.

ASSESSMENT OF RIGHTING REFLEXES

Neck Righting Reflex

Turning head to one side, the whole body turns to that side. It is seen at birth and is strongest at 3 months.

Labyrinth Righting Reflex

It enables the child to lift the head first in a prone position and later in a supine position. This reflex is strongest at 10 months.

Body Righting Reflex

Body righting reflex is responsible for sitting and then later standing. Most of the righting reflexes that provide stability to the voluntary motor development such as sitting, standing do not develop well in children with cerebral palsy.

DEVELOPMENTAL DOMAINS

There are five domains of development: Gross motor, fine motor, personal–social, language and cognitive milestones. Developmental history will elicit history pertaining to age at attainment of each developmental milestone

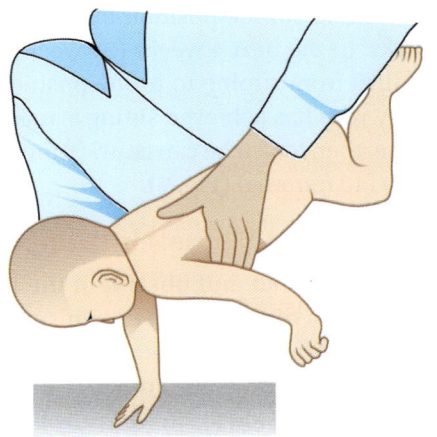

Fig. 4: Parachute reflex.

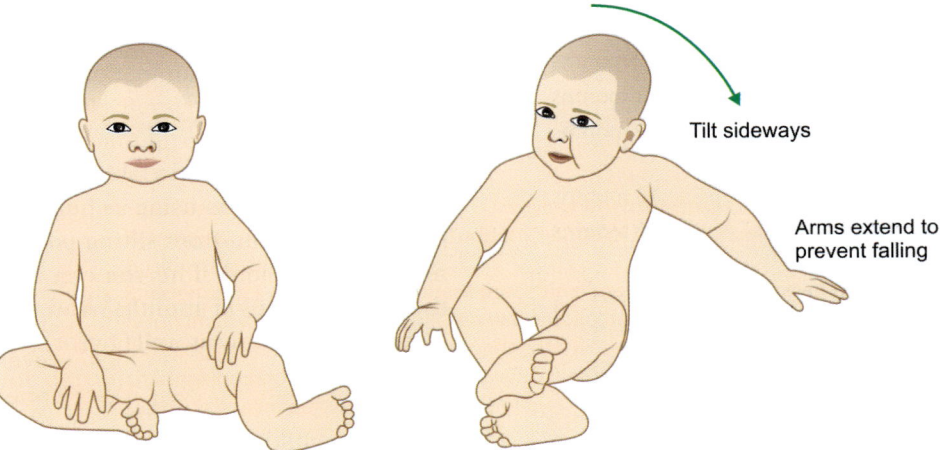

Fig. 5: Propping reflex.

in specific domains. The developmental examination would confirm the observations based on the history to arrive at the probable developmental age in the child in each domain. Hence, developmental examination supplements the developmental history. Let us see each domains of the development.

Gross Motor Milestones

Gross motor milestones refer to development of motor milestones for locomotion. Apart from eliciting the history of attainment of motor milestones, we must observe the child for his gross motor skills **(Table 1)**. The major milestones in gross motor domain are depicted in the following text.

Pull to Sit

When pull to sit, there will be slight head lag at 12 weeks, and there will be no head lag by 20 weeks. He can lift his head when approached by someone to lift him (24 weeks) and by 6 months, he can spontaneously lift his head.

Prone Position

Make the infant lie on a prone position and observe the movement. If the baby can lift the head momentarily (4 weeks) or sustained (8 weeks), head above the plane (12 weeks), head and chest above the plane supported with elbow flexed (12 weeks) or extended elbow (24 weeks) **(Fig. 6)**. He can start turning from prone to supine position by this age of 24 weeks. In the next 4 weeks (28 weeks), he could turn from supine to prone position. If the baby who has achieved sitting is made to lie prone, then look if he can crawl (9 months) or creep (10 months) **(Fig. 7)**.

Sitting

Make the infant sit and observe if the baby can sit with or without his/her own support. Accordingly, the developmental age can be determined **(Fig. 8)**. For example, if the child can pivot while made to sit, we know that his developmental age in gross motor milestone is at least 10–12 months. If the child is already walking and running, it is presumed that he has already achieved mature sitting, then we can skip this part of examination.

Pull to Stand

The child may be offered a table or a chair and encouraged to get up using its help. Look for his ability to stand from sitting position (10 months). Also, look if he/she can cruz over the furniture (10–11 months) and walk few steps independently as well (1 year) **(Fig. 9)**.

Run

Watch the child run around to see if he can run broad-based (13 months), run and jump

TABLE 1: Gross motor milestones.

Gross motor	Expected age at attainment
Head control	3 months
Turn from prone to supine	6 months
Turn from supine to prone	7 months
Sitting with support	8 months
Sitting without support	9 months
Standing with support	10 months
Cruising around the furniture	11 months
Walk few steps without support	12 months
Broad-based gait	13 months
Can run, jump over the furniture	18 months
Walk steps two up two down	2 years
Walk steps one up two down	3 years
Walk steps one up and one down	4 years
Skip on both feet	5 years
Skip on one foot	6 years

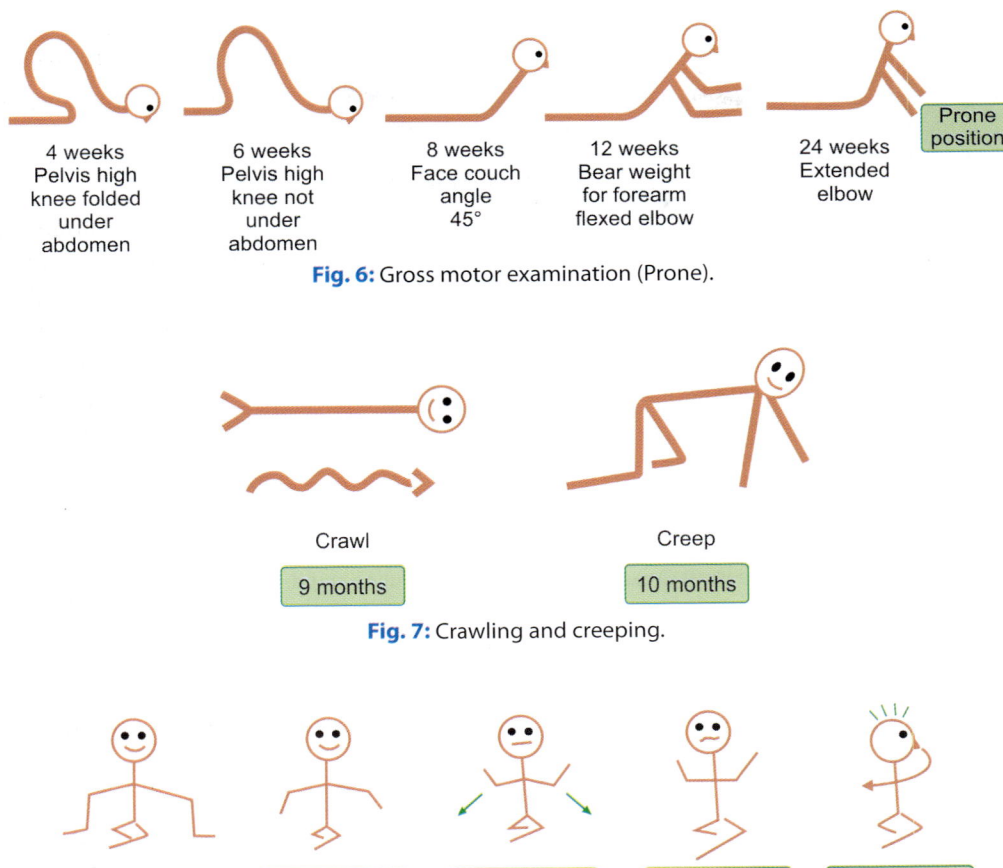

Fig. 6: Gross motor examination (Prone).

Fig. 7: Crawling and creeping.

Fig. 8: Gross motor examination: Sitting.

on the furniture (18 months) or run front and back (24 months) **(Fig. 10)**. Ask the child to walk upstairs and downstairs to see whether he can do it with one foot per step, or he uses two feet per step. He can stand on one foot by 3 years and can hop on one foot by 4 years.

Fine Motor Milestones

Fine motor skills involve use of hands and upper extremity to explore the environment for manipulation **(Table 2)**.

Cubes

When cubes are offered to the baby, look at the grasp of the cube **(Fig. 11)**. He attains ulnar grasp by 6 months, radial palmar grasp by 7 months, scissor grasp (four fingers on one side and thumb on other side) by 8 months, radiodigital grasp (first two fingers on one side and thumb on the other side) by 8–9 months and mature pincer grasp by 10 months. Hand-to-mouth transfer begins at 24 weeks and by 28 weeks the child can

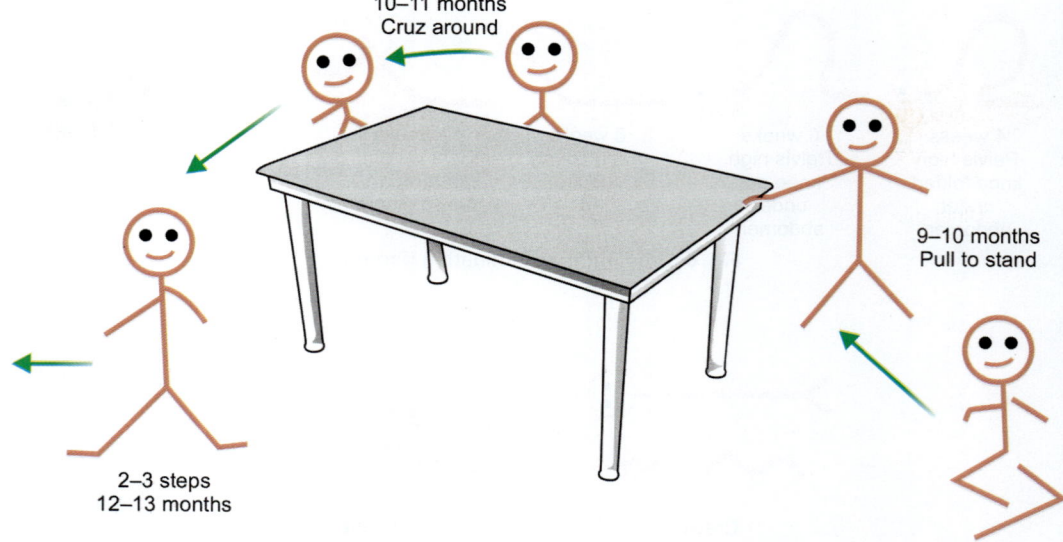

Fig. 9: Gross motor examination: Pull to stand.

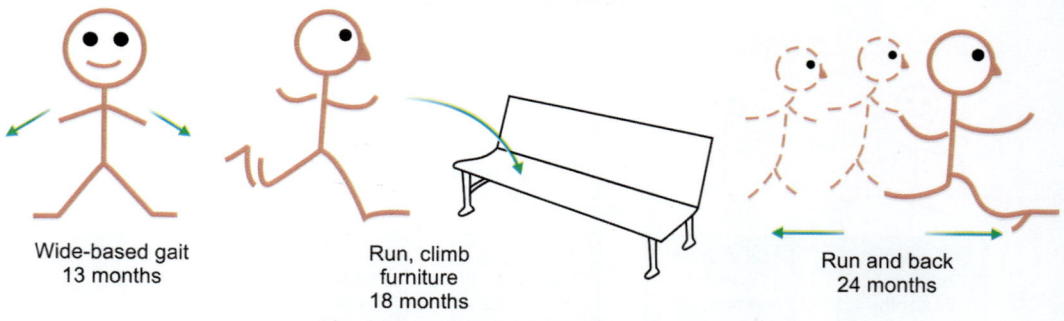

Fig. 10: Gross motor assessment: Running.

TABLE 2: Fine motor milestones.	
Fine motor milestone	**Age at attainment**
Closed hands	4 weeks
Open hands and holds the object placed on the hand	12 weeks
Stares at the offered object as if trying to grab but overshoots	16 weeks
Reaches for object using both the hands (bidextrous grasp)	20 weeks
Ulnar grasp (grasps using ulnar border of the hand), can transfer from one hand to other, retain one object when another was given	6 months
Radial grasp (grasps using radial border of the hand)	8 months
Scissor grasp (four fingers on one side and thumb on other side)	9–10 months
Mature pincer grasp	10 months

CHAPTER 2: Developmental History, Examination, and Analysis

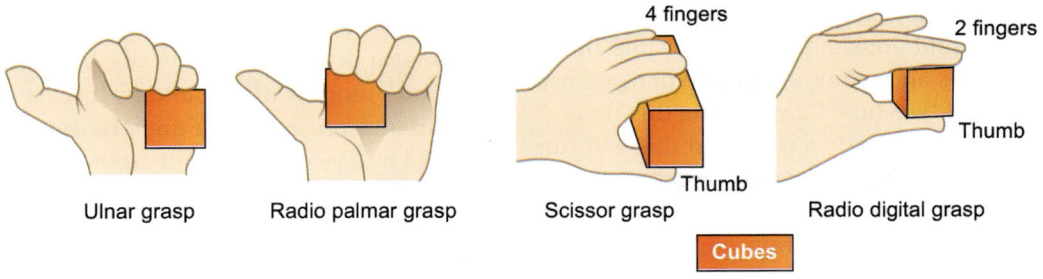

Fig. 11: Fine motor grasp cubes.

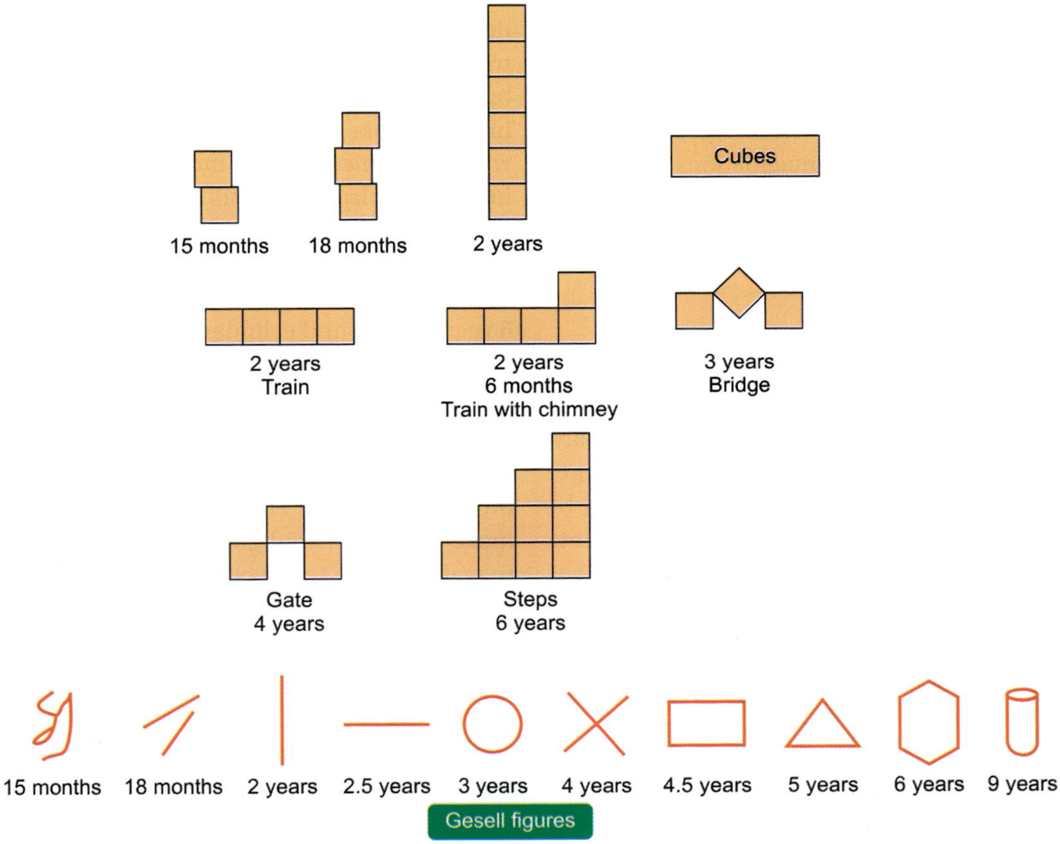

Fig. 12: Fine motor examination using cubes.

transfer the cube from one hand to other hand. He retains one cube when next is offered by 6–7 months. He can match a cube with another cube by 36 months. A 13-month child will cast the cubes, casting usually stops by 15 months. He can make a tower of 2 by 15 months, 3–4 by 18 months, 6–7 by 2 years, 8 by 2.5 years, and 9 cubes by 3 years of age **(Fig. 12)**. He can make a train by 2 years, add a chimney to the train by 2.5 years, can imitate a bridge by 3 years, gate by 4 years, steps by 6 years of age.

Remember that when you provide cubes to the child, look at the way the child holds the cubes and manipulates it. When you ask the child "see how I am making this train..." "see we have made a train and this will run chuk chuk chuk...." Now dismantle it and give all the cubes to the child and ask the child "now you make the train and make it run chuk chuk chuk..." This is called imitation where the child makes the train based on memory of how you made the train. If you show him a train that is already made and give him another set of cubes and tell the child to make this kind of train, then this is called copying. While copying child will have to use his own imaginations as to how I could make this train. Copying skills develop 6 months later than imitating skills. So, a child can imitate train by 2 years and copy train by 2.5 years.

Pellet

When offered with a pellet, 40-week baby starts with index finger approach. Gradually, the child starts picking with index finger bent and thumb (inferior pincer grasp) by 9 months before developing a complete pincer grasp by 10 months **(Fig. 13)**. It is important to be vigilant that child should not swallow the pellets. Keep a count of number of pellets in your box.

Book

He can turn two to three pages of a book at a time by 18 months of age, and by 2 years of age, can turn one page at a time. He can put his socks by 2 years of age and dress/undress by 3 years of age.

Pencil

Initially the child will hold the pencil by a cylindrical grasp (12 months), then will develop digital grasp (2–3 years), and finally tripod grasp (5–7 years) **(Fig. 14)**. A 15-month baby can imitate scribble, 18 month child can imitate strokes on the paper when offered with the pencil. By 24 months of age, he imitates vertical stroke and by 2.5 years, can imitate a horizontal stroke. He can copy a circle by 3 years, cross by 4 years, rectangle by 4.5 years, triangle by 5 years, diamond by 6 years of age, and cylinder by 9 years. These are called as Gesell figures **(Fig. 12)**.

Draw a Man Test

Tell the child (>3 years) to draw your father on this page. Keep encouraging the child to make the man. Avoid guiding the child what to make next. A 3-year child can make one to two parts, 4 year child can make three parts, 5 years child can make six to 7 parts, 6 years child can make up to eight parts.

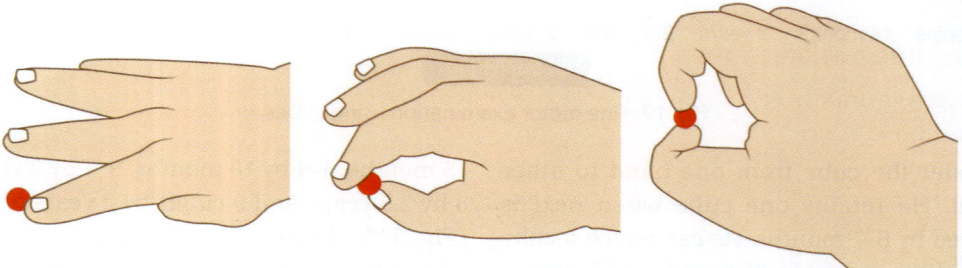

Fig. 13: Approach to a pellet showing Index finger approach, inferior pincer grasp and mature pincer grasp.

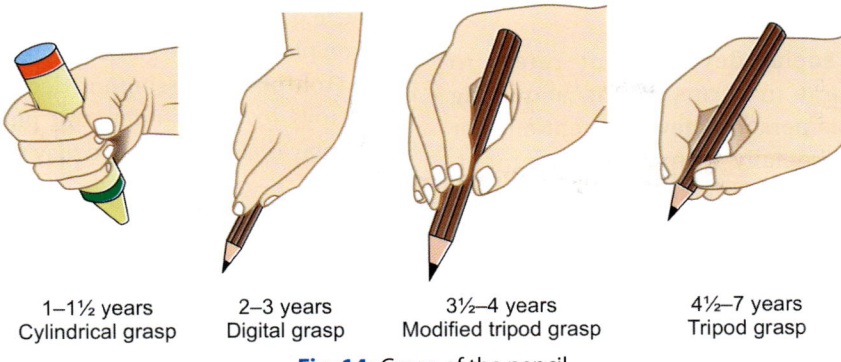

| 1–1½ years | 2–3 years | 3½–4 years | 4½–7 years |
| Cylindrical grasp | Digital grasp | Modified tripod grasp | Tripod grasp |

Fig. 14: Grasp of the pencil.

TABLE 3: Language milestones.

Language milestones	Age at attainment
Begins to vocalize	4–6 weeks
Begins to say gaga, ah goo	12 weeks
Laughs aloud, squeals with delight	4 months
Razzing (blowing between lips)	5 months
Monosyllables (ma, da, ka)	6 months
Vocalize to call	7 months
Bisyllables (mumum, dada)	8–9 months
Begins to imitate sounds, may speak one word with meaning, responds to "no"	9–10 months
Two to three words with meaning, he can imitate the sounds of dog, cat, crow	1 year
Jargon speech	15 months
10 words' vocabulary	18 months
Simple sentences using 2 words	2 years
Three-worded sentences	3 years
Four-worded sentences and story-telling, use of past tense	4 years
Use of future tense	5 years

Language Milestones

Language milestones consist of preverbal communication and subsequently verbal communication. We can observe the preverbal communication skills such as vocalizing sounds, laughing aloud, and vocalizing to call the parents. We can communicate with the child to note the verbal output and ability to use appropriate words, and sentences. We are concerned when the child does not speak a single meaningful word by 15 months, and a meaningful phrase of two words by 24 months. These can be considered as red flags for language developmental milestones. It is essential to observe the language milestones as parents often overestimate the language acquisition by their child when asked on history **(Table 3)**.

Social Milestones

Personal social development refers to development in terms of his acquiring skills for his personal development and for interacting socially with the environment. It is essential to understand the difference between social development skills that lead to social interaction with surroundings and cognitive skills that determine the intelligence of the child. For example, knowing that this is my toy is cognition, asking the mother to give me that toy by use of appropriate gestures is social skill.

When children play with toys looking at the way other kids are playing with their toys, this kind of play is called parallel play which develops by 24 months. This is followed by joint play where children jointly perform a task, e.g., building a mud house. Many children play imitative games such as doctor–patient role plays, dressing and decorating the Barbie toys, teacher–student role play games. Such a play is called imitative play **(Table 4)**.

Adaptive Milestones

Adaptive milestones mean how the child is able to adapt to the environment. We can observe how the child is feeding self. Offer a biscuit to the mother and tell her to give him. A 6-month baby can feed self with a biscuit and will develop chewing. Then offer him cup and spoon. A 15-month child can use the spoon with some spilling and 18 months can feed from a cup without any spilling. One can observe the way the child puts on his clothes and removes them. Look at the way

TABLE 4: Social milestones.

Social milestones	Age at attainment
Social smile	4–6 weeks
Vocalizes	8 weeks
Squeals with delight	3 months
Laughs aloud	16 weeks
Recognize mother, show interest in surroundings, watch people moving around	4 months
He imitates, acts like tongue protrusion or coughing	6 months
Smiling at mirror image	7 months
Search for dropped object, stranger anxiety	9 months
Respond to "NO"	32 weeks
Pulls at mother's clothes, repeats performance laughed at, imitates pat a cake and waves bye-bye	9 months
Laughs at mother when she puts an unusual object on her head	11–12 months
Plays a simple ball game	1 year
Asks for object by pointing and can indicate wet pants	15 months
Domestic mimicry and is dry by day	18 months
Parallel play	24 months
Knows full name and gender	30 months
Knows gender	3 years
Right left discrimination	4 years
Knows his age	5 years

he buttons and unbuttons his shirt, he wears his shoes and tie his shoelaces. He is usually dry by day by 18 months. Around 50% are dry by night by 2 years, 75% by 3 years, and 90% by 5 years **(Table 5)**.

Cognitive Milestones

Cognitive milestones refer to acquiring intelligence. Knowing shapes, colors, sizes, identifying pictures, and naming the pictures are all cognitive milestones. Parents are often concentrating on these cognitive skills. It is essential to differentiate these milestones from social milestones. For example, a child may understand that biscuits are kept in that jar in the kitchen, but he may not communicate verbally (language milestone) or by non-verbal gestures such as mature finger pointing by making a sustained eye contact with the mother (social milestones). This often happens in children with autism spectrum disorder.

Vision Assessment

The vision assessment precedes the formal developmental evaluation. A red ring is often used for visual fixation and tracking. A 4-week baby will regard the red ring, 6-week baby will fix and follow-up to 90° and 12-week baby can follow-up to 180° **(Fig. 15)**.

Hearing Assessment

The hearing regard must be always tested in absence of visual cue. A bell, if often, is used for hearing regard. It is expected that 3-month baby will turn to the sound, 6-month baby

TABLE 5: Adaptive milestones.

Adaptive milestone	Age at attainment
Chewing	6 months
Cup feeding with spilling	1 year
Spoon feeding with some spilling	15 months
Can feed from cup without spilling	18 months
Can zip and unzip his garments and take off his clothes	2 years
Can wash his hands and can brush his teeth with some assistance	2.5 years
Dress fully, can unbutton, independently can eat, can put his shoes but need help with shoelaces	3 years
Can button his shirt, tie shoelaces, can wash his face and hands	4 years
Can independently dress and bath himself	5 years

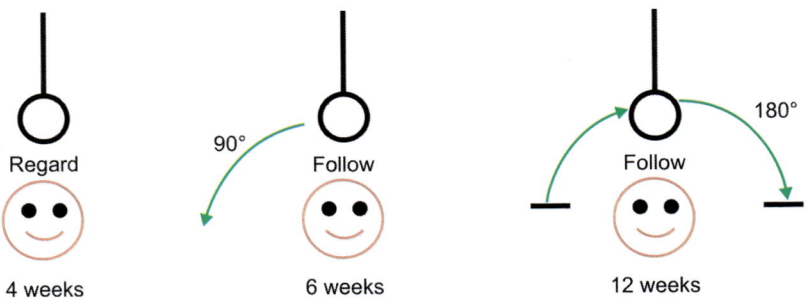

Fig. 15: Visual assessment milestones.

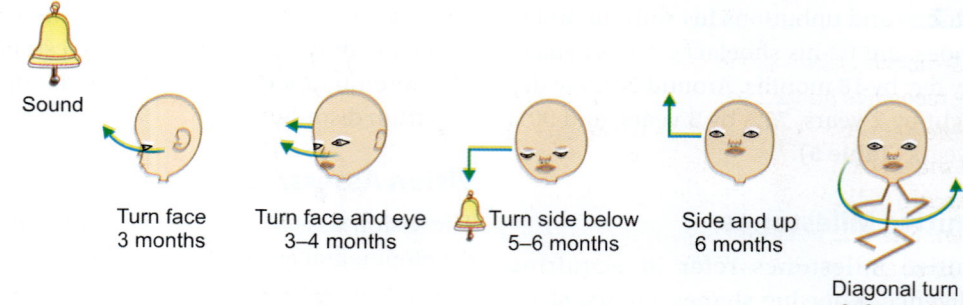

Fig. 16: Murphy's sequence of hearing.

can turn when sound is from side and up and a 9 month baby can turn to the direction of sound in a diagonal manner (Murphy's sequence) **(Fig. 16)**.

Case 1

A 2-year-old child presented was not able to speak till now. He can walk and run in the house. He can feed himself well without any spilling using a spoon. He can understand and recognize few colors and shapes. He does not respond to verbal commands. His vision is intact.

Assessment of developmental history:

Milestones	Attained milestone	Developmental age
Motor	Can run and can walk 2 steps per step while climbing up and down	24 months
Fine motor	Feeding without spilling using spoon	18–24 months
Cognition	He can recognize few colors, can match shapes	30 months
Language	No cooing	<3 months
Social	He engages in domestic mimicry and is dry by day	24 months

Assessment on developmental examination:
- *Gross motor:* You observed the child walking upstairs and downstairs with two steps per foot. This confirms the developmental age determined by the history.
- *Fine motor:*
  - He can build tower of six to seven cubes when offered cubes
  - He can imitate a horizontal line when offered a pen and white paper
- *Social:* You observed a good eye contact; he looks at a pointed object but does not respond when commanded verbally.
- *Language:* You observed that he was mute and had no cooing as well.
- *Cognition:* When asked by gestures, he can point to at least two to three pictures in a picture book but his response to verbal commands is poor.

Hence, the developmental assessment by history and examination points to developmental dissociation. Developmental age of this child is 24 months against chronological age of 24 months in gross motor, fine motor, cognitive, and social milestones; also, there was marked delay in language milestone (developmental age of <3 months) and hearing response.

Final interpretation: Hearing loss with language impairment

CHAPTER 2: Developmental History, Examination, and Analysis

Case 2

An 18-month child presents with inability to smile, recognize parents, nor is the child able to hold the neck. She keeps her hand open. There is no meaningful eyes contact. She responds to hearing and stops her activity briefly when spoken. She has multiple episodes of sudden jerks since the age of 12 months.

Assessment of developmental history:

Milestones	Attained milestone	Developmental age
Motor	No neck holding	Less than 3 months
Fine motor	Hands open	4 weeks
Cognition	No meaningful response	Less than 1 month
Language	No cooing	<3 months
Social	No social recognition	Less than 3 months

Assessment on developmental examination:
- **Gross motor:** On pull to sit, there is complete head lag. On prone position, the pelvis is high, but legs are not folded under the abdomen.
- **Fine motor:** hands are open and grasp reflex persisting.
- **Social:** No meaningful response
- **Language:** No cooing
- **Cognition:** No meaningful response
- **Vision:** Probably affected
- **Hearing:** Probably intact

Hence, the developmental assessment by history and examination points to developmental delay in all the domains with developmental age of <3 months against chronological age of 18 months.

Final interpretation: Global developmental delay with developmental age of <3 months against chronological age of 18 months.

KEY MESSAGES

- Primitive reflexes must disappear for the mature advanced postural reflexes to appear during the normal development of the baby.
- There are five domains of developmental assessment—gross motor/fine motor, language, social, cognitive, and adaptive milestones.
- Developmental history needs to be correlated with developmental examination and the discrepancy if any must be recorded.
- Developmental examination must be performed when the child is cheerful, well fed and parents or the caregivers are present during the assessment.
- Based on the last attained milestone, the developmental age is calculated approximately and compared with chronological age.

CHAPTER 3: Examination of Central Nervous System

INTRODUCTION

Examination of central nervous system is challenging in children. The components of examination include higher mental function examination, cranial nerve (CN) examination, motor system examination, sensory system examination, cerebellar examination, and meningeal signs.

HIGHER MENTAL FUNCTION EXAMINATION

It is extremely challenging to perform higher mental function (HMF) assessment in children when compared to adults. It is often difficult to fit HMF examination of children into adult protocols. It needs to be tailored according to age and development of the child. Many clinicians and students often get confused between cognitive development assessment and assessment of HMF. It is essential to remember that cognitive (intelligence) assessment is just one component of HMF. Most of HMF assessment in infants and young children is based on observation rather than formal methodical assessment. Components of HMF are summarized in **Flowchart 1**.

Consciousness

Consciousness refers to awareness of self and environment. Is the child responding appropriately to visual, auditory, and tactile stimulus from the surrounding? Does the child respond to verbal commands? If yes, then the child is conscious. There can be several alterations in the consciousness: Delirium, minimally conscious state, persistent vegetative state, coma, and brain death. For our convenience, we can divide

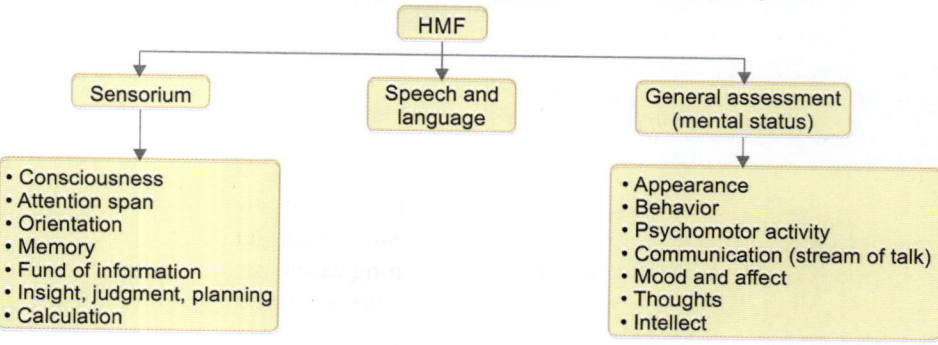

Flowchart 1: Components of higher mental function (HMF).

TABLE 1: States of altered consciousness.

	Conscious	Minimally conscious state	Persistent vegetative state	Coma	Brain death
Wakefulness	Preserved	Preserved	Preserved	Absent	Absent
Awareness	Preserved	↓↓	Absent	Absent	Absent
Sleep–wake cycle	Preserved	Preserved	Preserved	Absent	Absent
Brainstem reflexes	Preserved	Preserved	Preserved	Preserved	Absent

consciousness into wakefulness (eye open/closed), awareness (of self/surrounding), and sleep–wake cycle (preserved or absent). Various states of consciousness are summarized in **Table 1**.

Minimally conscious state:
- Altered consciousness with consciousness being unstained, and intermittent
- Communication is minimal during minimally conscious state.
- Child could vocalize rather than give meaningful speech.
- There is no emotional connect, but reflex smile or cry may be preserved.
- Child cannot follow any verbal commands but can orient to sound.
- He/she can exhibit occasional visual fixation/following
- Motor response to pain (localizes) and occasionally posturing to painful stimulus

Persistent vegetative state:
- No evidence of consciousness or any communication
- No evidence of emotional response
- No response to verbal command but may startle to loud noise
- No visual fixation/following but opens eyes intermittently
- No voluntary motor response, only reflex movement
- Sleep–wake cycle is preserved.

Coma:
- No evidence of consciousness
- No communication
- No emotional response
- No response to verbal command
- No visual response (eyes closed)
- Sleep–wake cycle not preserved
- Brainstem reflexes preserved

Locked-in syndrome:
- Fully conscious
- Communication only by vertical eye movement/blinking
- Emotions expressed in full range
- He/she responds with eye movement to auditory stimuli
- Motor function impaired with double hemiplegia

Delirium (acute confusional state):
- It is a transient, acute confusional state characterized by global impairment of sensorium.
- It is a state of disorientation, small attention span, vivid delusions, disconnected thoughts, and agitation.
- It is usually secondary to toxic, metabolic, or endocrine derangement.

Other terms to describe the states of consciousness like lethargy, obtundation, and stupor are generally avoided, but their meaning would be useful if someone uses it:
- *Lethargy:* No awareness but on arousal he gives appropriate response

- *Obtundation:* No awareness; on arousal, he gives confused response
- *Stupor:* No awareness or arousal, arousal only to vigorous stimulation

Assessment of Consciousness

Consciousness can be assessed using Glasgow coma scale (GCS), FOUR (Full Outline of UnResponsiveness) score, or AVPU (Alert, Voice, Pain, Unresponsive) scale. Anatomical structures for consciousness include medial hemispheric wall, diencephalon, midbrain tegmentum, and basal forebrain **(Fig. 1)**. Examination of an unconscious patient is discussed in **Chapter 11** (approach to a child with altered sensorium).

Glasgow coma scale: GCS has three components: Eye opening score, motor score, and verbal score. The minimum score is 3 (not 0) and maximum score is 15 **(Table 2)**. It is widely used in emergency setting. While scoring each component, the best scores need to be assessed and recorded. For example, if the eye opening is not spontaneous (E1), then it must be assessed by response to voice (E3) and response to touch or pain (E2) before assigning a score of E1 to the patient. GCS has limited use in intubated or paralyzed children where the verbal component and motor component of GCS are difficult to assess. In such situations, FOUR scores are more useful.

FOUR score: FOUR scores are useful for monitoring sensorium in intensive care unit (ICU) patients who are intubated. FOUR

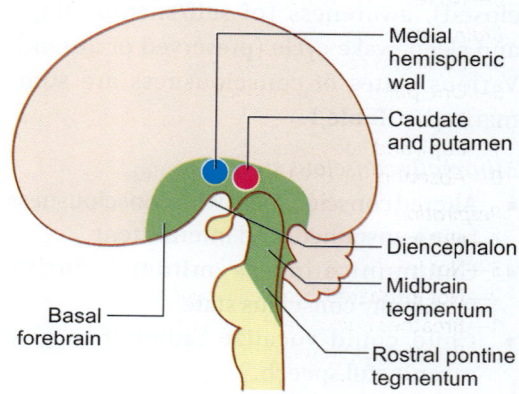

Fig. 1: Structures for consciousness.

TABLE 2: Glasgow coma scale.		
	Adult	**Children**
Eye opening	4—Spontaneous 3—To verbal stimuli 2—To pain 1—No response	Spontaneous eye opening To loud noise To pain No response
Verbal response	5—Oriented 4—Confused 3—Inappropriate 2—Incomprehensible 1—No response	Smiles, coos, cries Irritable, cries Inappropriate crying Grunts, moans No response
Motor response	6—Spontaneous 5—Withdraws to touch 4—Withdraws to pain 3—Abnormal flexion 2—Abnormal extension 1—No response	Obeys commands Localizes pain Withdraws pain Flexion to pain Extension to pain No response

BOX 1: FOUR score.

Eye response:
4—Eyelid open, tracking or blinking to command
3—Eyelid open, not moving
2—Eyelid closed, open to loud voice
1—Eyelid closed, open to pain
0—Eyelid remain closed with pain

Motor response:
4—Thumbs-up, fist or peace sign
3—Localizing to pain
2—Flexion to pain
1—Extension to pain
0—No response to pain

Brainstem reflexes:
4—Pupil and corneal reflex present
3—One pupil wide and fixed
2—Pupil or corneal absent
1—Pupil and corneal absent
0—Absent pupil corneal cough reflex

Respiration:
4—Not intubated, regular breathing
3—Not intubated, Cheyne–Stokes breathing
2—Not intubated, irregular breathing
1—Breathes above ventilator rate
0—Breathes at ventilator rate

scores have four components: Eye opening, motor response, brainstem reflex, and respiration **(Box 1)**. The minimum FOUR score is 0 and the maximum score is 16.

AVPU Score: It is useful only in the triage setting. Its components include:
- *A:* Awake
- *V:* Responds to verbal stimulation
- *P:* Responds to painful stimulation
- *U:* Completely unresponsive

Attention Span

Attention span is best tested in children using the digit span test **(Fig. 2)**. In the digit span test, we start with two digits, then increase it to three digits, four digits, five digits, and then finally six digits while testing the digit forward test. We record the number of digits that the child can repeat correctly. After testing

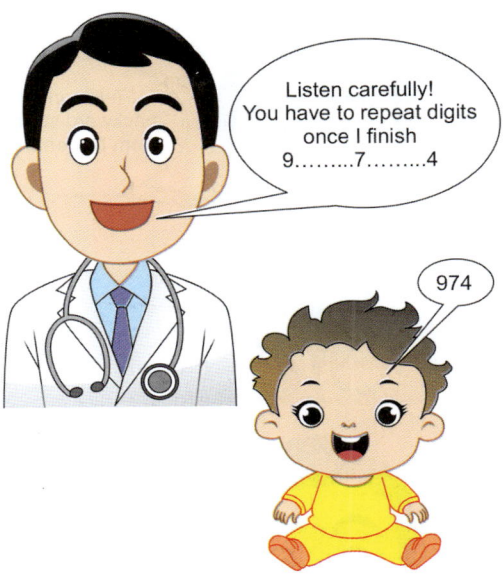

Fig. 2: Digit span test.

the digit forward, we again start with two digits and ask the child to repeat backward. It is essential to be very slow while speaking the digits so that immediate memory is not tested. The child may be instructed, "I will tell few digits, listen carefully and repeat them". The child may be asked to repeat "four ... seven ... nine ..."; if the child is able to repeat correctly, then ask him/her to repeat "nine ... seven ... four ...", and so on.

Example of digit span:
- 49
- 974
- 7294
- 69149
- 804624

Numbers must not follow any predictable sequence like 1, 3, 5, 7 (or) 1, 2, 3, 4 (or) 2, 4, 6, 8 and so on. It is expected that a 6-year-old child can tell five digits forward and three digits backward. A 10-year-old child will be able to tell six digits forward and four digits backward. The attention can also be tested by asking the child to narrate the

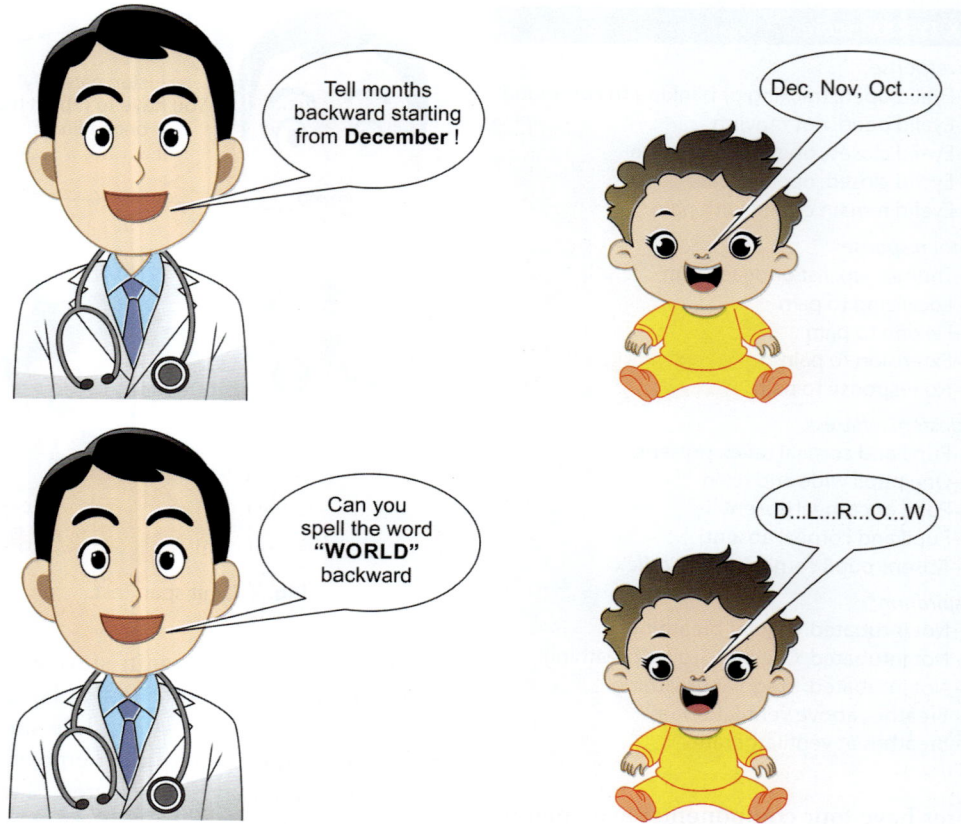

Fig. 3: Testing attention span.

months backward or telling the letters of word backward **(Fig. 3)**. Attention span is mediated by ascending reticular formation and pathways for consciousness.

Orientation

Test orientation if the patient is conscious and attentive. Orientation is tested to time, person, and place **(Table 3)**. Orientation and recent memory can be localized to medial temporal lobe structures **(Fig. 4)**. It is challenging to test orientation in infants and young children. If the baby is responding to the name, looking at the mother when asked, and looking eagerly at things in your clinic (it is a new place) then the baby is oriented.

TABLE 3: Orientation to person, place, and time.	
Person	• What is your name? • What is your last name/surname? • Who is this relative? • What is your gender?
Place	• Where are you now? • Which floor is this? • Which is this city? • Which is the state? • Which is the country?
Time	• Is it day or evening or night now? • What is the day today? • What is the date today? • Which month is this? • Which year is this?

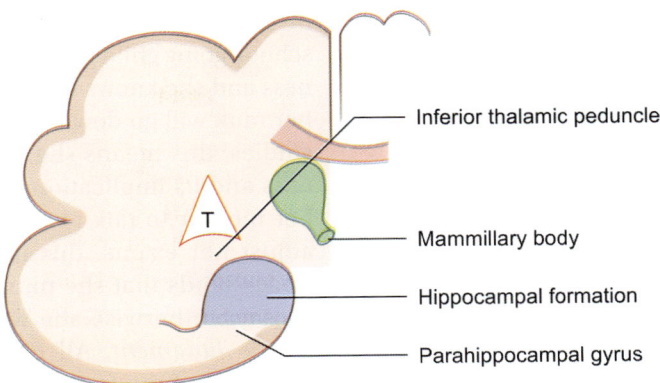

Fig. 4: Structures involved in orientation.

Memory

Recent memory often works together with orientation and attention span. When a sensory stimulus is given to the child, the stimulus gets registered and when asked the child can immediately repeat it. This information is stored temporarily (recent memory) and then it may be stored permanently (long-term memory). In most of the acute neurological conditions, recent memory is often more affected than long-term memory.

Recent Memory Testing

- Ask the child to remember three unrelated things, e.g., flat no 402; orange color; wooden table. Then ask the child to repeat the three things immediately (to check registration). Tell the child, "Remember them, I will ask you after some time". When you ask after some time, we test recent memory.
- Show him five objects and then hide these five objects in five different places in the room while the child is standing and watching (registration). After some time, ask the child to find out and give those five objects (recent memory).
- In an older child, you can ask the child to listen to a short story that you narrate. Ask the child to listen carefully (attention) and then after a few minutes, ask a few simple questions about that story (recent memory).

Long-term Memory

Simple questions can be used to test long-term memory:
- Which school do you study?
- What is your brother's name?
- What is your class teacher's name?

Anatomical localization to recent memory is the same as orientation (medial temporal lobe), whereas long-term memory is a function of the language cortex. In young infants and children, it may be challenging to assess memory but often the father and mother can tell you a few anecdotes to make you believe that his recent memory is good, for example,

- "My baby will search for his favorite toy in the place he left it last".
- "My baby will start smiling and will cuddle to grandmother even if she comes after 15 days".
- "He remembers where the broom is kept for his domestic memory".

Fund of Information

A child who is attentive and oriented with intact memory can accumulate a log of information provided to him. The fund of information would depend on which school he goes to, what medium he studies, and what kind of family support and environment is provided to the child. The questions need to be tailored accordingly. Some example questions include:
- Who is the chief minister of your state?
- Who is the president of India?
- Who is the prime minister of India?
- What is the capital city of your state?

The questions can be modified according to the background of the family.

Insight, Judgment, Planning, and Abstract Thinking

Insight, judgment, planning, abstract thinking, and motor sequencing are functions of the dorsolateral prefrontal cortex. If a school-going child gets admitted for some illness and she knows she will miss her exams, her rank will go down and she will miss her studies, this means she has *insight* into illness and its implications. If she then forces her mother to talk to her schoolteacher to adjust her exams, this is *planning*. If she understands that she must be admitted for 10 days, otherwise she will fall sick again, this is *judgment*. All these are executive functions of the frontal lobe. Most of these functions can be tested beyond 7 years of age **(Figs. 5A to C)**. Other tests include the following:
- Repeat quickly first-edge-palm sequence quickly. Try it yourself, remember do it fast!
- Can you quickly draw alternate square and triangle and connect them? See how long a child can make! **(Fig. 6)**. Try on a white paper, do it quickly it is a difficult task!

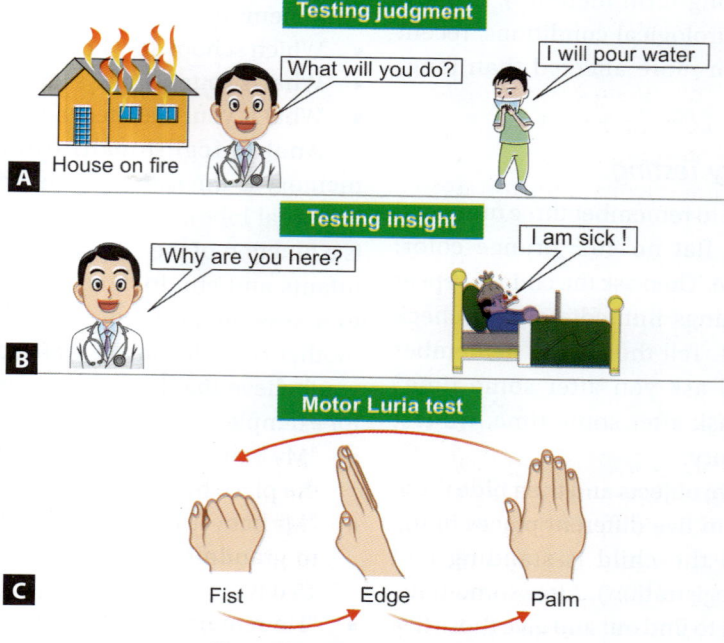

Figs. 5A to C: Testing judgment.

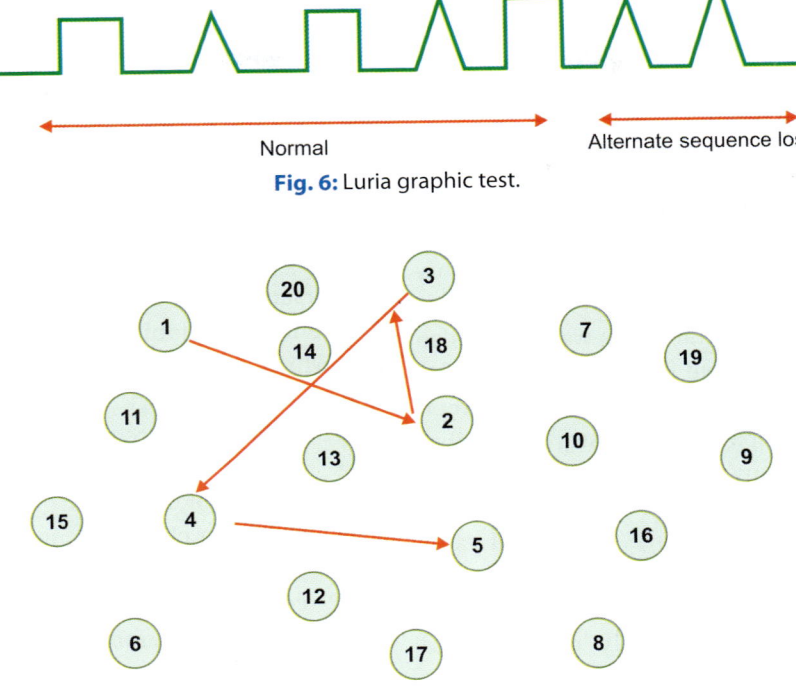

Fig. 6: Luria graphic test.

Fig. 7: Trail making test.

- Can you connect the numbers 1–10 in this trail? **(Fig. 7)**
- Tell me what is common between bananas and apples. (Both are fruits.)
- Tell me the difference between a shirt and pant? (One is worn at the top and the other at the bottom.)
- If the table is to leg, what is the car to? (Tyre)
- What is meaning of common proverbs? **(Fig. 8)**

Calculation

A 5-year-old child can do simple addition, 7 years can do subtraction, 8 years can multiply, and 9 years can do division. These are general milestones and there may be a lot of variations. For testing calculation, it is better to ask for an analogy instead of asking what is 2 + 2. This child might be able to

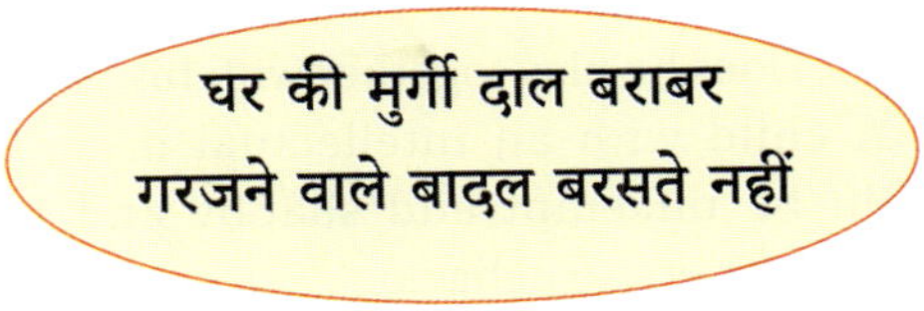

घर की मुर्गी दाल बराबर
गरजने वाले बादल बरसते नहीं

Fig. 8: Common proverbs.

answer with a rote memory as well. Examples of analogy:

- If I give you 2 apples, and your mother gives you 2 apples, how many will you have? (Addition)
- If I take back 1 apple from this lot, how many apples will be left? (Subtraction)
- If a worker is paid Rs 100 for 1 day and if he works for 5 days, how much should I pay him? (Multiplication)
- If a worker is paid Rs 100 per day and if you pay him Rs 500, how many days did he work? (Division)

- If the child can answer all these simple questions, then complex calculations can be tested on paper and pencil.

Calculation is a parietal lobe function and can be tested beyond 5 years of age.

Assessment of Mental Status

Despite normal memory, attention, orientation, and other executive functions, many children are still affected by their mental status. Hence, mental status well-being also needs to be assessed in older children. This assessment is usually performed to screen for associated psychiatric disturbances that often accompany neurological illnesses. This assessment may not be relevant in children younger than 7 years of age. The mental status assessment includes the following:
- *Appearance and behavior*
  - Is the child neatly dressed and combed?
  - Is there aggressive or disruptive behavior?
  - Does he play together with his peers?

A child with an intellectual disability might be unkempt and shabby and may exhibit aggressive behavior.
- *Psychomotor activity*
  - Is he hyperactive, restless, impulsive?
  - Is he lethargic or hypoactive?
- *Stream of talk*
  - Can the child talk and sustain a conversation?
  - How is the spontaneity in the speech?
  - Is the speech very rapid or is it slow?
  - Is the child able to add something meaningful to sustain the conversation?
- *Mood, affect, and emotion*
  - How has been your mood for the last few days?
  - Observe the affective response while talking to the child.
  - Observe the emotions while speaking to the child.

A child may say that I have been very tense and anxious in my mood over the last few days. You observe an anxious and tense look. This is an appropriate "affect" of the underlying mood. If while speaking to the child, you observe sudden crying/sudden laughing not appropriate to the content of the conversation, it is called emotional lability. This emotional lability is a pseudobulbar sign which is often observed in upper motor neuron (UMN) lesions.
- *Thoughts and perception*
  - Does the child have illusions, hallucinations, or delusions?
  - Does the child have any phobias or is he preoccupied with some body complaints?

Mirage is an *illusion*. Seeing snakes and reptiles (visual) or hearing God's voice or hearing someone else's voice (auditory) is *hallucination*. Yelling at a person, say doctor, that he is trying to kill him or trying to position him is a delusion. This is a false belief that reason cannot dispel.

Assessment of Language/Speech

The neuroanatomical basis of speech and language has been discussed in **Chapter 1**. The assessment of language has the following components:
- *Fluency:* It refers to how many words can the child use within a time frame. You can ask the child to tell as many words as possible that start with F, A, and S in 60 seconds. You can also ask the child to tell as many names of animals as he knows in 60 seconds.
- *Articulation:* Check for labials (Pa), linguals (Ta), and gutturals (Kha). Ask the child to say "Pa Pa Pa Pa", "Ta Ta Ta Ta", and

"Kha Kha Kha". If child is able to repeat appropriately, articulation is preserved.
- *Comprehension:* We can test comprehension using one or more of the following:
  - Ask the child to touch his nose or point to the door. (One-step command)
  - Now, "touch your nose and then point to the door". (Two-step command)
  - Now, "take this paper, fold it into half and put it on floor". (Three-step command)
  - "Can you point to the source of illumination in this room"? Then he points to tube light. (Semantic comprehension, which means he can understand meaning of instructions)
- *Naming:* It can be tested by asking him what this is:
  - Show him watch, comb, key.
  - See how promptly he replies and does he reply correctly?
- *Repetition:*
  - Can you repeat this phrase?
  - बिल्ली दूध पीती है।
  "No ifs and buts".
- *Reading:* You can ask older children to read heading, subheading, and then the first paragraph in a newspaper (Fig. 9). Look at the effort in reading and pronunciation of words.
- *Writing:*
  - Can you write your names, your address?
  - Now I will dictate, you write this sentence.

Disturbance in speech is summarized in **Flowchart 2**. Detailed discussion of types of dysarthria and aphasia can be read from **Chapter 1**.

Released Reflexes

Few reflexes are elicited in organic brain disease, for example, end stage of

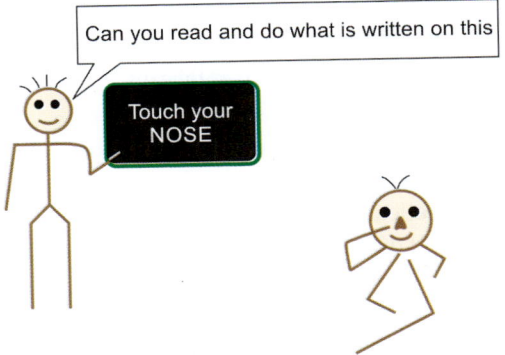

Fig. 9: Testing reading skills.

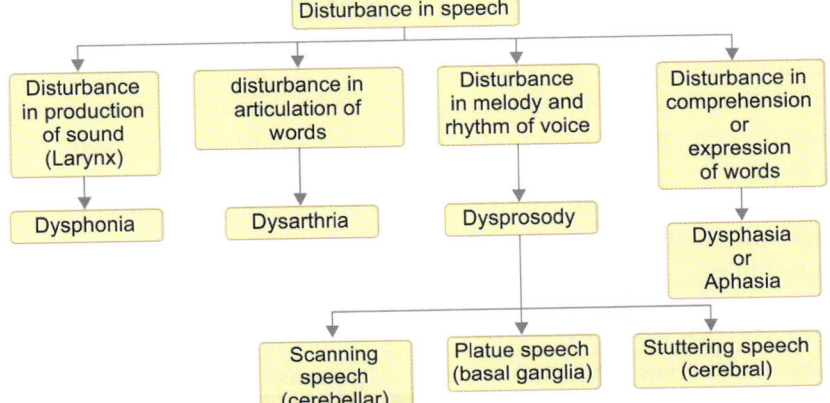

Flowchart 2: Approach to disturbance in speech.

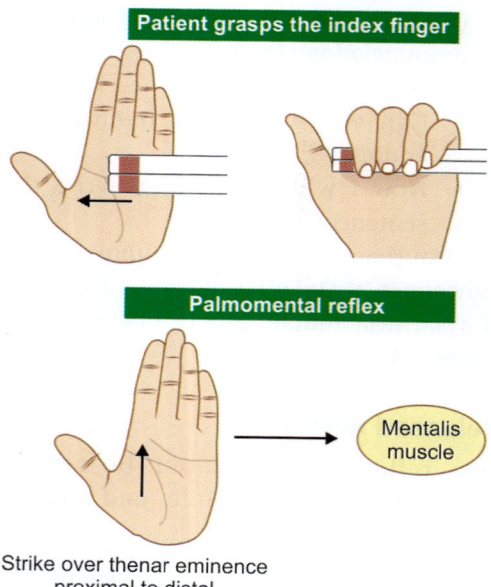

Fig. 10: Released reflexes.

neurodegenerative disease like subacute sclerosing panencephalitis (SSPE) **(Fig. 10)**. These reflexes may be normal in early infancy but must disappear subsequently.
- *Glabellar blink:* When you tap the glabella up to 10 times, normally the blinking response will be inhibited after a few taps. In organic brain disease, it may persist till 10th tap.
- *Snout reflex:* Ask the child to close eyes; when you press firmly over the philtrum, normally nothing happens. In organic brain disease, the upper lip may pucker.
- *Suck reflex:* With eyes closed, stimulating the lips from center to side may produce sucking reflex.
- *Grasp reflex:* Stimulation of thenar eminence will elicit reflex grasp of the stimulating fingers.

■ CRANIAL NERVE EXAMINATION

There are 12 cranial nerves (CN), and formal testing from the 1st to the 12th CN is often challenging in infants and young children **(Table 4)**.

Olfactory Nerve (CN I)

The olfactory nerve is usually not impaired in children. Recently, owing to coronavirus disease 19 (COVID-19) outbreak, anosmia (loss of smell) was recognized as a presenting feature. Other causes include upper respiratory tract infection, head trauma (occipital), and neoplasm in the frontal lobe. Assessment of smell can be done in cooperative children older than 2 years.

Ask the child to close his eyes and occlude one nostril using your hand. Present an aromatic smell familiar to children like toothpaste, chocolate, or vanilla flavor in front of another open nostril. If the child can "perceive" the smell, ask the child to "identify" the smell. Avoid pungent smells like onion or garlic as this will irritate and stimulate the trigeminal nerve instead of the olfactory nerve. Test the other nostril separately. Identification of smell may be difficult in young children. Look at facial expressions for perception of smell instead of asking the child to respond.

Optic Nerve (CN II)

The anatomy of the optic nerve and visual pathway has been discussed in **Chapter 1**. Components of optic nerve testing:
1. *Visual acuity:* Visual acuity in older children is tested using Snellen chart or Rosenbaum pocket vision screener. The Rosenbaum pocket vision screener is held at a distance of 14 inches. The child should be wearing his routine spectacles and each eye should be tested separately. Visual acuity in infants can be tested by ability to fix and follow familiar faces of parents. Optokinetic drum can also be used (there are free apps in google store

TABLE 4: Higher cortical functions.

Higher cortical function	What does it mean?	How to test?	Localization
Agnosia	Inability to understand the sensory stimuli even though sensory pathway and sensorium are intact	Ask the patient to close his eyes and touch his third finger. Ask him now to open his eyes. Ask him to touch the same finger in your hand (finger agnosia)	Association cortex or intracerebral connection (parietal lobe)
Agraphesthesia	Inability to recognize letters drawn on his hand	Use the blunt end of pen and write letter or number (1–10) in his hand with the patient eye closed. Now ask him what did you write?	Parietal lobe
Prosopognosia	Inability to recognize face in person or in photos	Show him a photo of his close relative or famous celebrity	Inferomedial temporo-occipital region
Asomatognosia	Inability to locate and identify one's body part	• Finger agnosia • Right–left discrimination • Touch your left ear with your right hand	Left angular gyrus
Hemispatial inattention	Failure to attend to entire left half of space	• Ask him to draw clock or wheels with spokes • He falls to draw left side	Right parietal lesion
Anosognosia	Unawareness of neurological defects	If you ask left hemiplegic patient "can you move your left hand?", he will say "Yes". "Is there any problem on your left side?" He says "No"	Parietal lesion, especially right side
Sensory inattention	Inattention to feel bilateral simultaneous stimuli	I may touch your one or both sides, you need to recognize it. Now close your eyes. Touch one or both sides of cheek, dorsum of hand, and feet	Right parietal lesion
Apraxia	Inability to perform a voluntary act even though motor and sensory sensorium are intact	• Show me how will you brush your teeth • Show me how will you comb your hair (ideomotor apraxia) • Can you copy this figure? (constructional apraxia) • Give him his shirt to wear (dressing apraxia)	Ideomotor (left parietal) construction dressing (right parietal lesion)

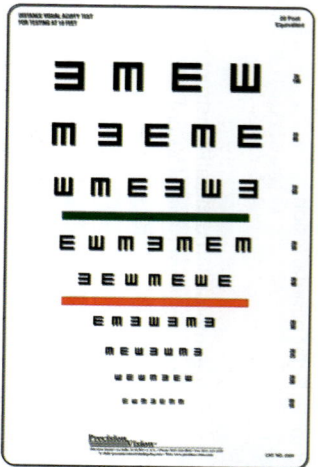

Fig. 11: Tumbling E chart.

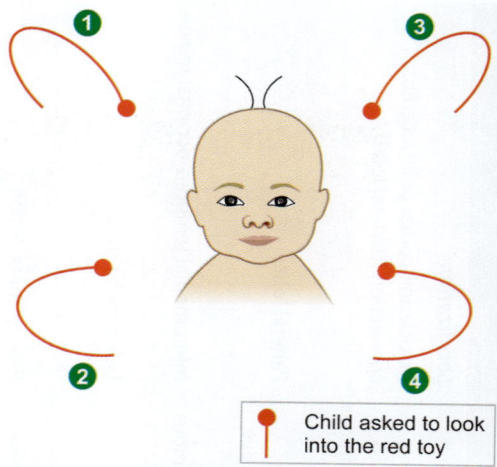

Fig. 12: Testing field of vision.

which you can download). We look for optokinetic nystagmus in the eyes of infants. In children older than 4 years, E-game can be used, where the child can be trained to point with his fingers on the open end of E. Different directions and sizes of E are presented to the child to assess his visual acuity **(Fig. 11)**.

2. *Field of vision:* Confrontation test is used for testing field of vision in older children. One examiner holds the toy and ask the child to look straight into the toy. This examiner sits 50 cm from the child. Another examiner brings a small (3 mm) red- or white-colored ball or toy from four quadrants standing behind the child while the first examiner is asking the child to look straight **(Fig. 12)**. Look for movement of eyes to look at red/white ball at four quadrants. Avoid giving instructions to the child to indicate when he sees the red ball/toy. He will keep seeing that only then! Testing field of vision in children is hence different from confrontation test used in older children. In conventional confrontation test, the examiner asks the child to keep focusing on his nose. The same examiner flickers his fingers across four quadrants and asks the child to indicate when he sees those flicking fingers. The defect of visual field testing is discussed in **Chapter 1**.

3. *Color vision:* It can be tested in older children using Ishihara cards **(Fig. 13)**. The other methods like color wool ball are not reliable (Holmgren wool test). Ishihara cards are also available free from Google play store.

4. *Fundus examination:* It involves examination of optic disc, macula, retinal vessels, and any other findings on retina. The optic disc is usually pale gray in color in infants and salmon colored in older children **(Fig. 14)**. Look at its margins (well defined or not), any hyperemia, or any hemorrhage. If the cup is deep, the disc may look pale at the center. In optic atrophy, the whole disc appears pale with decreased arterioles in the disc margin **(Fig. 15)**. In papilledema, there is elevation of disc-distended veins and lack of venous pulsations with blurring of

CHAPTER 3: Examination of Central Nervous System   67

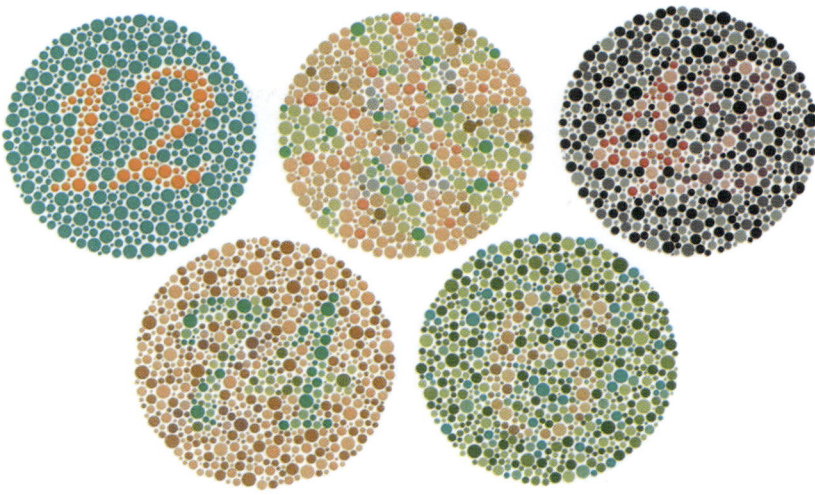

Fig. 13: Ishihara card.

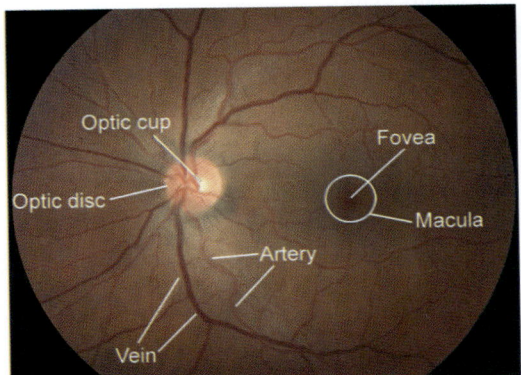

Fig. 14: Normal fundus.

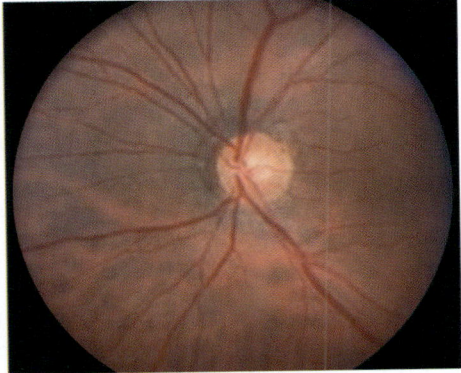

Fig. 15: Optic atrophy.

nasal margin and occasional hemorrhage around the disc **(Fig. 16)**. Comment on the retinal vessels (thick or thin), pulsatile (yes/no). One must also comment on macula and any other obvious findings like cherry red spot and pigmentary retinal changes.

5. *Pupils:* They must be observed in light. Look at shape, size, and reactivity to light. In optic nerve pathology like optic neuritis, when light is shown on normal eye, pupils constrict and when light is shown on affected eye both pupils dilate [relative afferent pupillary defect (RAPD)]

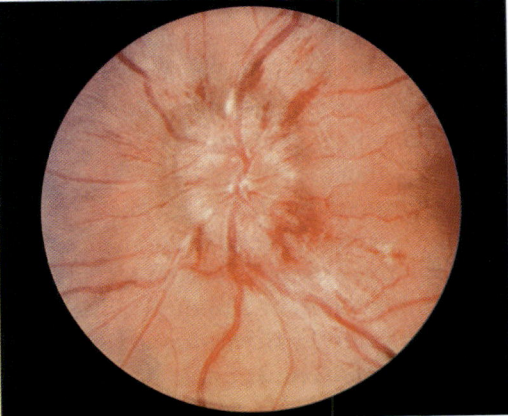

Fig. 16: Papilledema.

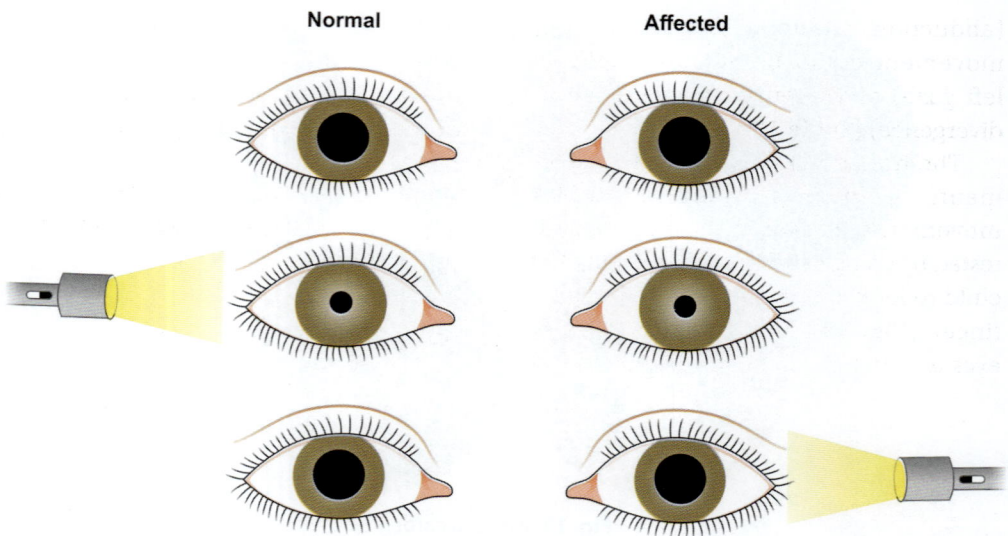

Fig. 17: Relative-afferent pupillary defect.

(Fig. 17). Pupillary reflex is usually presented in cortical blindness and is lost in pathology involving the anterior visual pathway.

Third, Fourth, and Sixth Cranial Nerves

The anatomical basis of ocular movement is discussed in **Chapter 1**. The examination of 3rd, 4th, and 6th CN is usually performed together. The following components are tested:

- *Alignment of eyes:* It is best tested using the Hirschberg test. Flashlight is shown on the eyes and the reflection of same is seen on the eyes **(Figs. 18A to C)**. We can note if there is any squint—is it latent or manifest squint. If it is manifest squint, then is it concomitant or paralytic squint. The terms esotropia, exotropia, paralytic, and concomitant squint are discussed in **Chapter 1**. Heterotopia (Esotropia or exotropia) must nerve be ignored in infants as the infants learn to suppress the image from the deviated eye which gradually leads to *amblyopia*. This may be prevented by patching the normal eye.

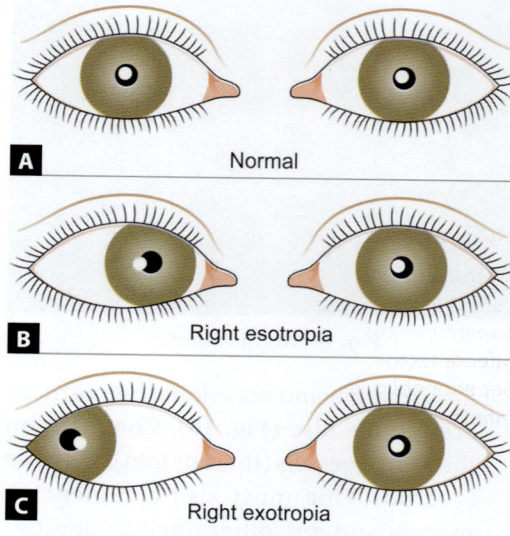

Figs. 18A to C: Alignment of eyes: (A) Normal; (B) Esotropia; (C) Exotropia.

- *Movement of eyes:* Movement of conjugate eyes is tested by asking the child to follow a figure of "H" **(Fig. 19)**. Movements that happen in one eye is called duction (abduction, adduction). Binocular eye movement could be version (right or left gaze) or vergence (convergence or divergence) **(Table 5)**.

The horizontal conjugate eye movements could be saccadic or pursuit movements. Saccadic movements are tested by using two fingers and asking the child to look alternatively at the wiggling finger **(Fig. 20)**. Pursuit movement of eyes is tested by asking the child to follow figure of "H", which is made in the air by the examiner. In a comatose patient, horizontal eye movement is tested by doll's eye movement (oculovestibular reflex).

- *Pupillary reaction:* Ask the child to look at a distant point in the dim room. Bring the flashlight slowly from the side; watch for direct light reflex on the eye where light is shown and indirect (consensual) light reflex on the opposite eye. Ensure that the child is looking at the distant point while bringing the light; otherwise accommodation reflex acts to constrict the pupils.
- *Accommodation reflex:* It consist of convergence and miosis when the child is asked to shift the focus from a distant object to nearby objects like your finger.
- *Ptosis:* Two muscles elevate the eyelid: Superior tarsal muscle (supplied by sympathetic pathway) and levator

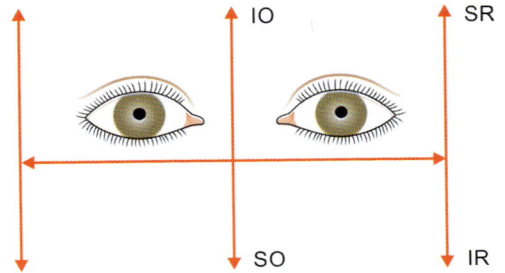

Fig. 19: Figure of "H". (IO: inferior oblique; SO: superior oblique; SR: superior rectus; IR: inferior rectus).

TABLE 5: Actions of individual extraocular muscles.			
Muscle	Primary action	Secondary action	Tertiary action
Medial rectus	Adducts	–	–
Lateral rectus	Abducts	–	–
Superior rectus	Elevates	Adducts	Intort
Inferior rectus	Depresses	Adducts	Extort
Superior oblique	Depresses	Abducts	Intort
Inferior oblique	Elevates	Abducts	Extort

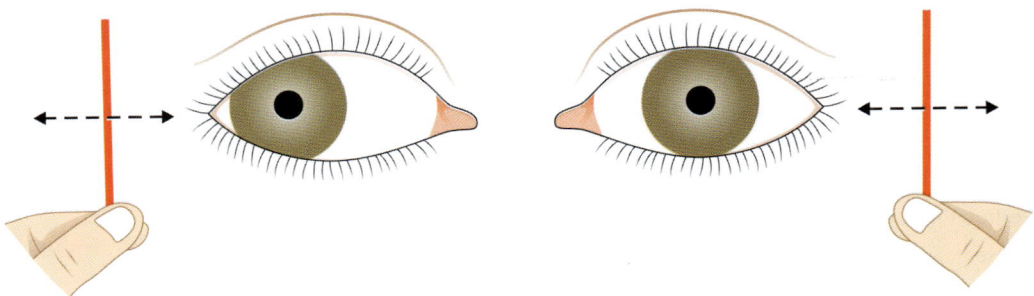

Fig. 20: Testing saccadic movements.

palpebrae superioris (LPS) muscle (supplied by CN III). If there is paralysis of LPS, then ptosis will worsen when the child is asked to look up. In contrast to a sympathetic pathway lesion, the eyelid will elevate on upward gaze. Ptosis can also be present in Bell's palsy owing to paralysis of frontalis muscle which inserts into eyebrow. Ptosis can also be seen in ipsilateral cortical lesion. Ptosis of myasthenia gravis can be alleviated using ice bag.

- *Nystagmus:* It is an involuntary, oscillatory rhythmic movement of eyeballs. Nystagmus can be a result of an ophthalmic cause (lesion in retina, media, or lens that interferes with vision), vestibular, cerebral, or brainstem tegmental etiology **(Table 6)**. Nystagmus can be physiological in the end gaze or while using optokinetic drum. It needs to be assessed under the following headings:
  - Is it horizontal, vertical, torsional? (Drug induced)
  - Is it pendular or jerk nystagmus?
  - What is the direction of fast component? (Jerk nystagmus)
  - What is the amplitude and rate of nystagmus?
  - Is it unidirectional (peripheral cause) or bidirectional (central cause)?

- *Other ocular movements:* Note must be made of other ocular movements like ocular bobbing, ocular flutter, and opsoclonus. These abnormalities in eyes are discussed in **Chapter 1**.

Trigeminal Nerve (CN V)

Motor component:
- Jaw movements include opening and closing mouth (lateral pterygoids), retraction (temporalis), and side-to-side movement (pterygoids). These jaw movements are supplied by trigeminal nerve.
- Look for wasting, any flattening of jaw line, deviation on opening the mouth, and any fasciculations.
- Feel for the masseter muscles (anterior border) and temporalis muscle.
- Test for side-to-side jaw movement against resistance. At baseline, the jaw is deviated to the weak side.

Sensory component: The trigeminal nerve carries the pain and temperature sensation over the face. Test for pain sensation over V1, V2, and V3 areas of trigeminal nerve **(Fig. 21)**.

Reflex: Jaw jerk
Ask the child to open the mouth slightly, place your index finger over the chin, and strike with narrow edge of hammer. Normally

TABLE 6: Difference between peripheral and central nystagmus.

	Peripheral nystagmus	Central nystagmus
Direction	Unidirectional away from lesion	Bidirectional or unidirectional
Pure horizontal nystagmus	(−)	(+)
Visual fixation	Inhibits nystagmus	No inhibition
Vertigo tinnitus	(+)	(−)
Causes	• Labyrinthitis • Meniere disease • Neuronitis	Vascular demyelinating neoplastic

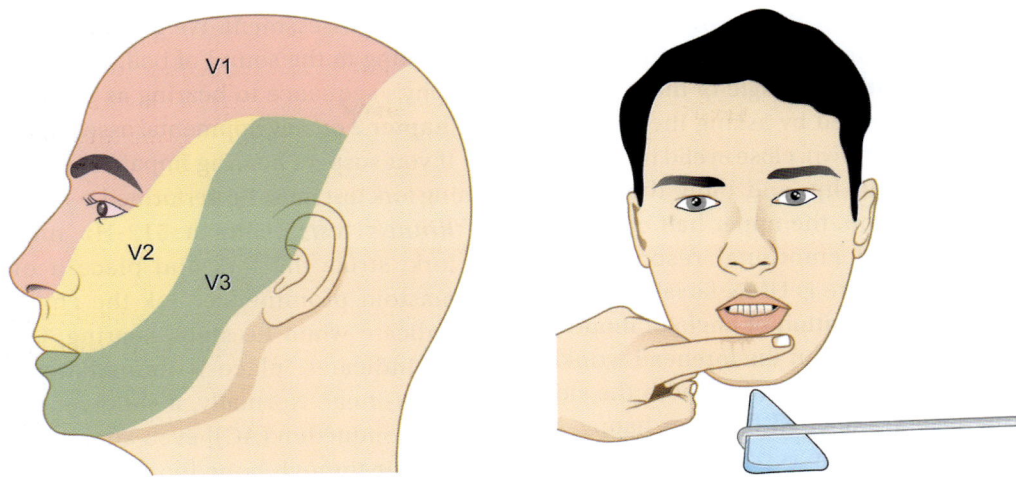

Fig. 21: Sensory component of trigeminal nerve.

Fig. 22: Testing jaw jerk.

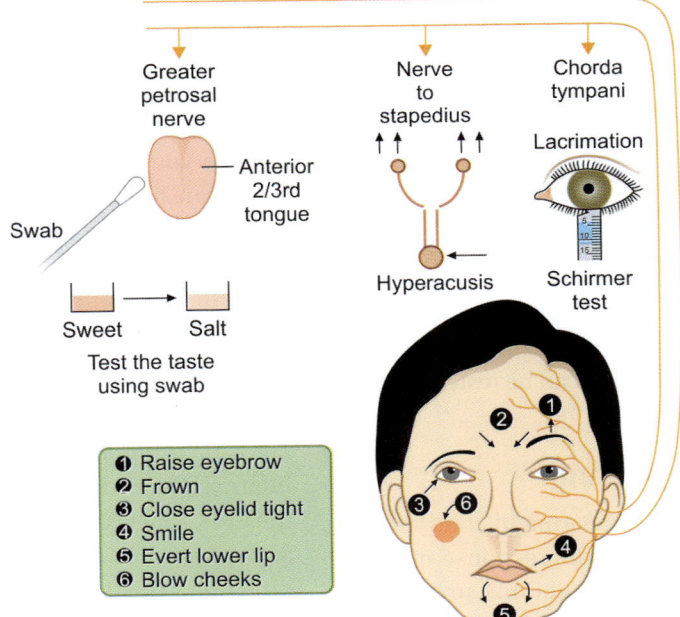

Fig. 23: Anatomy course of facial nerve.

it is absent. In a UMN lesion, the jaw jerk is elicited with closure of mouth when the hammer strikes the index finger placed over the chin **(Fig. 22)**.

Seventh Cranial Nerve

The course of seventh CN is depicted in **Figure 23**. The facial nerve testing includes looking for facial symmetry in terms of forehead folds, eyelid position, width of palpebral fissure, symmetry of nasolabial fold, and position of angle of mouth. Facial symmetry is tested by asking the patient to raise eyebrow, frown, close eyelid tight, smile, evert the lower lip, and blow the cheeks. In a UMN lesion, the upper half of the face is spared, and emotional responses are preserved. If there is UMN facial weakness, there will be deviation of angle of mouth to the opposite side, but the forehead wrinkles are symmetrically spared on both the sides of the face. If the child is sad or happy, his emotional response is preserved in a UMN lesion whereas in lower motor neuron (LMN) facial palsy, there is severe facial weakness and both volitional and emotional responses are affected. Bell's phenomenon is observed (one can see eyeballs turning up on attempted eyelid closure) in LMN facial palsy.

Apart from testing facial muscles, taste sensation from the anterior two-third of tongue can be tested using a swab. Test the sweet taste before testing the salt. Ask the child, "Did you taste something? How was it?" Avoid asking leading questions like "was it sweet or salt to taste?" Another component of facial nerve testing is testing for tear production which can be tested using Schirmer test.

Cochlear Nerve (CN VIII)

Bedside assessment of hearing in children is challenging. We look at the response of the child to whispering instructions provided from a distance of 6 and 15 cm. If the child does not respond to whispering instructions, conventional voice instructions may be provided from a distance of 15 and 60 cm. We can also look at the response of the child to rubbing of fingers near the ear. In case of infants, if he pauses for a while when a bell rings, it probably indicates intact hearing on bedside assessment. We can also look at the turning to the sound of bell. Remember Murphy's sequence to hearing as discussed in **Chapter 2** on developmental assessment.

If you suspect hearing impairment, then tuning fork test must be performed.

- *Rinne's test:* Using a 512-Hz tuning fork, strike the fork and place it over mastoid prominence. Ask the child to indicate when he stops hearing. Once he indicates, place it immediately in front of ear. Normally, a child can hear [air conduction (AC)] even after ceasing to hear through bone [bone conduction (BC)]. Normally, AC is better than BC. In conductive deafness, AC is decreased and BC is normal. In sensorineural hearing loss (SNHL), AC is decreased and BC is also decreased but AC is better than BC.
- *Weber test:* Place the tuning fork in forehead and ask the child, "In which ear can you hear better"? Normally, the child can hear in both ears equally. In conductive hearing loss, it is better heard in the affected ear. In SNHL, it is better heard in the healthy ear.

Vestibular Nerve Testing (CN VIII Testing)

- *Look for rotational nystagmus:* Hold the infant/child and spin clockwise. Look at the eyes. The eyes will turn anticlockwise and there will be nystagmus in a clockwise direction. This indicates the integrity of the vestibular nerve.
- *Rhomberg sign:* Ask the child to stand with open eyes and feet together with hands held horizontal to floor. Now observe for unsteadiness on closure of eyes **(Fig. 24)**. Swaying on closure of eyes indicates posterior column dysfunction and can be seen in a vestibular lesion.

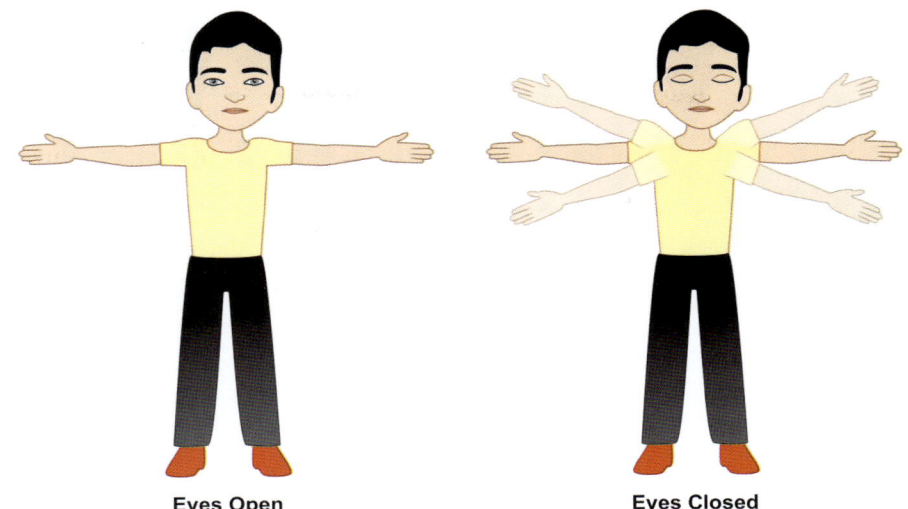

Fig. 24: Rhomberg sign.

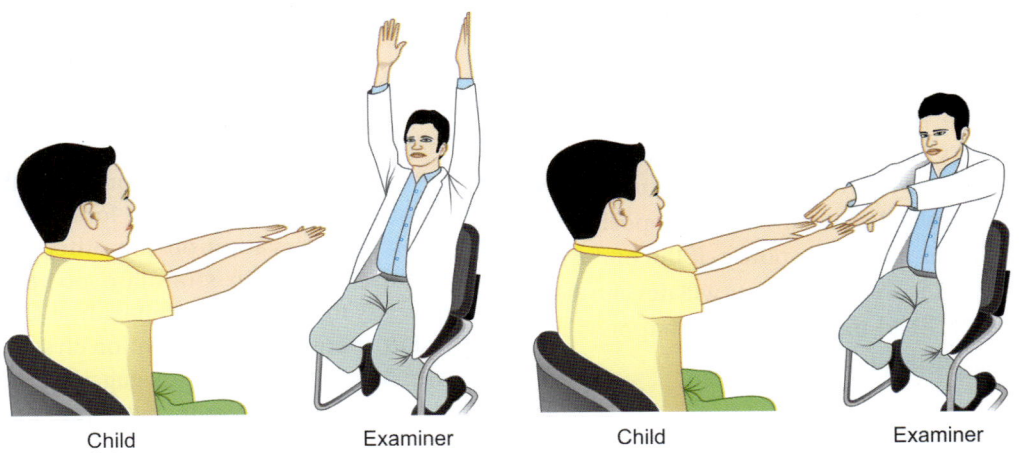

Fig. 25: Past-pointing.

- *Past pointing:* You sit in a chair with your arms held straight with palms facing up. Ask the child to sit in front of you with his arms held vertically up. Now ask the child to touch your right arm with right and left with left **(Fig. 25)**. If there is a right vestibular lesion, both arms of the child will sway away from midline and the child will be unable to touch the examiner's hand.

- *Cold caloric test:* 1 mL (conscious patient) and 5 mL (unconscious patient) of cold water is poured in the ear. One can notice that eyes are tonically deviated toward the side of stimulus, whereas nystagmus will be seen toward the opposite side **(Fig. 26)**. As we remember the mnemonic COWS (cold opposite; warm same side), here the direction refers to the direction of nystagmus.

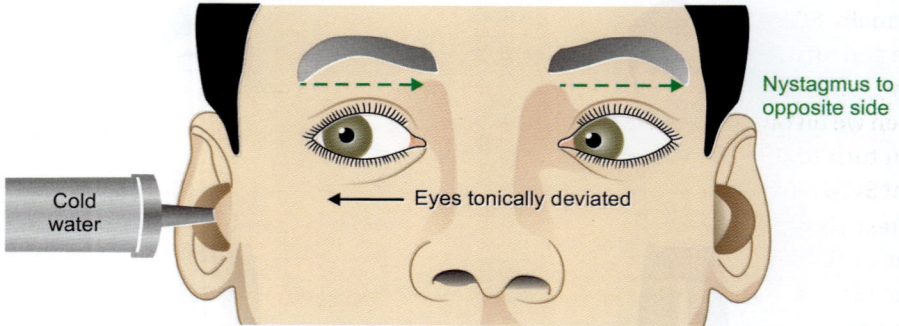

Fig. 26: Cold caloric test.

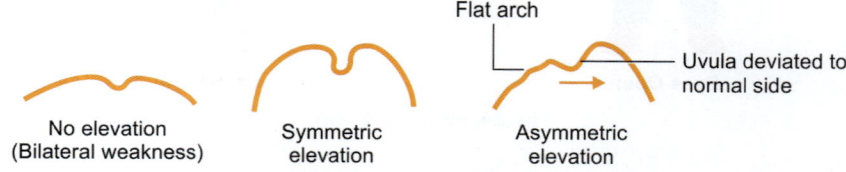

Fig. 27: Testing 9th and 10th cranial nerves.

- *Oculocephalic reflex (doll's eye reflex):* It is performed in infants and in an unconscious patient. Hold the head in midline and tilt the head to one side; the eyes will deviate toward the opposite side. This is normal response. If the brainstem reflex is absent, the eyes will deviate along with head movement as it happens in a brain-dead patient.

Ninth and Tenth Cranial Nerves

The 9th and 10th CN are tested using the following:
- Look at the pitch and quality of the spontaneous voice. Notice for any nasal twang.
- Test articulation in the speech by asking the child to say "Pa Pa Pa" (labials), "Tha Tha Tha" (linguals), "Kha kha Kha" (soft palate).
- Look for any difficulty in swallowing or pooling of secretion. Give a glass of water to drink.
- Ask the child to open the mouth and say "ahh". Look at the arch of the soft palate is there a symmetric elevation? **(Fig. 27)**
- Test for gag reflex. Touch one tonsillar pillar on one side and then look for the symmetric elevation on the other side. Remember not to stimulate posterior pharynx for testing gag reflex. In a UMN lesion, there will be no elevation on saying "Ahh", but it elevates on gag reflex. In children who are feeding well, and there is no dysarthria, one can avoid testing the gag reflex. Reserve this test as the last examination if at all you need to check because beyond this, the child becomes uncomfortable and loses cooperation.
- Taste sensation in the posterior one third of tongue is difficult to perform in young children.

Spinal Accessory Nerve (CN XI)

To test spinal accessory nerve, we need to test strength of sternocleidomastoid muscle (SCM) and trapezius muscle.

- Normally SCM, will tilt the head to same side and turn it contra laterally while head moves forward. We can feel it ourselves. When we tilt our head to the right side and then turn to the left side, we can feel our right SCM contracting.
- To test right SCM, you ask the child to turn to the left side and apply pressure over his left cheek and ask the child to resist that movement. Feel the right SCM contract.
- To test both SCM together, ask the child to flex the head. The examiner resists the movement at forehead and feel for both SCM.
- To test the trapezius, ask the child to shrug his shoulders and apply pressure down.

Hypoglossal Nerve (CN XII)

Movement of tongue can be tested by asking the child to protrude, retract, side–side, up–down and press tongue to cheeks. Genioglossus muscle turns the tongue to the opposite side on protrusion. This is similar to lateral pterygoid muscles (CN V) and SCM (CN XI). Hence, right genioglossus turns tongue to the left side. Right lateral pterygoids turn the jaw to the left side. Right SCM turns the head to the left side although it tilts on the same side. Remember, in unprotruded tongue, the patient can deviate tip to the normal side. However, when he protrudes, the normal genioglossus will contract and turn tongue to the paralyzed side. If it is an LMN lesion, same-side tongue will undergo atrophy and might exist fasciculations. While testing for hypoglossal nerve, we can also look for darting tongue (choreoathetosis). Summary of all cranial nerves is tabulated **(Table 7)**.

TABLE 7: Summary of cranial nerve.

Cranial nerve	What to see?
Olfactory	Perception and identification of smell
Second	Visual acuity, color vision, field of vision, fundus examination
Third Fourth Sixth	Alignment of eyes, eye movement (saccadic and pursuit), pupil size and reaction (direct, consensual, accommodation reflex), ptosis, nystagmus
Fifth	• *Motor:* Jaw deviation • *Sensory:* Sensation over face $V_1 V_2 V_3$ • *Reflex:* Corneal and jaw jerk
Seventh	• Facial symmetry • Taste sensation • Hyperacusis • Tear production (Schirmer test)
Eighth	• Hearing test • Rinne test/Weber test
Ninth Tenth	• Movement of palate • Gag reflex
Eleventh	Function of sternocleidomastoid muscle and trapezius
Twelfth	Position of tongue, deviation of tongue, fasciculations

■ MOTOR SYSTEM EXAMINATION

Bulk

- Bulk of the muscles needs to be tested by adequately exposing the muscles. Look for atrophy hypertrophy, asymmetry, or any visible fasciculations.
- Look at face, shoulder, pelvic girdle thenar, and hypothenar eminence.
- If the muscles had failed to develop, it is aplasia. If the muscle has failed to develop to its normal size, it is hypoplasia. If the muscle once had normal size but then lost its bulk, it is atrophy.
- Atrophy of the muscle could be due to an LMN lesion or could be disuse atrophy.

- In an LMN lesion, the atrophy is more evident in anterior horn cell pathology (generalized atrophy) and neuropathy (distal atrophy).
- True muscle hypertrophy is seen in congenital myotonia **(Fig. 28)**.
- Pseudohypertrophy is observed in Duchenne muscular dystrophy **(Fig. 29)**.
- Bulk of the muscle can be compared between two sides by measuring bulk around fixed points (e.g., in adults, fixed points could be 10 cm above/below olecranon and 18 cm above tibial tuberosity).
- Asymmetry of bulk is evident in chronic hemiplegia.
- Presence of special signs like valley sign **(Fig. 30)** and calf head on a trophy sign can be mentioned here.

Tone

- Tone is the baseline resistance of the muscle to passive flexion. Abnormalities of tone could be hypotonia or hypertonia (spasticity or rigidity) **(Flowchart 3)**.
- Tone in the flexor muscles is maintained by the lateral corticospinal tract whereas

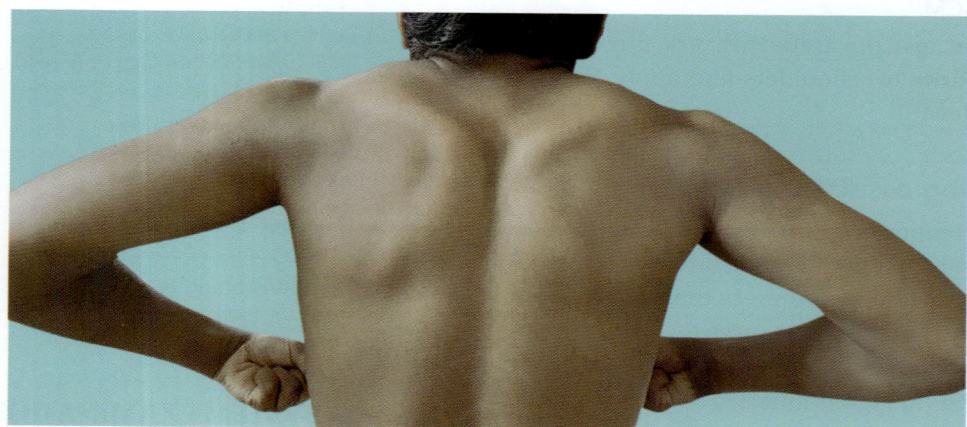

Fig. 28: Muscle hypertrophy.

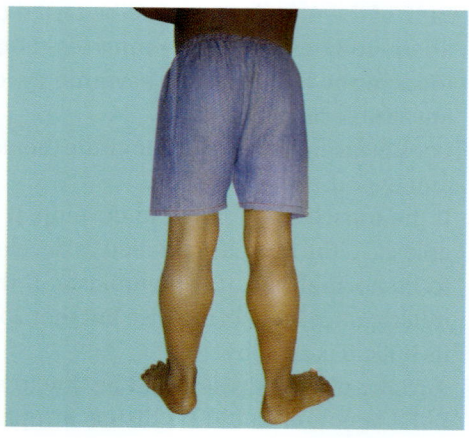

Fig. 29: Calf hypertrophy.

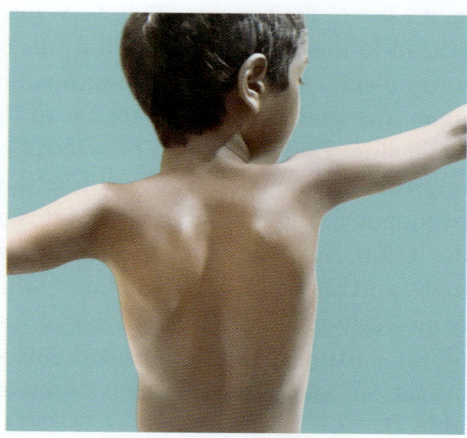

Fig. 30: Valley sign.

in the extensor muscles including back muscles, it is maintained by the anterior corticospinal tract.
- Rigidity can be cogwheel or lead-pipe type rigidity. Cogwheel rigidity is best tested by holding the child's hand in a handshake manner and feel for the resistance on passively pronating–supinating the child's forearm. You may ask the child to open and close the fist in the other hand (Froment's maneuver) (reinforcement phenomenon).
- Spasticity is a velocity dependent increase in the tone. Spasticity is best tested across elbow and knee by passive flexion–extension. Spasticity is felt as a catch followed by release (clasp-knife spasticity) **(Fig. 31)**. It can also be appreciated on dorsiflexion and plantar flexion at ankle joint.
- In spasticity, a selective group of anti-gravity muscles is involved (flexors of upper limb and extensors of lower limb)

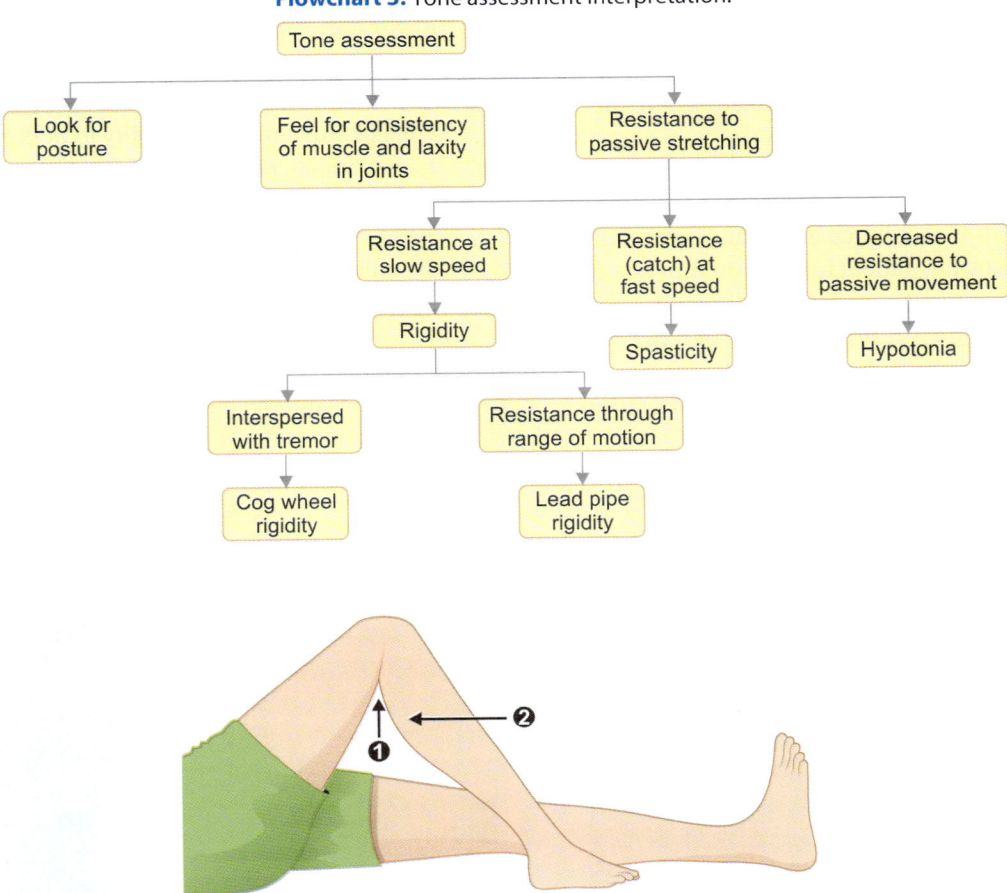

Check for resistance on flexion–Extension (2) while holding the knee joint (1)
Note: Movt (2) should be brick

Fig. 31: Testing tone.

whereas, in rigidity both against and antagonist are involved.
- Spasticity is velocity dependent, you do fast movement, you get a catch followed by release. If you do slow movement, you do not get any resistance. However, in rigidity the limb is tight irrespective of slow or fast passive movement.
- Spasticity is associated with brisk deep tendon reflex (DTR) and extensor plantar. Rigidity is associated with bradykinesia.
- Hypotonia can be tested using several maneuvers **(Flowchart 4)**.
- Movement disorders including dystonia and choreoathetosis result in variable tone (it looks increased during the activity and decreased when the child sleeps).
- Paratonia is not observed in children. It occurs in an adult patient with dementia. It is resistance equal in degree and range by the patient to each attempt of examiner to move a part in any direction.
- Tone examination across distal joints is challenging in the presence of contractures, e.g., ankle contractures.
- Myotonia refers to sustained contraction of muscle to the stimulus with delayed relaxation. It can be elicited in eyelid (open–close eyes), tongue (percussion over tongue depressor), and thenar muscle (percussion over thenar eminence).

Power Examination

Few general rules that we must remember while doing assessment of muscle power are as follows:
- Expose the muscle that needs to be tested.
- The line of muscle action must be against the gravity before we test the muscle power against resistance.
- Muscle action must be tested for full range of movement and ability to perform against gravity before applying resistance.
- Always stabilize the proximal joint while testing the muscle.
- All individual muscle power need not be tested in children. We often test the power of a movement across the joint rather than individual power testing. For example, we test for shoulder abduction rather than

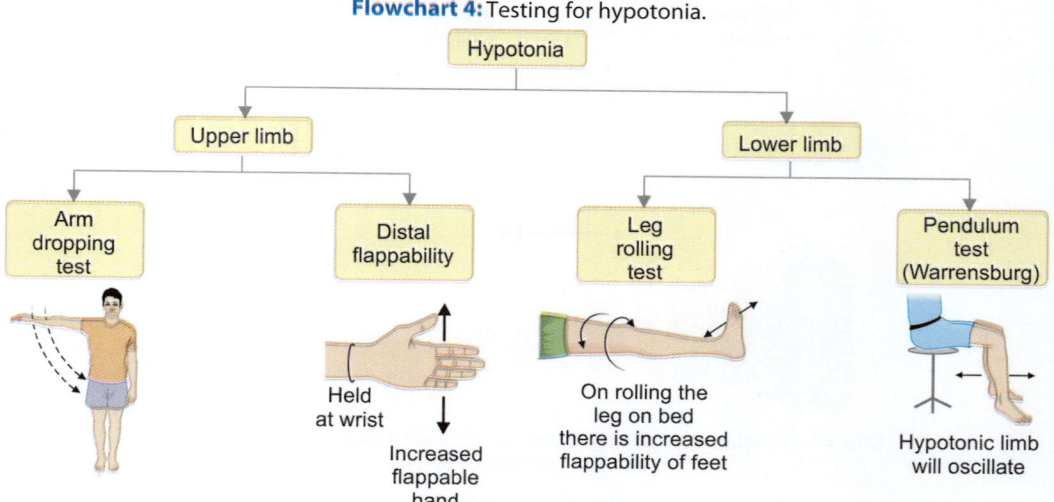

Flowchart 4: Testing for hypotonia.

individually testing deltoid muscle and supraspinatus muscle.
- All the muscles are not equally strong. Some of the muscles are more stronger than others. For example, wrist flexors are stronger than wrist extensors. Similarly, the neck extensors are stronger than neck flexors, elbow extensors are stronger than elbow flexors, finger flexors are stronger than finger extensors, hip extensors are stronger than hip flexors, knee flexors are stronger than knee extensors, and ankle plantar flexors are stronger than dorsiflexors. You can notice that antigravity muscles are stronger than their counterparts. To remember the above list, just imagine decerebrate posturing; all antigravity muscles contract together.
- Remember that muscle is strongest in its shortest length. Hence, biceps will be strongest in full elbow flexion and triceps will be strongest in full elbow extension. **(Figs. 32A and B)**.
- If you keep a strong muscle in its shortest length (triceps in elbow extension), it will be too strong to resist. So, even if there is minimal weakness, triceps can still manage in shortest length. This will miss subtle muscle weakness even if it is present. Hence, if we test triceps in full elbow extension, there is a high chance that we may miss power of 4/5 which would be erroneously reported as 5/5. Hence, strong muscles (antigravity muscles) must be tested in its longest length so that they are at disadvantage.
- Keeping this principle in mind, weaker muscles must be tested in its shortest length. For example, elbow must be flexed to test biceps muscle.
- Remember the longer the leverage from the joint (fulcrum), the higher is the chance that you can break the resistance. While testing children, the leverage could be mid-way rather than at end-point.
- There are two ways to check resistance in muscle power testing **(Fig. 33)**:
  1. *Fight resistance:* To test biceps in a patient, start from elbow extended to fully flexed; you apply resistance while he is performing this movement (you are fighting).
  2. *Break resistance:* To test biceps in a patient, keep the elbow fully flexed and ask him to maintain that position while you try to break the resistance by trying to extend the elbow.
- Apply resistance for at least 3–5 seconds.
- Remember breaking resistance is always better than fighting resistance except in biarticular muscles (hamstring, gastrocnemius). **Table 8** summarizes the grades of muscle power.

Remember: Test the weak muscle in its shortest length and then examiner can break or fight the resistance. Test the strong muscle in its longest length and then break or fight

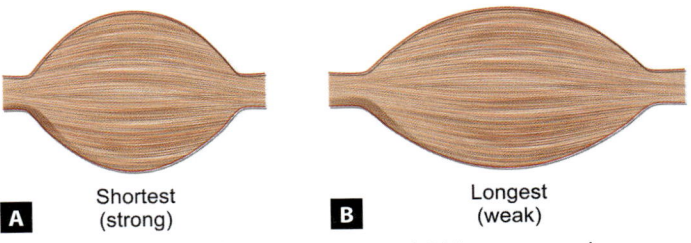

Figs. 32A and B: (A) Shortest and (B) longest muscle.

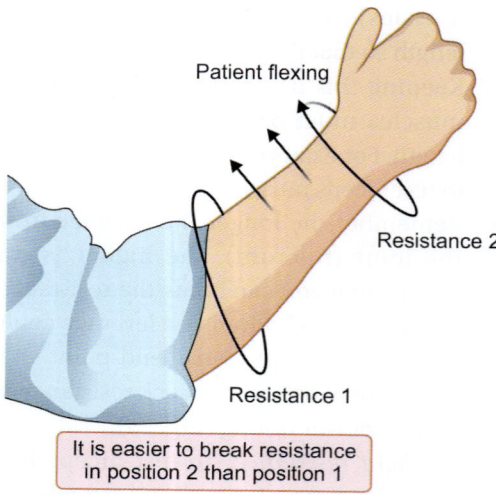

It is easier to break resistance in position 2 than position 1

Fig. 33: Fight versus break resistance.

TABLE 8: Grading of muscle power.

Grades	Description
5	Full ROM against gravity and maximum resistance
4	Full ROM against gravity and maximum resistance
3	Full ROM against gravity
2	Full ROM against gravity eliminates
1	Trace contractions, visible in muscle on an attempted movement
0	No flicker of contraction

(ROM: range of motion)

the resistance according to the position. The individual muscle power testing is discussed in the following text.

Neck Flexor and Extensor

Neck flexor is a weak muscle. Ask the child to lie supine and fully flex the neck (shortest length). Now ask the child to maintain that fully flexed posture and you try to extend it and the child resists that movement. If the child can resist the attempt of the examiner to extend, then the neck flexor power is 5/5 **(Fig. 34)**.

If the child can resist minimally but the examiner succeeds in extending the neck, power is 4/5. If the child is able to flex completely but cannot resist even minimal resistance and the examiner is able to very easily extend the neck, power is 3/5. If the child cannot flex the neck against gravity but is able to flex when made to lie on side-lying position (gravity eliminated), the power is 2/5. If even with gravity eliminated, the child cannot flex the neck, and there is just a small flicker of movement that does not cover full range of motion (ROM), then the power is 1/5. If there is absolutely no flicker, power is 0/5.

Neck Extensor

Neck extensor is a very strong muscle; in fully flexed neck, it is at its longest length and is at disadvantage **(Fig. 35)**. You fight resistance when the child tries to extend it. If the child succeeds, power is 5/5; if the child succeeds partly, power is 4/5. If the child is not at all able to fight the resistance that means you succeed, then place the child in prone position, ask him to extend the neck if full ROM against gravity power is 3/5. If on prone position, there is no full ROM, eliminate the gravity and ask child to lie on a lateral position. If there is now full ROM, power is 2/5; if not, power is 1/5 **(Fig. 36)**. Now you can understand that to grade muscle power, a child has to be placed in more than one position.

Shoulder Muscle Power

Ask the child to sit in a chair and ask him to move the arm forward–backward to the side and then over the head. Now you know that the power is at least 3/5 across all the muscles

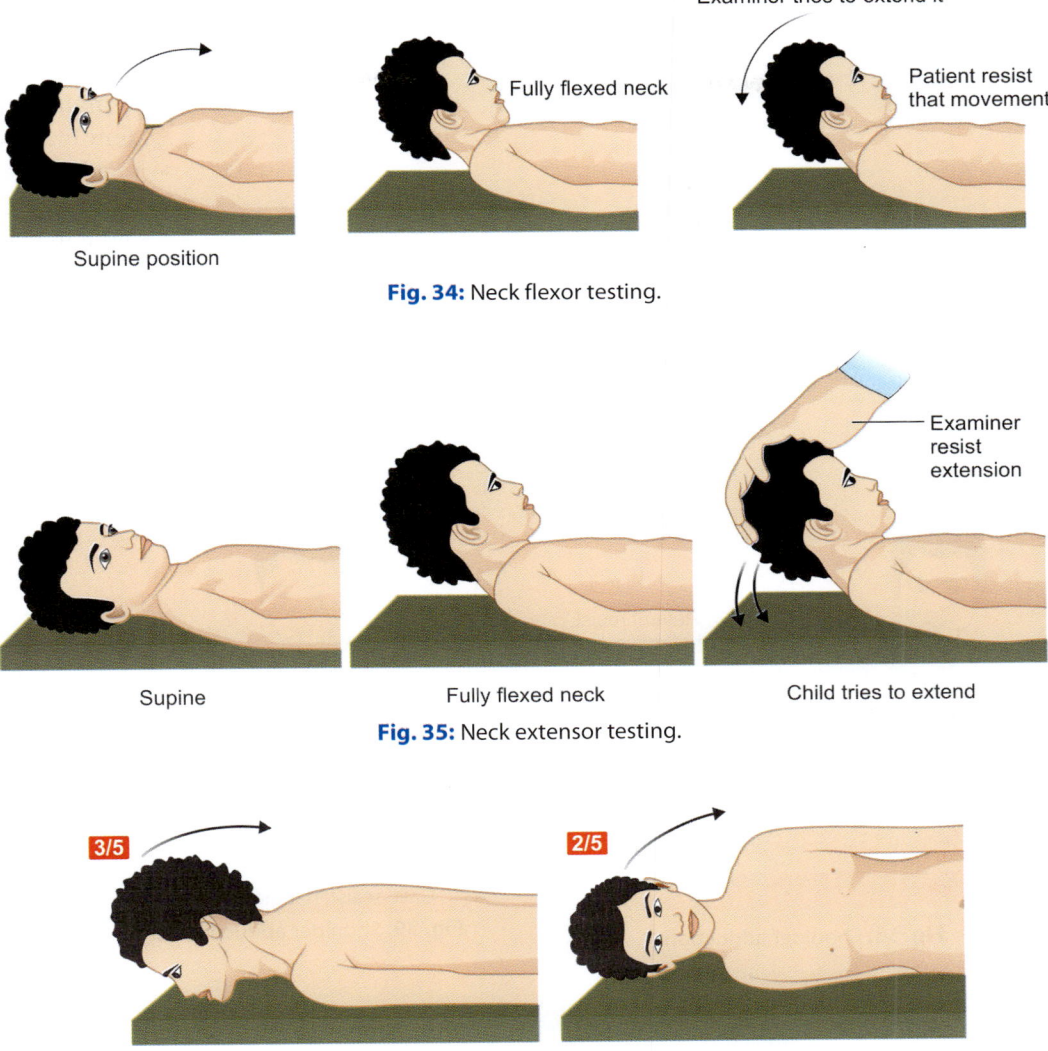

Fig. 34: Neck flexor testing.

Fig. 35: Neck extensor testing.

Fig. 36: Neck extensor muscle power testing.

of shoulder girdle. Now let us test individual movements keeping general principles in mind.

Shoulder Abduction
Shoulder abduction is done initially by supraspinatus and then by deltoid muscle to 90°. Deltoid muscle will be strongest in shortest length, that is, full abduction **(Fig. 37)**. The examiner asks the child to abduct the shoulder to 90° and maintain that posture while he tries to break the resistance. If the child succeeds in maintaining that 90° posture, then shoulder abductors' muscle power is 5/5.

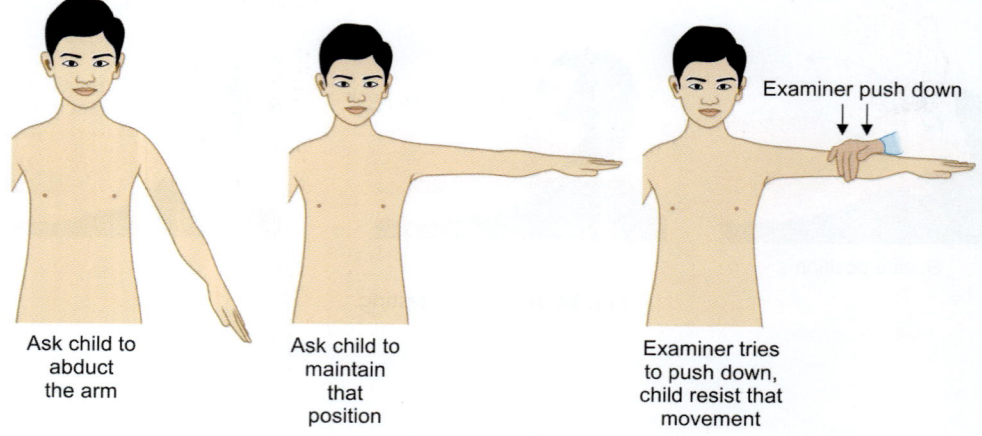

Fig. 37: Shoulder abduction.

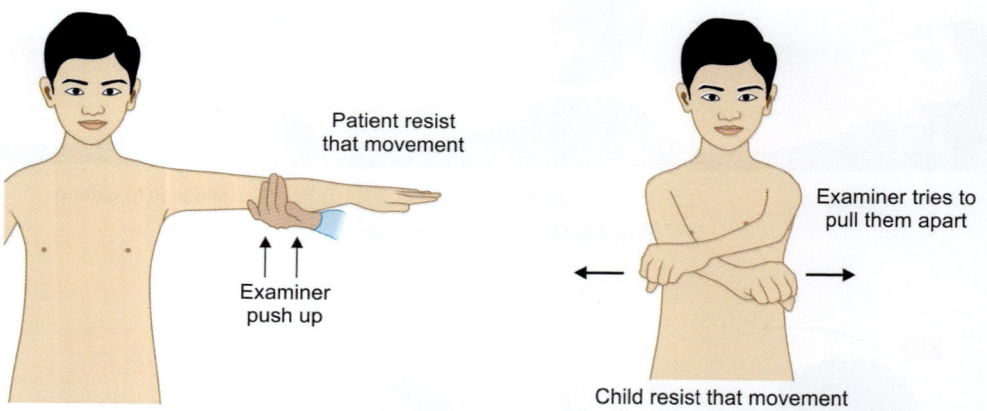

Fig. 38: Shoulder adduction.

Fig. 39: Shoulder abduction across chest.

Shoulder Adduction
Continuing with the same posture of 90° shoulder abduction, ask the child to adduct the shoulder when the examiner resists that movement by pushing the abducted shoulder upward. Shoulder adductors are stronger than shoulder abductors, so test them in longest length (fully abducted position) **(Fig. 38)**.

Shoulder Abduction Across Chest
Ask the child to extend the arms in front of the chest straight with his wrists crossed. The examiner tries to separate and instruct the child to resist this separation. Here we are testing pectoralis major **(Fig. 39)**.

Scapular Winging
Ask the child to extend both arms straight and push against the wall. Look for scapular winging (serratus anterior weakness). To test for trapezius weakness, ask the child to abduct both the arms to 90° with palm facing upward. Scapular winging in this position indicates trapezius muscle weakness **(Fig. 40)**.

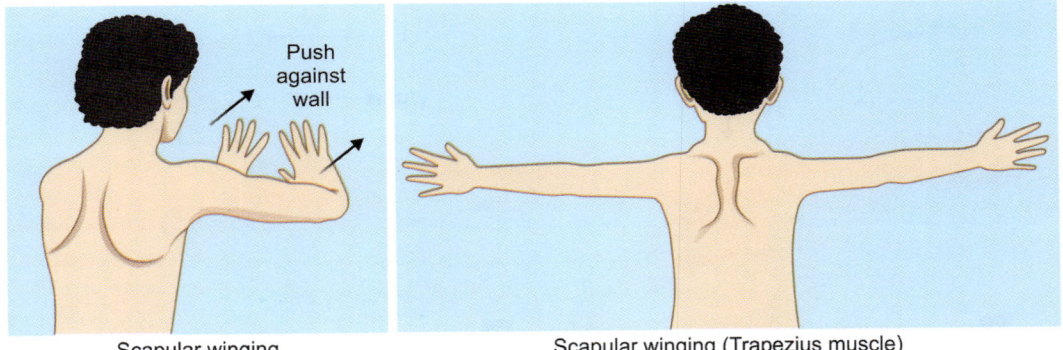

Scapular winging   Scapular winging (Trapezius muscle)

Fig. 40: Testing scapular winging.

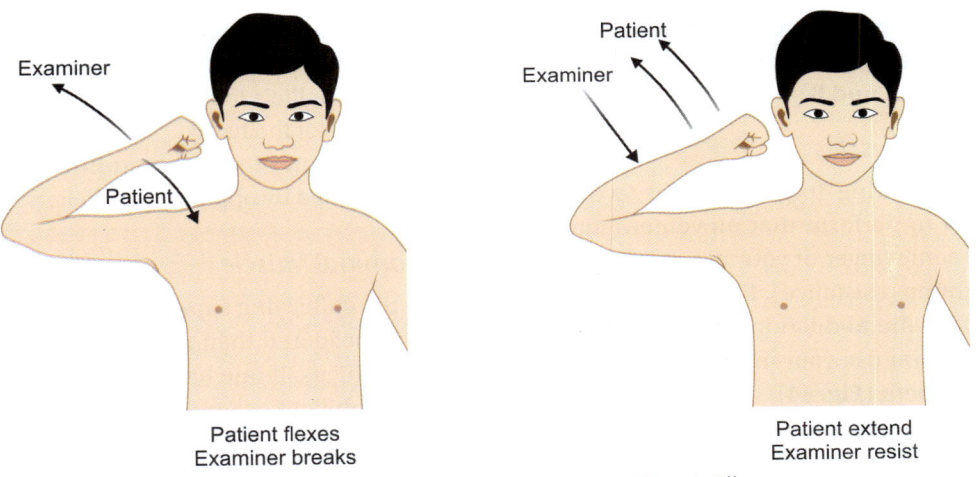

Patient flexes Examiner breaks   Patient extend Examiner resist

Fig. 41: Elbow flexor.   **Fig. 42:** Elbow extensor.

Upper Arm Muscles

Elbow Flexors

Ask the child to "show his biceps". Encourage him to fully flex his elbow and sustain that posture. The examiner holds the child's wrist and tries to break the resistance **(Fig. 41)**. If the child succeeds, then elbow flexor power is 5/5.

Elbow Extensor

The same posture as above, examiner holds the wrist and opposes extension of forearm by the child. Elbow extensor triceps is a strong muscle; hence, in fully flexed elbow, it is at disadvantage **(Fig. 42)**.

Forearm Muscles

Wrist Flexors

Place the child's supinated forearm on the table and ask him to make a fist and flex the wrist. The examiner tries to resist the movement of the wrist.

Wrist Extensor

Turn the hand, rest the forearm on the table pronated, dorsiflex/extend the wrist, and

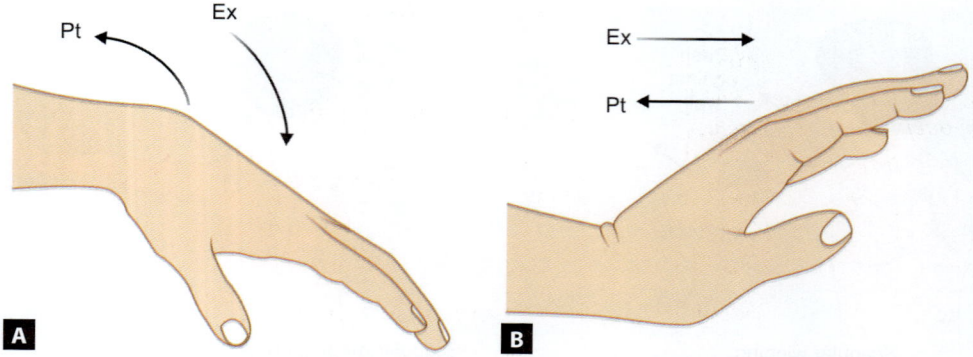

Figs. 43A and B: (A) Wrist flexion and (B) wrist extension. (Ex: examiner; Pt: patient)

ask the child to hold in that position. The examiner attempts to break the resistance **(Figs. 43A and B)**.

Finger Muscles

While testing finger muscles, we ask the child to perform that movement and using the same finger of your hand, give resistance (fighting resistance). For example, if you are testing the abduction of the index finger of child, you use your index finger to resist that movement **(Fig. 44)**.
- Try flexing your metacarpophalangeal (MCP) joints and extending the proximal interphalangeal (PIP) joints, it forms a figure of "L" (LUMBRICIALS)
- REMEMBER PAD (palmar interossei for adduction) and DAB (dorsal interossei for abduction)
- Flexion at PIP/DIP (distal interphalangeal joints) by FDP (flexor digitorum profundus)/FDS (flexor digitorum superficialis) (P comes before S).

Movement at Thumb
- Abductors of thumb are abductor pollicis brevis (APB)/abductor pollicis longus (APL). Abduction of thumb is perpendicular to the plane of the hand. Adduction is done by adductor pollicis.
- Extension of thumb (extensor pollicis longus and brevis) and flexion of thumb (flexor pollicis longus/brevis) are parallel to plane of the hand.
- Opposition of thumb and little finger is performed by opponens pollicis.

Abdominal Muscle

With the child lying supine, ask the patient to flex his head and then raise his legs. Look at the umbilicus. If one half above umbilicus is weak, umbilicus will pull up (Beevor's sign).

Movement at Hip Joint

Hip Flexion

Ask the child to sit on the chair and then stabilize his hip joint. Ask the child to lift the thigh up perpendicularly to the maximum possible distance and then ask the child to maintain it and the examiner tries to break that position. Remember that hip flexors are weak muscles so they will be strongest in full flexion; hence, we test hip flexors in full flexion of hip and the examiner attempts to break the resistance.

Hip flexion is better tested in sitting position rather than supine position **(Fig. 45)**. If power is <3/5, it means that the child is not able perform full ROM against

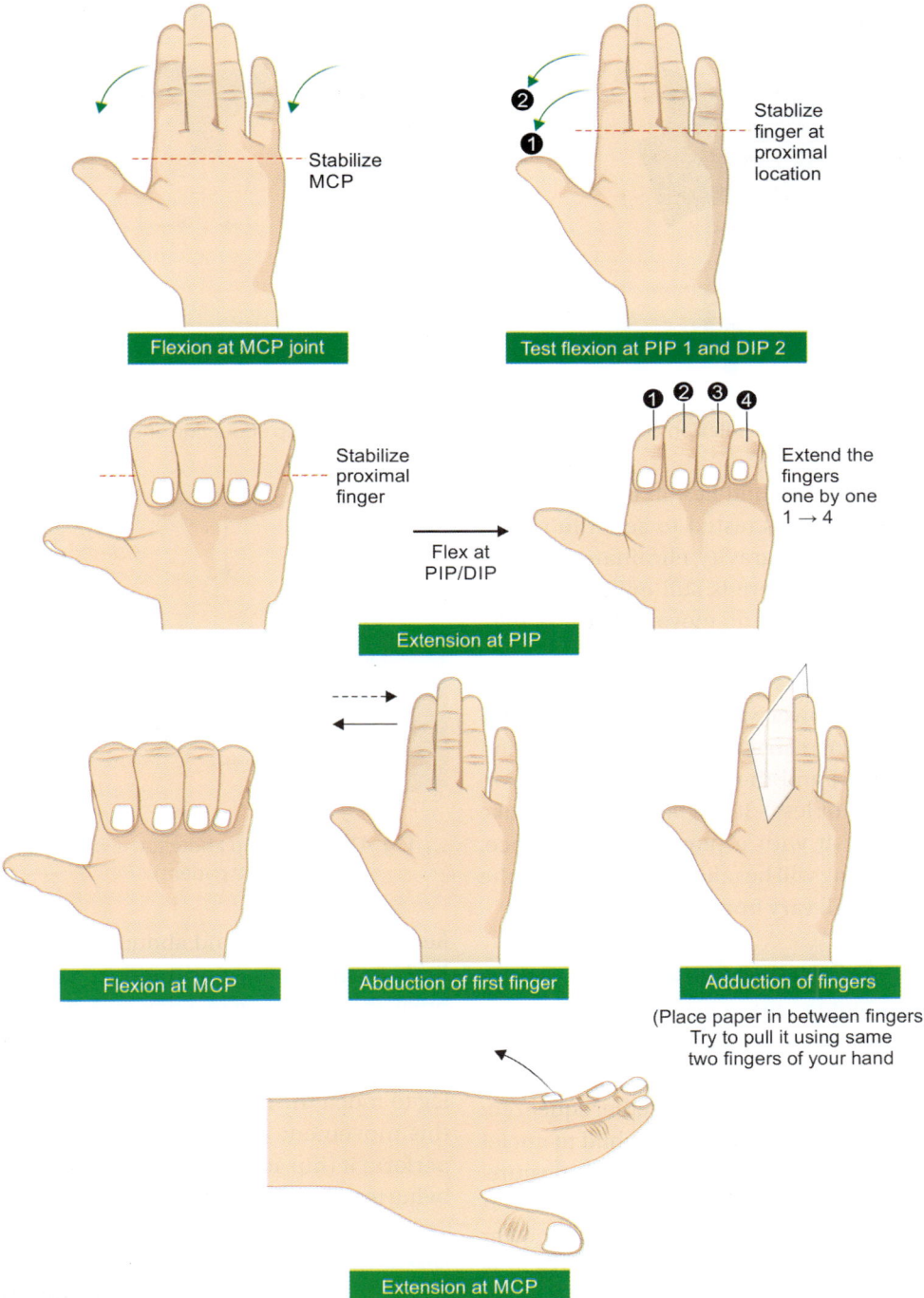

Fig. 44: Finger movement testing. (DIP: distal interphalangeal joint; MCP: metacarpophalangeal; PIP: proximal interphalangeal)

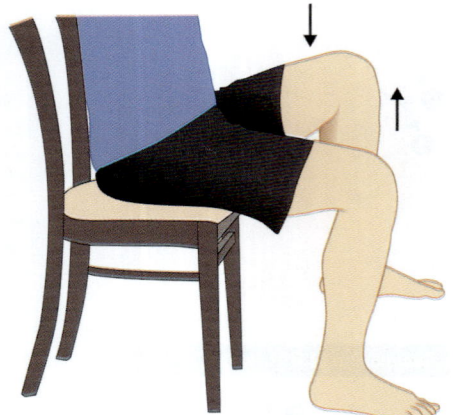

Fig. 45: Hip flexion testing.

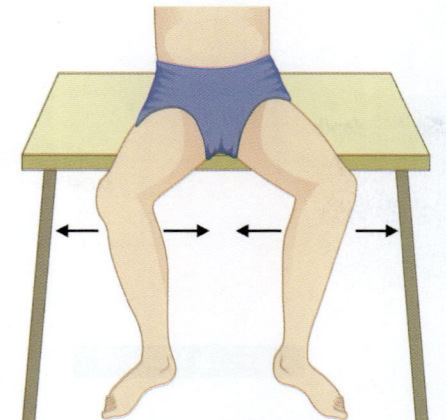

Fig. 46: Hip abduction and adduction.

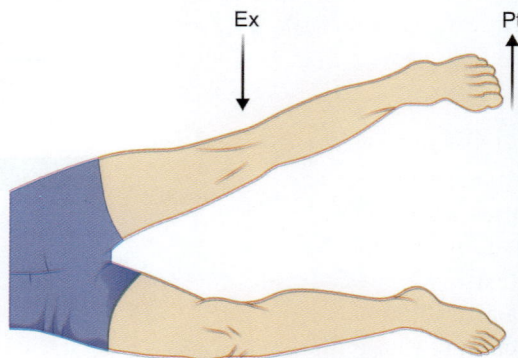

Fig. 47: Testing hip abductor. (Ex: examiner; Pt: patient)

gravity; then the child lies on lateral position and hip flexion is tested to see if full ROM is possible with gravity eliminated (power will be 2/5). If there is still only a flicker of movement (1/5) or no movement (0/5), then power can be graded accordingly.

If the child is nonambulatory, then you know that power will be less than 3/5; in that case, you can start from supine position (power 3/5) and then go to lateral position (power 2/5 or less). It will be difficult to make that child sit with a power of 3/5. Hence, power testing will be tailored according to the child and will vary from case to case.

Hip Abduction and Adduction

With the child is sitting, ask the child to abduct the thighs and you resist from the lateral side of knee (hip abduction) **(Fig. 46)**. Then ask the child to hold the knees together squeezed; you try to separate and ask the child to not let you succeed. Remember that in this posture, gravity is already eliminated, so if the child is not able to resist even minimally the power is 2/5 (rather than 3/5). In such a case, it is better to test hip adductors and abductors in lateral decubitus position **(Fig. 47)**. When testing left hip abductors, you ask the child to lie on his right side and abduct the left lower limb to maximum and hold it; you try to break the resistance in a downward direction and the child resists that movement. In this position, ask the child to adduct the right leg to touch the left leg. The examiner resists this movement while the child attempts to perform it (hip adductors of the right side are being tested) **(Fig. 48)**.

Hip Extensors

Ask the child to lie in prone position and lift the knee and hold it up in air. You try to place your hand in popliteal fossa and try to press

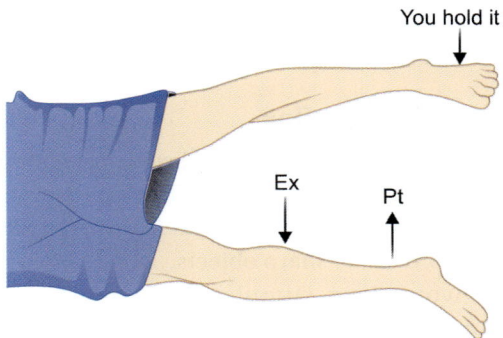

Fig. 48: Hip adduction. (Ex: examiner; Pt: patient)

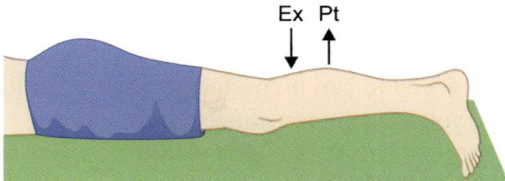

Fig. 49: Hip extensor. (Ex: examiner; Pt: patient)

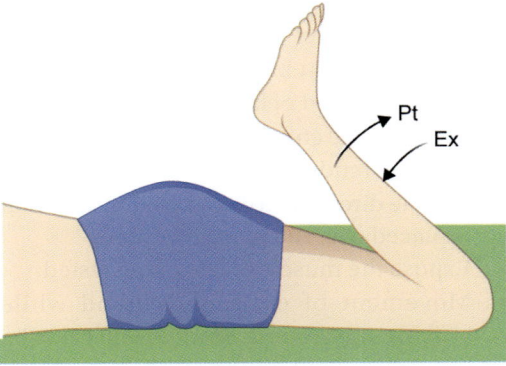

Fig. 50: Knee extensor. (Ex: examiner; Pt: patient)

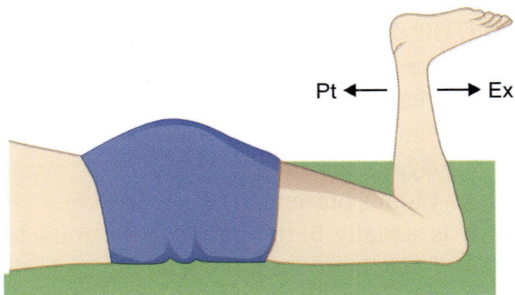

Fig. 51: Knee flexor. (Ex: examiner; Pt: patient)

knee back down and the child resists that movement **(Fig. 49)**.

Movement at Knee Joint

Knee Extensor

Quadriceps are extremely strong antigravity muscles. In full knee flexion, it will be stretched out maximally so that is the best position to test it. Hence, in prone position, a child is asked to flex knee completely. Now ask the child to extend the knee and you (examiner) fight the resistance **(Fig. 50)**. Knee extensors can also be tested in sitting position when the examiner resists extension of knee. However, a power of 4/5 or any subtle weakness may be missed in this position. While testing children, we also need to look at how cooperative the child is. These principles of muscle testing are applicable only to cooperative children. For example, to test knee extensors, it is ideal to test in prone position, but the child may not cooperate, then it is better to test in sitting position itself. Hence, the choice of position needs to individualized.

Knee Flexor

Hamstring muscle is best tested in prone position. Ask the child to maintain 90° at knee joint while you try to straighten it by grasping the ankle **(Fig. 51)**.

Movement at Ankle Joint

If the child can walk on toes, you know that plantar flexors are strong. If the child can walk on heels, you know that dorsiflexors are good. Plantar flexors are very strong muscles; it will be difficult to oppose them with your hands. Other movements like dorsiflexion inversion and eversion can be performed by the child and you fight the resistance.

Deep Tendon

Few general principles
- It is always better to use a heavier hammer than lighter ones.
- Always distract the child. Engage him in play while you bring your hammer. Kids are very scared of hammer.
- Reassure the child that it will not hurt him.
- Feel the tendon and do not strike on the muscle directly. Strike on your thumb that is placed over the muscle tendon.
- Expose the muscle that is being tested.
- Movement of examiner's hand while striking the muscle tendon must not be like drilling nail into the wall. There must be free movement at your (examiner) wrist joint rather than pecking movement.
- The movement must be sharp and crisp.
- DTRs can be graded as:
  0—Areflexia
  1—Hyporeflexia
  2—Normal
  3—Hyperreflexia
  4—Clonus present
- It is usually better to keep the muscle mid-way between full stretching and full flexion while eliciting DTR.
- Ankle clonus can be tested by gently and swiftly dorsiflexing the ankle. It results in well sustained (>5) or ill sustained (1–5) clonus.
- If DTRs are not elicitable despite correcting the method, one can attempt Jendrassik maneuver.
- If DTRs are very brisk, one can observe mass reflex; on eliciting knee jerk, there is ipsilateral hip adduction and contralateral knee extension and adduction.
- **Figure 52** summarizes the clinical examination of DTRs.

Superficial Reflex

- Ensure that the child is relaxed or sleeping while doing superficial reflexes (SR).
- Use a blunt object like a car key to elicit SR.
- Avoid use of sharp objects.
- Avoid deep stimulation. It must just indent the skin but not deep enough to cause pain.
- If SR are absent, it indicates spinal shock phase or a UMN lesion.
- SR include abdominal reflex, anal reflex, cremasteric reflex, and plantar reflex (**Fig. 53**).
- While eliciting planar response, both hip and knee must be extended and heel must rest on table (**Fig. 54**).
- Strike slowly starting from the lateral side and go up to the base of the first toe. It must take 3–5 seconds. Avoid quick jerky movement. This will result in withdrawal response rather than eliciting plantar response. If there is dorsiflexion of great toe with extension or fanning of other toes, it is labeled as extensor plantar responses or Babinski sign. If it is a severe UMN lesion, the above response may be accompanied with knee flexion with contraction of tensor facia latae muscle.
- If the first response to plantar is foot dorsiflexion irrespective of any toe movement, this is withdrawal response and needs to be repeated.
- Other methods of plantar response is depicted in **Figure 55**. It is a good idea to test these methods before concluding extensor plantar response.

Abnormal Movement

Description of hyperkinetic and hypokinetic movement disorder is discussed in **Chapter 17**.

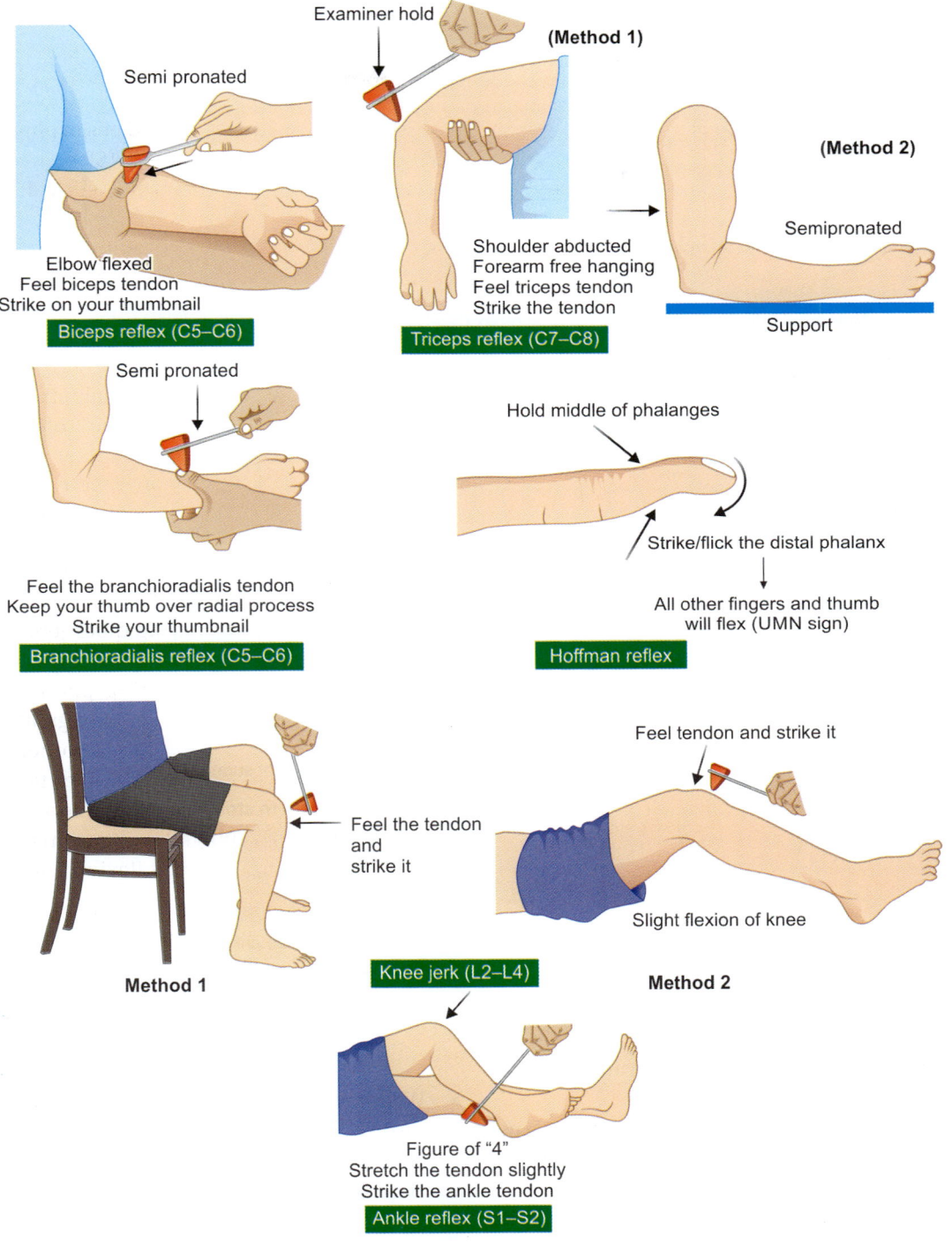

Fig. 52: Deep tendon reflex (DTR) testing.

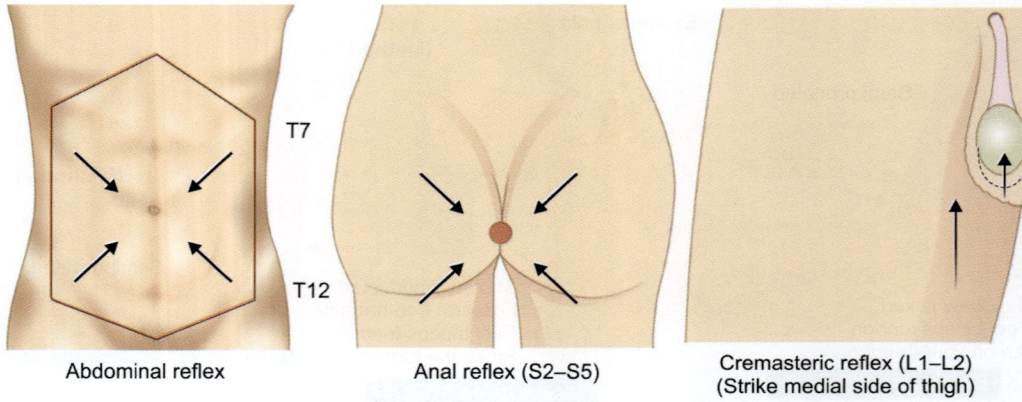

Fig. 53: Superficial reflexes (abdominal reflex, anal reflex, and cremasteric reflex).

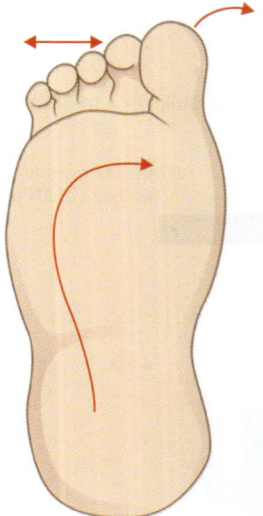

Fig. 54: Plantar response.

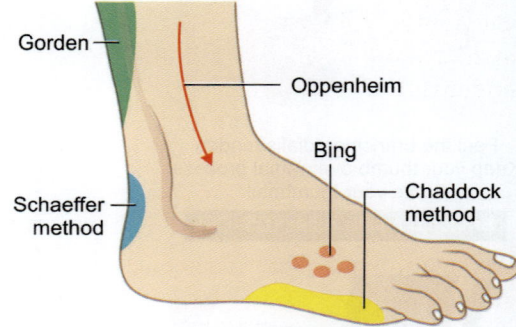

Other methods of superficial plantar reflex

Method	Where to strike?
Chaddock	Lateral side of feet strike
Bing	Multiple pin prick over dorsolateral foot
Gordon	Squeeze calf muscle
Schaeffer	Squeeze ankle tendon
Oppenheim	Press your knuckle down the shin

Fig. 55: Methods of plantar response.

Gait Examination

Gait examination in children includes the following tasks:
- Ask the child to sit on the floor and rise up.
- Stand erect with feet closed together.
- Stand on one foot at a time.
- Stand on toes.
- Stand on heels.
- Walk swiftly, stop abruptly, take quick turn.
- Tandem walk
- Hop on one foot.
- Run and come back.
- Stand with eyes closed and walk.

TABLE 9: Abnormalities of station.

Lesion	Abnormality in station
Cerebellar lesion	Stand on broad base, sway on affected side
Vestibular lesion	Unstable station with head tilt toward affected side, chin rotated to normal side, shoulder higher and in front in affected side
Pyramidal lesion	Hemiplegic station in which upper limb is adducted, elbow flexed, arm is pronated with cortical fisting of hands. Lower limb is extended at hip, knee and ankle
Parkinson	Stand in flexed posture with head and shoulder bent forward
Muscular dystrophy	Standing with abdomen out (lordotic posture)

Station

We look at the station, the way in which the child is standing. Normally, the child can stand erect with feet close together, head up, chest out, and abdomen in. The abnormalities in the station can provide a clinical clue to the underlying etiology **(Table 9)**.

Gait

There are two main phases of gait. The first phase is the stance phase (foot is touching the ground) and the other is swing phase (foot is away from the ground). Now start imagining that you have started walking on the floor. First you keep your right foot with heel (heels strike), then right foot becomes flat (foot flat), then there is a mid-stance (in which left foot starts the heel strike) followed by right heel off the ground and then the right foot pushes off with heel off the ground. This cycle from heel strike to push-off is stance phase which constitutes 60% of cycle. Now the left foot has started with its stance phase and the right foot is away from the floor (swing phase) where the right foot initially accelerates, then has mid-swing phase, and then decelerates before the next stance phase starts. Swing phases constitute 40% of the gait cycle.

If you have pain, you will prefer not to place that foot on floor (stance phase reduced). If you have dorsiflexor weakness, the swing phase will be affected as you cannot lift the foot off the ground. In spasticity and in extrapyramidal lesions, the swing phase will be affected.

Abnormalities of Gait

- *Muscular gait:* Patients with myopathy will have lordotic posture (abdomen-out) and will sway from one side to other side (waddling or duck-like gait). They will have difficulty in getting up from the floor; they will climb on their thighs and legs (Gower sign). They will walk broad based.
- *Neuropathic gait:* If there is paralysis of foot (common peroneal nerve) dorsiflexors, it causes foot drop. Hence with heel strike, there will be flat foot immediately in the stance phase. So, the child must lift the knee high to dorsiflex the foot and then when it falls on the floor, it would slap and produce a sound. Hence, this is also called high steppage or slapping gait. If there is tibial nerve palsy, it would result in heel-drop gait (patient can dorsiflex but not plantarflex). These two conditions can be detected by asking the child to stand on heels (test the dorsiflexor) and on toes (test the plantar flexor).
- *Sensory ataxic gait:* Here, the child has posterior column dysfunction; hence, there is loss of vibration and position

SECTION 1: Neurological Evaluation

TABLE 10: Localization of posterior column sensation.

Clinical feature of posterior column sensation	Site of lesion
One side of UL/LL and face spared	High cervical cord lesion
One side of UL/LL and face affected	Above medulla
Both sides affected; all DTR absent	Peripheral neuropathy
Both LL affected; DTR brisk	Cord lesion
All sensations lost	Radiculopathy
Vibration affected and joint position sensation	Vitamin B_{12} deficiency

(DTR: deep tendon reflex; LL: lower limb; UL: upper limb)

sense. The patient will walk looking at his own feet. The moment visual cue is lost, balance gets disturbed. The child sways on closing the eyes and has high steppage gait. The Rhomberg sign is positive **(Table 10)**.

- *Antalgic gait:* The child has limited weight bearing on the affected side. He will limp on the unaffected side. Hence, he has short stance phase and longer swing phase on the affected side. This gait abnormality is called antalgic gait.
- *Diplegic gait:* The child walks with a narrow base, shuffling gait, dragging both the legs with compensatory swaying of trunk. The feet seem to be stuck to the floor and the child walks as if walking deep through collection of rainwater.
- *Hemiplegic gait:* There is extension of knee joint and ankle joint with circumduction of lower limb on the affected side. The child makes a semicircle on the floor dragging the toe for moving forward. The ipsilateral arm is in hemiplegic posture (flexion at elbow with pronation, wrist, and finger flexion).
- *Cerebellar ataxic gait:* The patient has a wide broad-based stance and is clumsy, staggering with truncal titubation. He is unable to stand, walk, or take turns. He walks like an alcoholic or walks as if walking in a fast-moving bus.
- *Parkinsonian gait:* The patient walks with a stooped forward posture. He has difficulty initiating the steps. When he starts, he has short shuffling gait with decreased arm swing. He has difficulty in stopping; he takes turn en bloc and often freezes when encountered with an obstacle.

EXAMINATION OF SENSORY SYSTEM

The neuroanatomy, pathway, and localization can be read from **Chapter 1** before preceding to read this section. The main purpose of this section is to get familiar with performance of sensory system examination.

Testing Proprioception

We can sense the position of our own limbs and movement of the limbs (kinesthesia) even with our eyes closed. Thia is proprioception. This sensation is carried in posterior column of the spinal cord when it ascends on the same side till the high cervical region where it crosses to the opposite side **(Fig. 56)**. We can test for proprioception starting from distal joints and then proceeding to proximal joints.

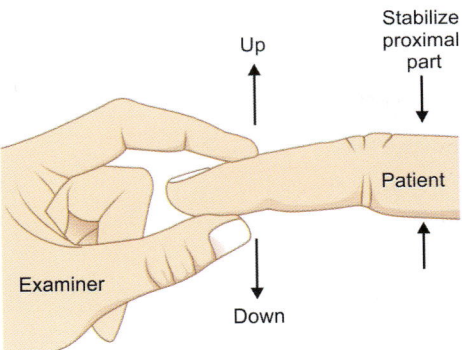

Fig. 56: Testing joint position sensation.

We hold the middle finger and stabilize the proximal joint. Apply force parallel to the plane of movement and move it little (avoid high amplitude movement). Move it slow (1–2 seconds). Instruct the child, "I will move your finger up and down", "This is up and this is down", "Up and down will not be sequential", "Once I stop you need to identify the position. Is it up or down", "Ok, let us start, close your eyes". Other ways to test proprioception include Rhomberg sign and look for pseudoathetosis **(Figs. 57A and B)**.

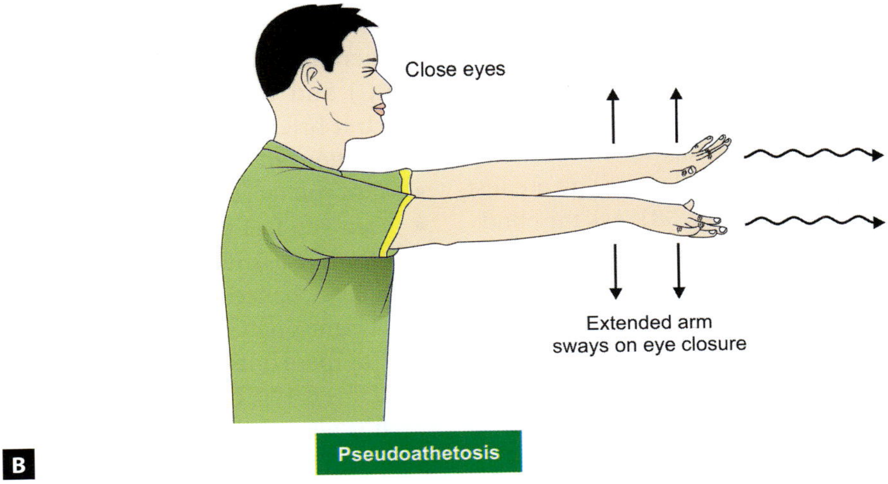

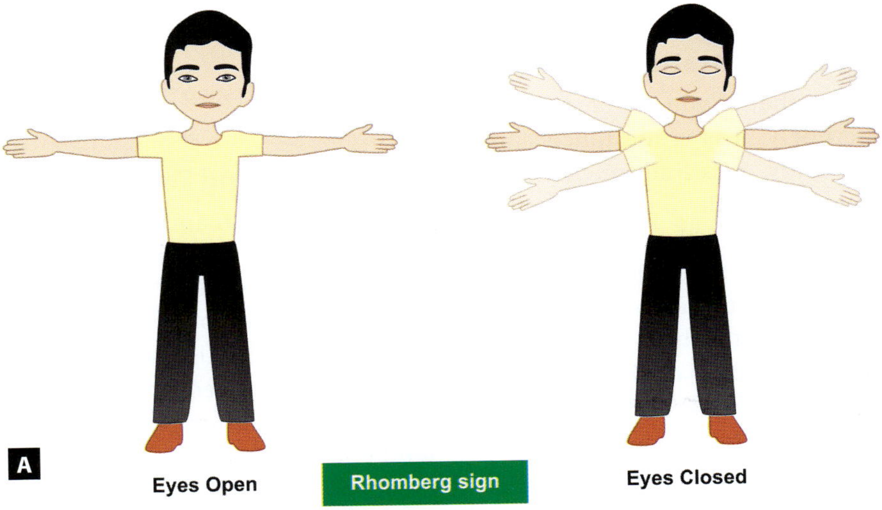

Figs. 57A and B: (A) Rhomberg sign and (B) pseudoathetosis.

Testing Vibration Sensation

The pathway is like proprioception. One can use a 128-Hz tuning fork to test vibration sensation. Strike the tuning fork against a firm surface and place it over bony prominence: Great malleoli, shin, anterior superior iliac spine, spinous process, PIP joints, wrist, and olecranon process. Ask/tell the child, "can you feel the vibration". Show it to the child how vibrating sensation feels before recording his response. Always test the vibration sense with eyes closed.

Testing Tactile Sensation

Many believe that if you touch a part of the body crudely, it is crude touch and if you touch lightly, it is fine touch. That is probably not correct. If you feel something has touched you, that feeling is crude touch. Now if you can feel that something round (shape) with soft texture has touched you, this appreciation is fine touch or discriminative touch. Touch sensation is carried by multiple pathways and there are a lot of variations in which is the pathway for fine and crude touch. In general, dorsal column is responsible for discriminative touch/tactile localization and anterior spinothalamic tract is for crude touch.

Use fine wisp of cotton to test tactile sensation. Remember to dab it over the area that you are testing. Do not drag it; avoid applying pressure. Prefer a nonhairy area. Ensure that the child's eyes are closed while you are testing tactile sensation **(Fig. 58)**. Ask the child;
- Can you feel the touch?
- Compare it to the other side. You may ask "if this is count of 100 on right side, how much is on left side?"
- Touch homologous area in sequence—do not touch it together or else the child will get confused.
- Preferably follow a dermatomal pattern.

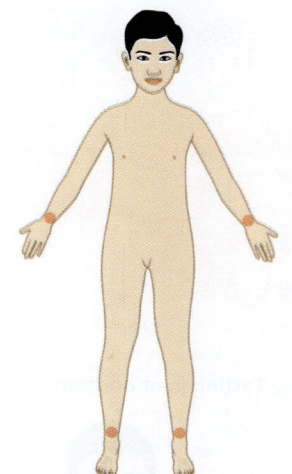

Fig. 58: Testing tactile sensation.

Testing Pain and Temperature

Sensations of pain and temperature ascend one to two levels higher and cross to the other side of the lateral spinothalamic tract. Cervical fibers are placed medial and sacral fibers are lateral. All fibers reach thalamus and then sensory cortex. To test pain, use a safety pin, ball pin, or toothpick. To test temperature, use a test tube. Testing pain must be reserved as the last part of examination. While testing for pain, use the same pressure everywhere. While testing temperature, fill a test tube with cold water (10°C) and then warm water (40°C) and touch it briefly (<2 seconds). Ask the child. Instructions to the child could be:
- Can you feel the pain?
- Can you feel the temperature? How is it? (DON'T ask if it is cold or HOT? There is a 50% chance that the child will be right) (Frame open-ended question.)
- Compare one side to other side.
- If this is 100, how much is this?

It is always good to follow a dermatomal pattern. The common patterns of sensory loss is summarized **(Fig. 59)**.

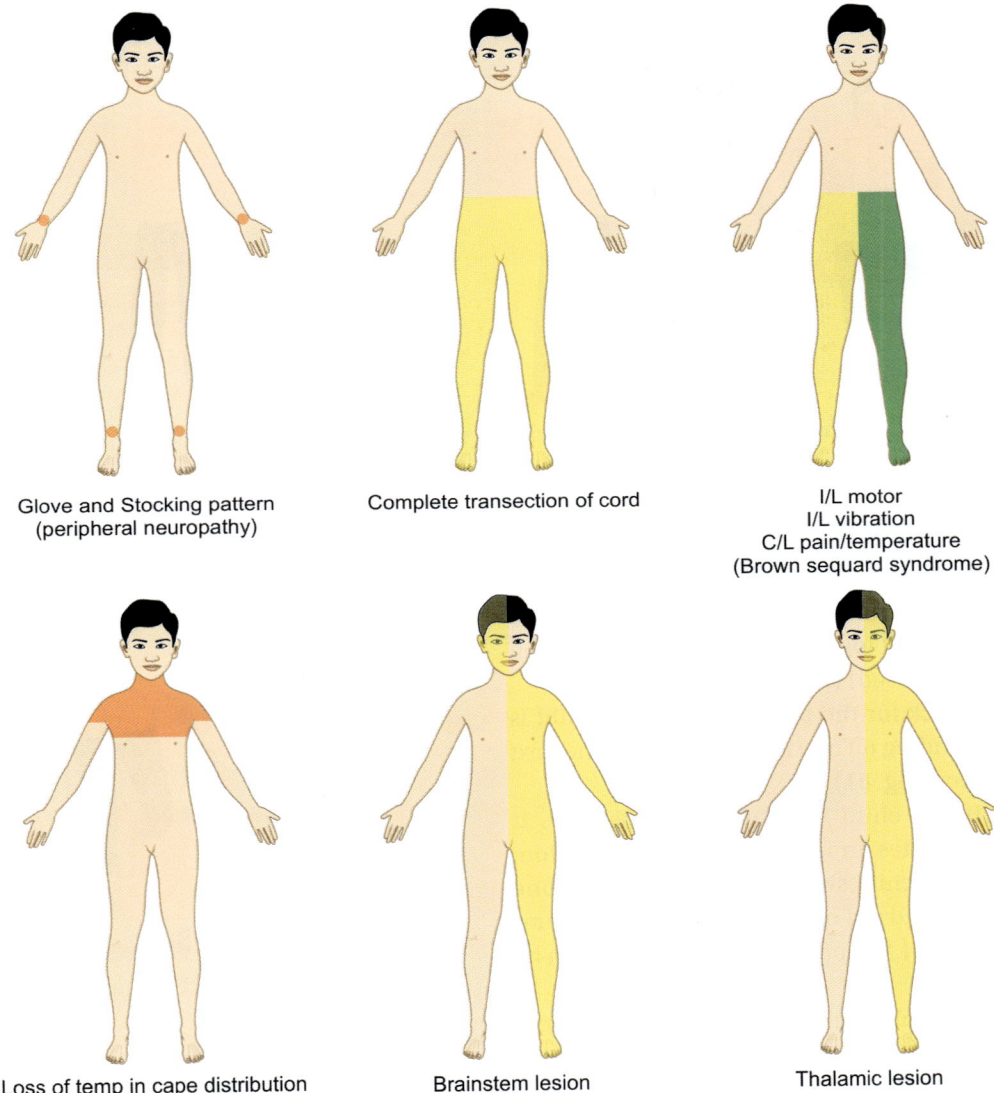

Fig. 59: Patterns of sensory loss.

Cortical Sensation

- *Two-point discrimination:* Use a compass, start from closed points and then gradually increase the distance. Ask the child to tell you when he can identify these two points separately. Check hands and then legs.
- *Stereognosis:* Give a 1-rupee coin and a 5-rupee coin in the child's hand with eyes closed. Ask the child if he can identify the object.
- *Graphesthesia:* Write a number 1–10 in the child's hand with his eyes closed. Ask him to identify the number.

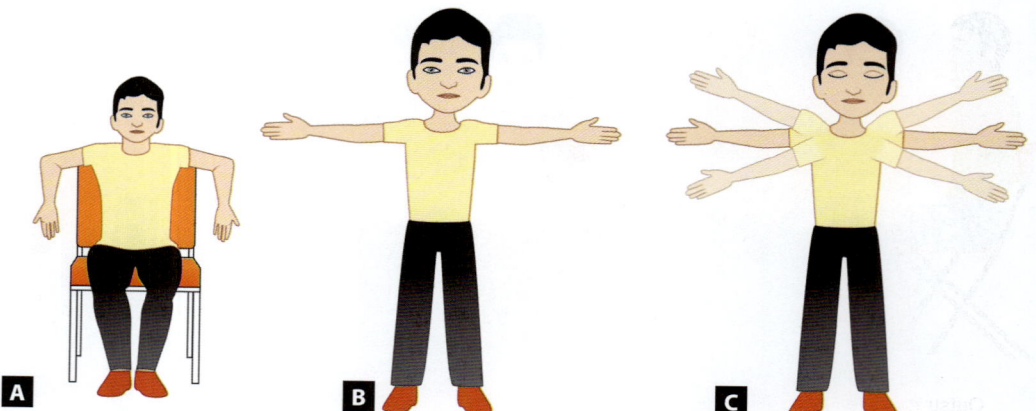

Figs. 60A to C: Testing balance: (A) Balance on sitting; (B) Balance on standing (eyes open); (C) Balance on standing (eyes closed) (Rhomberg sign).

EXAMINATION OF CEREBELLAR FUNCTION AND COORDINATION

- Look for balance while the child is sitting, with feet together on standing (eyes open and closed) **(Figs. 60A to C)**.
- Check for the balance while the child is standing on one foot and then on the next foot **(Fig. 61)**.
- If the child is swaying to one side, it indicates an ipsilateral cerebellar lesion. If the child sways when standing on one foot and not on the other foot, it indicates UMN/LMN paralysis of limb on which he sways.
- Past pointing (see vestibular nerve testing) can be performed to differentiate cerebellar from vestibular lesion.
  - If both arms drift toward one side, it indicates I/L vestibular lesion.
  - If there is outward drifting of one arm, it indicates I/L cerebellar lesion.
  - If both arms drift away from each other, it indicates B/L cerebellar lesion.
- It may be difficult to detect subtle weakness on one side (hemiparesis). To detect the same, you may ask the child to outstretch the arms/legs and hold it

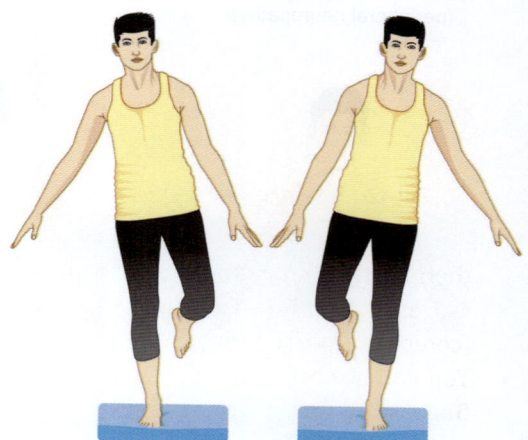

Fig. 61: Check balance on standing.

in that position for as long as possible with eyes closed. The affected side will start "drifting" in upper limb; the affected side will drift down and arm will pronate (pronator drift) **(Fig. 62)**.

- *Finger to nose test:* Ask the child to outstretch the abducted arm. Now ask the child to touch his nose. Repeat it quickly **(Fig. 63)**.
- *Finger to finger test:* Ask the child to touch your finger at position 1. If he is able to repeat, shift the finger to position 2 and

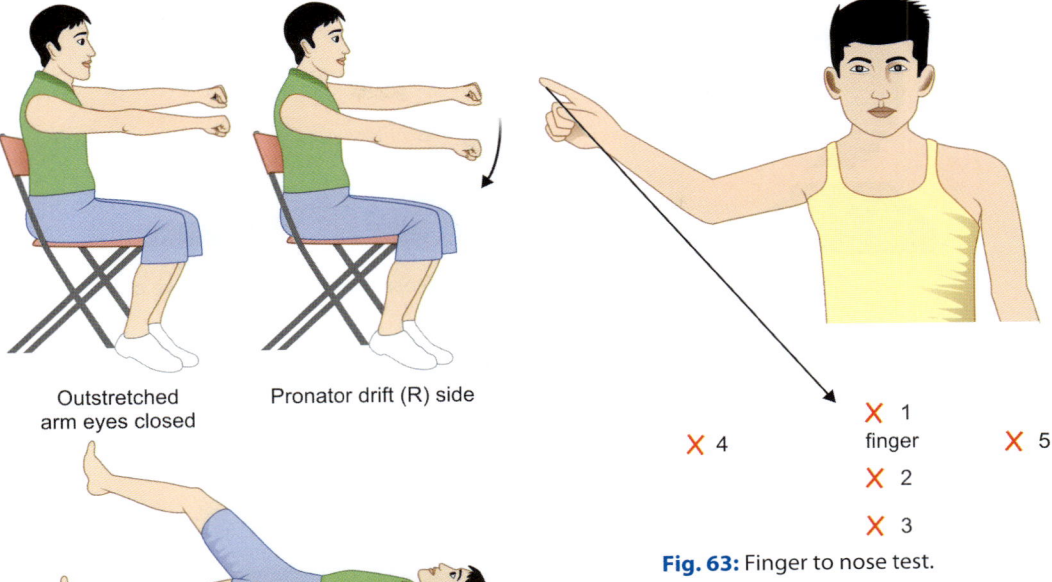

Outstretched arm eyes closed

Pronator drift (R) side

Hold leg in lying position

Fig. 62: Testing subtle hemiplegia.

X 4　　X 1 finger　　X 5
　　　　X 2
　　　　X 3

Fig. 63: Finger to nose test.

then to position 3. Avoid using position 4/5 as it does not truly test dysmetria (cerebellar dysfunction).
- You can also ask the child to touch your finger and then his nose (finger-to-nose test).
- In a cerebellar lesion, the child fails to reach the target (finger or nose) and stumbles to judge the distance (dysmetria).
- Heel to shin test also tests for coordination. If a child is able to use the right heel and slide run from top to bottom of his left shin, it indicates smooth coordination. If he is unable to perform, it indicates a right cerebellar lesion. Repeat it using the other side.
- Check for dysdiadochokinesia which indicates ability to perform rapid alternating movement. It could be rapid pronation–supination, opening and closure of hands, repeated tapping on floor with feet, rapid thumb–finger opposition from finger 2 to finger 5, and rapid alternate tapping with palm and dorsum of hand.

EXAMINATION OF MENINGEAL SIGNS

- Neck stiffness can be tested in supine position or with the child in sitting position. If the child is cooperative, you can ask the child to flex his neck so that the chin can touch his chest. Look at his eyes and facial expression. If he winces on pain, it indicates neck stiffness.
- In older children, you can passively flex the head in supine position so that the chin can touch the chest. If the child winces on pain, it again indicates neck stiffness. It is important to look at facial expressions and interpret.
- In uncooperative children, it is a good idea to bring the child's head to the edge of table. This will make the child

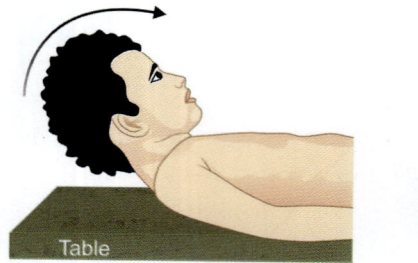
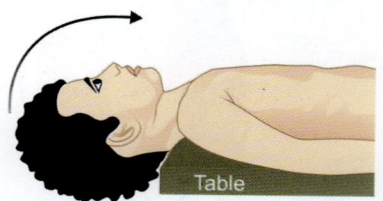

Fig. 64: Neck stiffness.

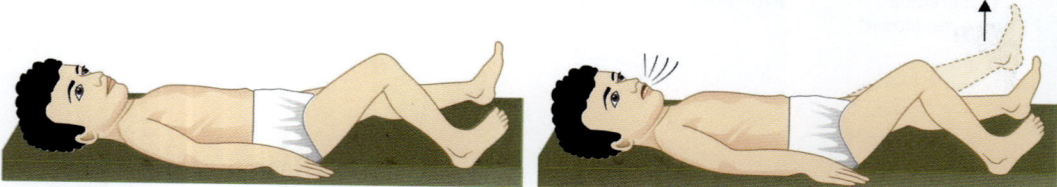

Fig. 65: Kernig sign.

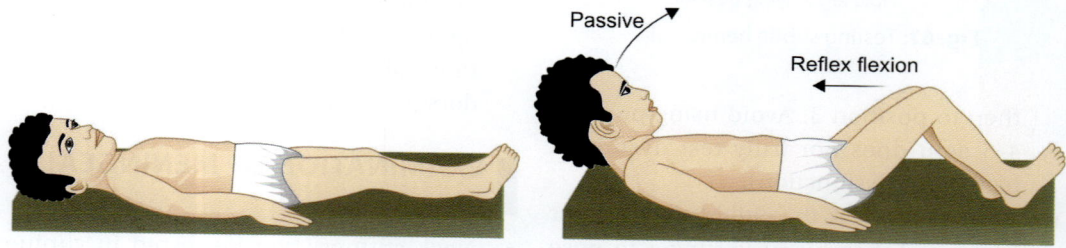

Fig. 66: Brudzinski sign.

uncomfortable, and the child would want to flex his neck so that he does not fall. You also want to flex the neck and see if there is stiffness. Hence, this posture will automatically remove voluntary resistance from the child so that if neck stiffness is seen, it is a true meningeal sign **(Fig. 64)**.
- Other signs of meningeal irritation include Kernig sign and Brudzinski sign.
- Passive extension of flexed lower limb will elicit pain (Kernig sign) **(Fig. 65)**.

Remember to look at the face and notice the wincing response.

- Reflex flexion of hip and knee on passive flexion of neck in supine position (Brudzinski sign) **(Fig. 66)**.

EXAMINATION OF SKULL AND SPINE

Concluding part of neurological examination is examination of skull and spine. Skull examination includes comment on fontanelle (open), closure/bony closure (anterior/posterior/temporoparietal), and sutures (well apposed/overriding in craniosynostosis). It could mention the shape of skull (dolichocephaly) scaphocephaly, trigonocephaly, and size of skull (microcephaly or normocephaly).

To perform spine examination and to feel for any spinal tenderness, you can ask the child to bend forward to touch his feet. Then run your thumb across the spine from top to bottom to look for any spinal tenderness. Presence of kyphosis/scoliosis must be commented on inspection of back in erect posture **(Fig. 67)**.

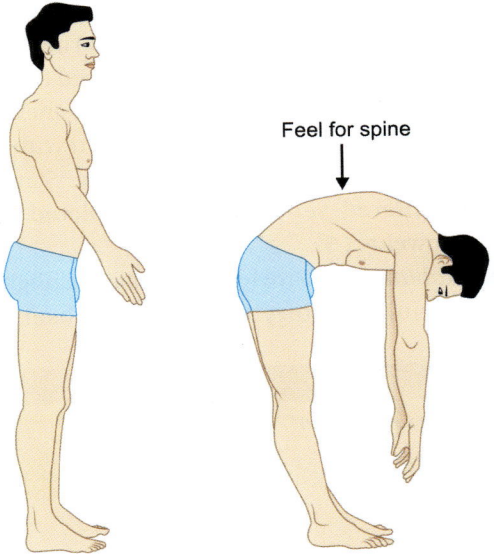

Fig. 67: Testing spine examination.

NEONATAL NEUROLOGICAL EXAMINATION

Observation

Observe the resting posture of the neonate. Normally by 32 weeks, we expect flexion of all limbs with adduction of thighs. Before 32 weeks, there will be flexion of arms but legs could be flexed or extended. If a 32-week-old baby lies in extended posture with abducted thighs and arms in flaccid posture, then we know that it is abnormal posture **(Figs. 68A and B)**. Also observe the cranial sutures and fontanelle **(Fig. 69)**. Feel for the sutures and their gap. Ideally, sutures should not admit the tip of a finger. Look for the shape of the skull. Normally, the head of preterm grows in an anteroposterior (AP) diameter more than biparietal diameter (BPD) (ratio of AP: BPD = 1.5).

Level of Alertness

There are four things to look for: State of alertness, habituation, consolability and cuddliness.
1. State of alertness is best assessed in between the feeds. Distinct change in alertness develops by 28 weeks, sleep–wake cycle is established by 32 weeks, baby remains alert by 34 weeks, and by

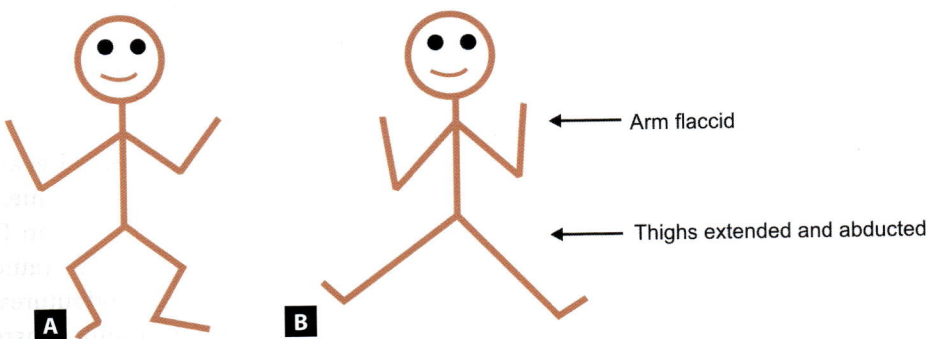

Figs. 68A and B: (A) Normal and (B) abnormal posture in a newborn.

36 weeks the child starts cycling during wakefulness. State of alertness can be commented using Prechtl neonatal behavioral scale **(Table 11)** or by Brazelton neonatal behavioral scale **(Flowchart 5)**. The stages in Brazelton neonatal behavior assessment scale include:

- *State 1:* Deep sleep, without movement, breathing regularly
- *Stage 2:* Light sleep, closed eyes, some corporal (body) movements
- *State 3:* Sleepy, eyes opening and closing
- *State 4:* Awake, opened eyes, minimal corporal movement
- *State 5:* Completely awake, strong corporal movement
- *State 6:* Cry

In a quiet awake state, the baby has smooth flowing movement and in bright light he blinks and avoids it and quietens on response to sound. Motor movements of the baby are quantified (normal or diminished) and quality is assessed (high level or low level). High-level movements are those that are nonstereotyped with a definitive latency and habituation. States of altered sensorium are depicted in **Flowchart 5**.

2. *Habituation:* Provide repetitive flashlight stimuli/auditory stimuli and observe

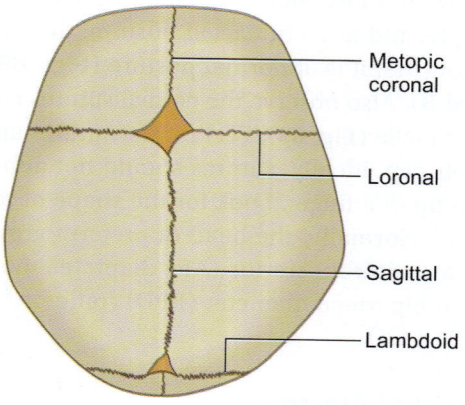

Fig. 69: Sutures of the skull.

TABLE 11: Prechtl neonatal behavioral scale.

State	Eyes open	Respiration regular	Gross movement	Vocalization
1	−	+	−	−
2	−	−	±	−
3	+	+	−	−
4	+	−	+	−
5	±	−	+	+

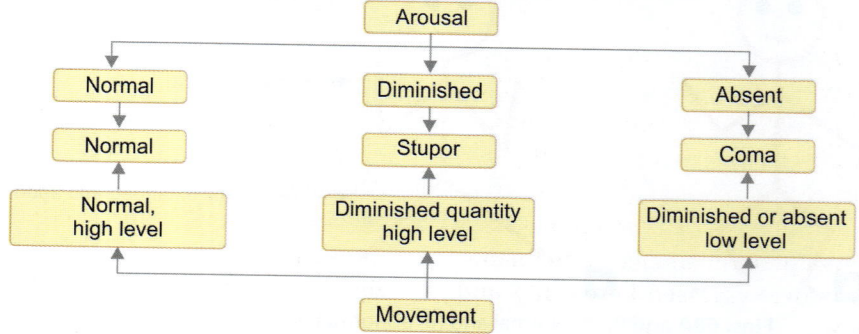

Flowchart 5: States of altered sensorium in newborn.

for blink/startle. Look for cessation of movement or breastfeeding. Normally, a term infant habituates after 3–5 stimuli. It is considered abnormal if it fails to initially respond or there is lack of habituation.
3. *Consolability:* Look for consolability after 15 seconds of crying:
   - Spontaneous
   - By talking
   - By putting hand on abdomen
   - By picking baby up
   - Unconsolable
4. *Cuddliness:* Assess the response of the baby to being held. Does he cuddle on being held.

Cranial Nerve Examination

- Olfactory nerve can be affected in the infant of a diabetic mother or in holoprosencephaly. We can look for grimacing response to cotton soaked in some peppermint extract.
- When a torch light is shown, a 28-week-old baby would blink to light; by 32 week, you can notice spontaneous roving eye movement; by 34 weeks, the baby can fix and follow; and by 36 weeks, he develops optokinetic nystagmus.
- Extraocular movements are best observed or can be tested by doll's eye maneuver (it appears by 28 weeks and disappears by 36 weeks).
- Pupils are reactive to light by 29–32 weeks. But it is difficult to elicit pupillary reaction owing to physiological photophobia. Hypoxic ischemic encephalopathy will result in decreased pupil reactivity.
- There is often minor dysconjugate eye position in preterm and few term infants. Squint is best assessed between 3 and 6 months.
- *Vision assessment in newborn:* One can look for optokinetic nystagmus. There is horizontal deviation in the direction of drum with nystagmus in the opposite direction.
- Facial sensation can be tested with pin prick (trigeminal nerve).
- Cessation of activity/breathing to clipping or ringing a bell is an indicator of intact auditory nerve.
- A term baby who is sucking and swallowing milk is presumed to have intact 9th and 10th CN.

Motor Examination

Posture and Tone

Posture can be graded and assessed **(Figs. 70A to D)**. Passive tone progresses in caudal to rostral direction with term infant having fully relaxed posture. Posture must be commented in a quiet alert stage of alertness. Passive tone can be assessed by flappability of extremity, scarf sign, arm recoil, and square window sign in upper extremity; popliteal angle and heel to ear in lower limb **(Table 12)**. Active tone is best assessed by testing neck flexion and neck extensor (pull to sit) **(Table 13)**.

Quality and Quality of Movement

- There are slow rotational components of limb movement at 28 weeks.
- There are symmetrical hip and knee flexion at 32 weeks and by 36 weeks these movements become stronger and alternating.
- After birth, there is writhing movement till 8 weeks, fidgety movement around 8–20 weeks, and then beyond 20 weeks, there are large amplitude swipe and swat movement.

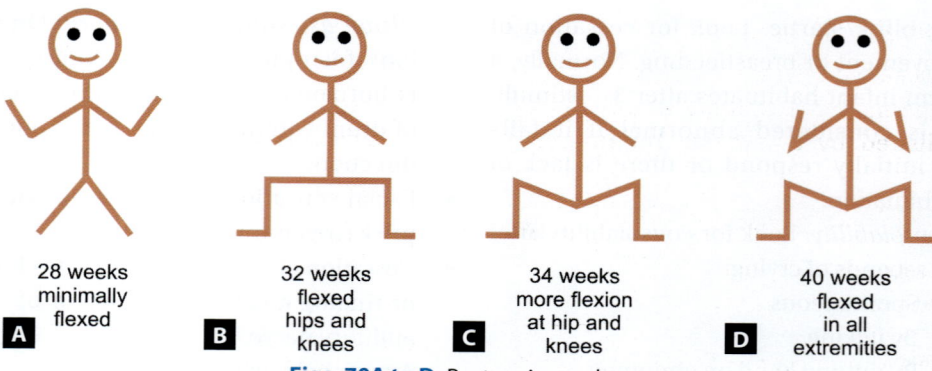

Figs. 70A to D: Posture in newborn.

TABLE 12: Passive tone assessment.

Method	What to do?
Arm recoil	Arms can be flexed to chest, hold it for 5 seconds, and then release to extension suddenly
Scarf sign	Arms can be placed across the chest by pulling it to opposite shoulder as if wearing a scarf
Popliteal angle	Thigh flexed on abdomen with one hand and with other hand you can straighten the leg by pushing on back of ankle till firm resistance
Heel to ear	Hold baby's feet in one hand; draw the leg toward ipsilateral ear to see how much resistance

TABLE 13: Active tone assessment.

Method	What to do?
Pull to sit	Starting from supine position, the baby is pulled by arms to siting position
Traction response	In supine position, pull the baby by both arms; normally, the baby's arms will flex as if resisting that traction
Ventral suspension	On ventral suspension, head is usually in midline and limbs flex against gravity
Horizontal suspension	Hold the infant by thorax (prone) without providing support to head or legs. Head rises intermittently and limbs flex against gravity

Deep Tendon Reflexes

Knee jerk can elicit crossed adductor response. Ankle clonus of 5–10 beats can be normal till 3 months of age.

Plantar Response

It can be extensor if elicited by the Babinski method by stimulating the lateral aspect of foot. Remember plantar grasp and nociceptive withdrawal can confound the interpretation.

Primitive Reflex

One can test sucking reflex, rooting reflex, grasp reflex, Moro reflex, crossed extensor response, and automatic walking response as a part of primitive reflex testing.

Sensory Examination

A 28-week-old infant can differentiate touch from pain, and response to pain is well established by 36 weeks. Hammersmith neonatal neurological examination and Amiel Tison neurological assessment are good objective ways to document neonatal neurological examination.

> **KEY MESSAGES**
>
> - Neurological examination in children is challenging and it consists of HMF, CN examination, motor system examination, sensory system examination, cerebellar signs, and meningeal signs.
> - HMF consists of COMA-PIFAC [Consciousness, Orientation, Memory, Attention span, Perception (spatial), Insight, Fund of information, Abstract thinking and Calculation].
> - Motor system examination consists of examination of gait (ambulatory) or posture (nonambulatory), tone, power, DTRs, SRs, and abnormal movement.
> - Sensory system examination consists of examination of posterior column sensation (vibration, fine touch, joint position, proprioception) and lateral spinothalamic sensation (pain and temperature).
> - Meningeal signs include neck rigidity, Kernig sign, and Brudzinski sign.

CHAPTER 4

Making a Clinical Neurological Diagnosis

■ INTRODUCTION

The chapter provides a broad outline on reaching a possible clinical diagnosis for neurological disorders in children. The clinical diagnosis is determined by three components—(1) history of neurological symptoms, (2) neurological examination, and (3) the possible neurological diagnosis. We must acknowledge that children are often not very cooperative for a detailed neurological examination. Hence, majority of information needs to be retrieved and interpreted from the clinical history. The examination must be focused to support or refute the possibilities raised from the history.

■ NEUROLOGICAL HISTORY

History is the most essential step in analysis of patient symptoms. It is considered that nearly 70–80% of diagnosis is made at the end of history. Neurological history includes analysis of presenting complaints, history to determine the extent of the neurological involvement and etiological history. Readers are suggested to refer to "Clinical Methods in Pediatrics" by Piyush Gupta for detailed description on history-taking in Pediatrics.

Presenting Complaints

Presenting complaint is the most essential aspect of history-taking and most crucial step for analysis. It is often revisited multiple times during the history of presenting illness and even at the end of examination. For instance, if we realize that child has right-sided hemiparesis on examination, we can go back to ask parents since when have they noticed paucity of movement of right upper and lower limbs. In such a case, "paucity of movement of right-sided upper and lower limbs" could be one of the presenting complaints. Presenting complaints often help in framing the possible hypothesis for the problem. There are no fixed rules as to how presenting complaints must be described as far as the course of entire illness appears congruent.

It is a good idea to use simple language and avoid medical jargons in presenting complaints. For example, "convulsion" is acceptable presenting complaint instead of "seizure." One may also prefer to use complaints like "an episode of abnormal body movement." However, we need to keep in the mind that abnormal movement could also mean any movement disorder such as chorea, dystonia, myoclonus, or seizure. Few examples of presenting complaints are provided in **Table 1**.

Ideally, a presenting complaint must depict the entire course of illness. For example, if a 10-year-old child has presented with one episode of seizure, his presenting complaint would be "one episode of convulsion 2 days back." In such a case, we would start thinking of causes of first unprovoked seizure in a 10-year-old boy, which would be like neurocysticercosis,

TABLE 1: How to frame presenting complaints based on the neurological history?

History	Presenting complaints
A 10-year-old child presented with sudden onset of weakness of right upper limb and lower limb with deviation of face for last 2 days. He was admitted in the hospital. He developed an episode of convulsion on the day of admission and subsequently developed altered sensorium for next 3 days. You are examining the patient on day 5 of illness	• Sudden onset weakness of right side of body with deviation of face to left side for last 5 days • One episode of convulsion on 3rd day of illness • Altered consciousness for last 3 days
A 5-year-old boy presented with complaints of weakness of both lower limb for last 10 days with urinary retention for last 5 days. On examination, he has severe pallor and is severely malnourished. Mother also mentioned that he has lost significant weight in last 6 months. He does not eat anything and has fever on and off	• Fever on and off with loss of weight and appetite for 6 months • Weakness of both lower limb for 10 days • Retention of urine with inability to pass urine for last 5 days
• A 2-year-old boy presents with global developmental delay, spasticity involving all the four limbs, small head, and multiple episodes of convulsions since 6 months of age • Current illness being fever, cough, and fast breathing for 5 days	• Inability to hold neck or speak any meaningful word till now • Tightness involving all the four limbs noticed since 6 months of age • Multiple episodes of convulsions since 6 months of age • Fever, cough, and fast breathing for 5 days
A 10-year-old boy presented with gradual loss of attained speech and drooling of saliva for 6 months. He has repeated falls with twisting of legs while walking. His speech has reduced clarity and is difficult to understand. He starts crying without any reason. He has become violent, started beating his siblings, often ends up breaking things at home	• Progressively increasing difficulty in speech with drooling of saliva for 6 months • Repeated falls with abnormal twisting of legs noticed for 6 months • Behavioral and emotional disturbances for 6 months

tuberculoma, and so on. However, if the same child has global developmental delay from beginning, suboptimal intelligence, and he has had three such previous episodes in last 2 years; our thinking changes altogether, and we will consider hypoxic-ischemic injury sequelae, perinatal stroke sequelae, or structural brain malformations as the probable etiology leading to these seizures. The presenting complaint in this child, thus, is better framed as:

- Delay in attainment of all milestones
- Four episodes of convulsions in last 2 years with the last (fourth) episode 2 days back

However, it is acceptable to present "one episode of convulsion 2 days back" as the presenting complaint and present "previous three episodes of convulsion" in the past history and "delayed development" in the developmental history. However, we need to ensure that all relevant negative histories pertaining to the entire illness must not be missed. While putting forward the presenting complaint, use the word "since" when you want to depict the onset of illness from one point of time, e.g., "multiple episodes of convulsions since 2 years of age" and "loss of attained milestones since 3 years of age."

Prefer the word "for" to depict the duration of one symptom, e.g., "fever for 5 days" and "altered sensorium for 2 days."

Chronology of Symptoms

The neurological history must be presented in a chronological order rather than mere elaboration of presenting complaints.

It should be like a story of clinical events that unfolds the illness as it progressed. The neurological history can be presented as in day of illness. For example, the *child was apparently well 4 days back when he developed fever. On day 2 of illness, he developed one episode of convulsion followed by altered sensorium. By day 4 of illness, he also developed weakness of right upper limb and lower limb.*

The course of events is best depicted diagrammatically to provide clarity during illness **(Fig. 1)**. In the example depicted in **Figure 1**, illness started with fever, which had subsided between 4th and 6th day of illness. Altered sensorium was seen postictal on day 2 of illness that improved by day 6. However, on day 6 of illness, fever reappeared, and child also developed paucity of movement of one side of body. Time of appearance of symptoms has a major impact in rearranging the clinical differentials. For example, if encephalopathy developed few days after a febrile illness, one would think of demyelinating pathology; whereas, one would think of viral encephalitis when encephalopathy is accompanied by fever.

Description of Neurological Complaints

Each neurological symptom needs detailed evaluation. For example, mere description of weakness of one side of body is probably not adequate. We need to know from the history whether it is proximal or distal predominant weakness, what is functional status, extent of neuromuscular weakness, i.e., which group of muscles are involved, whether it is a flaccid weakness or spastic weakness. Common neurological symptoms include headache, seizure/convulsion, weakness, wobbly gait, abnormal movement, or vision loss **(Table 2)**.

History of Extent of Neurological Involvement

In neurological cases, we need to decipher the extent of lesion or localize the neuroanatomical site. By extent of neurological involvement, we wish to decipher to what extent is central nervous system (CNS) affected in the child? Is it involving higher mental functions alone or is it affecting the cranial nerves, motor functions, sensory functions, or any urinary bladder functions as well? **Table 3** summarizes the points in neurological history that need to be elicited to determine the extent of neurological involvement.

Etiological History

Etiology of any neurological disease can fit into one of 7 categories: (1) Infective, (2) parainfectious/autoimmune/demyelinating,

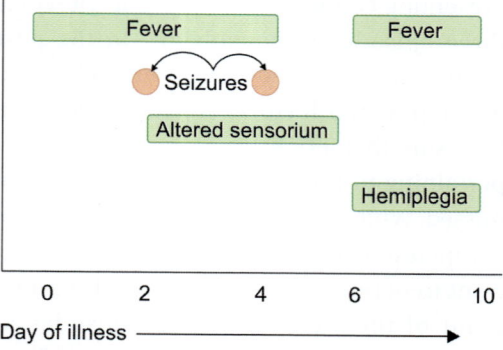

Fig. 1: Diagrammatic representation of history of neurological illness.

(3) vascular, (4) metabolic, (5) structural or space-occupying lesion, (6) traumatic, or (7) neoplastic. It is a good idea to keep such broad diagnosis such as infective, autoimmune, or demyelinating at this stage instead of labeling possibilities of tubercular meningitis, NMDA

TABLE 2: History-taking in common neurological symptoms.

Symptom	Description
Headache	- Nature of headache (dull aching and severe throbbing) - Location of headache (forehead, around eyes, occipital, and diffuse) - Duration of headache (approximate) - Frequency of headache (daily, weekly, and monthly) - Severity of headache (mild, moderate, and severe) - Activities during headache (whether he/she continues with his/her routine activities or prefers to sleep) - Any associated nausea and vomiting (projectile) - Any associated photophobia (irritation toward bright lights/prefers dark-room during the headache) or phonophobia (prefers silence and gets irritated when someone makes noise during his/her headache) - Need for medications and any response to them - Does the headache require school absenteeism
Convulsion	- Age at onset and presentation (neonate, infancy, and childhood) - Provocation factors (head trauma, fever, and preceding diarrheal illness) - Frequency of seizure (Is it the first episode?) - Preceding events (awake, sleep, playing, exercise, and following cry) - Presence of aura (somatosensory, auditory, visual, and abdominal) (child >5 years) - Ictal manifestations (motor, sensory, autonomic, cognitive, and behavioral) - Postictal period (postictal dizziness, loss of consciousness, and immediate return to normal)
Neurological weakness	- *Proximal upper limb:* Ability to lift arm to pick up an object in shelf, ability to comb hair, and ability to remove shirt by self - *Distal upper limb:* Ability to hold pen/any other object, clumsiness in holding objects, ability to button/unbutton shirt, ability to break *chapatti* into pieces - *Proximal lower limb:* Inability or difficulty to climb up/downstairs and ability to get up from the floor - *Distal lower limb:* Clumsiness while walking, repeated fall with twisting of ankles, and slipping of *chappals*
Wobbly gait	- Swaying while standing, inability to walk unassisted, overshooting of objects while trying to hold them and tremulous movement of hands while trying to reach for the object (*cerebellar ataxia*) - Stability of stance and gait but starts swaying when he closes his eyes (*sensory ataxia*) - Worsening of unsteadiness with sudden change of posture-like sitting from supine position (*vestibular ataxia*) - Sudden shock-like jerky movement preceding loss of stance (myoclonic seizures that result in unsteady gait as in children with subacute sclerosing panencephalitis) - Buckling of knees while walking (quadriceps weakness), twisting of ankles with child taking high steps while walking with feet thumping on the floor with repeated slippage of *chappals* (distal weakness of foot muscles as in hereditary motor sensory neuropathy)

Contd...

Contd...

Symptom	Description
Abnormal movement	• Is the pattern of movements normal (developmental movement disorder) or abnormal for age? • Are there excessive movements (hyperkinetic) or is there a paucity of movement (hypokinetic)? • Which part of the body is involved (mouth, face, head, neck, upper limb, and lower limb)? • Is the movement paroxysmal (sudden onset for brief period which may recur), continual (repeated and again), or continuous (without stop)? • Has the movement disorder changed over time (started with one movement and evolved to other movement types)? • Is the movement present over the rest/specific action/specific posture? • Do environmental stimuli or emotional stress modulate (increase or decrease) the movement disorder? • Does the movement abate with sleep? • Is the child aware of movement? • Can the movements be suppressed voluntarily? • Is the abnormal movement preceded by a premonitory sensation or urge?
Vision loss	Difficulty in reading letters written in black board, reading cricket scores in television, blurring or distortion of words, double vision (ophthalmoplegia), redness of eyes or eye discharge (conjunctivitis), haloes around bright light (glaucoma), headache (refractory error), floating spots (retinal detachment), pain in moving eyes (optic neuritis), not able to judge the periphery and bumps into objects (visual field defects)

TABLE 3: Identifying the extent of lesion and neuroanatomical localization, based on history.

Point covered to decipher extent of involvement	History to be elicited
Cortical functions	History of altered sensorium, seizures, and behavioral disturbances
Cranial nerve (CN) functions	History of difficulty in vision (CN 2); deviation of eyes, double vision (CN 3, 4, and 6); difficulty in chewing (CN 5); deviation of face, drooling of saliva (CN 7); difficulty in hearing (CN 8); nasal regurgitation of feeds, altered voice, difficulty in deglutition (CN 9 and 10)
Motor function	Wasting of any group of muscles, flabby limb (hypotonia) or tight limbs (hypertonia), paucity of movement of one side of both upper and lower limbs (hemiparesis) or both lower limbs (paraplegia), abnormal twisting postures (dystonia), abnormal flowing movements (chorea), abnormal writhing movements (athetosis), difficulty in maintaining balance (ataxia)
Sensory function	• History of tingling sensation, sensation of pins and needles • History of decreased sensation of touch or pain • "Walking on wool"-like sensation
Autonomic involvement	Retention of urine, dribbling of urine, excessive or lack of perspiration, and dizziness on sudden standing or getting up from lying down position
Features of raised intracranial pressure	Headache, vomiting (projectile), excessive irritability, head banging, and altered sensorium

(N-methyl-D-aspartate) encephalitis, and so on.

- Majority of infective etiologies will have ongoing fever.
- History of preceding febrile illness or vaccination followed by onset of neurological symptoms would point to demyelinating pathology.
- History of focal neurological deficits such as hemiparesis and cranial nerve pathology could point to vascular or structural pathology.
- Majority of babies with metabolic problems such as hypocalcemia would be asymptomatic in-between episodes. Metabolic disorders would also include hepatic (history of jaundice and bleeding), renal (oliguria and hematuria), hypoxic (history of prolonged ventilation and status epilepticus), and inborn errors of metabolism (consanguinity, recurrent abortions, and abnormal urinary odor).
- Presence of weight loss, fever, pallor, and lymphadenopathy would point to a neoplastic etiology.

Etiological history should ideally focus on cluster of symptoms rather than individual symptoms. For example, in case of a child with fever, seizure, and altered sensorium, it often becomes unnecessary to elicit history for other focus of infection such as burning micturition when neurological focus is leading.

Apart from a detailed neurological history, other relevant histories for neurological cases include treatment history, past history, birth history, developmental history, and family history. These play a pivotal role in analysis and arriving at the final diagnosis. Immunization history, nutritional history, and socioeconomic history also contribute to overall diagnosis.

FOCUSED NEUROLOGICAL EXAMINATION

In neurological practice, majority of cases are diagnosed based on the history. Neurological examination must be focused, as the child gives you very little window for examination. Hence, it is prudent that we already have in our mind as to what we want to examine in the child. Detailed neurological examination as in adults is not possible in children given the lack of cooperation. The present chapter only gives an overview of the neurological examination in children. This chapter does *not* intend to teach the correct method of examination. Refer to "Clinical Methods in Pediatrics" by Piyush Gupta for detailed description of performing neurological examination. A scheme of neurological examination is provided in **Box 1**.

BOX 1: Overall scheme of neurological examination in children.

- Mental status (appearance, behavior, communication, delusion/hallucination, and emotions) and higher mental function (consciousness, orientation, memory, attention span, spatial perception, insight, abstract thinking, fund of information, calculation, released reflexes, and specific individual lobe functions)
- Cranial nerve examination (I–XII)
- Motor system examination [gait (ambulatory)/posture (nonambulatory), bulk, tone, muscle power, deep tendon reflexes, superficial reflexes, and abnormal movement]
- Sensory system examination [lateral spinothalamic tract (pain/temperature), dorsal column tract (fine touch, vibration, and joint position), cortical sensation (two-point discrimination and tactile localization)]
- Cerebellar system examination
- Meningeal signs (neck rigidity, Kernig's sign, and Brudzinski's sign)
- Skull and spine examination (Macewen's sign and transillumination)

Purpose of Focused Examination

We need to use the limited time window in focused neurological examination rather than trying to focus on completion of examination. By the end of history, we had generated possible differential diagnosis in our mind. This needs to be kept in mind before one begins neurological examination. For example, in a child with chronic meningoencephalitis, we may not be able to examine most cranial nerves, sensory system, cerebellar system, and autonomic system that require cooperation of the patient. Examination of higher mental function is restricted to consciousness. Similarly, in a child with cerebral palsy, we need to use that limited time frame to examine the motor system that would aid in classifying the type of cerebral palsy and decide the management. In this case, detailed higher mental function evaluation, and examination of sensory system or cerebellar or meningeal signs might not be critical, although essential. Every child requires a detailed examination provided, there is no paucity of time and cooperation. However, priority in examination must be decided based on the differentials in the history.

Neurological Examination Performa

An one-page performa for neurological examination is suggested. This will ensure that key points in examination are never missed. It is a good idea to note down the points that you wish to focus in the examination while obtaining the history and analyzing it. With repeated use of this performa for every clinical examination, one will be able to perform the examination easily without missing any details. This will help in reaching the final diagnosis **(Table 4)**.

■ NEUROLOGICAL DIAGNOSIS

Analysis of symptoms after history and examination is the most crucial step in reaching the correct clinical diagnosis. The steps include providing an effective summary, framing clinical differentials, planning investigations on priority, and reaching a final clinical diagnosis. Investigations and management could be planned according to the possible etiology. Analysis of the history and examination could be done under following five heads:

1. Is the illness acute/subacute or chronic (duration of illness)?
2. Is the illness static or progressive (progression of disease)?
3. What is the extent of involvement (cerebrum, basal ganglia, cerebellum, cranial nerve, corticospinal tract, extrapyramidal tract, spinal cord, plexus, peripheral nerves, neuromuscular junction, and muscle)?
4. What is the most probable neuroanatomical site of localization?
5. What broad group of etiology could have led to this illness?

Duration of Symptoms

Duration of symptoms is a good starting point in analysis of symptoms and signs.

Process can be classified as *acute* (<14 days), *subacute* (14–30 days), or *chronic* (>30 days duration). These cutoff points are arbitrary, and there is no standard definition to classify the duration. Duration of symptoms is determined by the examining physician, based on synthesis and analysis of history obtained from the parents. In general, if current symptoms can be attributed to a significant past medical event, then this past event is considered a part of presenting complaints. For example, a 3-year-old child

TABLE 4: Neurological examination performa.

Mental status	Higher mental function	Cranial nerve examination

• Appearance
• Behavior
• *Communication:*
  – Comprehension
  – Articulation
  – Fluency
  – Repetition
  – Naming
  – Reading
  – Writing
• Delusion and hallucination
• Emotion
• *Frontal lobe function:*
  – Digit span test
  – Fist edge palm test
  – Trail making test
  – Stroop test
  – Go-no-go test
• *Parietal lobe:*
  – Ideational apraxia
  – Right left discrimination
  – Finger agnosia
• *Occipital lobe:*
  – Visual memory/ prosopagnosia
	• *Consciousness:*
	  – Wakefulness
	  – Awareness
	• *Orientation:*
	  – Time
	  – Place
	  – Person
	• *Memory:*
	  – Registration
	  – Recent
	  – Remote
	• *Attention span:*
	  – Digit forward
	  – Digit backward
	• *Perception (spatial):*
	  – Ability to draw clock
	  – Five-pointed star
	• Insight
	• Fund of information
	• *Abstract thinking:*
	  – Proverb
	  – Common/differences
	• Calculation
	• Released reflex
		I: Perception of smell
		    Identification of smell
		II: Visual acuity
		• Color vision
		• Field of vision
		• Fundus examination
		III/IV/VI: Alignment of eyes
		• Ptosis
		• Pursuit eye movement
		• Saccadic eye movement
		• Pupil size
		• Pupil reaction (direct/consensual/ accommodation)
		V: Motor: Jaw deviation
		• Sensation over face
		• Corneal reflex
		• Jaw jerk
		VII: Facial symmetry
		    Taste sensation (tongue)
		VIII: Hearing test
		    Tuning fork test: Rinne test/ Weber test
		IX/X: Movement of palate, uvula Gag reflex
		XI: Function of sternocleidomastoid/ Trapezius
		XII: Position of tongue deviation/ fasciculation

Motor examination	**Sensory examination**	**Cerebellar signs**

• *Gait:* Stance/steps (swing)
• *Posture:* Shoulder/elbow/ hand/trunk/hip/knee/ankle
• *Bulk:* Atrophy (focal/ generalized) hypertrophy
• *Tone:* Proximal UL/distal UL Proximal LL/distal LL
• *Power:* Across shoulder/elbow/ wrist
• Across hip/knee/ankle/neck flexor/neck extensor
• *Deep tendon reflexes:* Biceps, triceps, supinator, knee, and ankle jerk
• *Superficial reflex:* Plantar/ cremasteric/abdominal
• *Abnormal movement:* Chorea/ athetosis dystonia/ballismus/ myoclonus
	• Pain
	• *Temperature:*
	  – Warm
	  – Cold
	• Joint position
	• Light touch
	• Vibration
	• Romberg test
	• Two-point discrimination
	• Stereognosis
	• Graphesthesia
	• Tactile localization
		• Finger-nose test
		• Dysdiadochokinesia
		• Rebound phenomena
		• Heel to shin test
		
		Autonomic signs
		• Postural hypotension
		• Deep breathing test
		• Valsalva maneuver
		
		Meningeal sign
		• Neck rigidity
		• Kernig sign
		• Brudzinski's sign
		• Skull shape
		• Head size
		• Macewen's sign
		• Examination of spine

(LL: lower limb; UL: upper limb)

presents with wobbliness and instability of gait for last 10 days. There is a history of similar multiple episodes of wobbliness, each lasting for 4–7 days for last 2 years. In this case, duration of symptoms is 2 years rather than 10 days, and this should be considered as a chronic event. Here, our thinking process will include causes of intermittent–chronic ataxia rather than acute ataxia. While framing the presenting complaints, it is essential to have an overview of illness rather than framing only the chief complaint.

Is the Disease Static or Progressive?

If clinical symptoms or signs are improving with time, the process is considered *static*. If the child is gaining new milestones as the time is progressing, then it is also a static insult. Loss of attained developmental milestones or worsening of neurological symptoms with time will be considered a progressive illness.

Static insult to a developing brain could be prenatal [maternal drug intake and maternal TORCH (toxoplasmosis, others—syphilis, hepatitis B, rubella, cytomegalovirus, herpes simplex) infection], natal [hypoxic-ischemic event, prematurity, neonatal jaundice (kernicterus), neonatal meningitis, and neonatal seizures] or postnatal (trauma, meningitis, and hypoxic damage). Children who suffer a static insult often present with developmental delay and/or tone abnormalities including spasticity or extrapyramidal manifestations such as dyskinesia, and dystonia.

It is essential to recognize *pseudoregression* where a new contracture, worsening dystonia, and new-onset epilepsy could lead to loss of attained motor or cognitive milestones. For example, a child with spastic quadriplegic cerebral palsy who had attained neck holding, started smiling and cooing, could lose all these attained milestones, if he develops epileptic spasm. This condition of epileptic spasm is considered an epileptic encephalopathy where abundance of epileptiform discharges contributes to additional cognitive decline over and above what could have resulted from the structural lesion in the brain. In this case, once the spasm gets treated, the child will restart gaining milestones. Hence, this will not be considered a progressive disorder.

Extent of Involvement and Neuroanatomical Localization

Extent of involvement determines the extent to which the disease process has involved the central nervous system.

- Presence of encephalopathy, behavioral problems, and seizures could indicate *cortical involvement*.
- Presence of abnormal movements including choreoathetosis, dystonia, and ballismus would indicate involvement of *extrapyramidal* or *basal ganglia* involvement.
- Presence of ataxia, incoordination, hypotonia, and nystagmus would point to cerebellar involvement.
- Involvement of *corticospinal tract* is indicated by the presence of hypertonia (clasp knife spasticity), hyperreflexia, and extensor plantar response.
- Cranial nerve involvement with presence of ipsilateral hemiparesis would point to *lesion above the brainstem*.
- Crossed hemiparesis (ipsilateral cranial nerve palsy and contralateral hemiparesis) would point to *brainstem lesion*.
- Cranial nerve involvement (VIth and/or VIIth nerve palsy) in presence of features of raised intracranial pressure would point to supratentorial pathology (intracranial space-occupying lesion) resulting in false localizing signs such as bilateral VIth or VIIth cranial nerve palsy.

- Involvement of bladder and bowel is crucial among those with suspected *spinal cord involvement*.
- Involvement of sensory system (positive and negative sensory symptoms) and autonomic system (postural hypotension and excessive or lack of sweating) could help in localization of lesion in *peripheral nervous system*.

Presence of signs of raised intracranial pressure (bradycardia, hypertension, irregular respiration, papilledema, and unequal pupil) must be recorded. Symptoms of herniation syndromes including unequal pupil size, decerebrate or decorticate posturing, and abnormal respiration also need to be noted. Based on the extent of involvement, site of localization can be identified. It may be often difficult to identify a single site of lesion based on the cluster of symptoms and signs. In such cases, diffuse or multifocal neurological illness including metabolic or demyelinating pathology need to be considered.

What is the Etiology?

Neurological illness needs to be classified into one of seven categories: (1) Infective, (2) parainfectious/autoimmune/demyelinating, (3) vascular, (4) metabolic, (5) structural or space-occupying lesion, (6) traumatic, and (7) neoplastic. Clinical clues to the above-mentioned etiologies have been explained above under the section of etiological history.

■ CASE VIGNETTES

Case 1

A 10-month-old girl was brought with complaints of repeated episodes of fever, cough, and fast breathing since birth. She remains floppy and is unable to hold the neck. She has attained good social, cognitive, and language milestones appropriate for age. On examination, she had tachypnea and tachycardia. Chest examination revealed fine crepitations. Cardiovascular examination was unremarkable. The baby was alert, active with no evident cranial nerve palsy. Tongue fasciculations were evident. Motor examination revealed flaccid weakness involving all the four limbs with complete head lag. Examination also revealed hypotonia and absent deep tendon reflexes in all the limbs, and plantar response was absent. Rest of the systemic examination was normal.

Analysis of Symptoms

- It is a *chronic process* (considering the motor delay and floppiness since beginning), which predisposes to recurrent respiratory tract infection. However, child has presented with acute respiratory tract infection. Hence, it is an acute illness on underlying chronic process.
- It looks like a *static illness* (as the child was gaining motor milestones with age).
- *Extent of involvement:* Cognition and higher mental function appears to be preserved. There appears to be no cranial nerve involvement. There is flaccid motor weakness involving all four limbs. The respiratory muscles are possibly weak leading to repeated respiratory tract infection. Ocular and bulbar muscles are spared.
- *Neuroanatomical localization:* Presence of isolated motor delay, floppiness, hypotonia, and areflexia suggests a peripheral nervous system involvement. Absence of extensor plantar response is against an upper motor neuron involvement. Intact cognition is also against central nervous system pathology. Peripheral nervous system includes anterior horn cell, peripheral nerve, neuromuscular junction, and muscle. Possible *neuroanatomical site of lesion*

is anterior horn cell, since presence of fasciculation is highly specific for anterior horn cell involvement.
- *Etiology:* Etiology is likely to be genetic or metabolic. Floppiness since birth is unlikely to be infective, parainfectious/autoimmune, structural, or traumatic in origin. Common genetic or metabolic etiology affecting anterior horn cell resulting in floppiness from birth would include spinal muscular atrophy and Pompe disease. In absence of fasciculations, however, one could have also considered congenital myopathy, congenital muscular dystrophy, congenital myasthenic syndrome, possibility of congenital myotonic dystrophy, and early-onset hereditary motor sensory neuropathy.

Interpretation and Probable Diagnosis

This 10-month-old baby with floppiness since birth with recurrent respiratory tract infection had presented with a fresh episode of acute respiratory tract infection. She had peripheral hypotonia (hypotonia with areflexia), fasciculation with preserved cognition. The likely neuroanatomical site of lesion is anterior horn cell. The etiology could be a genetic condition such as spinal muscular atrophy or metabolic disorder such as Pompe disease that affects anterior horn cell. Points in favor/against of these conditions are shown in **Table 5**.

Case 2

A 10-year-old boy presented with sudden onset of altered sensorium for 3 days. There was preceding history of fever and loose stools 10 days back that lasted for 2–3 days. Currently, there is no history of fever. There was no preceding seizure prior to onset of encephalopathy. His anthropometric parameters were age appropriate. His general physical examination was unremarkable. Neurological examination showed minimally conscious state with no cranial nerve palsy. Pupils were normal sized and reactive. There were no tone abnormalities, reflexes were normal, no abnormal movement, plantar were extensor. There were no meningeal signs. Rest of the systemic examination was unremarkable.

Analysis to Reach a Diagnosis

- It is an acute neurological illness (duration of symptoms of 3 days).
- *Static or progressive:* Not applicable (distinction into static or progressive illness is usually not applicable in acute neurological illness as most of the acute illness are progressive till appropriate treatment is instituted).
- *Extent of involvement:* The sensorium of the child is affected (minimally conscious state) with sparing of cranial nerve and no motor or sensory deficits. Absence of motor deficits points to

TABLE 5: Points in favor/against of spinal muscular atrophy and Pompe disease.

Differentials	Points in favor	Points against
Spinal muscular atrophy	Peripheral hypotonia, tongue fasciculation, and repeated respiratory tract infection	No family history
Pompe disease	Peripheral hypotonia, tongue fasciculation, and repeated respiratory tract infection	No cardiomegaly (apex at 4th intercostal space) and no hepatomegaly

sparing of pyramidal tracts, and absence of abnormal movement points to sparing of extrapyramidal tracts and cerebellum. Considering that cranial nerves are completely spared, this means that brainstem is intact and there are no impending signs of herniation or features of raised intracranial pressure. Absence of meningeal signs indicates no meningeal involvement. The most likely site of involvement is cortical gray matter.
- *Etiology:* Considering that there was preceding febrile illness prior to onset of encephalopathy, a strong possibility of parainfectious/demyelinating/autoimmune pathology looks more likely. Other possibilities include—(1) Infective process (but there is no ongoing fever, no meningeal signs), (2) vascular: either arterial ischemic or venous thrombotic (but there is no cranial nerve palsy, no hemiparesis, and no focal deficits), or (3) metabolic process (but prior development normal, acute presentation, no history suggestive of hypoxic insult, and no other systemic illness). There is no history suggestive of neoplastic and traumatic etiology.

Interpretation and Different Diagnosis

This 10-year-old boy presented with acute encephalopathy following a febrile illness. There are no focal neurological deficits (cranial nerve palsy or motor/sensory deficits). The likely neuroanatomical site of lesion is gray matter and the etiology is likely to be parainfectious/demyelinating. Demyelinating process that presents with acute encephalopathy is likely to be acute disseminated encephalomyelitis (ADEM). The other differentials would include metabolic encephalopathy such as hepatic encephalopathy (but no jaundice), toxic encephalopathy (need to probe further history for possible toxic exposure), and hypoxic encephalopathy (but no hypoxia and no status epilepticus). It is difficult to attribute to other inborn errors of metabolism, especially considering the prior development was normal, no previous episodes of crises, and well-thriving child with normal anthropometric parameters. This could have been secondary to postictal state (but no history of seizure) or post-traumatic (but no history of trauma to head). Other differential would obviously include acute viral encephalitis had there been ongoing fever. Considering these thoughts, ADEM appears to be most probable clinical diagnosis.

Case 3

An 11-month-old boy presented with complaints of inability to hold neck for last 1 month and excessive irritability and startle response to loud noise noticed for 1 month. There is no history of seizure. Vision and hearing are preserved. There is tightness of all four limbs with paucity of movement. Child is now bedridden and remains irritable with no meaningful response. He had an uneventful neonatal period with normal development till 10 months of age. Examination reveals macrocephaly, signs of spasticity, brisk reflexes, and extensor plantar response. There are no abnormal movements such as chorea or dystonia.

How will you analyze to reach a diagnosis?

Analysis to Reach a Diagnosis

- *Duration:* It is subacute-to-chronic process considering 1-month duration.
- *Static or progressive:* It looks like a progressive disorder considering the loss of attained motor and cognitive milestones and clinical condition worsening with time.

- *Extent of involvement:* Presence of excessive irritability raises the possibility of raised intracranial pressure or possible gray matter involvement. However, lack of meaningful eye contact and meaningful response increases the probability of gray matter involvement. Presence of spasticity, brisk reflexes, and extensor plantar response points to pyramidal tract involvement. Absence of abnormal movements probably rules out extrapyramidal involvement. Based on these constellations of signs, there is possibility of both white matter and gray matter involvement.
- *Etiology:* There is obvious neuroregression involving motor and/or cognitive milestones. This is associated with pyramidal tract involvement [spasticity, brisk deep tendon reflex (DTR), and extensor plantar]. Presence of macrocephaly without fever should arise the suspicion of genetic or metabolic process. Lack of history of trauma rules out traumatic etiology. No history of febrile illness or immunization prior to onset of neurological symptoms makes parainfectious process unlikely.

Interpretation and Differential Diagnosis

This 11-month-old boy presented with a progressive genetic/metabolic neurodegenerative disorder (because of history of neuroregression). Age of presentation, presence of macrocephaly, hyperacusis, and pyramidal tract involvement is highly indicative of Tay-Sach disease. Other differential diagnoses are discussed in the chapter on approach to a child with developmental regression **(Chapter 14)**.

Case 4

A 12-year-old boy presented with difficulty in standing and walking, which progressed to involve the upper limbs for the last 3 days. The child has severe pain in the legs, and he is bedridden. There is no involvement of respiratory, bulbar, or ocular muscles. He has normal sensorium with no signs of any cranial nerve palsy. There is global areflexia and mute plantar.

How will you approach this case?

Analysis to Reach the Diagnosis

- *Duration:* It is an acute neurological illness considering 3-day history.
- *Static or progressive:* It is not applicable; however, it appears to be a progressive neurological illness with onset of weakness in lower limbs.
- *Extent of involvement:* Weakness of lower limb, trunk, upper limb with sparing of neck flexors, and neck extensors muscles. There is no involvement of respiratory, bulbar, or ocular group of muscles (sparing of cranial nerves). There is no involvement of sensorium or any cranial nerve involvement (sparing of central nervous system and brainstem).

  Considering ascending paresis from lower limb to upper limb with areflexia, mute plantar, radicular pain, and sparing of bladder, all suggest peripheral nerve involvement most likely polyradiculoneuropathy. Muscle involvement is ruled out by mute plantar and areflexia. Spinal cord involvement from cervical region in a spinal shock stage can also have these manifestations.
- *Etiology:* The cause could be parainfectious/autoimmune. Infectious causes are unlikely considering absence of fever.

Traumatic causes again are unlikely owing to lack of history of trauma. Vascular causes are unlikely to cause polyradiculoneuropathy, although they can result in spinal cord lesions that are patchy (present case could have diffuse involvement).

Interpretation

This 12-year-old boy presented with acute flaccid quadriparesis with features of possible peripheral nerve involvement. This could have been most likely secondary to a parainfectious pathology like Guillain–Barré syndrome. Other differentials for this condition would include acute poliomyelitis (but no asymmetry and no patchy involvement), transverse myelitis (but no bladder involvement, no specific sensory level, and difficult to explain radicular pain that is better explained by polyradiculopathy), traumatic neuritis (but no history of trauma, quadriparesis is very difficult to be explained). Hence, we are probably dealing with diagnosis of Guillain–Barré syndrome.

KEY MESSAGES

- It is challenging to reach at a clinical diagnosis in pediatric neurology unless a systematic history-focused examination followed by an analysis is performed.
- It is prudent to determine the extent of neurological involvement and possible neuroanatomical site of localization before arriving at the possible etiology.
- Children allow only a limited time for neurological examination; hence, the examination must be focused based on the history.
- Neurological diagnosis may be summarized under duration of symptoms, static or progressive illness, extent of involvement, probable neuroanatomical site of lesion, and most probable etiological diagnosis.
- Investigations must be planned based on the clinical diagnosis and differentials raised rather than by presenting symptoms alone.

Neuroimaging

COMPUTED TOMOGRAPHY OF BRAIN

Procedure

The patient is asked to lie down on the computed tomography (CT) table in supine position. The tube rotates around the patient in the gantry. Precautions should be taken to avoid irradiation to orbit (lens). It is performed at an angle parallel to the base of the skull **(Fig. 1)**. The slice thickness is between 5 and 10 mm for a routine head CT.

Principles

Computed tomography works on the principles of ionizing radiation. The patient is passed between a source of X-rays and a series of detectors. In general, the atoms with higher density have a greater ability to attenuate (stop) X-rays, while those with lower density have lesser ability to attenuate X-rays. *Hyperdense* means that structure is brighter compared to brain parenchyma, whereas *hypodense* means that it is darker compared to brain parenchyma. These attenuation intensities are computerized into numbers called Hounsfield units (HU) or CT numbers **(Table 1)**. So, the structures that have higher HU, like bone, will be able to attenuate the rays better, thus appearing brighter on a CT scan. Hence, the bone looks white and air looks black. Hypodensity on CT brain can be

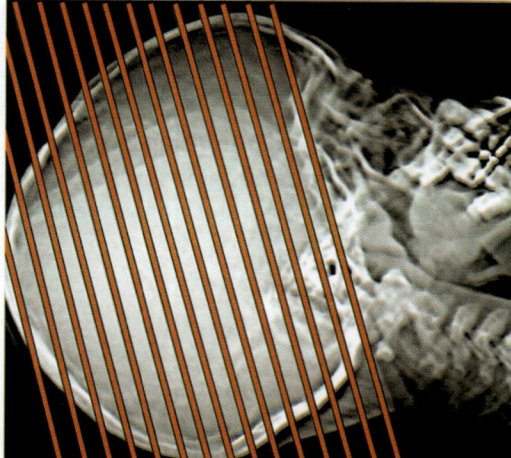

Fig. 1: Computed tomography (CT) head performed parallel to the base of the skull.

TABLE 1: Appearance of various tissues on computed tomography (CT) brain.

Tissue	How will it look on CT scan?
Bone, calcification, and metallic objects	Bright white
Acute blood	White
Subacute blood	Light gray
Muscle	Light gray
Gray matter	Light gray
White matter	Medium gray
Cerebrospinal fluid	Black
Air and fat	Dark black

focal as in arterial ischemic stroke (Fig. 2) or it could be diffuse as in global hypoxic injury where there is loss of gray matter–white matter differentiation (Figs. 3A and B). Other than infarction, edema, neoplasms, and cysts will also appear hypodense (dark) on CT scan. Contrast material, acute blood, and calcification will look hyperdense (bright)

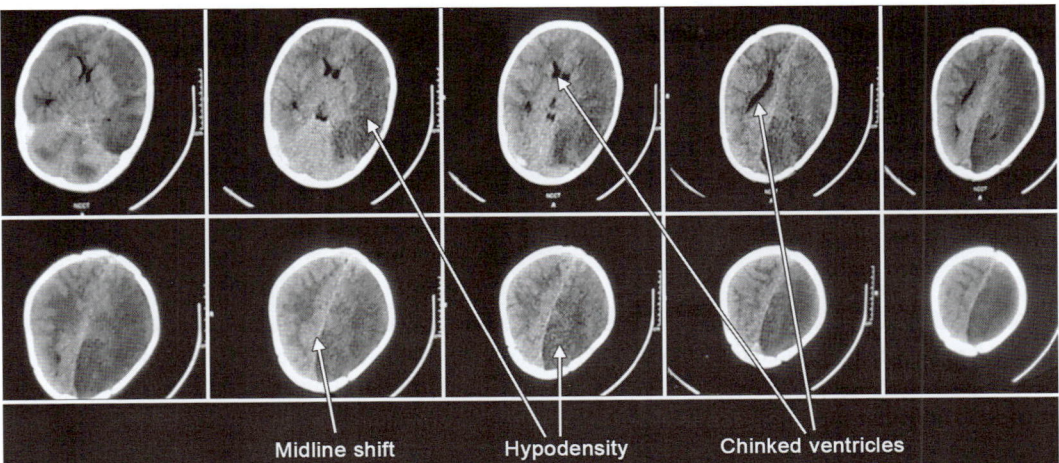

Fig. 2: Diffuse hypodensity involving left cerebral hemisphere with midline shift. Notice that ventricles on the same side are not visible, whereas they are dilated on the opposite side. These findings are suggestive of ischemia involving left anterior and middle cerebral artery.

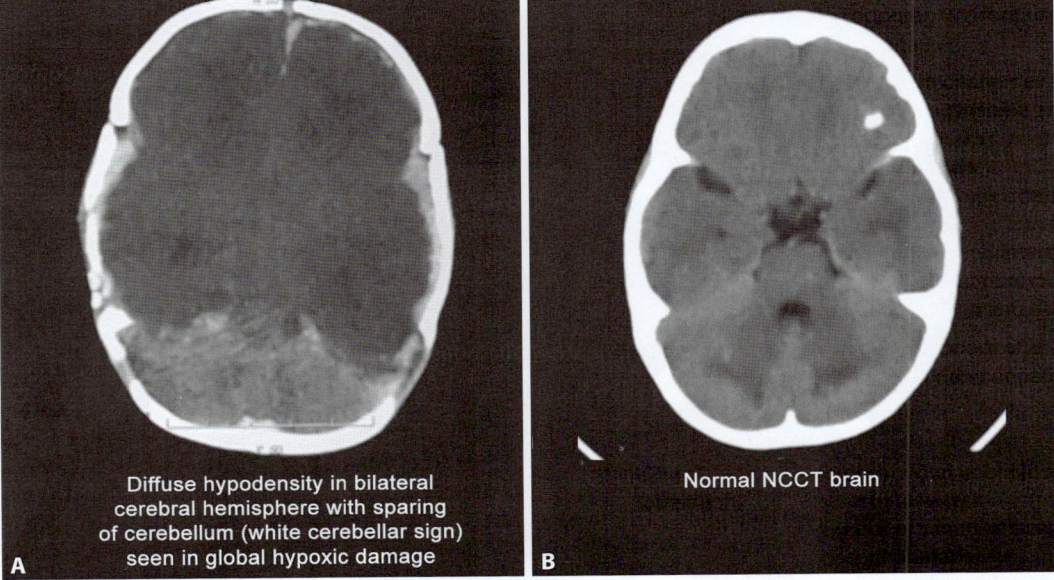

Figs. 3A and B: (A) Computed tomography (CT) brain showing global hypoxic injury (white cerebellar sign) when compared to normal CT scan (B), there is loss of differentiation of white matter and gray matter, ventricles are small and shrunken, and cistern spaces are effaced suggestive of cerebral edema. (NCCT: noncontrast CT)

on CT scan. Common causes of intracranial calcifications include neurocysticercosis, TORCH (toxoplasmosis, other agents, rubella, cytomegalovirus, and herpes simplex) infection, tuberous sclerosis, and Sturge–Weber syndrome (tram track calcification).

Interpretation of CT Brain

We should be able to recognize basic structures on CT brain **(Figs. 4 and 5)**. It is important to identify the cisterns—suprasellar cistern, quadrigeminal cistern,

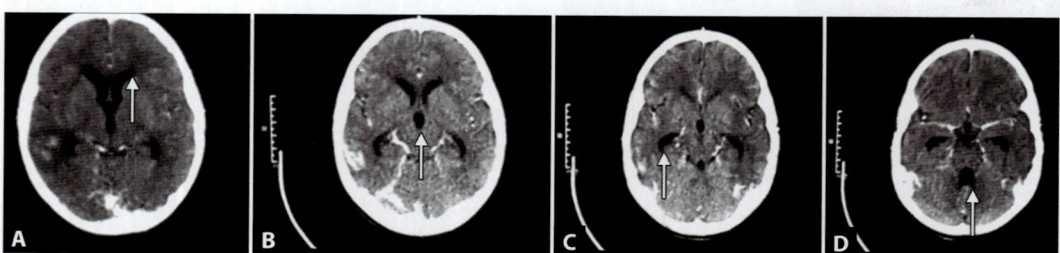

Figs. 4A to D: Axial computed tomography (CT) brain showing (A) lateral ventricle (frontal horn), (B) third ventricle, (C) temporal horn of lateral ventricle, and (D) fourth ventricle.

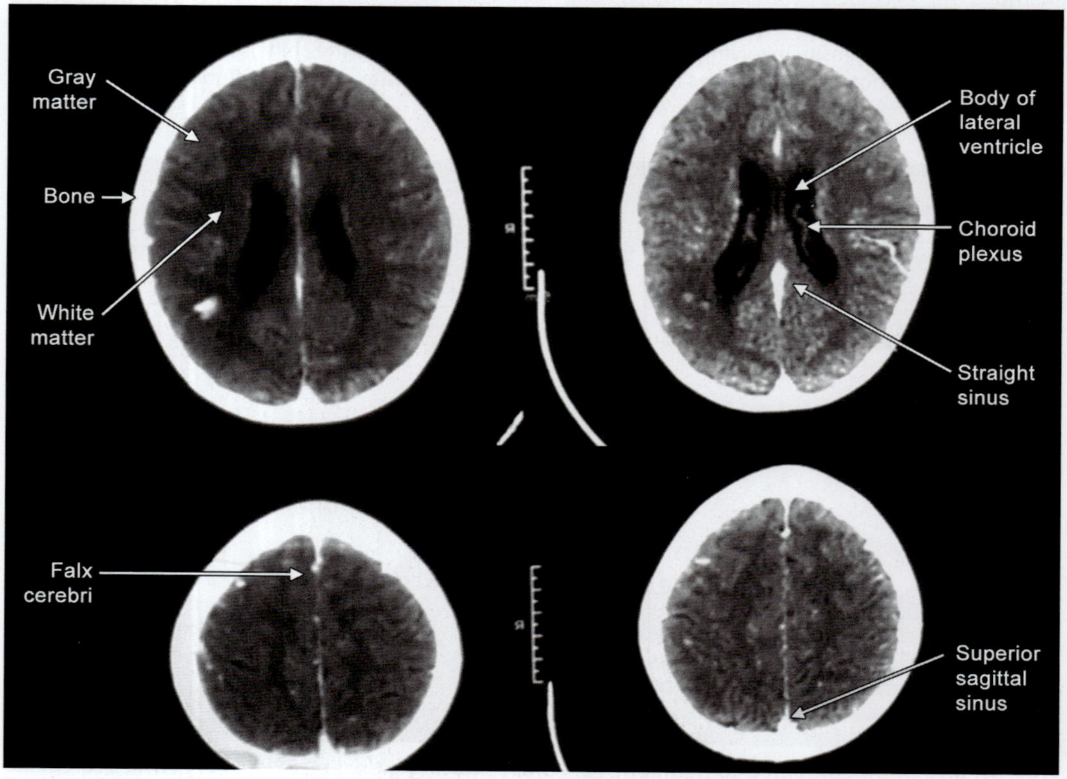

Fig. 5: Axial computed tomography (CT) brain showing gray matter, white matter, and venous sinus.

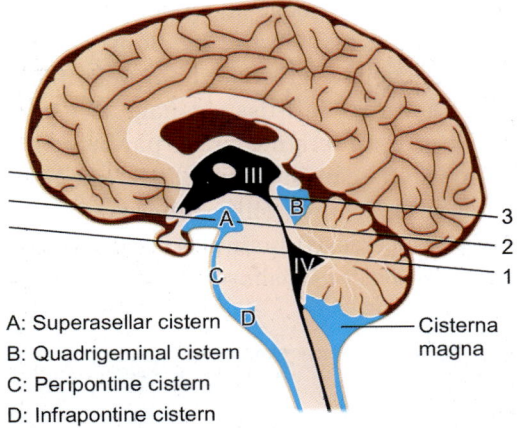

A: Superasellar cistern
B: Quadrigeminal cistern
C: Peripontine cistern
D: Infrapontine cistern

Cisterna magna

Fig. 6: Cisterns of the brain evident on sagittal view. (III: third ventricle; IV: fourth ventricle; axial sections on CT scan are taken at the levels 1, 2, 3)

> **BOX 1:** Advantages and disadvantages of computed tomography (CT) brain.
>
> *Advantages:*
> - It is a short procedure and can be performed quickly
> - It clearly shows acute and subacute hemorrhages into the meningeal spaces and brain
> - It shows bone (and skull fractures) to advantage
> - It is less expensive than MRI
> - It can appreciate calcifications
>
> *Disadvantages:*
> - It does not clearly differentiate between acute or subacute infarcts or ischemia or brain edema
> - CT is not useful for white matter and gray matter differentiation
> - It exposes the patient to ionizing radiation

ambient cistern, peripontine cistern, and infrapontine cisterns **(Fig. 6)**. While reading a CT brain, it is advisable to follow few steps so that important details are not missed:
- Compare the right and left sides of brain
- *Midline:* Look for midline shift
- *Look at anatomy:*
- *Brain tissue:* Gray matter, white matter, and lesion
  - *Cerebrospinal fluid (CSF) spaces:* Ventricles, basal cisterns, sulci, and fissures
  - *Skull and soft tissue:* Scalp swelling, fractures, sinuses, orbit, and intracranial air
- *Subdural window:* To look for subdural collection.

Clinical Relevance

The advantages and disadvantages of a CT scan are summarized in **Box 1**. Radiation exposure is one of the major concerns with a CT scan. In neonates and infants with open anterior fontanel, ultrasonography can be useful in diagnosing germinal matrix

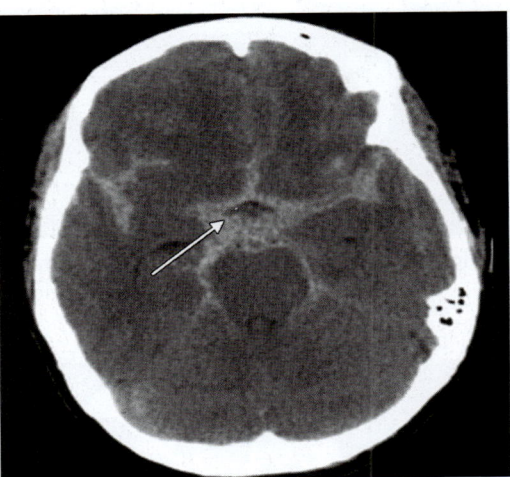

Fig. 7: Noncontrast computed tomography (CT) brain showing subarachnoid bleed (white arrow), which appears bright (hyperdense).

hemorrhage, intraventricular bleed, and enlarged ventricular size as in hydrocephalus.

Figure 7 shows a noncontrast CT scan of a patient with altered sensorium. Note that the bone is white, brain parenchyma is gray, and the bright signal in the subarachnoid space indicates subarachnoid hemorrhage.

You need to remember that contrast would also look hyperdense in subarachnoid spaces **(Figs. 8A and B)**. Hence, any hyperdense subarachnoid space would indicate either subarachnoid bleed on a noncontrast scan or normal to enhanced contrast enhancement on a contrast scan. CT scan is good for bone fractures and for assessment of temporal bone, orbits, and sinuses. We would often see a soft-tissue image and a bony image on a CT head **(Figs. 9A and B)**. Bony window image is good to screen for bony deformities and fractures. Soft-tissue image is useful to see the underlying brain parenchyma. Contrast CT scan is useful to delineate ring-enhancing lesions (like tuberculoma or neurocysticercosis), brain abscess, neoplasm, and arteriovenous malformation.

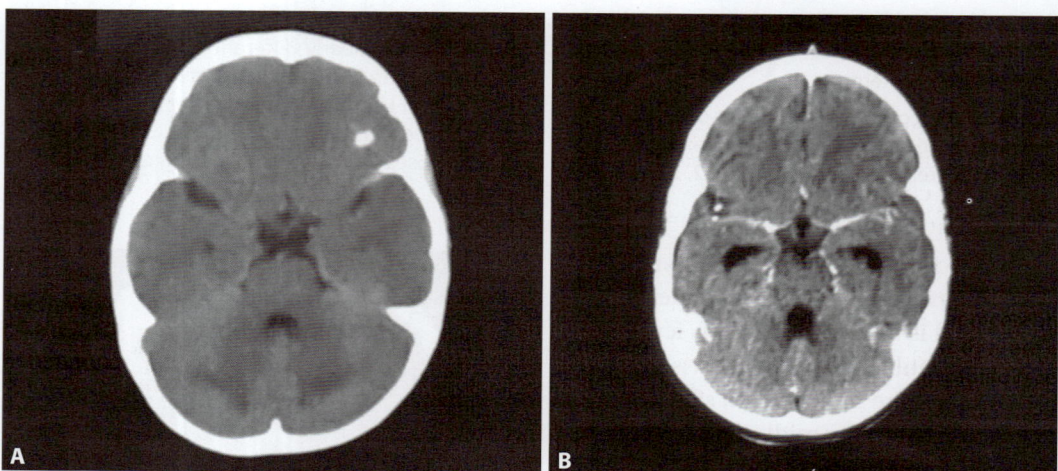

Figs. 8A and B: (A) Noncontrast computed tomography (CT) scan; (B) Contrast-enhanced computed tomography (CECT).

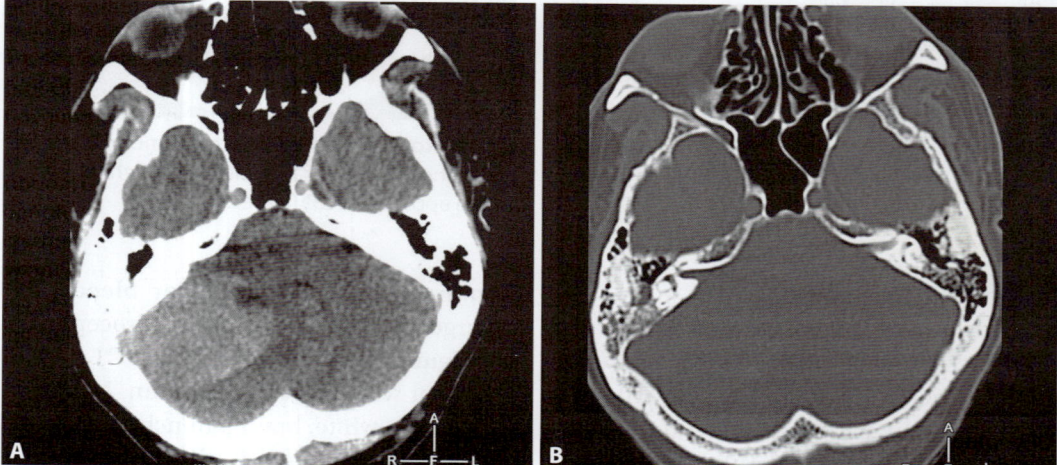

Figs. 9A and B: (A) Soft-tissue image and (B) bony window image of computed tomography (CT) head.

Hydrocephalus is difficult to differentiate from cortical atrophy as both of them result in dilated ventricles. Brain atrophy as a result of *ex vacuo* dilatation leads to dilated ventricles. Points that favor hydrocephalus are presence of periventricular ooze, fullness of sulci, effacement of gyri, and dilatation of temporal and frontal horns of lateral ventricle while brain atrophy results in prominent sulci and gyri and basal cisterns are open.

MAGNETIC RESONANCE IMAGING BRAIN

Magnetic resonance imaging (MRI) works on the principle of hydrogen ion that is a positively charged proton present in water (H_2O) that can induce magnetic field. The patient is positioned in an MRI scanner, and this forms a strong magnetic field around the area to be imaged. Field strength of magnet is measured in Tesla, which can range from 0.2 to 7 Tesla. Conventional MRI machines are usually 1.5 Tesla. Different tissues are identified by different rates at which excited atoms return to baseline. On MRI, we use terminologies like hyperintense (bright) and hypointense (dark), whereas on CT scan, we use hyperdense (bright) and hypodense (dark). Two tissues (bone and air) will be dark in all the MRI sequences. A major advantage of MRI brain over CT brain is better resolution of brain structures and lack of ionizing radiation. But MRI brain is costly and time consuming. Calcifications and blood are better identified on CT scan and may often be missed on MRI. How tissues look in CT and MRI brain have been summarized in **Table 2** along with common pathologies and their appearance **(Table 3)**.

T1-weighted Image

Fat, subacute hemorrhage, and gadolinium contrast appear bright whereas bone, CSF, water, and ligament will appear dark on

TABLE 2: Tissue characteristics on computed tomography (CT) and magnetic resonance imaging (MRI).

	T1 image	T2 image	CT scan
Bone	Dark	Dark	Bright
Air	Dark	Dark	Dark
Fat	Bright	Less bright	Dark
Water	Dark	Bright	Dark
Brain	Anatomic	Intermediate	Intermediate

TABLE 3: Common pathologies on computed tomography (CT) and magnetic resonance imaging (MRI) brain.

	T1	T2	CT scan	Enhancement
Infarct	Dark	Bright	Dark	Subacute
Bleed	Bright unless very fresh or very old	Bright unless very fresh or very old	Bright	No
Tumor	Dark	Bright	Dark unless calcified	Yes
Demyelinating plaque	Dark	Bright	Dark rather often isodense	Acute

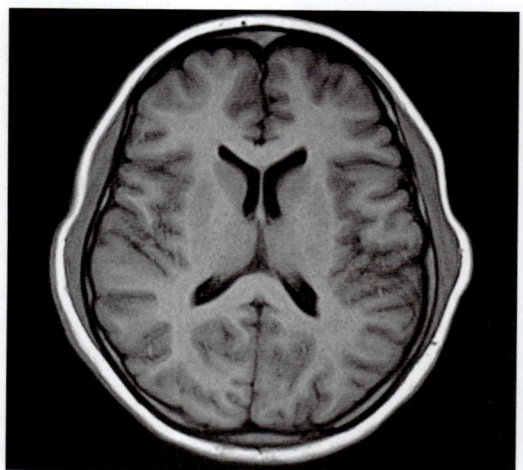

Fig. 10: T1-weighted axial image of magnetic resonance imaging (MRI) brain.

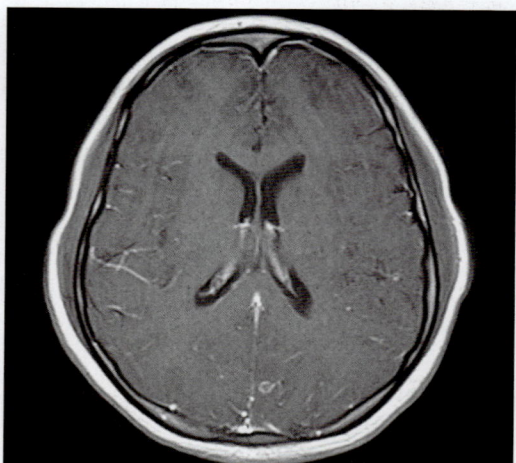

Fig. 11: T1-weighted contrast axial image of magnetic resonance imaging (MRI) brain.

T1-weighted images **(Fig. 10)**. Calcifications and flow voids have no signal intensity and could be missed on T1. Gray matter will look gray, white matter will look white, and CSF will look black on T1-weighted image in fully myelinated brain. This is similar to the appearance of gray matter (gray in color) and white matter (white in color) on a CT scan. We expect myelination to be complete by 2 years of age. T1-weighted image is useful for anatomy and to look for the effects of contrast enhancement. Cortical malformation or heterotopias are better visualized on T1 and T1 inversion recovery sequences. Contrast images are always seen on T1-weighted images. T1-weighted images are not suitable to delineate intraparenchymal lesions that are better appreciated on T2/FLAIR (fluid-attenuated inversion recovery) sequences.

Contrast T1-weighted Image

Gadolinium-DTPA (gadopentetic acid) is the most common contrast agent used in MRI. When a contrast is injected, it is first seen in sagittal sinus, then the vessel gets filled, and then it leaves the vessels and reaches the defective tissue **(Fig. 11)**. A breach in blood–brain barrier will result in contrast meningeal enhancement. Contrast scans are useful to diagnose infective pathologies like brain abscess, meningitis, tuberculomas, and brain neoplasms.

T2-weighted Image

In T2-weighted images in a fully myelinated brain, gray matter looks gray, white matter looks dark, and CSF looks bright (in contrast to T1 image) **(Fig. 12)**. CSF, slow-flowing blood, bleed, and cyst will look bright on a T2-weighted image. Vesicular stage of neurocysticercosis will look bright in the center, whereas tuberculoma will have caseous material in center and hence will look dark on a T2-weighted image **(Fig. 13)**. Cortical bone and deoxyhemoglobin will look dark on a T2-weighted image. Air, blood, and calcification will have no signal changes. Any tissue with increased water content such as edema, tumor, infarct, infection, and subdural collection will look bright on T2-weighted images. Eyes look bright (white) on T2 (clue to identify the image T2).

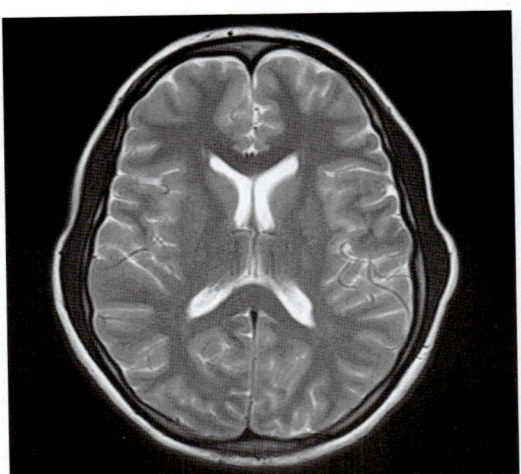

Fig. 12: T2-weighted axial image of magnetic resonance imaging (MRI) brain.

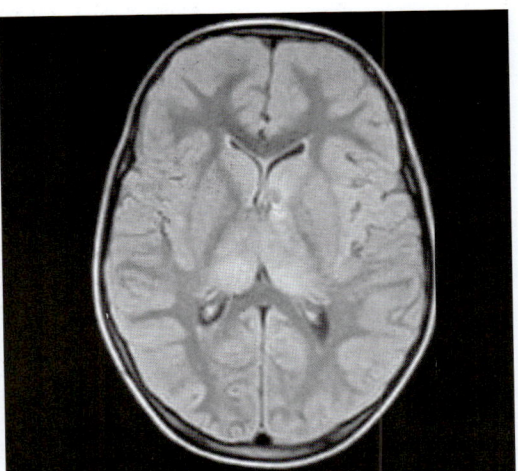

Fig. 14: Normal T2 FLAIR axial image of magnetic resonance imaging (MRI) brain.

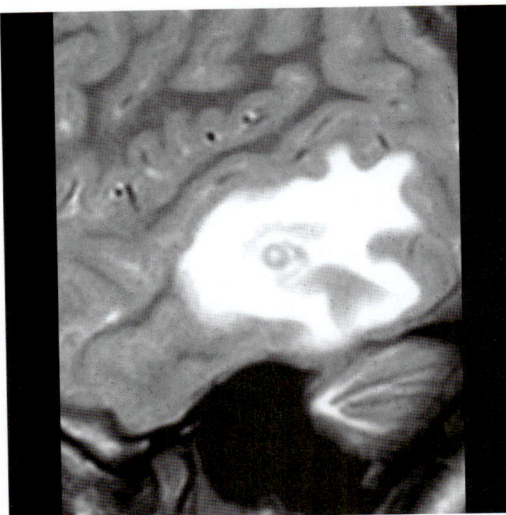

Fig. 13: T2-weighted image revealing a small lesion with hyperintense (bright) core with surrounding perilesional edema suggestive of neurocysticercosis.

FLAIR Sequence

FLAIR sequence is basically a T2-weighted image in which CSF signal is suppressed **(Fig. 14)**. This makes other lesions prominent in brain, especially the one that is close to ventricles like periventricular leukomalacia, infarct, and demyelinating plaque. FLAIR images are very good to differentiate between gray and white matter. To delineate lesions located in fatty tissue like orbit or neck, short tau inversion recovery (STIR) sequences are useful.

Gradient-recalled Echo

Gradient-recalled echo (GRE) image is essentially a T2 image that is useful for detection of blood and calcium **(Figs. 15A and B)**. Both calcification and hemorrhage will show "blooming effect" on GRE sequences. Blooming means it will look larger and darker than what is actually present. Susceptibility-weighted image (SWI) is a gradient sequence, which accentuates the paramagnetic properties of deoxyhemoglobin useful to detect microbleeds and calcium. SWI images are useful in detection of vascular malformation, venous thrombosis, and neoplasms with hemorrhage. Thrombosed sinus contains deoxyhemoglobin, which can be readily detected on SWI **(Figs. 16A to C)**.

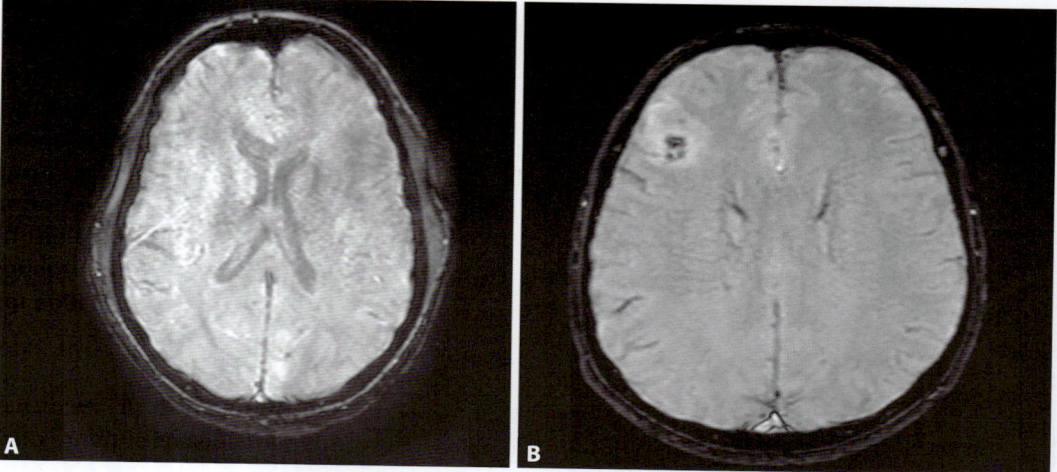

Figs. 15A and B: (A) Normal gradient-recalled echo (GRE) image and (B) GRE image with blooming effect.

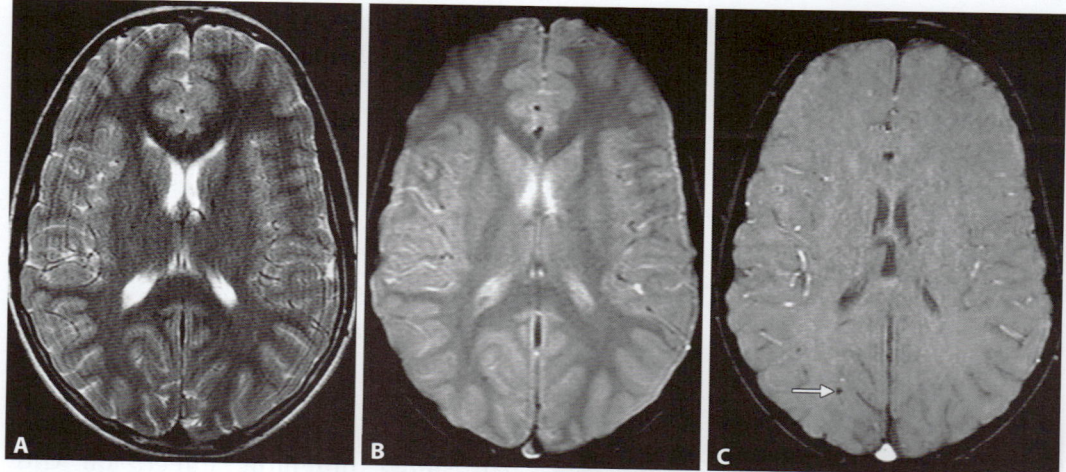

Figs. 16A to C: (A and B) T2-weighted images and (C) susceptibility-weighted image (SWI) that reveal a small cavernoma (arrow) (also note that lesion is not clear on **Figures 16A and B**).

Diffusion-weighted Imaging and Apparent Diffusion Coefficient Map

Diffusion-weighted imaging (DWI) measures the magnitude of random Brownian movement of water molecule within a particular tissue. Areas where the tissue is infarcted will demonstrate *restricted diffusion*, which appears bright on DWI images and corresponding areas look dark on apparent diffusion coefficient (ADC) map **(Figs. 17A and B)**. This needs to be differentiated from phenomena of *T2 shine through* in which DWI might look bright as in T2 images, but there is no restricted diffusion in the ADC map.

Restricted diffusion may indicate acute infarction resulting from cytotoxic edema.

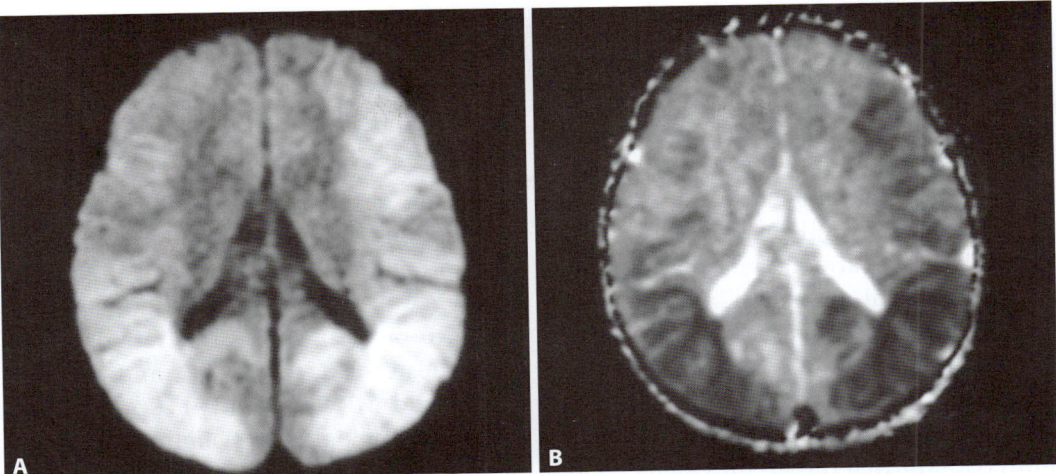

Figs. 17A and B: Diffusion-weighted images (DWIs) showing diffusion restriction in bilateral parieto-occipital area, which appears (A) bright on DWI image and (B) dark on apparent diffusion coefficient (ADC) map.

Abscess, hemorrhage, certain neoplasms, and some acute demyelinating lesions may demonstrate diffusion restriction. Brain abscess also shows restricted diffusion and low ADC coefficient that improves with treatment. Among the benign cystic lesions, the arachnoid cyst shows no diffusion restriction. Necrotic tissue such as high-grade glioma might also demonstrate restricted diffusion.

MAGNETIC RESONANCE SPECTROSCOPY

Magnetic resonance spectroscopy (MRS) measures the biochemical changes in the brain metabolites like lactate, lipid, myoinositol, N-acetyl aspartate (NAA), creatine, and choline. Lactate indicates hypoxic and metabolic insult, lipid indicates brain injury, NAA is an indicator of neuronal injury, creatine is a brain energy marker, and myoinositol is marker of astrocyte injury.

Lactate doublet peak at 1.3 ppm indicates ischemia or mitochondrial disorder. NAA is absent in a destructive lesion, whereas it is elevated in Canavan disease. Choline peak (3.2 ppm) is elevated in membrane disruption seen in lymphoma, demyelination, or axonal shearing. Myoinositol and choline peaks are seen in neonates; they decrease as the brain matures. Raised lactate to NAA ratio and reduced NAA peak are indicators of perinatal asphyxia.

DIFFUSION TENSOR IMAGING

Injury to white matter across the fiber is called *anisotropy*. Diffusion tensor imaging (DTI) is a technique to determine the location, orientation, and anisotropy of white matter tracts in the brain. Its use is limited to localization of tumor in relation to white matter tracts and to track the localization of white matter lesion. This imaging helps neurosurgeons in planning surgery. Color coding is used to depict white matter tracts—red for right-to-left fibers, green for anterior-to-posterior fibers, and blue for superior-to-inferior fibers.

MAGNETIC RESONANCE ANGIOGRAPHY

Magnetic resonance angiography (MRA) is useful for assessment of cerebral vasculature including evaluation for the etiology of intracranial hemorrhage (aneurysm and arteriovenous malformations), acute ischemic stroke (arterial stenosis, moyamoya disease, arterial dissection, and sickle cell vasculopathy), and to ascertain the vascular supply of brain tumors. Techniques used to perform MRA include time of flight (TOF), phase contrast (PC), and contrast-enhanced MRA (CE-MRA). It reveals the caliber of both anterior circulation and posterior circulation. In contrast to conventional invasive digital subtraction angiography (DSA), MRA is noninvasive and does not involve risk of radiation exposure or possible vascular injury as expected with invasive angiography. Anterior circulation consists of internal carotid artery that divides into anterior and middle cerebral artery. In the posterior circulation, two vertebral arteries join to form basilar artery that divides into right and left posterior cerebral artery, which joins the anterior circulation to form circle of Willis **(Fig. 18)**.

MAGNETIC RESONANCE VENOGRAPHY

Magnetic resonance venography (MRV) is useful noninvasive investigation to evaluate the intracranial venous system to look for evidence of sinus thrombosis. Techniques used to perform MRV are similar to MRA and these include TOF, PC, and contrast-enhanced MRV (CE-MRV). Conventional catheter angiography (venous phase) has been considered gold standard to diagnose venous sinus thrombosis. Sagittal sinus joins both transverse sinuses to form sigmoid sinus **(Fig. 19A)**. Vein of Galen **(Fig. 19B)** drains into straight sinus **(Fig. 19B)** that drains into sigmoid sinus. Presence of dense collaterals **(Figs. 19C and D)** could indicate thrombosis of venous sinus. Although flow gaps in MRV often indicate underlying venous sinus thrombosis, they can be absent in up to 30% of normal nondominant transverse sinus. Hence, caution must be exercised to interpret the findings of transverse sinus thrombosis

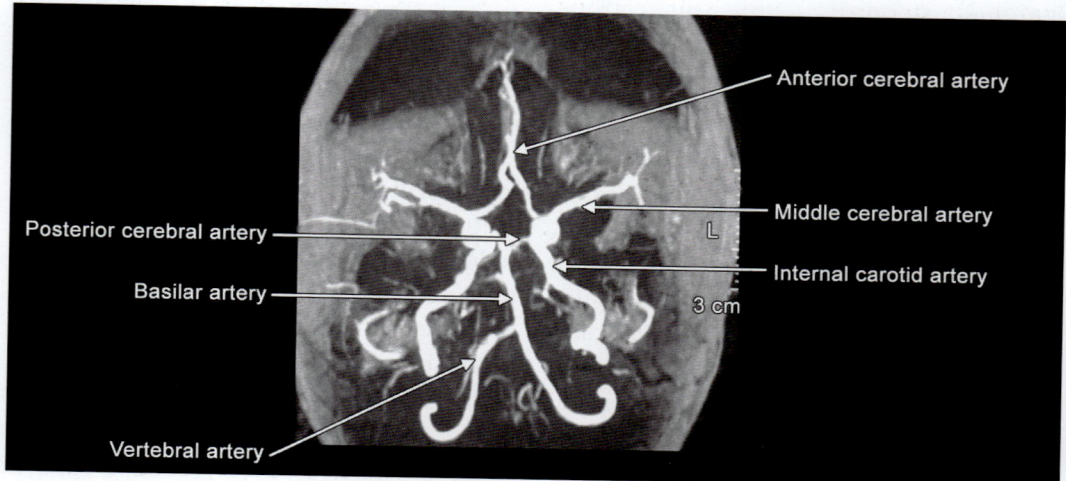

Fig. 18: Structures evident on magnetic resonance angiography (MRA).

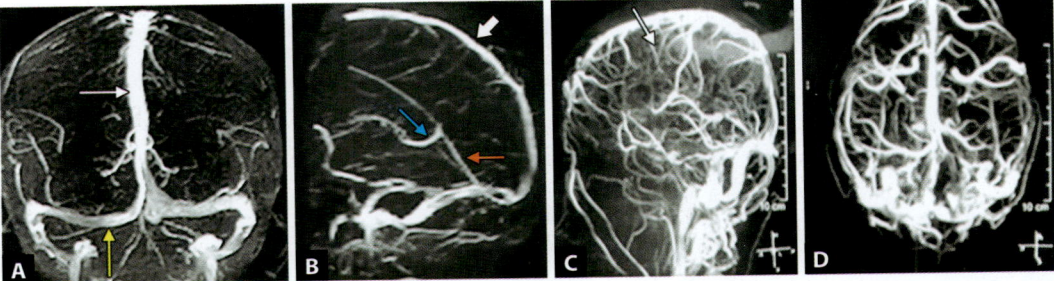

Figs. 19A to D: Magnetic resonance venography (MRV) showing (A) patent sagittal (white arrow) and transverse sinus (yellow arrow) and (B) vein of Galen (blue arrow) and straight sinus (red arrow). There are dense collaterals in (C) and (D) suggestive of venous sinus thrombosis.

(nondominant side) on MRV alone. Similarly, hypoplastic left transverse sinus can also result in flow gaps on MRV. Imaging artifacts, anatomical variants, and pathology are often difficult to differentiate on MRV. Hence, MRV is used in conjunction with other findings on MRI brain and clinical context.

NORMAL MYELINATION OF BRAIN

Myelination begins in the 5th fetal month and continues till 2 years of age. It progresses from caudal to cephalad, central to peripheral, dorsal to ventral, and posterior to anterior. Structures that are myelinated at birth include posterior limb of internal capsule, middle cerebellar peduncle, tegmentum pontis, ventrolateral thalamus, pyramidal tracts, and optic nerve/chiasma/optic tract **(Fig. 20)**. Myelination is best appreciated on T1-weighted image till 1 year of age beyond which T2-weighted image is good to monitor for myelination. Any myelinated structure will look hyperintense or bright on T1-weighted image and dark on T2-weighted images. By 2–3 months, the anterior limb of internal capsule and splenium of corpus callosum; by 6 months, the genu of corpus callosum; and by 8 months, subcortical white matter will be myelinated (look bright) on T1-weighted image **(Fig. 21 and Table 4)**.

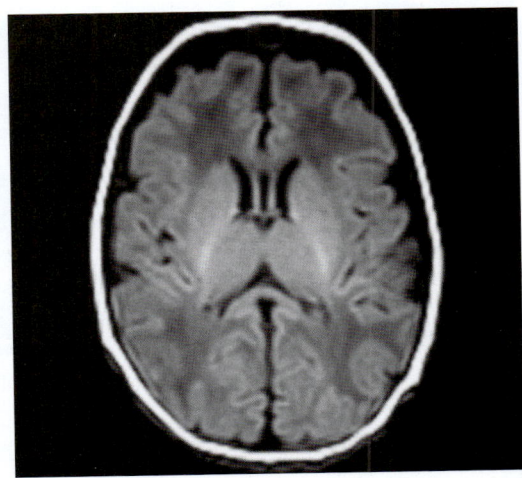

Fig. 20: Normal newborn T1-weighted MRI showing bright signal on posterior limb of internal capsule indicating normal myelination.

If myelin is not developed, then it is termed *hypomyelination*. Hypomyelination is observed in conditions like Pelizaeus–Merzbacher disease (PMD), Cockayne syndrome, and Salla disease. If myelination gets delayed, for example, if splenium of corpus callosum is not myelinated till 6 months of age, then such pattern will be considered as *delayed myelination*. To label it as delayed myelination, we need serial MRI scans at a minimum interval of 6 months to demonstrate that myelination is proceeding further. Many children with developmental

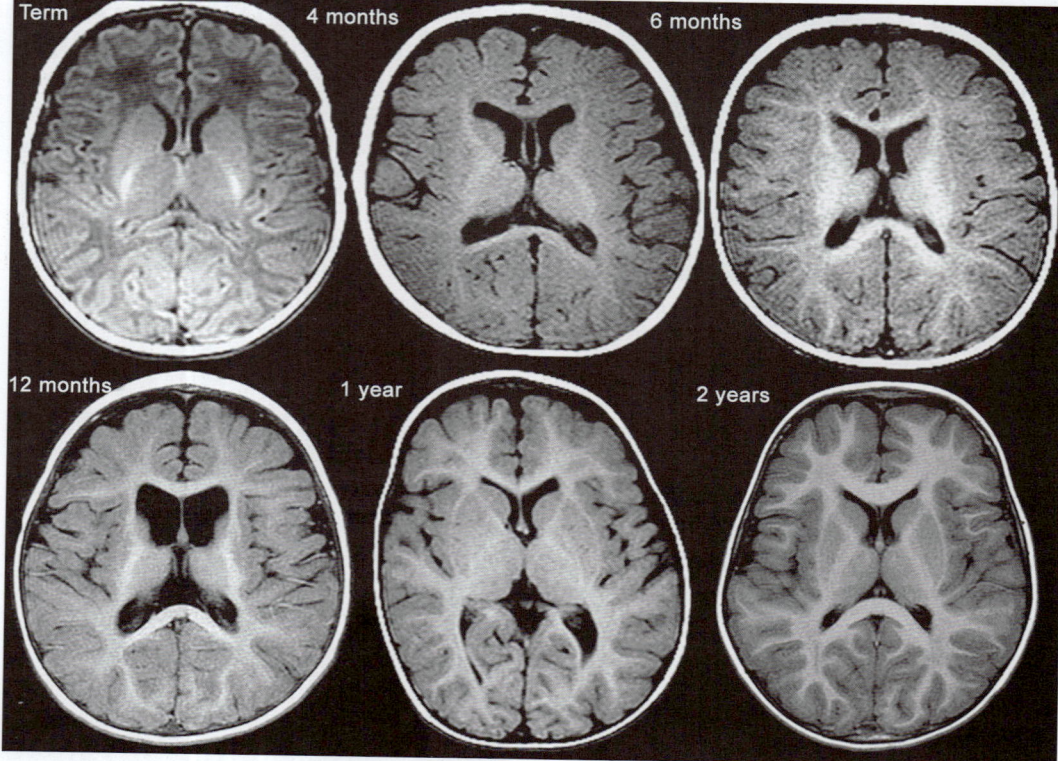

Fig. 21: Progression of myelination after birth.

TABLE 4: Sequence of myelination in the brain.	
Myelinate before	**Myelinate after**
1. Brainstem and cerebellum	Cerebrum
2. Basal ganglia and thalamus	Deep white matter
3. Posterior limb of internal capsule	Anterior limb or internal capsule
4. Splenium of corpus callosum	Genu of corpus callosum
5. Corona radiata	Subcortical region

delay, inborn error of metabolism, and chromosomal disorders have delayed myelination. Whereas, if at any point of time, the structures that are supposed to be myelinated at birth are still not myelinated or there is no progress of myelination in the serial MRI scans performed at 6 monthly gaps, it is more likely to be a hypomyelinating disorder. Delayed myelination is a nonspecific radiological finding in comparison to hypomyelinating disorders. Neuroanatomical structures that need to be recognized by clinicians are highlighted in **Figures 22A to C**.

■ CASE VIGNETTES

Case 1

- *Clinical features:* A 2-year-old boy presented with gait difficulties. He was born premature with delayed cry at birth.
  He required neonatal intensive care unit (NICU) stay for 3 days. Examination shows spasticity more evident in both the lower limbs.

- *Neuroimaging:* MRI brain reveals T2 FLAIR hyperintensity with volume loss **(Figs. 23A and B)**.
- *Analysis:* The clinical features and neuroimaging suggest *spastic diplegia* secondary to prematurity and perinatal asphyxia. The diagnosis correlates with findings of periventricular leukomalacia on MRI brain.

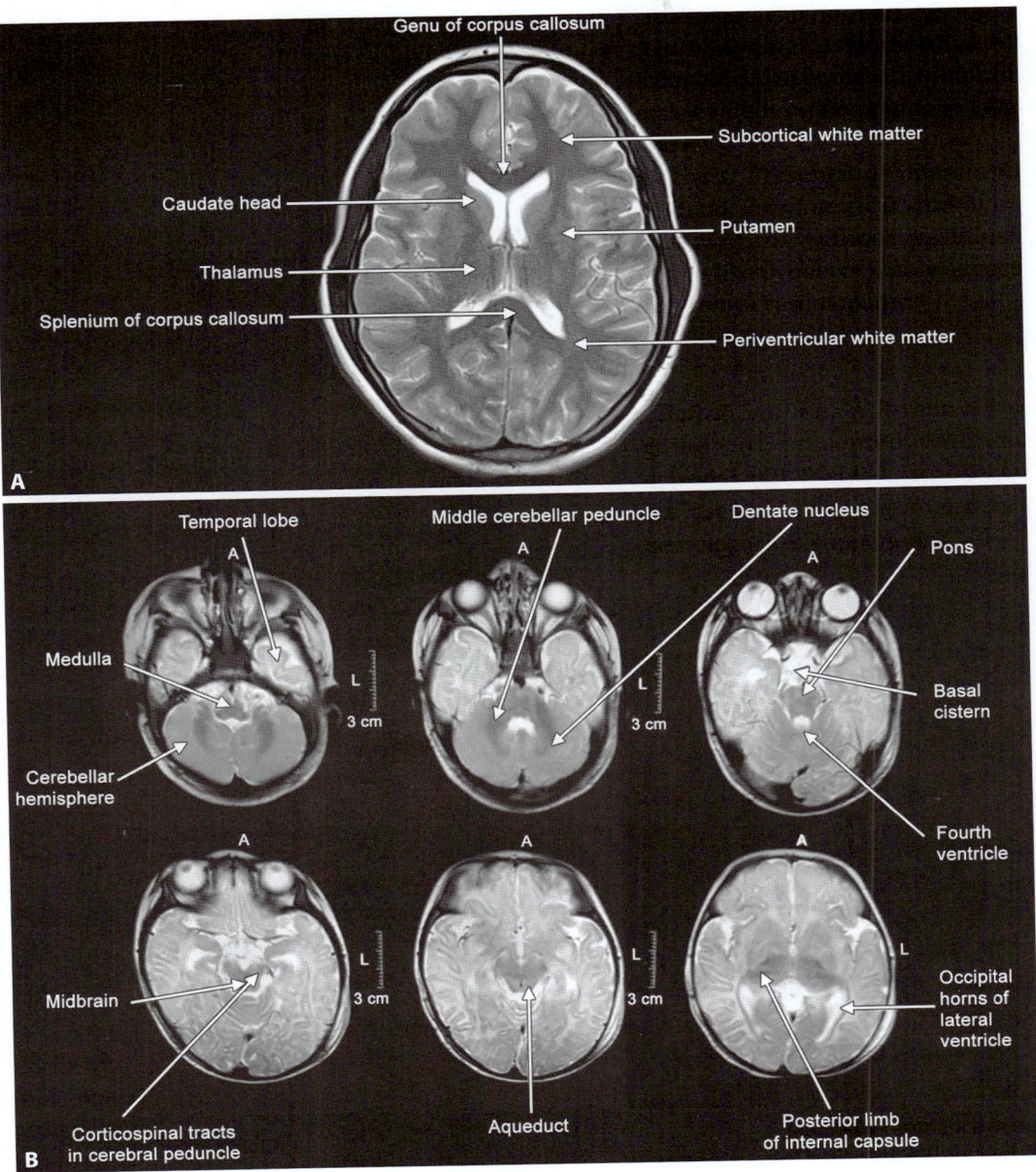

Figs. 22A and B

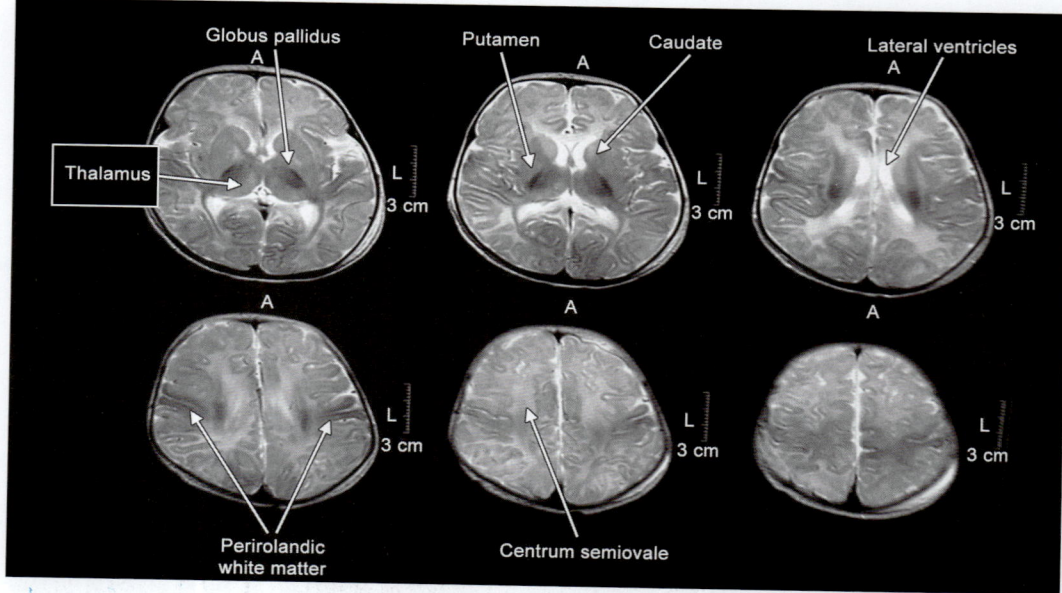

Fig. 22C
Figs. 22A to C: Common neuroanatomical structures on magnetic resonance imaging (MRI) brain.

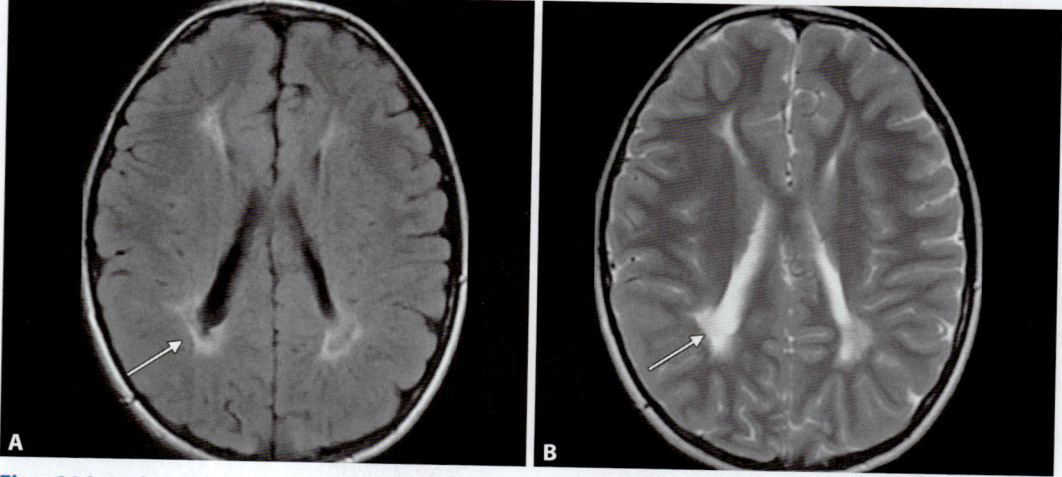

Figs. 23A and B: Magnetic resonance imaging (MRI) brain showing periventricular signal changes and gliosis (arrow) evident on (A) FLAIR (fluid-attenuated inversion recovery) image and (B) T2 weighted image suggestive of periventricular leukomalacia (arrow).

Case 2

- *Clinical features:* A 10-year-old girl presented with high-grade fever for 20 days, altered sensorium for 10 days, and multiple episodes of seizure 7 days back. Examination revealed a cachectic child with signs of raised intracranial pressure with meningeal irritation.
- *Neuroimaging:* MRI brain T1-contrast image shows multiple ring-enhancing

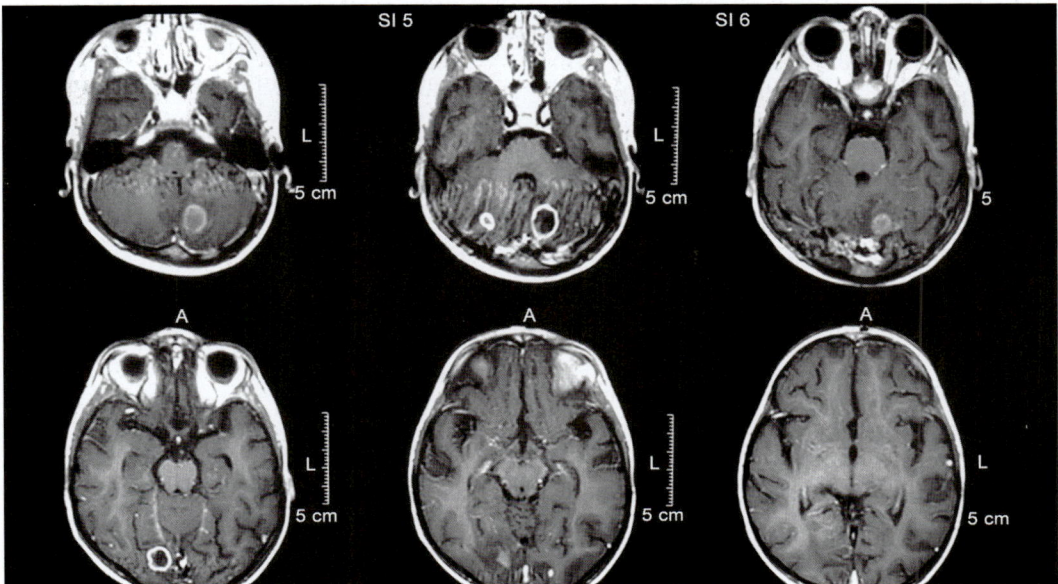

Fig. 24: Multiple ring-enhancing lesions in the infratentorial region evident on T1 contrast magnetic resonance imaging (MRI) brain suggestive of tuberculoma.

lesions in posterior fossa with evidence of basal exudates **(Fig. 24)**.

- *Analysis:* Presence of prolonged fever, meningeal signs, and neuroimaging findings of multiple ring-enhancing lesions could suggest a possibility of tubercular meningitis with multiple tuberculoma.

Case 3

- *Clinical features:* A 3-year-old child presented with global developmental delay, hearing impairment, and generalized dystonia. Examination reveals microcephaly, signs of malnutrition, and generalized dystonia.
- *Neuroimaging:* MRI brain T2-weighted images show bilateral symmetrical hyperintensity in globus pallidus (arrows) **(Fig. 25)**.
- *Analysis:* Combination of developmental delay, hearing impairment, and dystonia with neuroimaging evidence of bilateral globus pallidus involvement is highly suggestive of diagnosis of bilirubin encephalopathy sequelae.

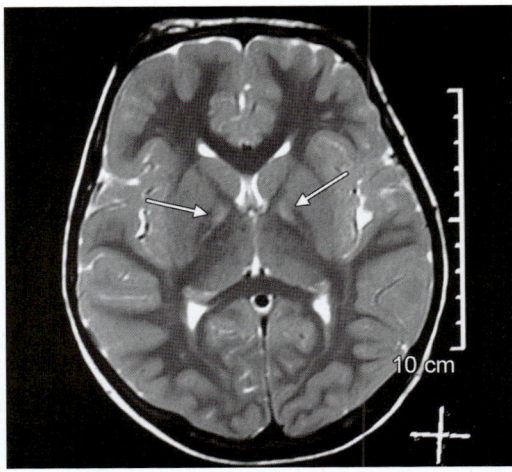

Fig. 25: Magnetic resonance imaging (MRI) brain T2-weighted image showing bilateral symmetrical hyperintensity in globus pallidus (arrows) suggestive of kernicterus sequelae.

Case 4

- *Clinical features:* A 7-year-old boy presented with recurrent episodes of hemiparesis involving both right and left sides in the last 6 months. Examination reveals right-sided hemiparesis with right facial palsy with normal sensorium.
- *Neuroimaging:* Asymmetrical bilateral infarcts on MRI brain with bunch of collaterals evident on angiography **(Figs. 26A and B)**.
- *Analysis:* Presence of infarcts that are bilateral, asymmetrical, and of different ages with or without past history of stroke-like events is highly suggestive of moyamoya vasculopathy.

Case 5

- *Clinical features:* A 6-year-old schoolgoing girl presented with multiple episodes of left-sided focal seizures for the last 1 year. She has an unremarkable neurological examination.
- *Neuroimaging:* FLAIR coronal images reveal atrophy of right hippocampus suggesting a possibility of mesial temporal sclerosis **(Fig. 27)**.
- *Analysis:* Presence of refractory left focal seizures appears secondary to right-sided mesial temporal sclerosis (structural epilepsy). If the child does not improve with antiepileptic drugs, she is a good candidate for epilepsy surgery.

Case 6

- *Clinical features:* A 4-year-old boy presented with multiple episodes of right-sided focal seizure for the last 3 months. He had a history of focal status epilepticus at the age of 18 months. He subsequently developed right-sided hemiparesis, which persists till now.
- *Neuroimaging:* Serial imaging shows unilateral cerebral edema at the age of 18 months followed by atrophy on the ipsilateral side done at the age of 4 years **(Figs. 28A to C)**.

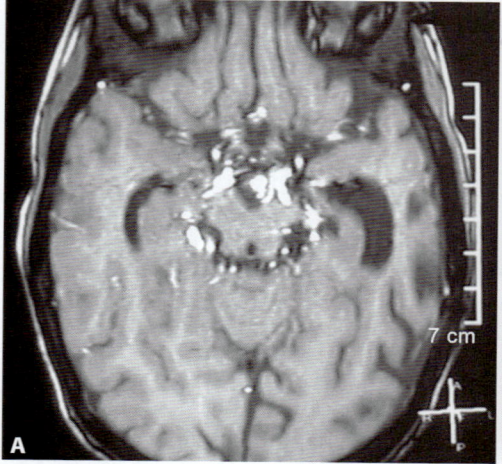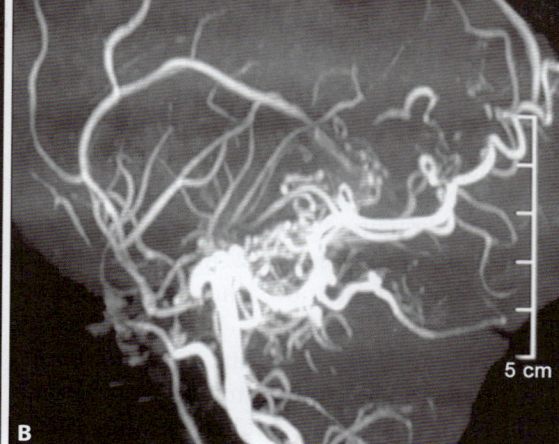

Figs. 26A and B: Magnetic resonance imaging (MRI) brain T1 contrast image (A) reveals bunch of vessels clustered in base of brain with MR angiography (B) showing occlusion at distal internal carotid artery with a bunch of collaterals (puff of smoke appearance) suggestive of moyamoya vasculopathy.

CHAPTER 5: Neuroimaging   135

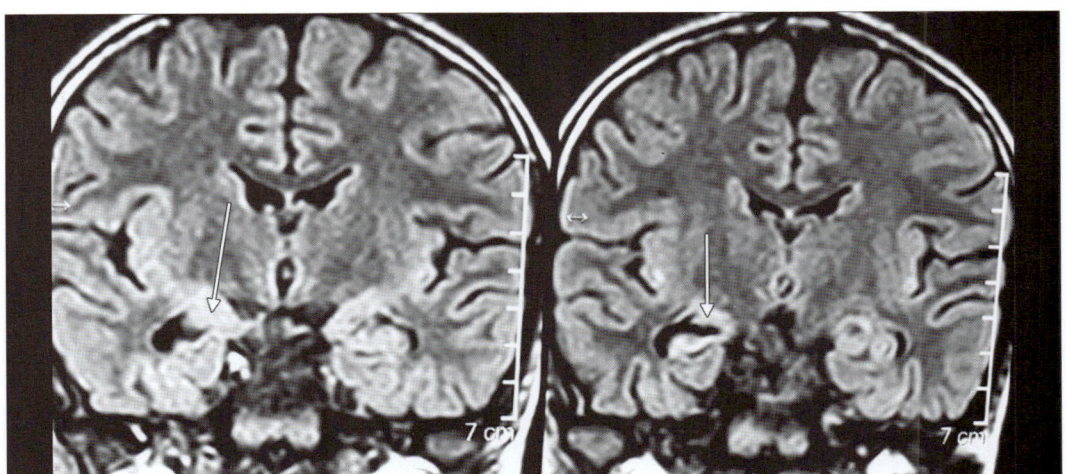

Fig. 27: Magnetic resonance imaging (MRI) brain T2/FLAIR (fluid-attenuated inversion recovery) coronal image reveals bilateral (right > left) gliosis of mesial temporal structures suggestive of mesial temporal sclerosis.

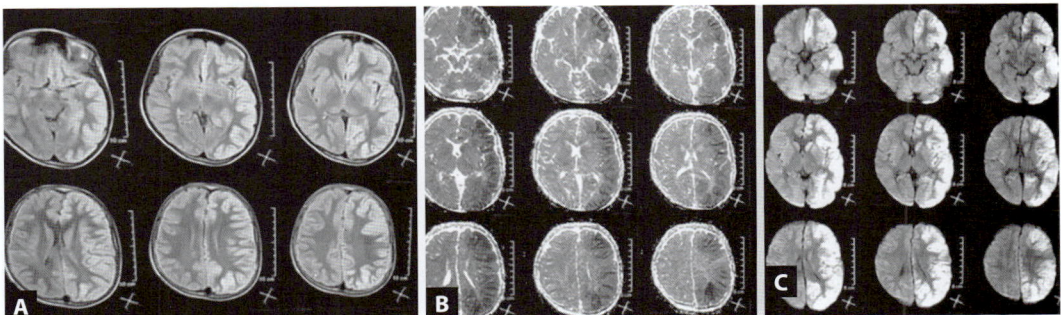

Figs. 28A to C: Magnetic resonance imaging (MRI) brain T2/FLAIR (fluid-attenuated inversion recovery) images showing hyperintensity along left hemisphere with prominent gyrus (A) with diffusion restriction evident as dark signals in ADC map (B) and corresponding bright signal across the left hemisphere in diffusion-weighted images (DWI) (C). These findings could be consistent with diagnosis of acute stage of hemiconvulsion–hemiplegia–epilepsy syndrome.

- *Analysis:* Patient first developed hemiconvulsion, then he developed hemiplegia, and now he has focal epilepsy on the same side with contralateral cortical atrophy. The sequence of hemiconvulsion, hemiplegia, and subsequent epilepsy is suggestive of diagnosis of hemiconvulsion–hemiplegia–epilepsy syndrome.

Case 7
- *Clinical features:* A 6-year-old boy presented with sudden onset of right-sided hemiparesis and right focal seizure. He was encephalopathic on examination.
- *Neuroimaging:* MRI brain reveals arterial ischemic stroke with hemorrhagic transformation **(Figs. 29A and B)**.

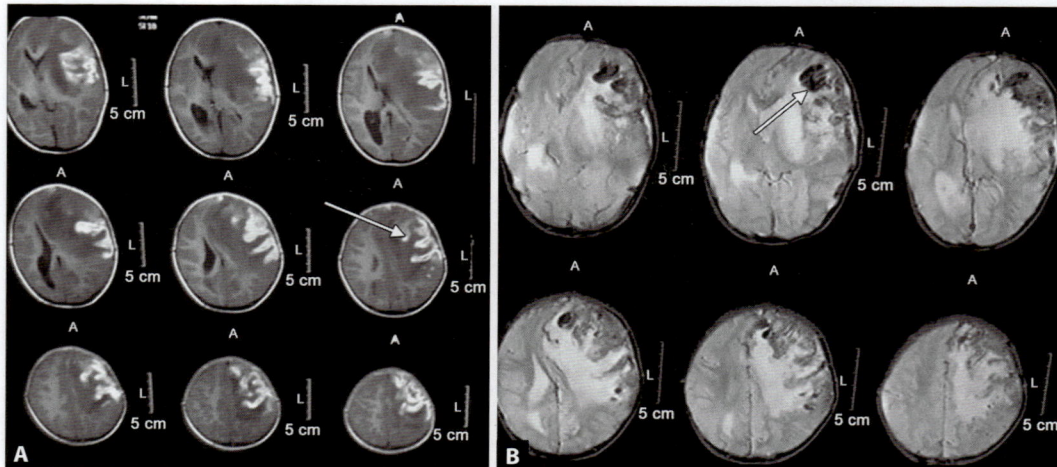

Figs. 29A and B: Magnetic resonance imaging (MRI) brain reveals T1 (A) hyperintensity along the gyrus (cortical ribbon sign) (arrow) along with underlying hypointense signal with midline shift. On gradient-recalled echo (GRE) images (B), blooming effect (arrow) is evident in the corresponding area suggestive of hemorrhagic transformation of arterial ischemic stroke.

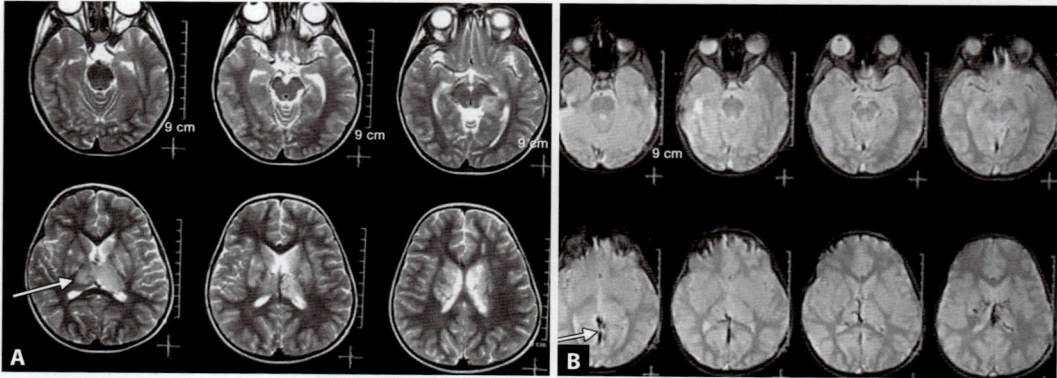

Figs. 30A and B: Magnetic resonance imaging (MRI) brain T2 images reveal symmetrical bilateral hyperintensity in thalamus, striatum (arrow) (A). Susceptibility-weighted images (SWIs) (B) show prominent straight sinus (arrow) suggestive of possible thrombus. These findings suggest deep venous sinus thrombosis.

- *Analysis:* Sudden onset of focal neurological deficit with neuroimaging evidence of arterial ischemic stroke is highly suggestive of vasculopathy.

Case 8

- *Clinical features:* A 3-year-old child presented with loose stools and vomiting for 3 days followed by flurry of seizure and encephalopathy. Examination reveals signs of raised intracranial pressure (bilateral sixth nerve palsy, hypertonia, and hyperreflexia).
- *Neuroimaging:* MRI brain findings **(Figs. 30A and B)** are highly suggestive of venous sinus thrombosis.

CHAPTER 5: Neuroimaging | **137**

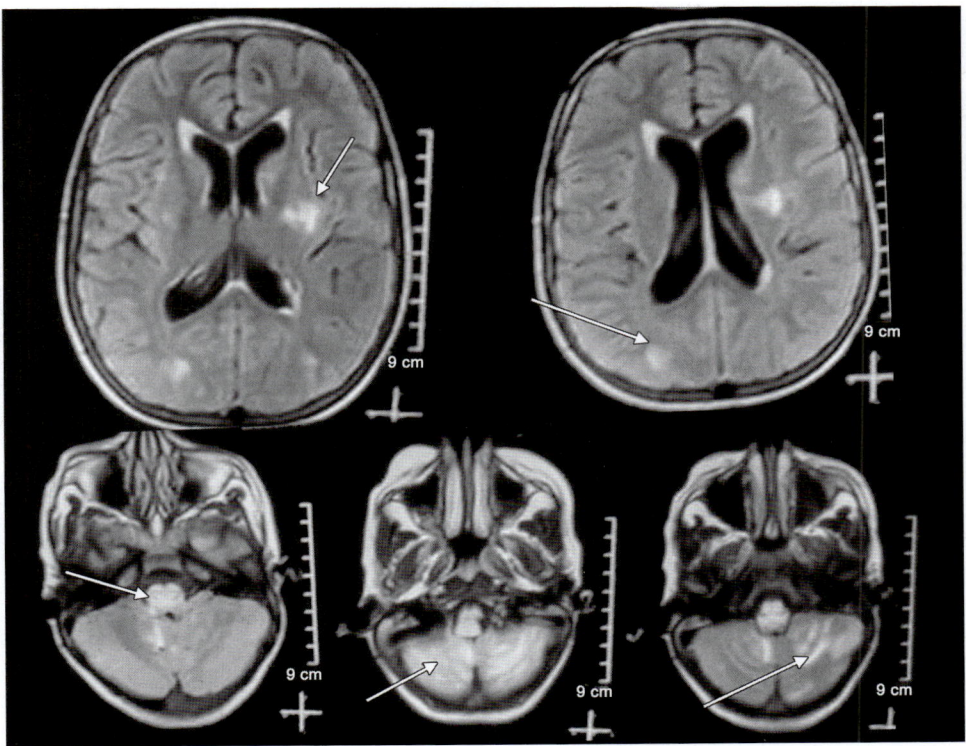

Fig. 31: Magnetic resonance imaging (MRI) T2 FLAIR (fluid-attenuated inversion recovery) images showing multiple patchy hyperintensity (white arrow) involving brainstem, cerebellum, subcortical, and periventricular white matter suggestive of acute disseminated encephalomyelitis (ADEM).

- *Analysis:* Dehydration is a risk factor for thrombosis. Hence, sudden onset of encephalopathy in a baby subsequent to diarrheal illness must raise a suspicion of venous sinus thrombosis. Neuroimaging findings also correlate with clinical possibility.

Case 9
- *Clinical features:* A 10-year-old boy presented with history of sudden onset of seizures and encephalopathy. He had a history of febrile illness lasting for 3 days, a week ago.
- *Neuroimaging:* MRI brain reveals features suggestive of acute disseminated encephalomyelitis (ADEM) **(Fig. 31)**.

- *Analysis:* Encephalopathy in a child following a febrile illness must raise suspicion of postinfectious/autoimmune etiology. Considering the neuroimaging findings of patchy and asymmetrical lesions, a possibility of ADEM could be entertained.

Case 10
- *Clinical features:* A 3-year-old boy presented with global developmental delay and refractory seizures. Examination revealed microcephaly and spasticity.
- *Neuroimaging:* MRI brain T1 inversion recovery (good modality for structural lesions) reveals pachygric-agyric cortex (red arrow) with evidence of nodular

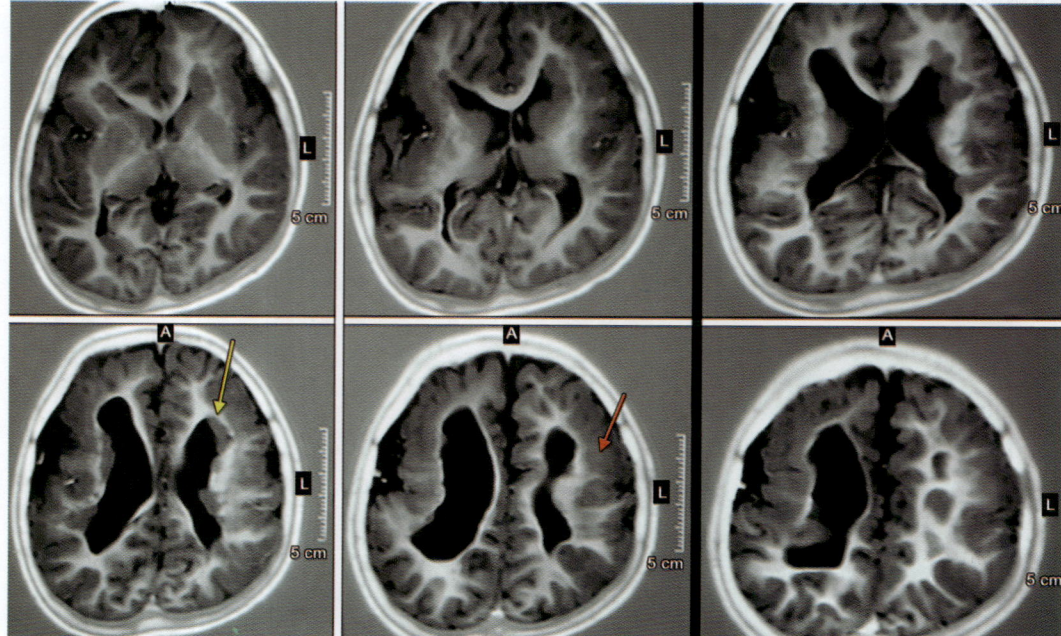

Fig. 32: MRI brain T1 inversion recovery images revealing cortical dysplasia with agyric-pachygyric cortex (red arrow) with heterotopias (yellow arrow).

heterotopias (yellow arrow). One of the ways to identify inversion recovery images is to look at gray background; most of other sequences have black background **(Fig. 32)**.

- *Analysis:* Presence of global developmental delay, microcephaly, and seizures must always consider cortical structural malformation as a possibility, especially when supported by neuroimaging findings.

KEY MESSAGES

- Restrict the use of CT head to only children with head trauma and where we desire to look at orbit, temporal bones, or to look for any intraparenchymal calcifications considering the risk of radiation exposure.
- MRI brain has a better resolution of brain structures and lack of radiation exposure, but it is time consuming and requires the cooperation of the child or procedural sedation.
- Contrast MRI is useful among suspected infective (brain abscess and neurocysticercosis) and inflammatory disorders (demyelinating). MRA is useful to delineate arterial vasculature and MRV is useful for suspected sinus venous thrombosis.
- T1-weighted images are useful for anatomy, T2/FLAIR-weighted images are useful to delineate the abnormal structure, SWI is useful for calcification/bleed, DWI/ADC maps are useful to ascertain diffusion restriction (cytotoxic edema), and STIR images are useful for describing lesions within fatty structures such as orbit.
- The appearance of structures is compared to brain parenchyma. On T2 image, anything that looks brighter than parenchyma (such as CSF, fluid, and cyst) is called hyperintense and anything that looks darker (such as bone and subacute bleed) is called hypointense.

6. Neurophysiologic Evaluation

ELECTROENCEPHALOGRAPHY

Principle of Electroencephalography

Electroencephalography (EEG) is a useful electrophysiological investigation for evaluating a child with a paroxysmal event. It measures the electropotential difference between two points on the scalp, caused by ion trafficking. Potential differences between electrodes are amplified and the net signal from each amplifier is displayed on a monitor to provide a graphic record. EEG signals are generated by the summation of excitatory and inhibitory synaptic potentials from large, vertically oriented pyramidal neurons located in layer III, V, and VI. These EEG signals are synchronized by subcortical structures such as thalamus and brainstem reticular formation. Sleep spindles are considered a result of this thalamocortical phenomenon. It is a noninvasive, readily available, and relatively cheap investigation to study the neuronal dysfunction and abnormal cortical excitability.

Technical Aspects

The electrodes made of gold or silver discs (silver chloride) are placed at standard points over scalp with a conductive paste. The International 10–20 system (10 and 20% gap between electrodes) is used for electrode placement. Pediatric EEG routinely requires the placement of 21 electrodes on the scalp with fewer electrodes (minimum of 12 electrodes) in neonates and young infants. Additional channels of electrocardiogram and respiration are recommended to record physiologic artifacts. Electrodes are named according to the underlying area of the brain—FP: frontopolar; F: frontal; P: parietal; T: temporal; and O: occipital. Central electrodes are abbreviated as zed (z) [Fz (frontocentral), Cz (central), Pz (parietocentral)] and referential electrodes include postauricular (A1 and A2). The odd numbers (Fp1, F3, P3, C3, T3, T5, T7, and O1) depict the left side of the hemisphere and even numbers (Fp2, F4, P4, C4, T4, T6, and O2) for the right side. These electrodes are either fixed to the scalp using conductive paste or electrodes fixed onto a head cap are used.

Patient Preparation

The scalp should be clean and dry. The patient should be instructed to continue antiepileptic drugs as prescribed. They can take their routine breakfast on the day of the appointment. Routine EEG recordings usually last for a minimum of 30 minutes including hyperventilation for 3 minutes and intermittent photic stimulation at 1–30 Hz (**Fig. 1**). Continuous long-term EEG recordings are particularly useful for presurgical evaluation for epilepsy surgery.

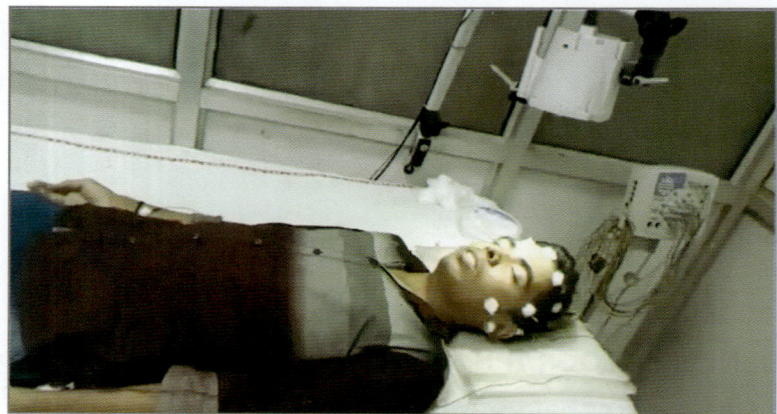

Fig. 1: Photic stimulation administered during electroencephalography (EEG) recording.

In children <5 years, EEG is performed only during the sleep considering excessive movement artifacts during the wakeful state. Moreover, sleep EEG provides vital information on the maturation of the brain.

Sleep-deprived EEG protocol requires 4–6 hours of sleep deprivation. Children >3 years of age could be kept awake until midnight and woken up at 5:00 AM on the morning of the test. Triclofos (20 mg/kg/dose), melatonin (2–6 mg/dose), or clonidine (0.05–0.2 mg) can be used for sedation. Intravenous midazolam should *not* be used to induce sleep due to its suppressive effect on epileptiform discharges. In addition to sleep deprivation, the yield of EEG can be increased by repeat recording, prolonging the duration of recording, increasing the number of channels during the procedure, simultaneous video recording, and recording both awake and sleep state.

Activation Procedure

Infants, young children, and children with suspected focal epilepsies require sleep EEG record. Sleep EEG is essential for the diagnosis of epileptic encephalopathy with continuous spike waves during slow sleep (CSWS). EEG in the wakeful state is useful to detect generalized epilepsy. Activation procedure includes *hyperventilation* (3 Hz pattern in absence epilepsies), and *intermittent photic stimulation* (4–6 Hz generalized epileptiform discharges in Juvenile myoclonic epilepsy). Other activation procedures are indicated for specific conditions such as fixation off sensitivity (late-onset occipital lobe epilepsy), precipitation by a trigger (e.g., video watching) in reflex epilepsies, and suggestion to precipitate paroxysmal nonepileptic events.

Electroencephalography Requisition

An EEG requisition form from clinician must consist of the basic demographic profile (name, age, gender, telephone number, or email), type of seizure, the frequency of seizure, age at onset, an indication of EEG, neuroimaging findings, any previous EEG if done, and nature of antiepileptic drugs. The neurophysician can decide on the EEG protocol based on clinical diagnosis—awake EEG record with hyperventilation and photic stimulation or sleep EEG record.

Electroencephalography Interpretation

Abnormalities in EEG could be categorized into—(1) *background abnormalities* and (2) *abnormal epileptiform discharges*.

The background gives information about the neurologic state of the child. The normal awake record consists of posterior dominant α-rhythm (4–10 Hz) with reactivity to eye closure (children >8 years, have 9–10 Hz). Similarly, sleep background consists of sleep markers of non-REM sleep such as sleep spindles, vertex waves, and K-complexes.

Epileptiform discharges have distinct waveforms classified as spikes (<70 ms) or sharp wave (70–200 ms). EEG findings in common self-limited epilepsies **(Table 1)** and epileptic encephalopathy **(Table 2)** in children are summarized.

Pitfalls of Electroencephalography

- Surface EEG can be normal in few epileptic children, especially those with remote and deep location of epileptogenic lesion like interhemispheric area, mesial and basal cortex.
- Few genetic types of epilepsy such as benign familial neonatal epilepsy and benign familial infantile epilepsy can have normal interictal EEG.
- Epileptiform discharges are found in 0–5.6% of normal healthy children and 0.5% of adults without any event of a seizure.
- EEG can be abnormal in approximately 5.7–59% of children with autism spectrum disorder without any clinical seizures.
- There is a lot of variability and subjectivity involved in reporting pediatric EEG.
- The most common error in pediatric EEG reading include misinterpreting movement artifacts, hypnagogic hypersynchrony during hyperventilation and normal sleep markers including vertex waves, and K complexes as epileptiform **(Fig. 2)**.
- Benign epileptiform variants such as wicket waves, benign epileptiform transients of sleep (BETS), and rhythmic mid-temporal theta bursts of drowsiness (RMTD) can mimic epileptiform discharges to a naïve reader.
- It is not surprising to see normal awake EEG record in children with suspected rolandic epilepsy, structural focal epilepsy, or CSWS. These abnormalities are detected only on sleep EEG record. Among those with suspected childhood absence epilepsy and juvenile myoclonic epilepsy, hyperventilation and photic stimulation during awake EEG record are mandatory.

Importance of Clinical Information

Electroencephalography is an adjunct to clinical evaluation and findings on EEG need to be interpreted in the clinical context.

Indications of EEG and indications for not using EEG are summarized in **Table 3**. Diagnosis of epilepsy should not be reached solely based on EEG findings. A wrong diagnosis of epilepsy has widespread social implications apart from side effects of antiepileptic drugs and restriction of physical activities. EEG is often abused in evaluation of a child with abnormal paroxysm to differentiate epileptic from nonepileptic event. It was observed that overinterpretation of EEG abnormalities including focal slowing and generalized and focal epileptiform discharges has often led to syncope being misdiagnosed as epileptic seizures. Similarly, if a baby has a history that clearly suggests breath-holding spells, there is no role of EEG to support this clinical diagnosis. Common

SECTION 1: Neurological Evaluation

TABLE 1: Self-limited epileptic seizures and syndromes.

Epilepsy	Clinical features	EEG pattern
Neonatal onset		
Benign neonatal seizure (5th day fit)	Unilateral focal clonic seizure on 4–6th day of life in healthy neonate	Normal or discontinuous EEG background with focal or multifocal abnormalities. Focal rhythmic theta activity with sharp waves (theta pointu alternans) can be seen in 60% of babies
Benign familial neonatal seizure	Focal clonic seizure with occasional apneic spells on day 2 or day 3 of life, persist longer in otherwise healthy neonate	Normal background or theta pointu alternans
Infantile onset		
Benign myoclonic epilepsy in infancy (BMEI)	Myoclonic jerk for 1–3 seconds in developmentally normal child; onset 4 months to 3 years	Normal EEG background with generalized spike and polyspike discharges
Childhood onset		
Childhood absence epilepsy	Frequent absence seizures in school-going child; can be precipitated by hyperventilation	Normal background with 3–4.5 Hz generalized spike wave discharge with frontal dominance
Benign epilepsy with centrotemporal spikes	Seizures during sleep with orofacial motor signs, speech arrest, sialorrhea, and unilateral sensory symptoms	Normal sleep background, with sharps/spike waves in centrotemporal region with a tangential dipole
Early-onset childhood occipital epilepsy (Panayiotopoulos syndrome)	It occurs in sleep with ictal vomiting and autonomic features	Normal EEG background with multifocal and occipital spikes
Late-onset childhood occipital epilepsy (Gastaut syndrome)	Visual hallucinations and colored circular patterns	Runs of rhythmic occipital spikes and sharp waves seen during eye closure called "fixation off" sensitivity. It disappears when eyes are open and fixating at an object "fixation on"
Adolescent		
Juvenile absence epilepsy*	Speech and behavioral arrest without aura. May have automatisms	3–4 Hz spike and wave and polyspike wave discharges
Juvenile myoclonic epilepsy*	Myoclonic jerks in morning, GTCS, and absences	4–6 Hz bilateral polyspike wave and spike slow wave discharges; accentuation by photic stimulation
Nocturnal frontal lobe epilepsy	Focal hypermotor seizures during sleep	Runs of bilateral frontal spike and sharp waves

*May require lifelong antiepileptic medications.
(EEG: electroencephalography; GTCS: generalized tonic–clonic seizure)

TABLE 2: Clinical and electroencephalography (EEG) features of epileptic encephalopathy.

Age	Clinical phenotype	Interictal EEG features	Background abnormality	Epileptiform abnormalities
Neonatal onset				
Ohtahara syndrome	Tonic spasm	BS in wakefulness and sleep	Bursts of high-voltage slow waves: 2–3 seconds suppression: 3–5 seconds	Intermixed multifocal spikes
EME	Erratic fragmentary myoclonus	BS in sleep, may disappear in awake	• Burst 1–3 seconds • Suppression 2–10 seconds	Multifocal spikes
Infantile onset				
Migratory focal seizures (previously MPSI)	Multifocal clonic autonomic	Migrating epileptiform discharges	Normal to discontinuous	Migrating or multifocal epileptiform discharges
West syndrome	Epileptic spasms in clusters, after waking up from sleep	Hypsarrhythmia Classical or modified	Chaotic, high amplitude, and asynchronous slow waves	Multifocal spikes and polyspikes
Dravet syndrome	• Recurrent febrile and afebrile seizure • Myoclonic, atypical absence, and focal seizures	May be normal initially for 1–2 years	Slow diffuse	Generalized, focal or multifocal discharges
Childhood onset				
MAE (Doose syndrome)	Myoclonic—atonic, absences, tonic clonic, tonic	Doose rhythm photosensitive	Normal or Doose rhythm (rhythmic parietal theta activity)	Burst of 2–5 Hz generalized spike and polyspike waves
LGS	Tonic seizures, atypical absences, myoclonic seizures	2–2.5 spike wave discharges and PFA	Diffuse slow, absence of sleep markers	2–2.5 spike wave discharges PFA
CSWS	GTCs during sleep, atypical absence, atonic, myoclonic	Frontocentral continuous spike wave	Awake normal Sleep: diffuse slow wave	1.5–2.5 Hz spike wave discharges; activation during sleep; up to 85%
LKS	Seizures in 70% Autistic regression	Temporoparietal spike wave	Awake normal Sleep: diffuse slow wave	Continuous temporoparietal spike wave

(BS: burst suppression; CSWS: continuous spike and wave during sleep; EME: early myoclonic epilepsy; GTC: generalized tonic clonic; LGS: Lennox–Gastaut syndrome; LKS: Landau–Kleffner syndrome; MPSI: migrating partial seizures of infancy; MAE: myoclonic astatic epilepsy; PFA: paroxysmal fast activity)

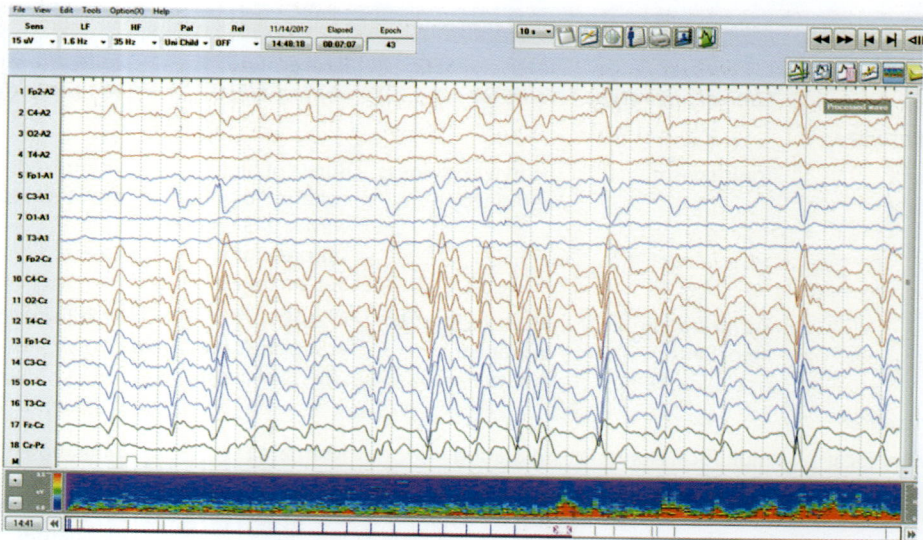

Fig. 2: Normal sleep electroencephalography (EEG) record showing K complexes.

reasons for misinterpretation include poor expertise for EEG interpretation, lack of good-quality EEG recording, inappropriate indication leading to poor yield of EEG, and absence of clinical correlation. Indications of EEG have been summarized in **Table 3**. **Table 4** provides a template of composition of an EEG report.

Characterization of Type of Seizure and Syndromic Diagnosis

Electroencephalography abnormalities are broadly divided into background abnormalities and abnormal epileptiform waveforms. Background abnormalities include diffuse slowing, asymmetric slowing, discontinuous background, and electrodecremental response. Group of disorders with discontinuous EEG background where epileptiform activities contribute to encephalopathy or nonattainment of milestones is called epileptic encephalopathy. This includes early myoclonic encephalopathy, Ohtahara syndrome **(Fig. 3)**, West syndrome **(Fig. 4)**, Lennox–Gastaut syndrome **(Fig. 5)**, and Landau–Kleffner syndrome. There are signature EEG features to diagnose epileptic encephalopathies as these conditions have treatment implications.

Interictal epileptiform discharges can be categorized into focal or generalized based on the morphology of epileptiform discharges and organization of background activity. Generalized spike and spike-wave discharges with normal interictal background activity are observed in childhood/juvenile absence epilepsy (CAE/JAE) **(Fig. 6)**, epilepsy with myoclonic astatic seizures (Doose syndrome), juvenile myoclonic epilepsy (JME), and epilepsy with eyelid myoclonia (Jeavons syndrome). There are a group of self-limited epilepsies with focal stereotyped spikes wherein the focal spikes can be seen with normal interictal EEG background **(Fig. 7)**. This includes Rolandic epilepsy **(Fig. 8)**, Panayiotopoulos syndrome, and benign occipital epilepsies. Children with structural lesion such as neurocysticercosis,

TABLE 3: Uses and abuses of electroencephalography (EEG) in pediatric epilepsy.

Indications for EEG in pediatric practice	When not to use?
EEG helps in differentiating epileptic from nonepileptic clinical event. Video EEG with capture of ictal event is useful adjunct to support clinical possibility of epileptic event	To exclude a diagnosis of epilepsy, since epilepsy is largely a clinical diagnosis
To classify the type of epilepsy into focal or generalized epilepsy and diagnosis of various electroclinical epilepsy syndrome	To monitor the progress of epilepsy with EEG (*Note*: In children with epilepsy, new-onset clinical features such as cognitive decline or behavioral issue warrants fresh EEG to rule out NCSE)
Video EEG monitoring with spell capture is vital to localize the epileptic focus in case of focal epilepsy	To monitor the efficacy of antiepileptic drugs (AED) in epilepsy, except in infantile spasm, LKS, CSWS, or absence epilepsy where there could be no change with AED (*Note*: Valproate and benzodiazepines can decrease the spike burden.)
To characterize the type of epileptic syndrome based on cluster of clinical seizure semiology, age at onset, and EEG findings	Intracranial space-occupying lesions include stroke without any history of seizures or raised intracranial pressure to form the basis of starting prophylactic AED.
It helps clinician to decide on tapering AED after a seizure-free interval and to predict possible relapse after tapering antiepileptic drug	Clinical history that clearly suggests paroxysmal nonepileptic event such as shuddering spells, gratification, and syncopal attacks
To guide about the etiology in a case of meningoencephalitis, e.g., periodic lateralized epileptiform discharges (PLEDs) in case of herpes simplex encephalitis	
To diagnose NCSE in case of prolonged coma after status epilepticus or encephalopathy of unknown etiology	
In children with cognitive or language regression even without seizures, it is indispensable to rule out epileptic encephalopathy like CSWS and LKS	
To prognosticate an epileptic disorder, e.g., periodic complexes and triphasic waves in a sick patient in ICU is suggestive of poor prognosis. Also, presence of epileptiform discharges predicts seizure recurrence in epilepsy	
Ancillary test for documentation of brain death	

(AED: antiepileptic drug; CSWS: continuous spike wave in sleep; LKS: Landau–Kleffner syndrome; NCSE: nonconvulsive status epilepticus;)

glioma, or vascular lesion can also have focal epileptiform discharges. Children with subacute sclerosing panencephalitis can have periodic epileptiform discharges **(Fig. 9)**. One can predict structural abnormality based on focal slowing **(Fig. 10)**.

TABLE 4: Essential components of electroencephalography (EEG) report.

Parts of report	Description	Sample EEG report
History	Clinical history, indication, medication, and imaging findings	A 10-year-old boy with multiple episodes of left focal seizure with normal MRI
Technical details	• Number of electrodes (21-channel electrodes) • Electrode placement technique (10–20 system) use of filters (1.6–70 Hz) • Sensitivity (7–10 µV) • Duration of recording (20–30 minutes)	21-channel electrodes were placed using 10–20 system. Record lasted for 30 minutes
	Use of premedication must be documented. State of the patient: Awake, sleep, drowsy, or comatose must also be mentioned	Child was awake and cooperative during the record. HV and PS were performed.
EEG description	Background electrocerebral activity *Normal awake:* As posterior dominant rhythm with reactivity to external stimuli *Normal sleep:* Presence of sleep markers and preservation of sleep architecture in sleep record	Background activity consists of 9–10 Hz, 60–80 µV posterior dominant reactive rhythm
	Abnormality in background described in terms of: • Frequency and voltage • Continuous or intermittent • Location (right or left) • Topography (frontal, parietal, temporal, or occipital)	There was intermittent delta (2–3 Hz and 60–90 µV) slowing in right temporal region
	Epileptiform discharges are described in terms of: • Morphology (spike, sharp, spike wave, and polyspike) • Frequency (Hz) • Voltage, location, pattern (run, rhythmic, and periodic) • Incidence (rare, intermittent, occasional, frequent, and continuous) or preferably quantification and duration of abnormality	There were frequent runs of spike wave discharges (3.5–4.5 Hz, 150–250 µV) arising from right temporal region that lasts for variable duration of 3–5 seconds. These discharges occupy almost 60% of EEG epochs. HV and PS did not augment the discharges
Impression	Normal or abnormal; if abnormal: Background abnormality and epileptiform discharges	Abnormal EEG record suggestive of right temporal epileptiform discharges with background slowing
Clinical correlation	• Focal slowing could indicate underlying structural lesion • Lack of organized background could indicate encephalopathy • Suggestions for sleep record and comparison with previous EEG should be mentioned	Possibility of underlying structural lesion needs to be explored

(HV: hyperventilation; PS: photic stimulation)

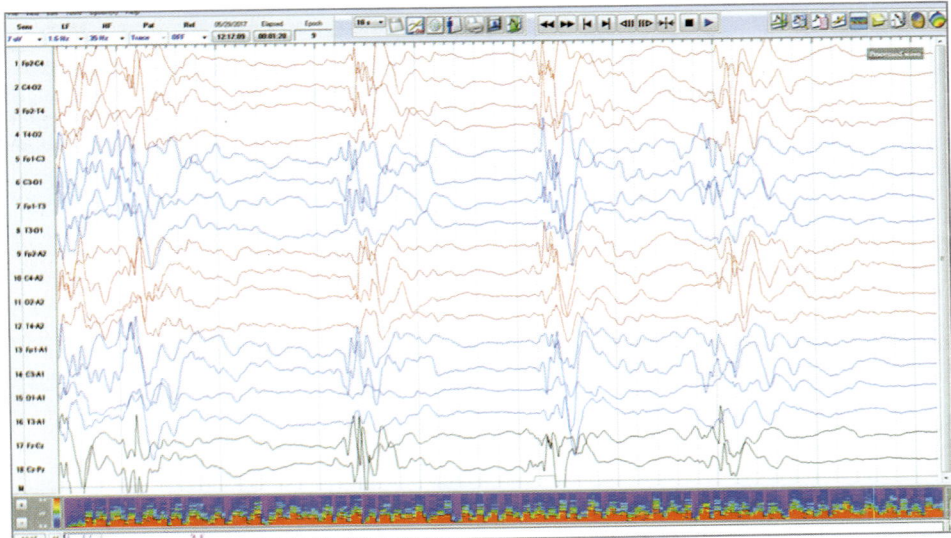

Fig. 3: Electroencephalography (EEG) showing burst suppression in a child with Ohtahara syndrome.

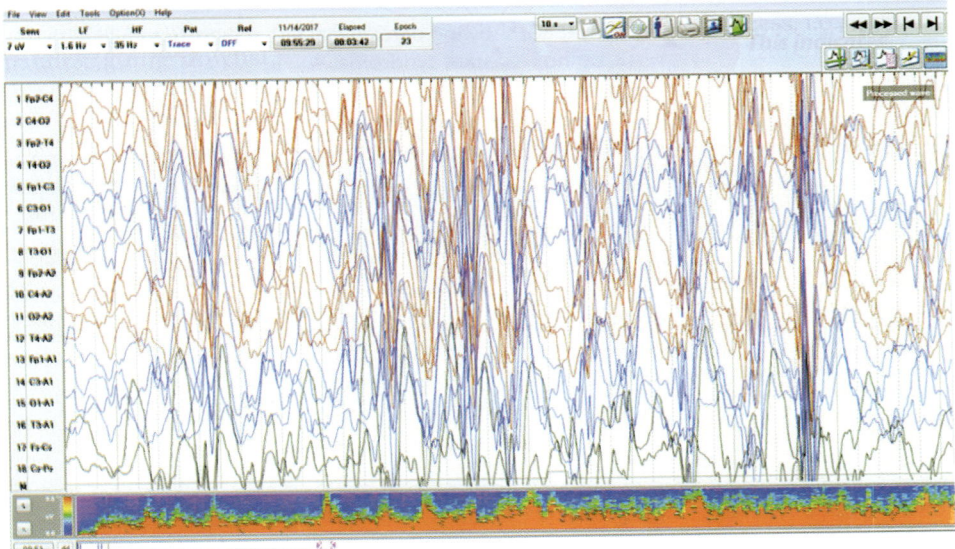

Fig. 4: High-voltage, chaotic epileptiform discharges suggestive of classical hypsarrhythmia.

Common Abnormalities in Electroencephalography

- In a child with *first episode of unprovoked focal seizure*, a sleep-deprived EEG record would be useful. Both awake and sleep records are essential to detect and improve the yield of picking up focal epileptiform abnormalities.
- In a child with episode of *status epilepticus*, febrile status epilepticus, or focal febrile

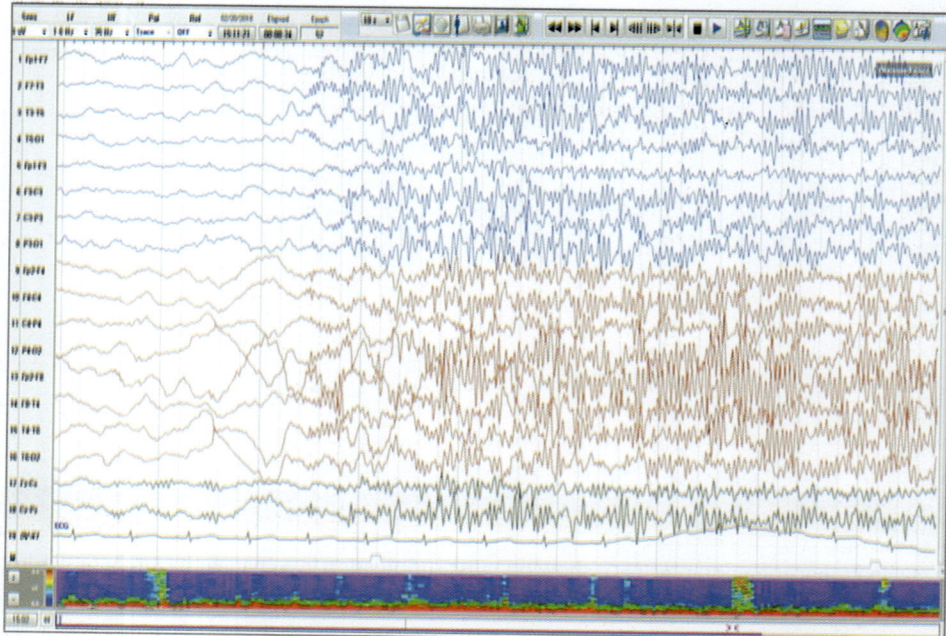

Fig. 5: Electroencephalography (EEG) showing paroxysmal fast activity in a child with Lennox–Gastaut syndrome.

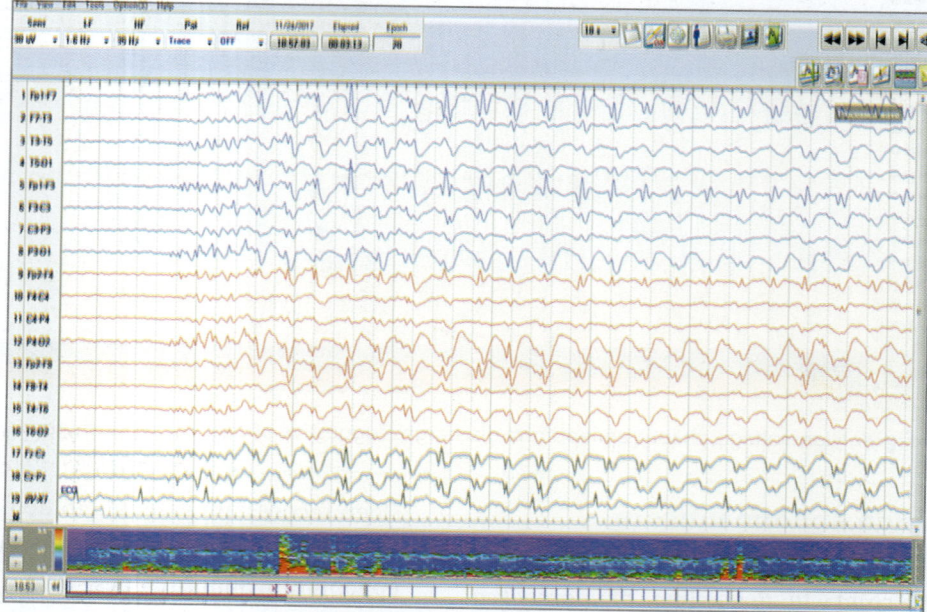

Fig. 6: Electroencephalography (EEG) showing generalized epileptiform discharges in child with juvenile absence epilepsy.

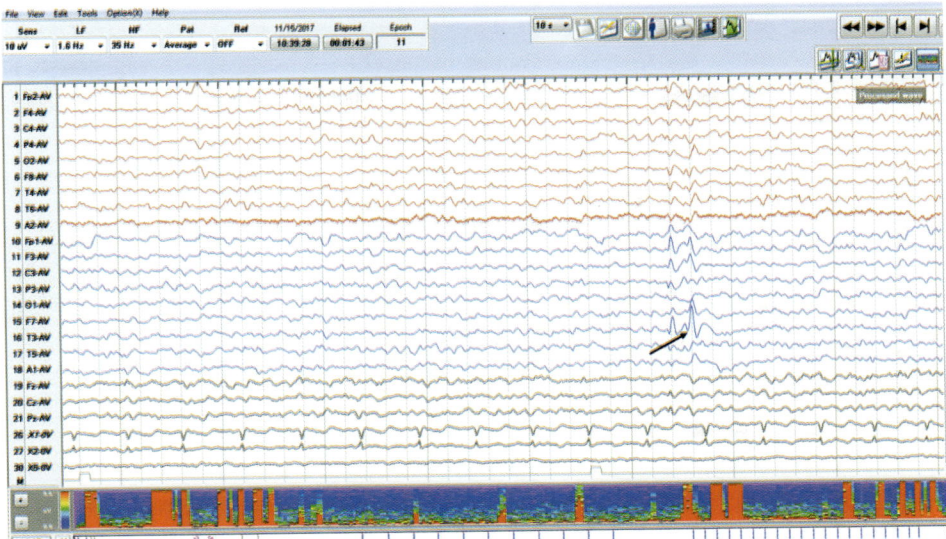

Fig. 7: Electroencephalography (EEG) showing left temporal epileptiform discharges (arrow).

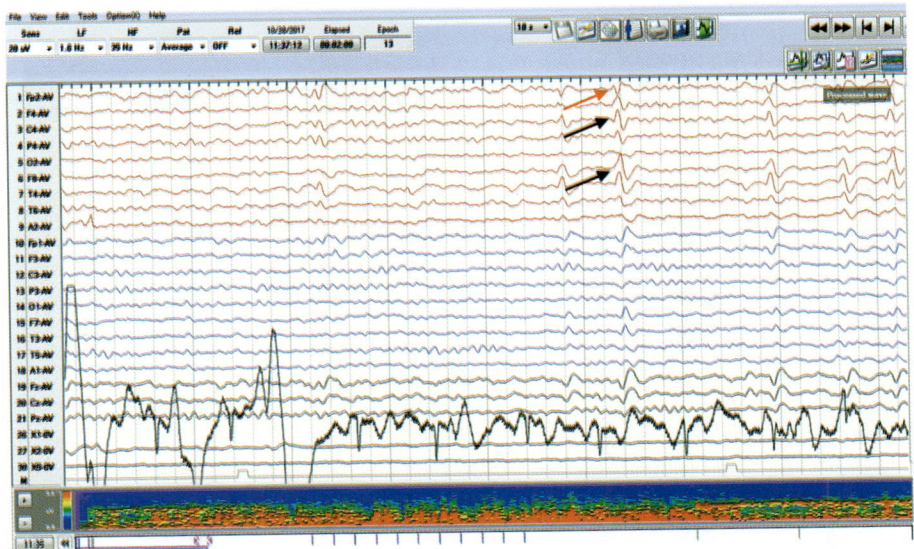

Fig. 8: Electroencephalography (EEG) showing right centrotemporal epileptiform discharges (black arrows) with tangential dipole (red arrow) suggestive of Rolandic epilepsy.

seizures, it would be ideal to get sleep EEG record to look for possible temporal discharges arising from hippocampal injury.

- In a child with suspected *absence seizures*, awake EEG record with good hyperventilation would be ideal to pick up 3-Hz generalized spike wave discharge.

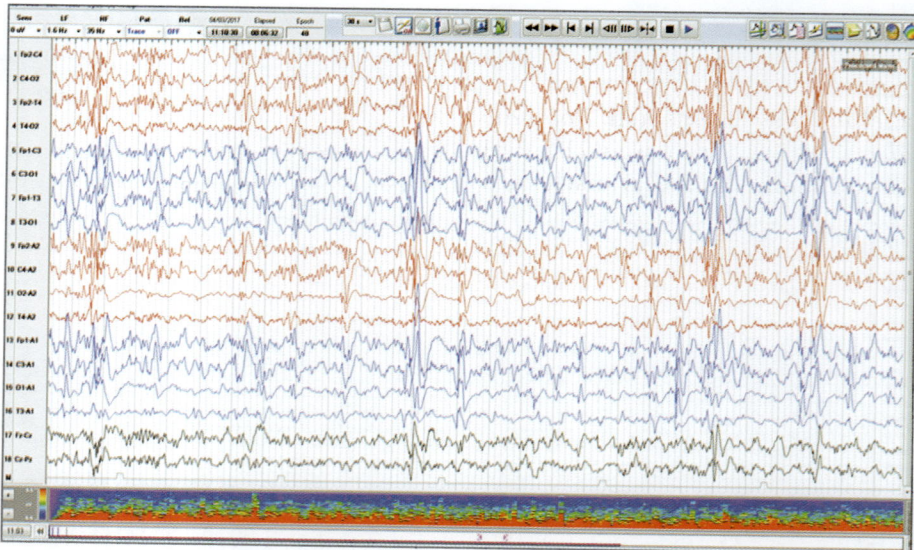

Fig. 9: Periodic interictal epileptiform discharges in a child with subacute sclerosing panencephalitis (SSPE).

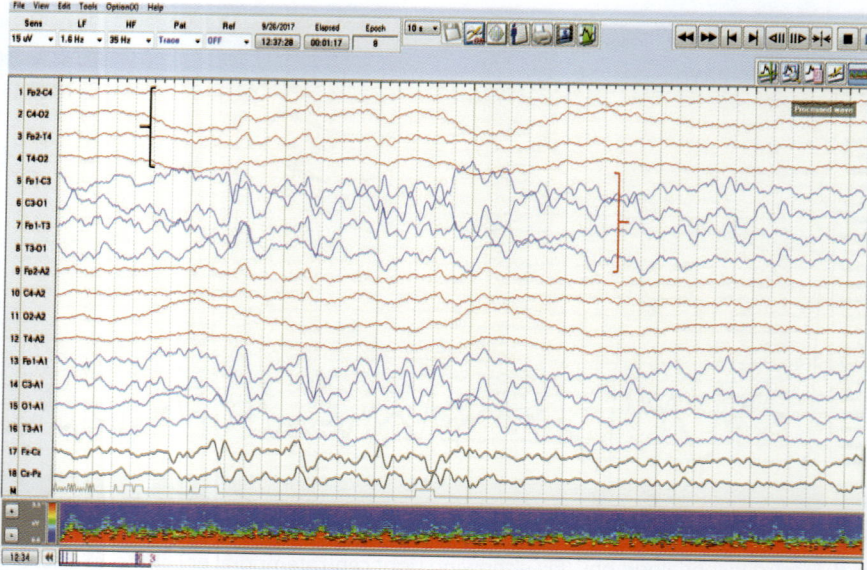

Fig. 10: Electroencephalography (EEG) showing right hemispheric slowing (black curly bracket) evident when compared to left hemisphere (red curly bracket) suggesting an underlying right hemispheric lesion.

Similarly, in a child with suspected Juvenile myoclonic epilepsy, 4–5-Hz generalized spike wave discharges are evident on photic stimulation.

- In a child with *suspected occipital seizures* based on semiology of visual hallucinations, awake EEG record with fixation off sensitivity is required.

- In a child with *West syndrome*, a sleep EEG record would often reveal hypsarrhythmia or modified version of hypsarrhythmia.
- In a child with suspected *Rolandic seizures*, sleep EEG record would be ideal to look for centrotemporal discharges with or without tangential dipole, which might be missed on an awake EEG record.
- In a child with *developmental delay and epilepsy*, new onset of unexplained encephalopathy or behavioral problems warrants a sleep EEG to look for evidence of CSWS.
- In a child with well-controlled structural or *focal epilepsy*, a normal sleep EEG record is essential before deciding to taper the antiepileptic drug.
- In a child with status epilepticus, with persistent unexplained encephalopathy following convulsive status epilepticus, an ambulatory EEG is required to look for nonconvulsive status epilepticus (NCSE).

EVOKED POTENTIALS

Brainstem-evoked Auditory Potential

Evoked potentials refer to electrical activity in response to specific stimulus such as auditory, visual, or somatosensory. This electrical response is recorded from the surface of the scalp. In auditory evoked potentials, a sound passes through the external and middle ear to reach cochlea where auditory potentials are generated. It travels through cochlear nerve, cochlear nucleus, superior olivary complex, lateral lemniscus, inferior colliculus, and medial geniculate body to finally reach auditory cortex **(Fig. 11)**. This electric response called brainstem-evoked auditory potential (BEAP) tests the integrity of pathway from cochlea to auditory cortex and is used for assessment of hearing in newborns and older children.

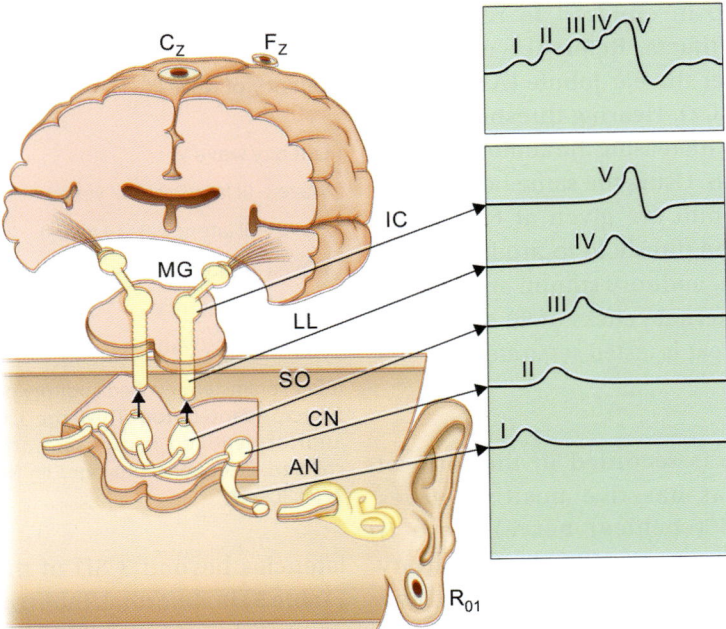

Fig. 11: Origin of brainstem-evoked auditory potentials (BEAP) waveforms. (AN: auditory nerve; CN: cochlear nucleus; SO: superior olivary nucleus; LL: lateral lemniscus; IC: inferior colliculus)

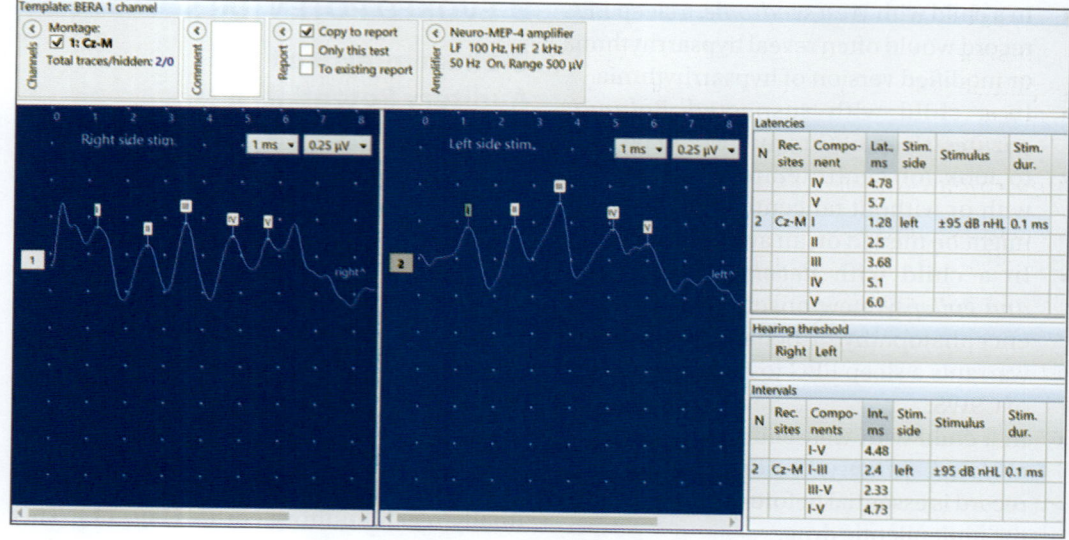

Fig. 12: Normal brainstem-evoked potentials.

Procedure

The BEAP is recorded in a quiet room with an ambient temperature of 28°C. It is preferably done in sleep in children to reduce the movement artifacts. Reference electrodes are placed over the ear lobule (A1/A2) and in the vertex (Cz). Hearing threshold is first determined by increasing the auditory stimuli from 0 to 50 dB. Using the same headphone, repetitive stimuli are given at 60 dB and 75 dB above the threshold to produce BEAP. By convention, auditory stimuli are given in the form of alternate clicks of 90 dB (11 per second). Each ear is tested separately.

Waveforms

The response is recorded in the form of waveform that has five positive waves (I–V)—wave I (cochlear nerve), wave II (cochlear nucleus), wave III (superior olivary complex), wave IV (lateral lemniscus), and wave V (inferior colliculus). The waveform is analyzed in terms of latency and amplitude of the waveform **(Fig. 12)**. Prolongation of latencies beyond 3 SD of the normal data **(Table 5)** is abnormal. Interpeak latencies are more prolonged in children when compared to adults. Interpeak latencies of I–III represent auditory nerve and caudal brainstem and

TABLE 5: Normal values of interpeak latencies and amplitude of wave V/wave I ratio.

BEAP parameters	Girls	Boys
Latency of wave I	1.64 (4–7 years); 1.61 (8–14 years)	
Latency of wave III	3.61 (4–7 years); 3.72 (8–14 years)	
Latency wave V	5.48	5.61
Wave I–III latency (4–7 years)	1.97	2.06
Wave I–III latency (8–14 years)	2.01	2.11
Wave I–V latency	3.87	3.98
Wave III–V latency	1.88	1.88
Amplitude V/I ratio	1.74	

(BEAP: brainstem-evoked auditory potentials)
Source: Adapted from Thivierge J, Cote R. Brainstem auditory evoked response: normative values in children. Electroencephalogr Clin Neurophysiol. 1990; 77(4):309-13.

interpeak latencies of III–V represent rostral brainstem and midbrain. The ratio of amplitude of wave V/wave I is normally more than 0.5.

Abnormalities in Waveforms

If the BEAP shows prolongation of wave I–III latencies with relatively normal wave III–V latencies, it possibly indicates a brainstem structural pathology. Extra-axial brainstem tumor such as acoustic neuroma shows prolongation of wave I–III and I–V interpeak latencies, whereas intra-axial brainstem tumors shows prolongation of III–V and I–V latencies. Prolongation of both wave I–III latencies and wave III–V latencies indicates a diffuse pathology such as demyelination (e.g., multiple sclerosis). In addition, it is clinically useful in postsurgical patients of posterior fossa tumor to see the integrity of waveforms. It is also useful for prognosis of posttraumatic and anoxic coma, especially absence of wave III to wave V indicates a poor prognosis. Absence of wave I can indicate peripheral auditory nerve damage. Factors known to influence BEAP latencies and amplitude include age, gender, temperature, stimulus rate, and stimulus intensity, anthropometric variables. It is not influenced by sleep, coma, or sedation.

Visual-evoked Potentials

Principle

Conduction in visual pathway from retina to striate occipital cortex is assessed by visual-evoked potential (VEP). It is based on cortical response to a patterned (*patterned VEP*) or unpatterned (*flash VEP*) visual stimulus. It is a function of the central visual pathway. *Checkerboard pattern reversal* is the most commonly used patterned visual stimulus for VEP. In this method, black and white boxes are flipped at a rate of 2–4 Hz (2–4 per second). Patterned VEPs are more sensitive and specific for abnormalities of visual pathway when compared to flash VEP. However, in uncooperative children and those who are unable to focus on the light, flash VEP is commonly used.

Waveforms

In VEP, negative polarity is designated as N and positive polarity is designated as P. Low-rate stimulation of patterned VEP typically produces a V-shaped wave. It has three components—N1 or N75, P1 or P100, and N2 or N145. Initial negative wave (N1) is followed by positive wave (P1), which is followed by N2 (second negative wave).

The majority of clinical interpretation of patterned VEP is restricted to P100 latencies and to a lesser extent P100 amplitude. Impairment anywhere along the visual pathway will affect P100. In general, demyelinating lesions such as optic neuritis affect P100 latencies; whereas, ischemic, compressive, or toxic lesions will affect P100 amplitude **(Figs. 13A and B)**.

In flash VEP, there are six waves labeled as wave I–VI. There is lot of individual variations in the latencies of these peaks. Hence, the utility of flash VEP is restricted to elicitation or no elicitation of response. There are no normative data for flash VEP latencies. Electrodes are placed as per the international 10–20 system (Oz, O1, and O2 electrodes).

- Prolonged P100 latencies with reduced amplitude are surrogate markers of optic nerve lesions such as optic neuritis and multiple sclerosis.
- Larger amplitudes of N1-P1 and P1-N2 are observed in children with migraine.
- Visual-evoked potential is a good indicator of subclinical visual impairment. This is specifically useful in determining the

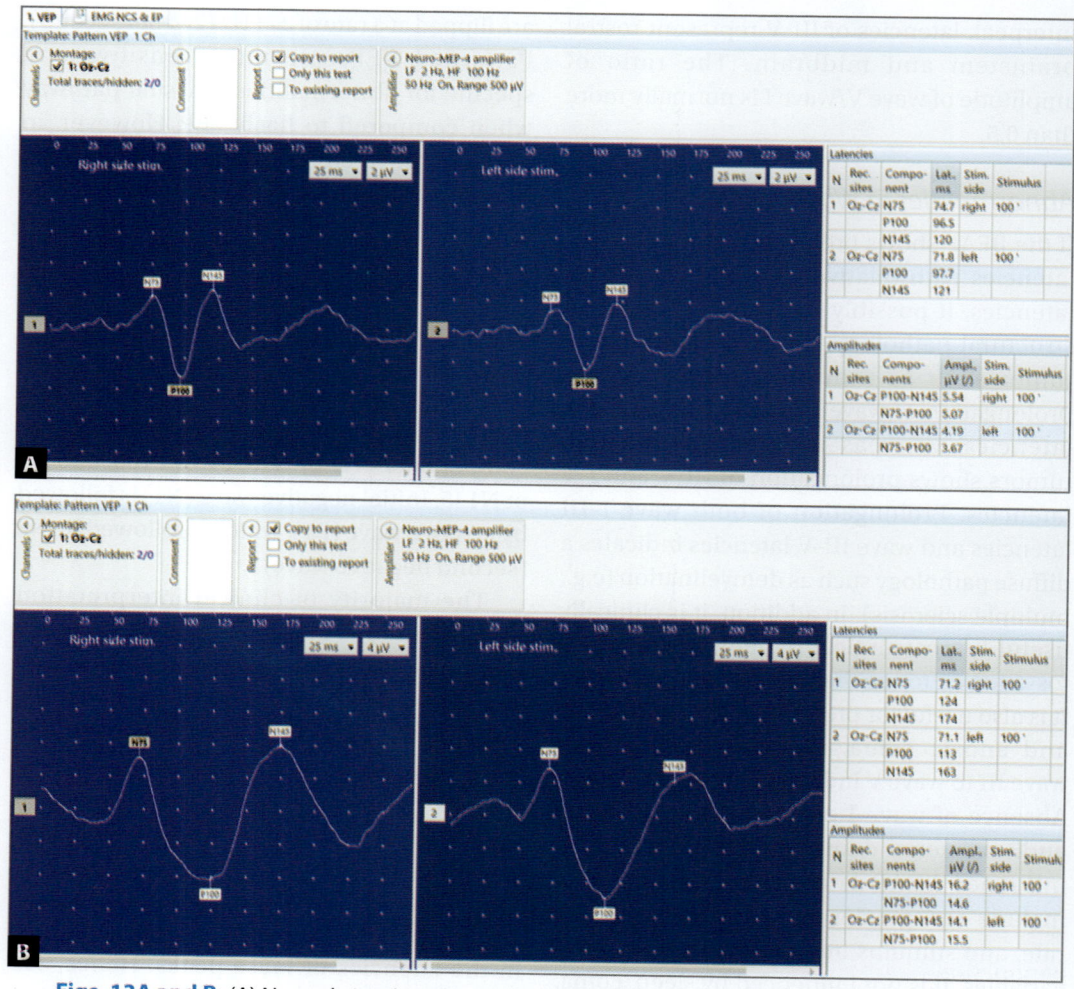

Figs. 13A and B: (A) Normal visual-evoked potential (VEP) with N75, P100, and N145 waveforms; (B) Prolonged P100 latencies (P100 latency = 124 msec).

need for surgical intervention among those with benign raised intracranial pressure.
- It is also useful in diagnosis of neurodegenerative disorders such as neuronal ceroid lipofuscinosis (NCL).
- Newer methods such as multifocal VEPs are useful to detect small abnormalities in optic nerve pathway. Normal VEP response in a patient with suspected nonorganic or psychogenic blindness supports the clinical diagnosis.

Abnormalities in VEP waveform can be detected even with normal optic pathway as in conditions with uncorrected refractory errors, amblyopia, and excessive fatigue. VEP is, thus, a noninvasive, simple, low-cost method for diagnosis of abnormalities of visual pathway.

Somatosensory Evoked Potentials

Electrophysiological response of nervous system to electric stimulation of somatic

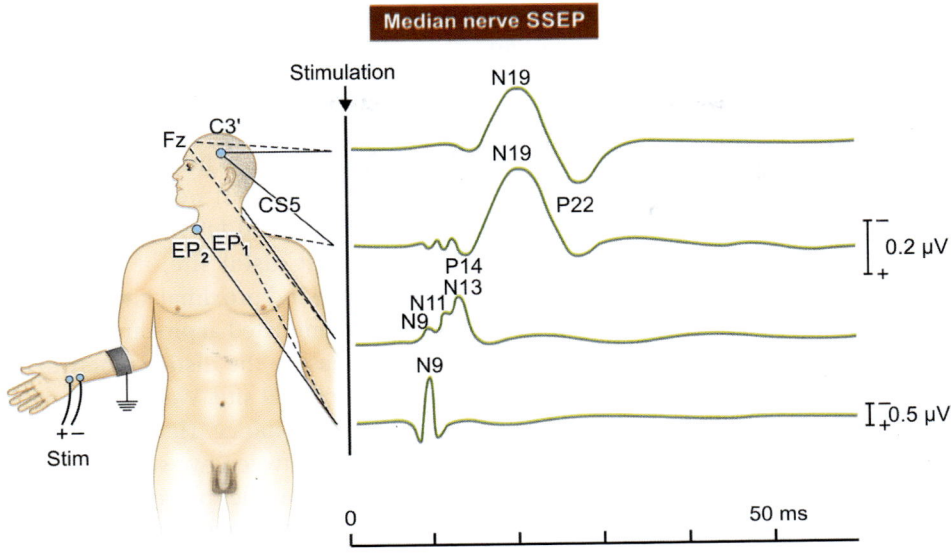

Fig. 14: Somatosensory-evoked potential (SSEP) generated on stimulation of median nerve.

peripheral nerve is called somatosensory-evoked potential (SSEP). On stimulation of mixed motor and sensory nerves such as median nerve (2–4 Hz, 100–500 repetition, 0.2–2-ms duration), there will be orthodromic conduction to the muscle to generate compound muscle action potential (CMAP) and there will be antidromic conduction along sensory Ia fibers to spinal cord. It reaches and ascends along the dorsal column, decussate at the level to medulla, ascend to contralateral thalamus to finally reach parietal sensory cortex.

This response along the sensory pathway can be recorded from the scalp using C3 and C4 electrodes with Cz, Fz acting as reference electrodes (cortical SSEP), cervicomedullary junction at cervical spine (brainstem SSEP) or along the Erb point (N9) and on antecubital fossa **(Fig. 14)**. This response can be tested in the lower limbs in the tibial and peroneal nerve. Hence, on testing upper limb nerves, integrity of dorsal column is tested and on testing lower limb nerves, additional integrity of spinocerebellar pathway is also tested. It is largely influenced by noise and muscle artifacts.

Dorsal column loss is suspected when there is >50% decrease in amplitude and >10% increase in latency. SSEPs are resistant to sedation and most of anesthetic agents but are sensitive to hypoxic damage. Hence, absence of SSEP following a hypoxic event in intensive care unit (ICU) will predict a poor outcome.

■ NERVE CONDUCTION STUDY

Physiology

Electrophysiological study of peripheral nerve is called nerve conduction study (NCS). NCS can study only peripheral large (α) myelinated motor and sensory fibers. Motor response to electrical stimulus is summated as CMAP and sensory response as sensory nerve action potential (SNAP). An electric stimulus on the nerve depolarizes the nerve fibers. As the stimulus strength increases, more and more fibers will be recruited till it reaches a maximum, beyond which increasing the stimulus strength does not affect the CMAP/SNAP. We usually give supramaximal stimulus to reduce the technical variability.

Procedure

The electrode that is used to stimulate is called stimulating electrodes. The stimulus is provided at one distal site **(Fig. 15; S1)** and one proximal site **(Fig. 15; S2)**. The motor response is recorded by two surface electrodes placed over the muscle (active electrode) and its tendon (reference electrode). These electrodes are called recording electrodes. A ground electrode is placed between the stimulating and recording electrode for zero voltage reference.

Motor Nerve Conduction Study

Upward deflection in electrophysiology is negative and downward deflection from baseline is positive. When a motor nerve is stimulated, the time interval between stimulation and first negative deflection in the CMAP is called *latency*. If the nerve was stimulated at distal site, it is called distal latency (DL) and proximal latency (PL) when nerve was stimulated at proximal site **(Fig. 16)**. We can measure the distance between distal site and proximal site. We know that velocity is time upon distance. Hence, once we enter the distance between two stimuli, the velocity or rather the conduction velocity (CV) can be determined. The maximum amplitude of the CMAP is also recorded.

Amplitude is the height of the negative peak from baseline, area is the area under negative waveform, and duration is time from start of negative peak to return to baseline.

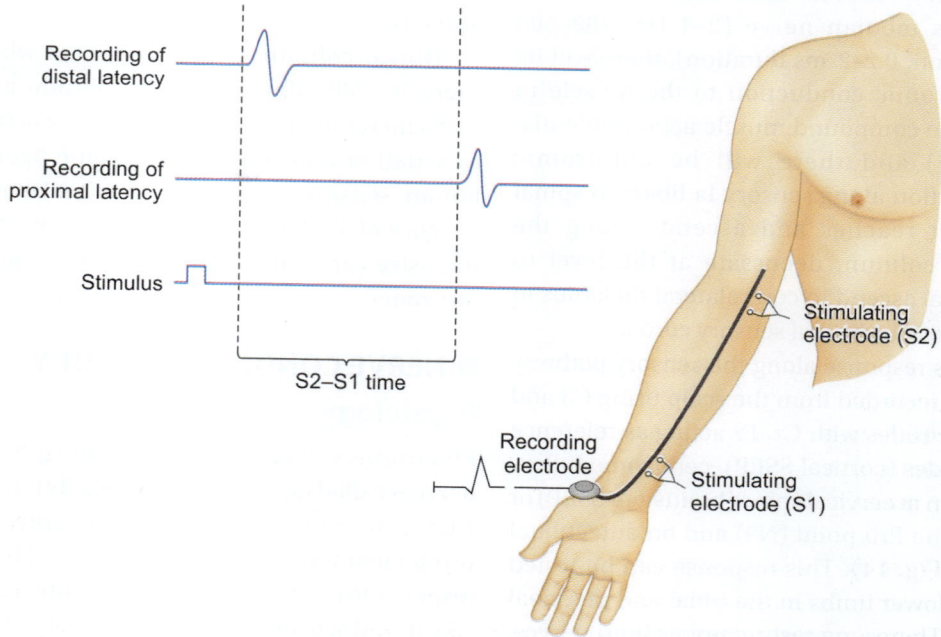

Fig. 15: Procedure of nerve conduction study along with waveforms.

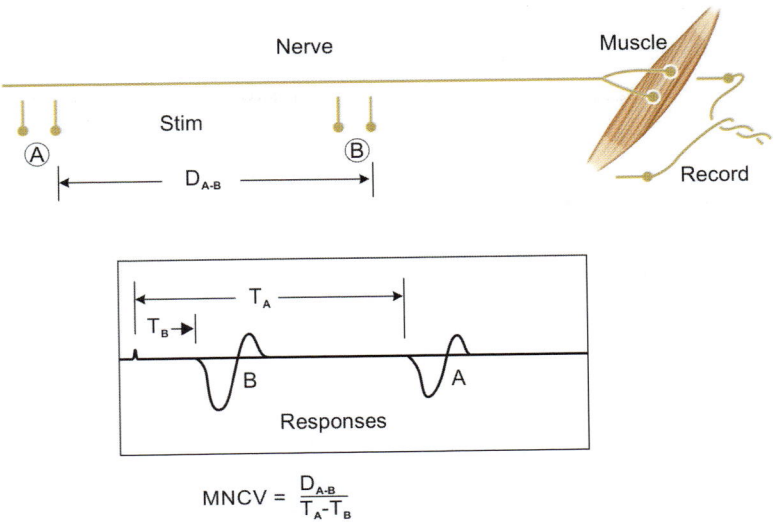

Fig. 16: Basic motor nerve conduction. (D: distance; T: time; A: proximal site; B: distal site)

$$MNCV = \frac{D_{A-B}}{T_A - T_B}$$

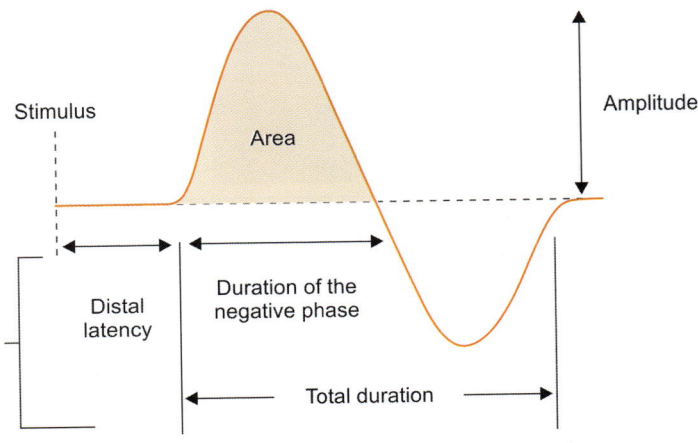

Fig. 17: Parameters of nerve conduction study.

Hence, we have three main parameters—compound muscle action potential or amplitude (CMAP), CV, and DL **(Fig. 17)**. We usually test median nerve, ulnar nerve in the upper limb, and peroneal nerve and tibial nerve in the lower limb **(Table 6 and Fig. 18)**.

Sensory Nerve Conduction Study

We know sensations move from distal to proximal. There are no synapses in the peripheral nerve. It ends in dorsal root ganglia.

If we stimulate the sensory nerve at distal site and record it proximally, it is called *orthodromic conduction*. However, if we stimulate the nerve proximally and record this distally, it is called *antidromic conduction*. It is technically much easier to do antidromic conduction rather than orthodromic conduction study while performing sensory NCS. There is a stimulating electrode and a recording electrode. The distance between the two is measured to calculate CV. Amplitude

TABLE 6: Commonly performed motor nerve conduction study in upper and lower limbs.

	Distal stimulation	Proximal stimulation	Muscle
Median	Wrist (PL/FCR)	Elbow	Abductor pollicis brevis
Ulnar	Wrist (medial to FCR)	Elbow (medial epicondyle)	Abductor digiti minimi
Peroneal	Ankle	Knee (fibular head)	Extensor digitorum brevis
Tibial	Ankle (Behind medial malleolus)	Knee (popliteal fossa)	Abductor hallucis

(FCR: flexor carpi radialis; PL: palmaris longus)

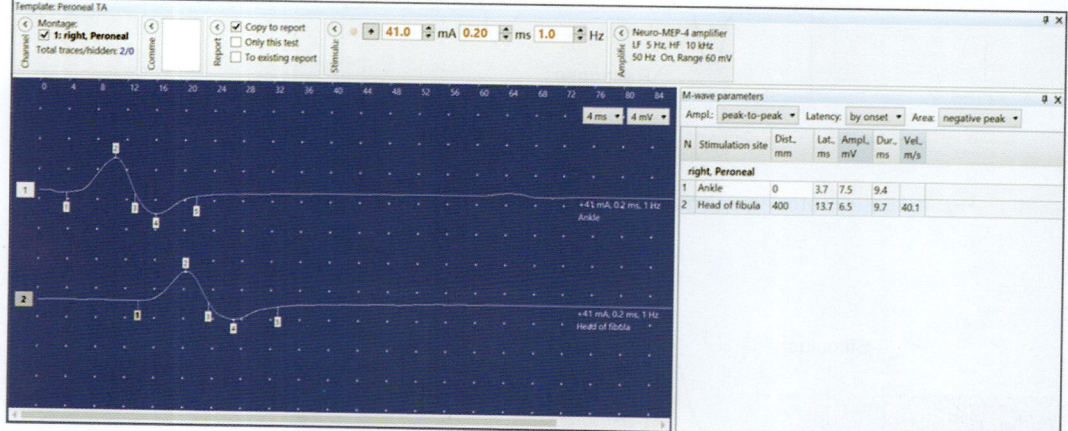

Fig. 18: Motor nerve conduction study in common peroneal nerve.
Note: Distal latency is 3.7 ms, conduction velocity is 40.1 m/s, and amplitude is 7.5 mV on distal stimulation and 6.5 mV on proximal stimulation representing normal values.

(SNAP), latency, and CV of sensory nerve are measured. Notice here that there is single stimulating electrode in sensory NCS vis-a-vis two electrodes in motor NCS.

Clinical Applications

It is very important to note that only largest and fastest conducting fibers (fine touch, vibration, and position sense) are tested by NCS. Hence, in small fiber neuropathy despite symptoms of burning and tingling sensations, the sensory NCS can often be normal. Another important note is that sensory NCS will not test conduction beyond dorsal root ganglion **(Fig. 19)**. Hence, in a preganglionic lesion (between the spinal cord and dorsal root ganglion), the sensory NCS can be normal. However, if there is a postganglionic lesion (beyond dorsal root ganglion), NCS will be abnormal. This is relevant information in congenital Erb palsy where a preganglionic lesion might reveal normal NCS, although the baby has severe motor weakness and segmental areflexia. Commonly tested sensory nerves include median nerve, ulnar nerve, and sural nerve **(Fig. 20)**.

F-Wave

When you throw a stone in a pond of water, you get a string of waves that hits the

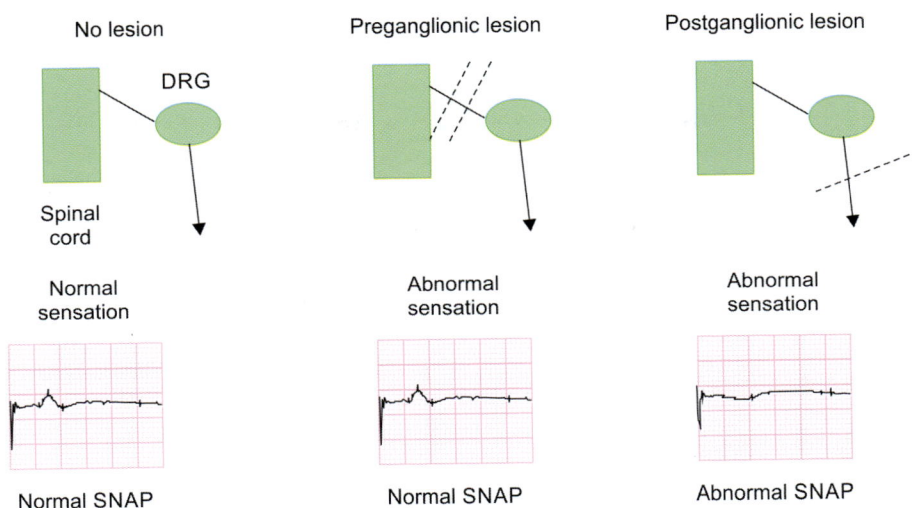

Fig. 19: Sensory nerve conduction study results in a preganglionic and postganglionic lesion. (DRG: dorsal root ganglion; SNAP: sensory nerve action potential)

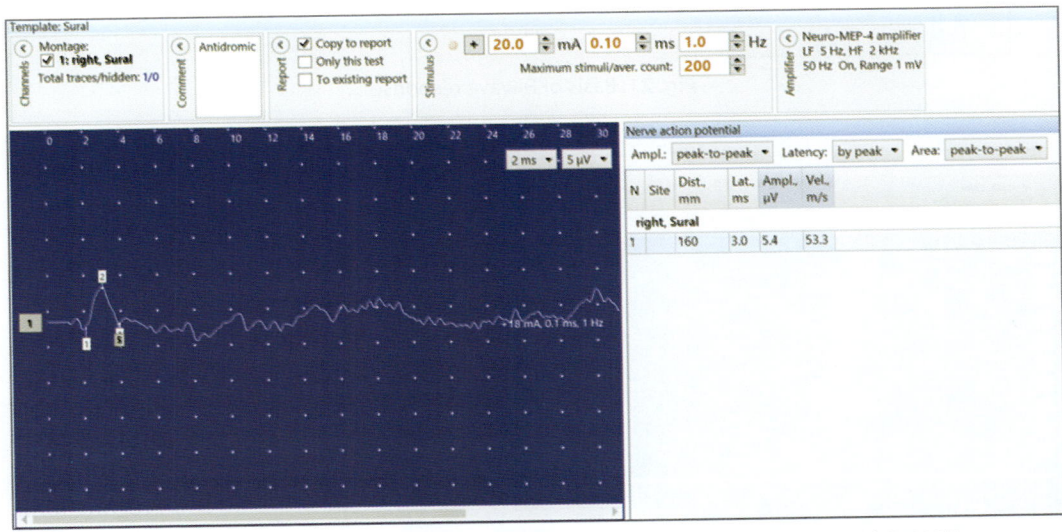

Fig. 20: Normal sural nerve sensory response [sensory nerve action potential (SNAP)].

boundary wall and gets back with smaller waves back to center. Similarly, when an electric stimulation is given to a motor nerve, there is orthodromic conduction to muscle (which generates CMAP) and there is antidromic conduction along the motor nerve to spinal cord followed by return along the same motor nerve orthodromically to the muscle to generate a very small waveform called F-wave **(Fig. 21)**. Hence, F-wave is *not* a true reflex. It is a good indicator of proximal peripheral nerve root lesion **(Fig. 22)**.

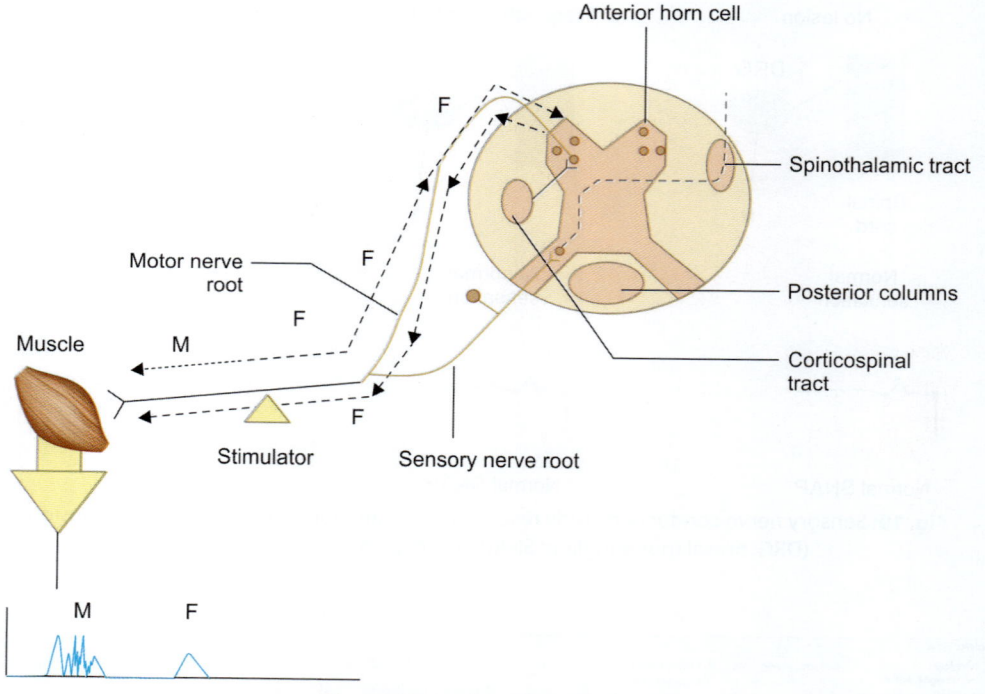

Fig. 21: Basis of F-wave response.

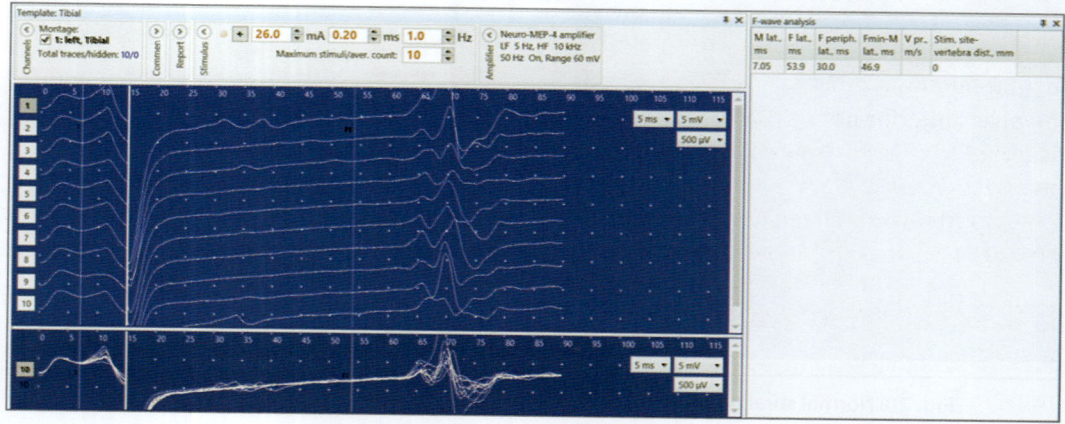

Fig. 22: F-wave response in tested tibial nerve in a child with early stage of demyelinating polyneuropathy.
Note: Prolongation of minimal F-wave latency to 53.9 ms.

This F-wave is extremely useful in diagnosis of early demyelination, which involves only proximal nerve roots before involving entire peripheral nerves.

H Reflex

H reflex is initiated with a submaximal electric stimulus delivered for prolonged period. Such stimulus over the skin stimulates

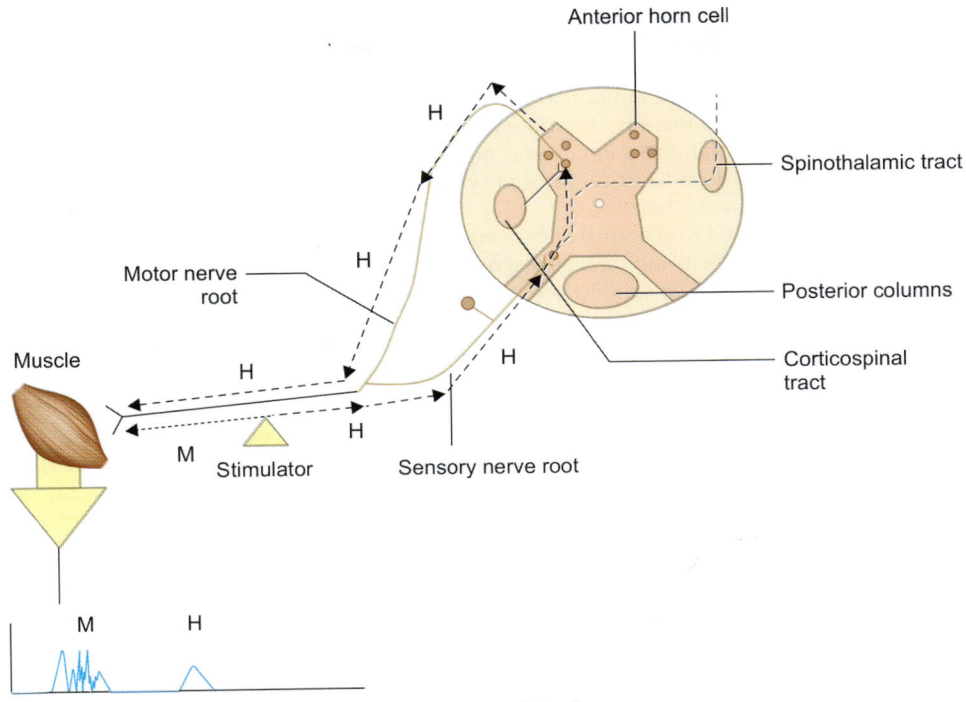

Fig. 23: Basis of H reflex.

Ia afferent sensory fibers, which in turn stimulate anterior horn cell to generate motor action potentiation. This is a true reflex as it involves anterior horn cell **(Fig. 23)**. H reflex is useful to determine the integrity of S1 root in radiculopathy.

Important tips related to nerve conduction study (NCV) are summarized in **Box 1**.

■ ELECTROMYOGRAPHY

Electrical activity recorded directly from the muscle is called electromyography (EMG). Its utility is limited in pediatrics. EMG is used to differentiate neurogenic from myogenic cause of weakness **(Table 7)**. It is useful for neuropathies and in localizing the site of lesion in plexopathies. It can be useful to see signs of recovery in traumatic neuropathies in terms of reinnervation potentials. It is a painful investigation, seldom used in this era of molecular genetics and limited cooperation from children. A disposable concentric needle is inserted into the muscle to record this electrical activity.

Components of EMG Record

There are three components of EMG recording—(1) spontaneous activity, (2) motor unit action potential (MUAP), and (3) interference pattern.

Spontaneous activity:
- Normally, a relaxed muscle is silent; this resting activity is called *spontaneous activity* of the muscle.
- In case of denervation, the resting muscle becomes hypersensitive and discharge spontaneously. These discharges are recorded as *fibrillations*. It is not only seen in acute and chronic denervation,

BOX 1: Basic facts on nerve conduction study.

- Nerve conduction study always tests myelinated nerve fibers. Unmyelinated fibers conduct very slowly and make no significant contribution to CMAP/SNAP
- Amplitude indicates axonal integrity; distal latency and conduction velocity indicate integrity of myelin. Myelin helps to conduct the impulse faster, whereas axons determine how strong will be the impulse. So, axonal loss will reduce the amplitude whereas myelin loss will result in increased distal latency and decreased conduction velocity
- CMAP amplitude reduction with normal or marginally increased latency and normal or marginally decreased conduction velocity indicates axonal neuropathy
- Prolonged latency with reduced conduction velocity with or without marginal reduction in amplitude implies demyelinating pathology. Amplitude will be decreased in demyelinating pathology only if there is "conduction block" or "temporal dispersion" or secondary axonal loss **(Fig. 24)**
- Normally, waveform of distal stimulation and proximal stimulation are nearly identical. The amplitude of a proximal stimulated waveform is less than a distal stimulated waveform. If there is >20% decline in the amplitude of proximal stimulation when compared to amplitude of distal stimulation, it indicates "*conduction block*". Conduction block always implies acquired demyelination **(Fig. 25)**
- When proximal waveform has longer duration (by >30%) and smaller amplitude (by >20%) but same area when compared to distal stimulated waveform, then this is called *temporal dispersion*. This indicates segmental demyelination **(Fig. 26)**
- F-wave latency is a surrogate marker for integrity of proximal nerve roots. Prolonged F-wave latency indicates proximal demyelinating pathology
- Abnormality in nerve conduction can be classified based on:
    - Whether *motor* or *sensory* or both are affected?
    - *Type:* Whether it is primarily axonal or demyelinating neuropathy?
    - *Number of affected nerves:* Is it mononeuropathy or polyneuropathy?
    - *Site:* Does it involve predominantly lower limb nerves and/or upper limb nerves?

(CMAP: compound muscle action potential; SNAP: sensory nerve action potential)

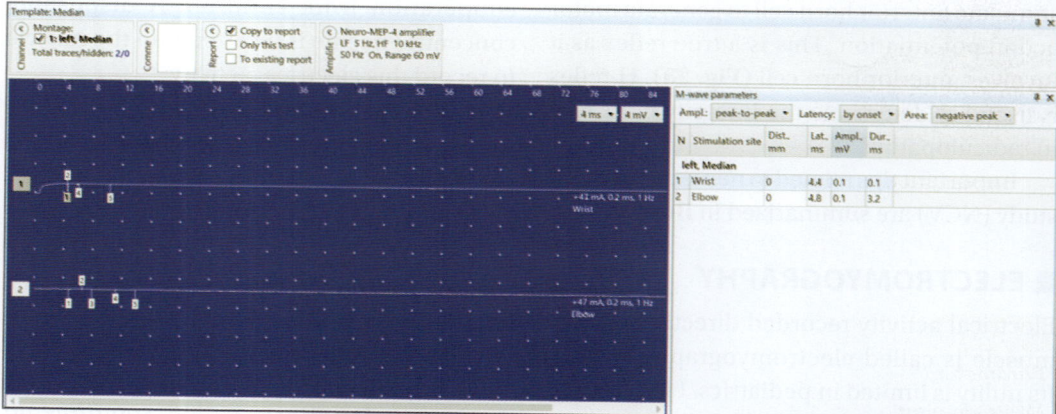

Fig. 24: Nerve conduction study showing markedly reduced (0.1 mV) compound muscle action potential (CMAP) amplitude suggestive of motor axonal neuropathy.

but also seen in dystrophic process and inflammatory muscle disease.

- *Fasciculations* are isolated discharges that are large and complex; they occur at irregular interval **(Fig. 27)**. It can be seen in motor neuron disease, spinal muscular atrophy, and other radiculopathies and neuropathies.

CHAPTER 6: Neurophysiologic Evaluation   163

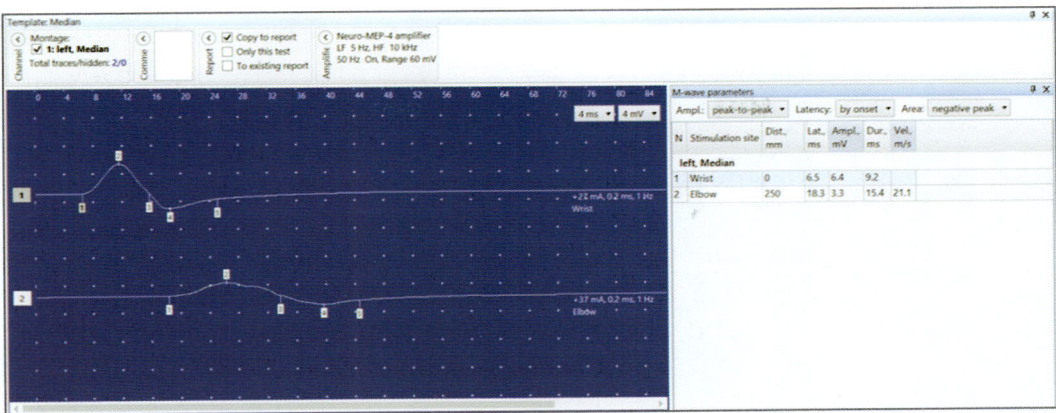

Fig. 25: Nerve conduction study showing prolonged distal latency (6.5 msec) with reduced conduction velocity (21.1 m/s) with temporal dispersion (flat looking wave) in the proximal stimulated waveform (wave 2).

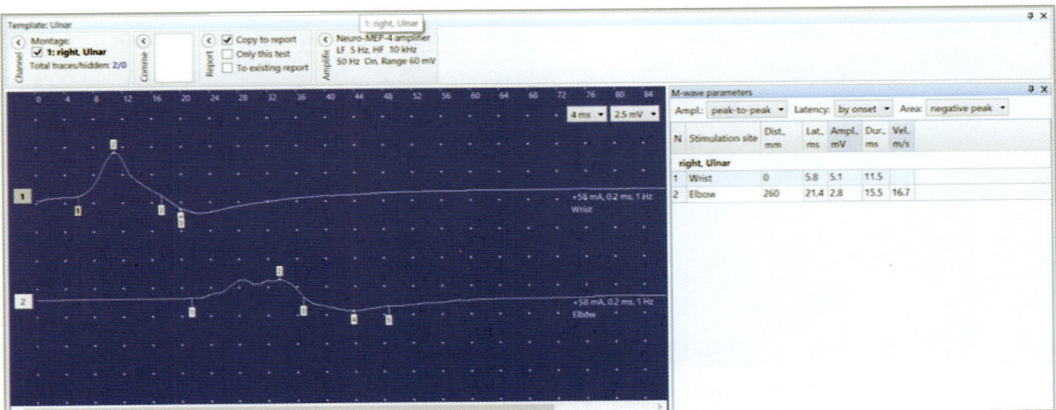

Fig. 26: Nerve conduction study showing drop in the compound muscle action potential (CMAP) amplitude in proximally (2.8 mV) stimulated waveform (wave 2) when compared to distally (5.1 mV) stimulated waveform (wave 1) suggestive of conduction block.

TABLE 7: Differentiating features of myopathic and neuropathic involvement.

Parameter	Myopathic pattern	Neurogenic pattern
MUPs amplitude	Reduced	Increased
MUPs duration	Shorter	Normal; increased in chronic
Spontaneous activity	Present	Fibrillations, positive sharp wave; normal in acute stage
Recruitment pattern	Early and excessive	Reduced

(MUPs: motor unit potentials)

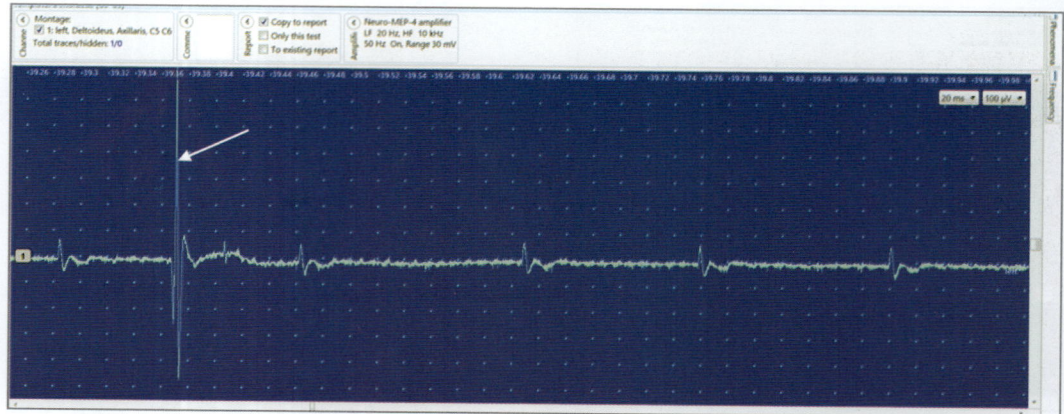

Fig. 27: Electromyography (EMG) showing fasciculation (arrow) in the tested deltoid muscle.

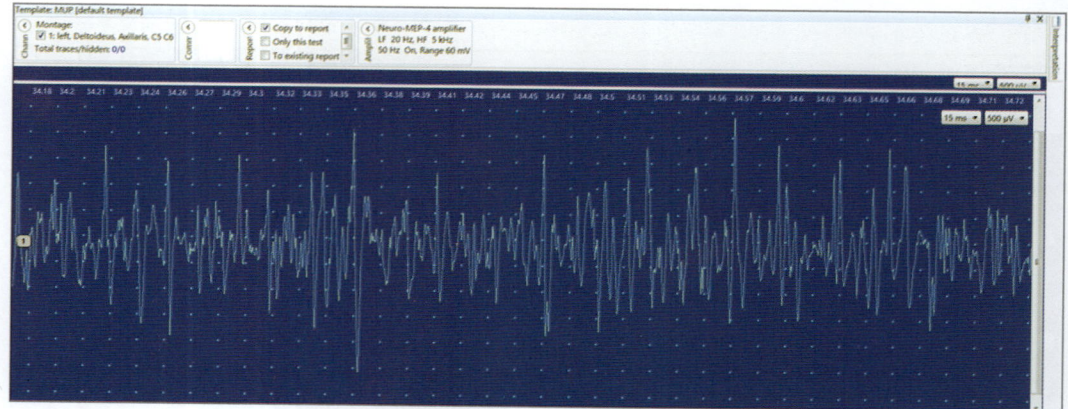

Fig. 28: Normal electromyography (EMG) recruitment pattern.

- *Myotonia* is another abnormal spontaneous activity observed in myotonic dystrophy, congenital myotonia. Myotonia has variable amplitude and frequency giving a sound of "dive bomber" on EMG.

Motor Unit Recruitment

Motor unit recruitment is assessed by asking the patient to minimally activate the muscle. By this action, few motor units are recruited, which is reflected in EMG as motor unit potentials (MUPs). Its amplitude, duration, number of phases, and firing rate are computed. Normally, MUPs have 3–4 phases, duration of 10 ms and amplitude of <2 mV **(Fig. 28)**. When a patient is making full efforts to activate the muscle, large number of motor units is recruited simultaneously. These motor units interfere with each other and are called as *interference pattern*.

- In primary muscle disease, with minimal efforts, large number of motor units is recruited. This phenomenon is called *early recruitment*. MUPs are small (<0.5 mV) and shorter duration.

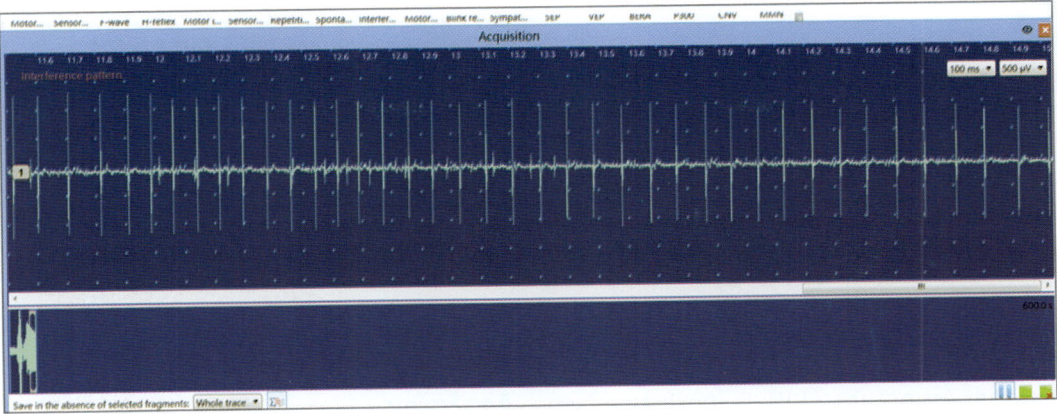

Fig. 29: Electromyography (EMG) showing neurogenic pattern of recruitment with motor unit potentials (MUPs) showing large amplitude, normal duration MUPs with reduced recruitment.

- In neurogenic process, there is *reduced recruitment* with large amplitude motor units **(Fig. 29)**. Reduced recruitment can also occur with minimal cooperation and upper motor neuron lesion. Hence, caution must be exercised before reduced recruitment is attributed to purely neurogenic process.

- If the MUPs are of normal morphology and there is reduced recruitment, despite good efforts, and there is no spontaneous activity, it indicates possibility of conduction block. However, if the patient develops fibrillations, it indicates secondary axonal loss.

KEY MESSAGES

- Electroencephalography must not be ordered to exclude a diagnosis of epilepsy, as epilepsy is largely a clinical diagnosis.
- Electroencephalography is useful to classify the type of epilepsy into focal or generalized epilepsy and for the diagnosis of the various electroclinical epilepsy syndromes.
- Brainstem-evoked potential tests the integrity of the pathway from the cochlea to the auditory cortex and is used for assessment of hearing in newborns and older children.
- Visual-evoked potential tests the conduction in the visual pathway from retina to striate occipital cortex and is assessed in terms of P100 latency.
- Nerve conduction study tests myelinated motor and sensory nerves and can be normal in patients with small fiber neuropathy and preganglionic lesions.

CHAPTER 7

Cerebrospinal Fluid and Tissue Diagnosis

■ LUMBAR PUNCTURE

Lumbar puncture (LP) is performed to analyze cerebrospinal fluid (CSF). It is performed in lateral decubitus position with knee chest position or in the sitting position in older children. Sufficient flexion of spine is essential to expose the interspinous or intervertebral space. All aseptic precautions are exercised. LP is done at L3–L4 level at the level of superior iliac crest. Topical anesthesia is not routinely used before the procedure, but it may decrease the pain, thus facilitating a successful procedure especially in infants. Eutectic mixture local anesthetics (EMLA) and 1% lidocaine are the most commonly used local anesthetic agent. A 22-gauge LP needle is often used for LP. The needle is inserted perpendicular to the plane of back with bevel of the needle parallel to sagittal plane.

Back pain and postprocedure headache are the two most common complications of LP. Risk of cerebral herniation is high among those with raised intracranial pressure secondary to intracranial pathology like brain abscess. Hence, it would be prudent to delay the procedure till features of raised intracranial pressure (ICP) settle or after neuroimaging has ruled out intracranial space-occupying lesion. However, it is safe in benign raised intracranial pressure, as the pressure raise is uniform across both cerebral and spinal subarachnoid space.

■ CEREBROSPINAL FLUID

Anatomy

Cerebrospinal fluid is produced by choroid plexus of lateral ventricles, third ventricle and fourth ventricle. CSF flows from the two lateral ventricles through foramen of Monro to the third ventricle. Subsequently, through aqueduct of Sylvius, it reaches the fourth ventricle (*see* **Figure 25, Chapter 1**). Fourth ventricle is connected to subarachnoid space through foramen of Luschka (two lateral) and foramen of Magendie (median). CSF flows between the pia mater and arachnoid mater in the subarachnoid space over the cerebral convexities where it finally gets absorbed by arachnoid granulations, and then into venous circulation. Around 20% of CSF flows to spinal subarachnoid space. Brain floats in the CSF and it provides buoyancy, reducing brain weight effectively by >75%. It also serves as a conduit for nutrition and chemicals to intercellular spaces.

Physiology

The choroid plexus is composed of single layer of epithelial cells with tight junctions that form the blood–brain barrier (BBB). Total volume of CSF is around 150 mL; whereas, in neonates, it is around 40–60 mL. Rate of CSF production is 0.3 mL/min. CSF is reformed 3–4 times in a day, making CSF production to be around 500 mL/day.

Normal CSF pressure is around 70–180 mm H_2O. Values above 250 mm H_2O are considered as increased and values below 60 mm H_2O are considered as intracranial hypotension. CSF pressure is measured by manometer using a three-way stopcock. During measurement of CSF pressure, child's back should be held in a straight posture. If CSF opening pressure is high, CSF should be removed slowly and should stop once CSF pressure drops to 50% of its opening pressure (guarded procedure).

Appearance

Normally, CSF looks clear. It will be xanthochromic when there is bilirubin (above 10–15 mg/dL) secondary to old subarachnoid bleed or if the leukocyte count is >1,000 cells/mm^3. Red blood cells (RBCs) from subarachnoid bleed hemolyze to release hemoglobin that gets converted to oxyhemoglobin, methemoglobin, and bilirubin. Presence of fresh blood in CSF is suggestive of either a traumatic tap or subarachnoid hemorrhage. This could be clarified by collecting the CSF samples in three consecutive tubes. Traumatic CSF clears up after first or second tube collection, whereas in subarachnoid bleed, it would persist in all the three tubes.

Cerebrospinal Fluid Cytology

Cerebrospinal fluid should be examined microscopically for cytology within the first hour of its collection, as the neutrophil count drops by more than 50% after 2 hours of collection. Normal CSF in children and adults can have 0–5 cells/mm^3 with predominance of lymphocytes whereas a newborn infant can have up to 10 cells/mm^3 with 60% polymorphs and 40% lymphocytes. In preterm infants, cell count to 30 cells/mm^3 can be considered normal.

Cerebrospinal fluid *pleocytosis* refers to increased CSF cell counts. The most common cause of neutrophilic CSF pleocytosis is bacterial infection of central nervous system (>250 cells/mm^3). Other causes of neutrophilic pleocytosis include acute stage of viral meningitis, tubercular meningitis, hemorrhage, after stroke, neurosurgical procedure, and status epilepticus. In viral meningitis and demyelinating pathology, cell counts are often around 10–100 cells/mm^3 with lymphocytic predominance. Apart from viral meningitis, lymphocytic pleocytosis is also observed in neuroborreliosis, subacute phase of bacterial meningitis, and polyradiculitis. In tubercular meningitis, CSF pleocytosis is usually around 100–500 cells/mm^3. CSF cell counts are often similar in ventricular and lumbar CSF. CSF eosinophilia can be seen in helminthic infections (*Taenia solium, Angiostrongylus,* and *Gnathostomata*), malignancies such as Hodgkin's lymphoma, and following drug reactions.

There are various formulae described for interpreting a traumatic CSF report. However, in general, we consider 1 leukocyte for every 1,000–1,500 RBCs. All said and done, *a traumatic CSF is a traumatic event* and it is difficult to have an accurate interpretation of a traumatic CSF. The best way is to repeat the LP after 48–72 hours.

Cerebrospinal Fluid Biochemistry

Cerebrospinal Fluid Protein

Choroid epithelial cells are bound by tight junctions and permit only small molecules to transfer from blood to CSF. BBB restricts the diffusion of protein from blood to CSF. Proteins reach CSF by passive diffusion across the BBB or by intrathecal synthesis of protein by central nervous system. The larger is the protein molecule such as IgM, lesser will be CSF concentration when compared to smaller proteins such as IgG but the gradient of CSF–blood concentration remains constant. If the blood IgG increases, CSF IgG level automatically increases, but the gradient remains constant. Hence, if there is an alteration or increase in CSF: blood gradient, it means there is an intrathecal production. For example, in children with suspected subacute sclerosing panencephalitis (SSPE), it is CSF:serum IgG antibody against measles virus that is important for diagnostic purpose. Four proteins are produced intrathecally in CSF: (1) Neuron-specific enolase (NSE) (neurons), (2) glial fibrillary acidic protein (astrocytes), (3) myelin basic protein (oligodendrocyte), and (4) ferritin (microglia). Decreased CSF flow rate because of reduced CSF production or restriction of CSF flow in subarachnoid space (meningitis) can also result in increase in the CSF protein. CSF:serum albumin quotient is a marker for BBB integrity.

The CSF protein is normally between 20 and 50 mg/dL. In healthy newborn infants, it can be as high as 170 mg/dL. In traumatic LP, CSF protein increases by 10 mg/dL for every 1,000 RBCs. Proteins are higher in the lumbar CSF compared to cisternal fluid. CSF proteins can be raised in infective (bacterial and viral meningitis), vascular (hemorrhage), inflammatory pathology [Guillain-Barré syndrome (GBS)] pathology, and following status epilepticus. In children with metabolic encephalopathies, CSF protein tends to be normal. Usually, CSF proteins are elevated beyond 100 mg/dL in bacterial meningitis; whereas in tubercular meningitis, they are elevated beyond 250 mg/dL.

Cerebrospinal Fluid Glucose

Blood glucose levels are estimated simultaneously. However, one should remember that it takes at least 2–4 hours for equilibrium of glucose in serum and CSF. The ratio of CSF–blood glucose is normally 0.6. Ratio <0.6 is called hypoglycorrhachia. In healthy term newborn infants, CSF–blood glucose ratio can be as high as 0.8. In a diabetic patient, sudden rise in blood glucose will be reflected in CSF after 2–4 hours. Hence, a ratio of 0.4 is often considered normal and a ratio <0.3 is considered abnormal. CSF glucose level will be low in a traumatic CSF. CSF glucose levels returns to normal limit within 36–48 hours of effective antibiotic therapy in children with meningitis. Hence, it is not useful for diagnosis of partially treated pyogenic meningitis.

Cerebrospinal Fluid Bacteriology

Cerebrospinal fluid Gram staining can reveal gram-positive cocci such as *Pneumococcus*, gram-negative bacilli such as *Escherichia coli* **(Fig. 1)**, gram-negative cocci such as *Meningococcus*, and budding yeast cells such as *Candida*. India Ink stain can be used to detect *Cryptococcus*; and Ziehl–Neelsen stain can be used to identify *Mycobacterium* **(Fig. 2)**. Wet mount preparations are useful for organisms such as *Acanthamoeba* causing chronic meningitis.

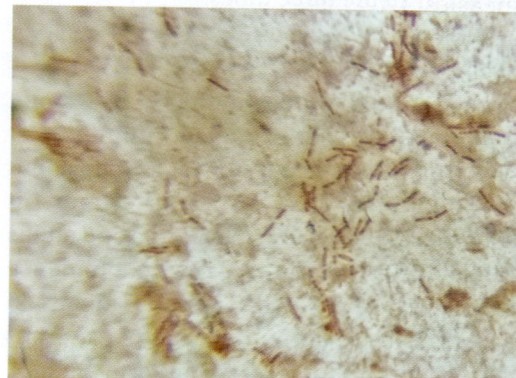

Fig. 1: Gram-negative bacilli on Gram stain of cerebrospinal fluid.

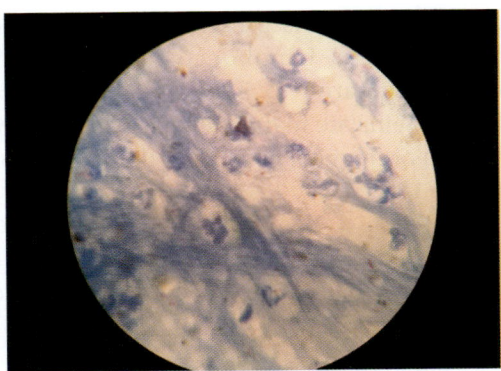

Fig. 2: Acid-fast bacilli on Ziehl–Neelsen staining.

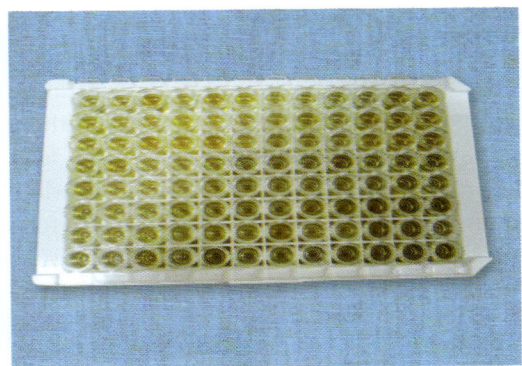

Fig. 3: Enzyme-linked immunosorbent assay (ELISA) kit.

The CSF polymerase chain reaction (PCR) can be done for detection of microorganisms including herpes simplex virus (HSV), cytomegalovirus (CMV), and *Mycobacterium tuberculosis* (TB-PCR). PCR looks for specific gene sequencing in microbial DNA. They are present before specific antibodies are generated, and they often persist after commencement of therapy. Hence, among children with meningoencephalitis, CSF for HSV PCR can remain positive for few days after commencement of empirical treatment with acyclovir. Antigen detection by ELISA is another sensitive method for detection of microbes **(Fig. 3)**. ELISA kits are available for detection of CMV, HSV, and measles. Organisms such as pneumococci and meningococci can be screened by latex agglutination test **(Fig. 4)**.

All CSF samples are cultured on MacConkey agar, blood agar, and chocolate agar and incubated in a candle jar at 37°C overnight. Colonies are identified after 48 hours of incubation. In cases where fungal infection is suspected, an additional Sabouraud dextrose agar is also inoculated.

Cerebrospinal Fluid Immunoglobulin

In a healthy individual, IgM antibodies are absent in CSF and only a small fraction of IgG

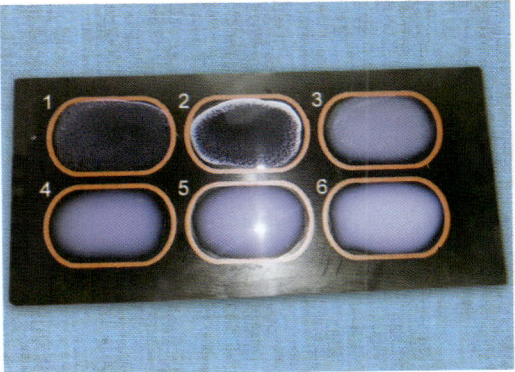

Fig. 4: Latex agglutination test to detect pneumococcal antigen in cerebrospinal fluid sample.
Note: 1 is positive control; 2 is positive test; 4 is negative control; and 3, 5, and 6 are negative.

reach CSF. CSF immunoglobulin IgG is largely derived from plasma by filtration across the BBB or by intrathecal synthesis. Breach of BBB results in leak of immunoglobulin into CSF. Hence, presence of raised CSF IgG level in isolation has no clinical relevance. However, detection of oligoclonal band in CSF is a surrogate marker for intrathecal synthesis as in multiple sclerosis and in other infections of CNS. Elevated IgG index with positive CSF oligoclonal bands are sensitive marker for diagnosis of multiple sclerosis in children.

Albumin is a low molecular weight protein and has high diffusibility. Hence, it can readily cross the BBB. CSF albumin concentration is a good indicator of transudation. If there is a systemic infection with intact BBB, IgG/albumin ratio will be higher in serum when compared to CSF. This will be obvious considering intact BBB, and inability of IgG to transudate-like albumin. In contrast, CSF IgG is produced by intrathecal synthesis and not contributed by plasma IgG level.

CONDITION-SPECIFIC CEREBROSPINAL FLUID ANALYSIS

Diagnosis of Meningitis

Diagnosis of bacterial meningitis is considered when there is either neutrophilic predominant CSF pleocytosis, raised CSF protein, low CSF glucose, positive Gram stain, or growth of organism in CSF culture. Within 48 hours of commencement of antibiotic, CSF glucose level normalizes, CSF protein may remain elevated, neutrophilic response is converted to lymphocytic response, CSF Gram stain will become negative, and culture would be sterile. Absence of organism on CSF Gram stain and sterile culture do not rule out pyogenic meningitis. In viral meningitis, CSF pleocytosis is present but to a lesser extent and is lymphocyte predominant when compared to bacterial meningitis. CSF proteins are marginally raised with near normal or marginally decreased CSF glucose **(Table 1)**.

Hypoxic–Ischemic Brain Injury

The CSF levels of creatine kinase (CK–BB) can increase within few hours of hypoxic damage to brain. CSF CK-BB level >20 IU/L is an indicator of severe hypoxic brain injury. Other CSF biomarkers for hypoxic brain injury include elevated CSF levels of NSE, S-100, and lactate. Markers of CNS damage include NSE (damage to neuron), myelin basic protein (damage to myelin), glial fibrillary acidic protein (indicator of gliosis), and gangliosides (marker of synaptic damage).

N-methyl-D-aspartate Receptor Encephalitis

The CSF samples are tested by semiquantitative cell-binding assay, which detects IgG antibody to NR1/NR2 subunit of N-methyl-D-aspartate (NMDA) receptor by indirect immunofluorescence. The report is often qualitative (positive or negative) based on intensity of detected immunofluorescence.

TABLE 1: Cerebrospinal fluid (CSF) findings in meningitis.

	Bacterial meningitis	Viral meningitis	Tubercular meningitis
Opening pressure	Elevated	Normal	Variable
TLC (in cells/mm³)	>1,000	<100	200–500
DLC	Neutrophilic predominance (lymphocytic in late stage)	Predominantly lymphocytic (neutrophilic in early stage)	Predominantly lymphocytic (neutrophilic in early stage)
CSF protein (mg/dL)	100–500	50–100	200–500
CSF:serum glucose	<0.5	>0.5–0.6	<0.5–0.6

(DLC: differential leukocyte count; TLC: total leukocyte count)

For positive results, antibody titers are often reported. Positive CSF for NMDA receptor antibody is diagnostic for NMDA receptor encephalitis. Apart from clinical response, antibody titers are often used to monitor the treatment response.

Subacute Sclerosing Panencephalitis

Measles antibody is tested by ELISA in the CSF sample. Majority of the laboratories have developed their own standards and cutoffs. Many of them adopt 1:625 antibody titers as their cutoff for significantly raised titers in CSF. Other methods include microneutralization test, complement fixation, hemagglutination inhibition, and immunofluorescence test. CSF shows raised gamma-globulin levels (above 10 µg/dL), which is often visible as oligoclonal band on agarose gel electrophoresis. Presence of oligoclonal band signifies production of gamma-globulin within CNS. Antimeasles antibody >1:256 in serum is considered positive. CSF:serum ratio of antimeasles antibody between 1:200 and 1:500 is considered normal. Ratio <1:128 is considered significant.

Hemorrhagic Stroke

The CSF levels of ferritin and hemosiderin can be useful surrogate marker in old subarachnoid hemorrhage, which is not picked up by routine CT scan, or in those with hemorrhagic transformation of arterial or venous stroke.

Guillain–Barré Syndrome

The CSF protein levels are increased beyond 40 mg/dL in three fourths of children with GBS within the 1st week of illness. They continue to increase till 3rd or 4th week of the illness. CSF is often acellular in the 1st week of illness but can show lymphocytic pleocytosis beyond the 1st week.

Inborn Errors of Metabolism

Neonates presenting with drug-resistant early-onset epileptic encephalopathy should be evaluated for pyridoxine-dependent seizures and folinic acid-responsive seizures. Infants with unexplained progressive extrapyramidal syndrome need evaluation for possible neurotransmitter disorders. Certain inborn errors of metabolism affecting central nervous system that can be diagnosed based on certain metabolite levels in CSF are listed in the following text. For collecting and transporting CSF samples for estimation of these metabolites, CSF should be stored in –70°C or in liquid nitrogen.

- Elevated CSF lactate (>20 mg/dL) and/or ratio of CSF:serum lactate (>0.91) are reliable marker of mitochondrial disease affecting central nervous system.
- Elevated CSF glycine level (normal value <20 µmol/L) and elevated CSF:plasma glycine ratio (normal value <0.02) are suggestive of nonketotic hyperglycinemia. Plasma amino acid levels are usually estimated simultaneously with CSF amino acid levels.
- Low levels of CSF serine (normal value 25–105 µmol/L) can suggest serine transporter deficiency. However, they can be decreased in disorders of folate metabolism and mitochondrial complex I deficiency.
- CSF glucose <35 mg/dL with CSF:serum glucose ratio <0.35 and normal CSF lactate is highly suggestive of CSF glucose transporter deficiency. This condition responds favorably to ketogenic diet.
- Disorders of biogenic monoamines including serotonin, dopamine, epinephrine, and norepinephrine are broadly

classified as neurotransmitter disorders. CSF should be tested for levels of biopterin, neopterin, 5-HTP (hydroxytryptophan), HVA (homovanillic acid), 5-HIAA (hydroxyl indole acetic acid), 3-OMD (ortho methyl dopa), and MHPG (3-methoxy-4-hydroxyphenylglycol) levels to diagnose various disorders of monoamine neurotransmitter disorders.
- Biogenic amines and pterins such as total neopterin and tetrahydrobiopterin are reduced in GTP cyclohydroxylase I deficiency causing dopa-responsive dystonia. This condition responds dramatically to levodopa supplementation.
- Elevated free gamma-aminobutyric acid (GABA) levels in CSF have been observed in GABA transaminase deficiency, succinic semialdehyde dehydrogenase deficiency, and glutaryl-CoA dehydroge-nase deficiency.
- *Others:*
  - CSF level of β-2 transferrin is a specific marker for CSF leak from nose, ear, or orbit.
  - Biomarkers including NSE and S-100 have been used as biomarkers for prognosis of patients with poststatus epilepticus and brain death.

■ MUSCLE BIOPSY

Site of Muscle Biopsy

Muscle biopsy is best obtained from the muscle that has moderate weakness rather than the muscle with severe weakness as the latter may have only fibrosis and fat in its tissue. The affected muscle can be screened using MRI muscle. However, in an acute disease such as suspected inflammatory myopathy, it would be wise to biopsy the most affected muscle. Most common muscle that is biopsied is vastus lateralis of quadriceps muscle. Other muscles include deltoid and biceps muscle. Open biopsy is always preferred over needle biopsy. The muscle where electromyography (EMG) has been performed or those muscles with trauma or intramuscular injections should be avoided for muscle biopsy. Muscle belly should be preferred over those parts of muscle near the tendons.

Procedure of Muscle Biopsy

After a written informed consent, pre-procedural sedation can be done with intravenous (IV) midazolam or ketamine. The site of muscle biopsy needs to be prepared with spirit and betadine followed by draping the site. An incision of 3–4 cm is given to the skin. Skin is retracted and fascia is incised. Muscle is held using an Allis forceps and cut free from the surrounding muscle on either side of the cylinder of muscle. The muscle sample should not be squeezed or damaged in any way during this procedure, so that artefact changes can be avoided. Firm pressure is applied to the biopsy site for 10 minutes after specimens have been obtained so that intramuscular bruising is reduced to a minimum. The skin is then sutured and covered with a protective sterile dressing. Finally, the specimens are transported in a vial rapidly to neuropathology laboratory.

Processing of Biopsy Sample

The muscle sample is clamped with a muscle clamp to avoid contraction artifacts. It is divided into three pieces: (1) The first piece is fixed in formalin for light microscopy; (2) the second piece is snap frozen in liquid nitrogen for histochemical and immunohistochemistry studies; and (3) the third piece is fixed in 3% glutaraldehyde for electron microscopy.

TABLE 2: Differences between type I and type II muscle fibers.

Characteristic	Type I	Type II
Contraction	Slow	Fast
Color	Red	White
Source of energy	Fats (lipids)	Glycogen
Respiration	Oxidative	Anaerobic
ATPase at pH 9.4	Light	Dark
ATPase at pH 4.3	Dark	Light
NADH-TR	Dark	Light
SDH	Dark	Light

(NADH-TR: nicotinamide adenine dinucleotide dehydrogenase-tetrazolium reductase; SDH: succinate dehydrogenase)
Note: Selective type I atrophy is seen in myotonic dystrophy, nemaline rod, and centronuclear myopathy; type II atrophy is seen following steroids, or disuse atrophy.

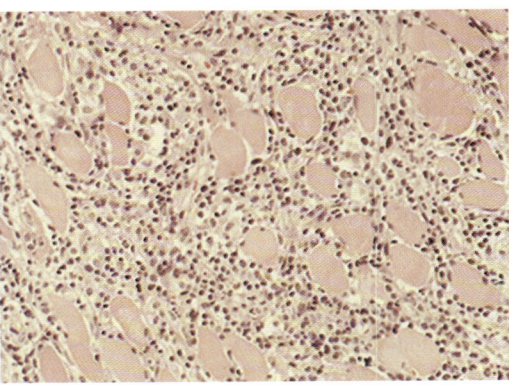

Fig. 5: Routine hematoxylin and eosin (H & E) staining showing inflammatory changes in inflammatory myopathy (dermatomyositis).

Main parameters that are assessed in a muscle biopsy sample received include integrity of fascicular architecture (deranged in dystrophic process), shape of muscle fibers (angular or rounded), size of muscle fiber (small or large), presence of fiber size variation (look for degeneration, atrophy, and hypertrophy), predominance of type of fiber (type I or type II), presence of active inflammation and perimysial or endomysial fibrosis **(Table 2)**.

- Routine histochemistry is useful for diagnosis of inflammatory myopathy **(Fig. 5)**, obvious mitochondrial abnormality, glycogen, and lipid storage abnormality. Stains used in routine histochemistry are enumerated in **Table 3**. Apart from routine hematoxylin and eosin (H & E) staining **(Fig. 6)**, other stains include nicotinamide adenine dinucleotide dehydrogenase (NADH) stain **(Fig. 7)**, and succinate dehydrogenase (SDH) stain **(Fig. 8)**.
- Immunohistochemical studies look for specific pathology involving proteins such as dystrophin (dystrophinopathy), myotilin (LGMD 1A), caveolin (LGMD 1C), dysferlin (LGMD 2B), emerin (EDMD), sarcoglycan (LGMD 2C-2F), laminin (merosin-negative CMD), β-dystroglycan (CMD), and collagen VI (Ullrich CMD).
- Electron microscopy is used for visualization of inclusion body, mitochondrial organelle, and sarcolemma.

Abnormal Findings on Muscle Biopsy

Normally, the muscles have polygonal appearance. Presence of small and angulated fibers involving both type I and type II fibers is suggestive of neurogenic atrophy. Presence of reinnervation is marked by grouping of atrophic fibers. Presence of fiber type variation with both atrophy and hypertrophy is highly suggestive of myopathic pattern. Atrophic fibers appear rounded in contrast to angulated atrophic fibers of neurogenic pattern **(Table 4)**, whereas hypertrophic fibers appear enlarged and split (split fibers). Presence of degenerating and regenerating fibers is classical pattern in muscular

TABLE 3: Common stains used in muscle biopsy.

Stain	Purpose
Hematoxylin and eosin (H & E) stain	Fiber size, connective tissue, presence of inflammatory cells, and storage material
Modified Gomori trichrome stain	Mitochondrial abnormality, collagen, and inclusions
ATPase (pH 4.3, 4.6, and 9.4)	To look for fiber type predominance, type I fibers look light, and type II fibers look dark on ATPase
Oxidative stains: NADH, SDH, COX stain	To detect mitochondrial pathology, dense rim of SDH staining suggests ragged red fiber
PAS staining	To look for glycogen storage
Oil red O	To look for fat globules

(COX: cytochrome oxidase; NADH: nicotinamide adenine dinucleotide dehydrogenase; PAS: periodic acid–Schiff; SDH: succinate dehydrogenase)

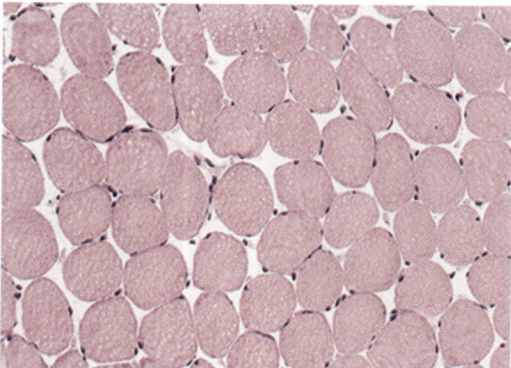

Fig. 6: Normal hematoxylin and eosin (H & E) staining of muscle.

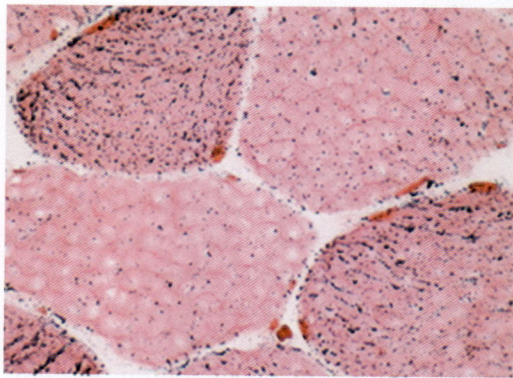

Fig. 8: Succinate dehydrogenase (SDH) staining for mitochondria.

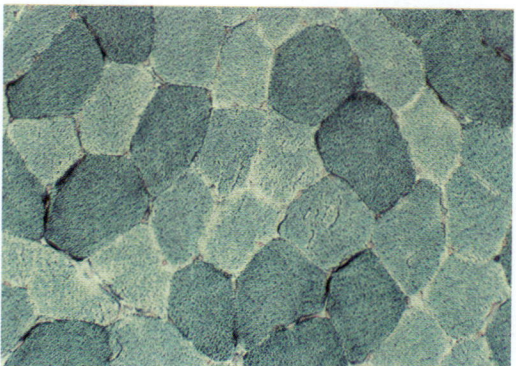

Fig. 7: Normal nicotinamide adenine dinucleotide dehydrogenase (NADH) staining.

dystrophy. Few features are diagnostic of specific diseases such as presence of ragged red fiber (mitochondrial myopathy), central core (central core myopathy), and increased number of internal nuclei with pyknotic nuclear clumps (congenital myotonic dystrophy).

- In *Duchenne muscular dystrophy*, routine H & E staining reveals degenerating fibers, regenerating fibers **(Fig. 9)**, increased internalized nuclei, and proliferation of endomysial connective tissue. Immunohistochemistry might reveal

TABLE 4: Differences between myogenic and neurogenic pattern.

Parameter	Neurogenic	Myogenic
Group atrophy, fiber type atrophy, fascicular atrophy, and target fibers	Present	Absent
Inflammation, degeneration, regeneration, and fiber splitting	Absent	Present
Interstitial fibrosis	Absent	May be present
Fiber shape	Angulated	Rounded

reduced or absent dystrophin around the sarcolemma membrane.
- In *congenital muscular dystrophy*, routine histology reveals myopathic changes and immunohistochemistry might reveal reduced collagen type VI suggestive of merosin-negative congenital muscular dystrophy.
- In *congenital myopathy* (inclusion body), in addition to myopathic changes on routine H & E stain, electron microscopy might be useful to look for filamentous inclusion bodies.
- In *myotonic dystrophy*, nuclear internalization can be seen **(Fig. 10)**.

Current Relevance of Muscle Biopsy

Once upon a time, muscle biopsy was considered diagnostic for various neuromuscular disorders. In the present era of genetic diagnosis, role of muscle biopsy is declining. For example, when genetic diagnosis of Duchenne muscular dystrophy is established by blood PCR or multiplex ligation-dependent probe amplification (MLPA), there is no need for muscle biopsy. Muscle biopsy is restricted only to those who were tested negative for DMD by MLPA or PCR. However, with advent of next generation sequencing (NGS), those who test negative for DMD by MLPA (79 exons) may be subjected to NGS to sequence all 79 exons of *DMD* gene before subjecting to muscle biopsy.

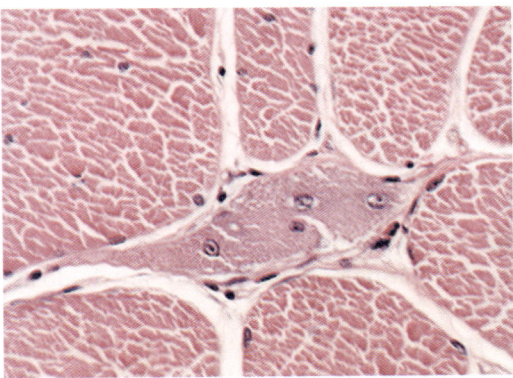

Fig. 9: Degenerating fibers in a child with Duchenne muscular dystrophy.

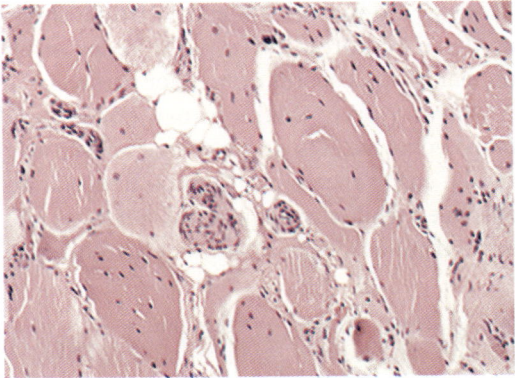

Fig. 10: Nuclear internalization in myotonic dystrophy.

There is rapid increase in the spectrum of clinical findings known to be associated with certain genotype. The textbooks are gradually replacing the classification of neuromuscular disorder based on histopathology to those based on genotyping. For example, classification of congenital myopathy based on pathology into disease such as central core disease and nemaline rod myopathy is now replaced with classification based on genetic defects such as mutation in *TUBBA4, CLN*, etc. This shift from neuropathology to genetics also has implications for genetic counseling of parents for the next pregnancy. May be in next few years, this section on muscle biopsy may only have historic importance.

NERVE BIOPSY

Nerve biopsy is a useful diagnostic tool for diagnosis of chronic peripheral nerve pathology including chronic inflammatory demyelinating polyneuropathy, amyloidosis, leprosy, Fabry disease, vasculitic neuropathy, mononeuritis multiplex, and few hereditary neuropathies that remain undiagnosed by genetic testing. Unlike muscle biopsy, which was largely used for genetic conditions, nerve biopsy is often used for acquired conditions. There are limited indications in children, as these acquired nerve pathologies often appear in adolescents or in older persons.

Sural nerve is the most commonly biopsied nerve. It is a pure sensory nerve and can be easily accessible. Caution needs to be exercised while dissecting sural nerve, as it is located anatomically close to saphenous vein. Other nerves that may be biopsied include obturator nerve and superficial radial nerve. There is minor concern of local permanent sensory loss following sural nerve removal. Hence, the procedure is limited to conditions, which remain undiagnosed despite extensive clinical, laboratory, and electrophysiological investigations.

SKIN BIOPSY

Skin biopsy is performed most commonly in the affected region or in the axilla. A punch biopsy needle is used to biopsy the skin. Indications of skin biopsy in pediatric neurology includes neuronal ceroid lipofuscinosis, Unverricht-Lundborg disease, galactosialidosis, mucolipidosis type IV, infantile neuroaxonal dystrophy, and Lafora disease. Lafora disease shows homogeneous perinuclear inclusions called Lafora body on skin biopsy. Skin biopsy from distal leg with quantification of linear density of intraepidermal nerve fibers is the reliable method for assessment of small fiber neuropathy. Dystrophin expression in smooth muscle of the skin may be useful for diagnosis of Duchenne muscular dystrophy. An ideal skin biopsy must be at least 3–4 mm in diameter and 6–8 mm in depth. Nuchal skin biopsy has been used for diagnosis of rabies.

KEY MESSAGES

- The CSF neutrophilic pleocytosis with raised CSF proteins (>100 mg/dL) with hypoglycorrhachia (low CSF sugar) supports the diagnosis of acute pyogenic meningitis.
- While interpreting CSF report after commencement of antibiotics, CSF glucose normalizes first followed by resolution of CSF pleocytosis followed by normalization of CSF proteins.
- Every effort must be made to establish the microbiological etiology in CSF using latex agglutination, PCR, ELISA, and other advanced techniques among children with infective meningitis.
- Apart from meningitis, CSF is useful in diagnosis of subacute sclerosing panencephalitis, autoimmune encephalitis, neurotransmitter disorders, and other inborn errors of metabolism.
- There is limited role of invasive investigations such as muscle and nerve biopsy in the era of advances in genetic and molecular diagnostics.

CHAPTER 8

Genetic Evaluation in Neurological Diseases

■ OVERVIEW

There is a rapid advancement of genetics in the present era. This chapter addresses the basic terminologies of genetics pertaining to pediatric neurology practice. The objective of the chapter will be to familiarize with newer genetic investigations—what to order, how to interpret, and what are the advantages and limitations of each genetic testing. Details of each genetic investigation are beyond the scope of this chapter.

■ INTRODUCTION

Human cell has 23 pairs of chromosomes with one derived from father and other derived from mother. There is only one deoxyribonucleic acid (DNA) in a single chromosome. Hence, there are two complementary copies of DNA derived from each parent. Approximately, there are around 20,000–25,000 total genes in the body. Each gene will have two complementary copies that are called *alleles*. Gene will have introns and exons. Exons are the part of gene that codes for a protein. Location or address of the gene is called *locus*. For example, survival of motor function gene (*SMN1* gene) (spinal muscular atrophy) is located on long arm of chromosome 5 (5q13.2). Hence, the locus of *SMN1* gene is 5q13.2. There will be two copies (alleles) of *SMN1*.

Based on expression of a trait, alleles can be *dominant* or *recessive*. If both alleles are identical, it is homozygous; if one is recessive and the other is dominant allele, then it is called heterozygous. Dominant traits show their effect when individuals have at least one copy of allele (heterozygous). In contrast, recessive traits express in homozygous state. Many of genes, especially intellectual disability genes are located on X chromosome. There are two X chromosomes; hence, two alleles for X chromosomes in females (XX) and one allele in males (XY), i.e., males are hemizygous for X chromosome alleles. For example, in Duchenne muscular dystrophy (*DMD* gene located on X chromosome), presence of one abnormal allele will result in manifestation in males (as they have single X chromosome, hemizygous) and carrier state in females (X_dX_D) (D is functional; d is defective). Hence, for X-linked diseases such as DMD, heterozygous females are carriers and hemizygous males are affected. Females can rarely manifest X-linked diseases as in Turner syndrome, X chromosomal structural defects and skewed X-inactivation.

Broadly, there are two groups of genetic disorders—chromosomal disorders and single-gene disorders. *Chromosomal disorders* are those that result from alteration in structure (deletion, duplication, and inversion) of whole or a part of the

TABLE 1: Broad classification of available genetic tests.	
Cytogenetic investigations (for chromosomal disorders)	**Molecular investigation (for single-gene disorders)**
• Karyotype • Fluorescent in situ hybridization (FISH) • Chromosomal microarray (CMA)	• Polymerase chain reaction (PCR) • Sanger sequencing • Next-generation sequencing (clinical exome/whole-exome/whole-genome sequencing)

chromosome. Examples are Down syndrome (Trisomy 21) and Cri-du-chat syndrome (5p microdeletion).

Single-gene disorders result from mutation of single gene that causes protein product to be altered or missing. Examples are neurofibromatosis (*NF1* gene) and spinal muscular atrophy (*SMN1* gene). Depending on the type of disorder, tests can be broadly divided into cytogenetic studies (for chromosomal disorders) and molecular genetic studies (for single-gene disorders) **(Table 1)**.

■ PLANNING THE TEST

Imagine whole genome to be a book.

If there are chapters that are missing (deletion, duplication, inversion of >5 Mbp), then we can consider *karyotyping*. Karyotype usually detects large deletion, duplications, and inversions of >5 Mbp depending on the resolution adopted and mosaicism; however, it cannot detect microdeletion and microduplication, lesser than the resolution of 5 Mbp. So, karyotype cannot detect if one or two pages of the book are missing.

If there is a single page that is missing and you probably know which page number is missing, then you should order FISH (fluorescent in situ hybridization) or MLPA (multiplex ligation-dependent probe amplification). FISH can detect only those mistakes, which it is trained to detect. For example, if FISH probes are designed for a specific DNA sequence on the chromosome (such as centromeric probes for chromosome 21 and 18), it can detect a defect only in that DNA sequence (it can detect only the centromeric region of chromosome 21 and 18). Similarly, we have locus-specific probes (e.g., 7q11.23 for William syndrome), subtelomeric probes (for the gene rich subtelomeric regions: 4p for Wolf–Hirschhorn), and whole chromosome paint. So, you need to suspect a condition or a group of condition, as there are specific FISH probes for aneuploidy and deletions. FISH can also detect mosaicism.

Multiplex ligation-dependent probe amplification (MLPA) will also detect alterations of DNA in a specific region of the genome. Hence, it is also trained to detect errors in few predecided pages, so it cannot detect if some other chapter has errors. The main advantage of MLPA is the lower cost and its ability to screen multiple areas of genome simultaneously. There are disease-specific MLPA probes, which can detect small deletions and duplication. It can detect any kind of alteration to say that this specific gene is defective or not. It can go to that section of the book and tell you if those pages are missing or not. But, it cannot differentiate whether it is a small or large deletion. It cannot tell you whether 2 pages are torn in that section (small deletion) or 10 pages (large deletion) are torn in that section of the book (exon); anyway you cannot read that section!

MLPA cannot diagnose point mutations (spelling mistakes in a page) in a gene. MLPA probes are available for conditions such as Duchenne muscular dystrophy and spinal muscular atrophy. So, you need to suspect a specific disease to order MLPA or FISH.

If you suspect that *few pages are torn or missing*, but you are not sure from where these pages are missing then consider *chromosomal microarray* (CMA). Microarray will detect copy number variations (CNVs). It can be considered a technique to study all the chromosomes at very high resolution (depending on the technique used). It can detect DNA gain or loss of size as small as 10 kb (depending on the platform used).

If you want to *detect spelling mistakes in a page that you know*, then consider *Sanger sequencing*. Here, all pages are intact, problem is spelling mistake in one or more pages (single gene disorders). You can sequence the entire gene to detect single base pair changes (point mutations, small deletions, insertions, and duplications). Sanger sequencing is the gold standard method for single gene disorders, but the technique is very costly and cumbersome for very large genes with multiple exons. Imagine proofreading every word of a page and that too we have 20,000–25,000 genes (chapters)! Hence, we use Sanger sequencing for disorders in small genes (where chapters are small) or common mutations (common pages where everyone makes a mistake), e.g., *HBB* Sanger sequencing in thalassemia, the common Aggarwal mutation for (c.320insC) megalencephalic leukoencephalopathy (MLC). Also, Sanger sequencing will help in confirming the diagnosis of mutations detected by the next-generation sequencing (NGS). So, you need to know the disease that you want to confirm, and then only Sanger sequencing is useful.

If you suspect *spelling mistakes in the entire section or few set of pages and you do not know where spelling mistakes could be* then we use the NGS technologies, which sequence the clinically important exome/whole exome/genome multiple times and align the sequence to a reference to detect the possible errors. For example, in a baby who has cryptogenic West syndrome (etiology is not clear, we presume genetic cause, so we do not know where the spelling mistake could be), where we do not know what genes would be affected, then based on the clinical clue, we can order *"clinical exome sequencing"*. As the name suggests, it will screen only disease-causing exons (around 6,000–7,000 known disease-causing exons). But, if you want to screen all the 22,000 coding regions (exons), then this is called *whole-exome sequencing*. If you want to screen both exons and introns, then it is called "whole-genome sequencing (WGS)". But it is most vital to know that the yield of these tests varies in different clinical conditions (around 30% in some neurological phenotypes to as high as 90% in genodermatoses). Once you detect the spelling mistake in a page, you go to that page and screen it properly (Sanger sequencing) before calling it the culprit. There is still a bunch of disorders where we will not get results with the above genetic testing because the underlying genetic etiology is not detected by the above tests. This includes the epigenetic methylation disorders such as Prader–Willi syndrome and Angelman syndrome; also, the triple repeat disorders such as Friedreich ataxia, myotonic dystrophy, Huntington chorea, fragile X syndrome, and spinocerebellar ataxia that requires triplet repeat primed polymerase chain reaction (TP-PCR) or southern blots.

GENETIC TESTS

Karyotyping

Karyotyping refers to ordered display of chromosome starting from 1 to 22 and sex chromosomes. Karyotype is useful for detection of numerical and gross structural chromosomal abnormalities including large inversion, duplication, deletion, aneuploidy, and mosaicism. Small submicroscopic alteration below 5 Mb size is not picked up by karyotype. It is good first-line screening investigation among children with unexplained global developmental delay/intellectual disability (GDD/ID); but nowadays, the gold standard and recommended first-line test is cytogenetic microarray.

Blood samples for karyotyping must be sent in heparinized vial. Blood lymphocytes are stimulated to multiply in a culture, these multiplying cells are arrested in metaphase by colchicine, cell membranes are broken, and cells are fixed and stained by Giemsa. Each chromosome is identified by the pattern of their staining. The report takes around 14–21 days. It is useful to detect structural chromosomal abnormalities such as Down syndrome (trisomy 21) **(Fig. 1)**, trisomy 13, Turner syndrome (45, XO), and Klinefelter syndrome (47, XXY).

Chromosomes have a centromere with a short arm (p) and a long arm (q). Each chromosome has a region, band, and a sub-band. Hence, if karyotype report mentions—46,XX, and del (22q14.2), it implies that there are 46 chromosomes with two X chromosomes, and there is deletion in chromosome 22 in the long arm (q), region is 1, band is 4, sub-band is 2 **(Fig. 2)**. Symbols used for karyotyping are listed and defined in **Table 2**.

Fluorescent in Situ Hybridization

Fluorescent in situ hybridization is useful for detecting a specific DNA sequence on a chromosome. To detect this specific sequence, DNA probe labeled with a

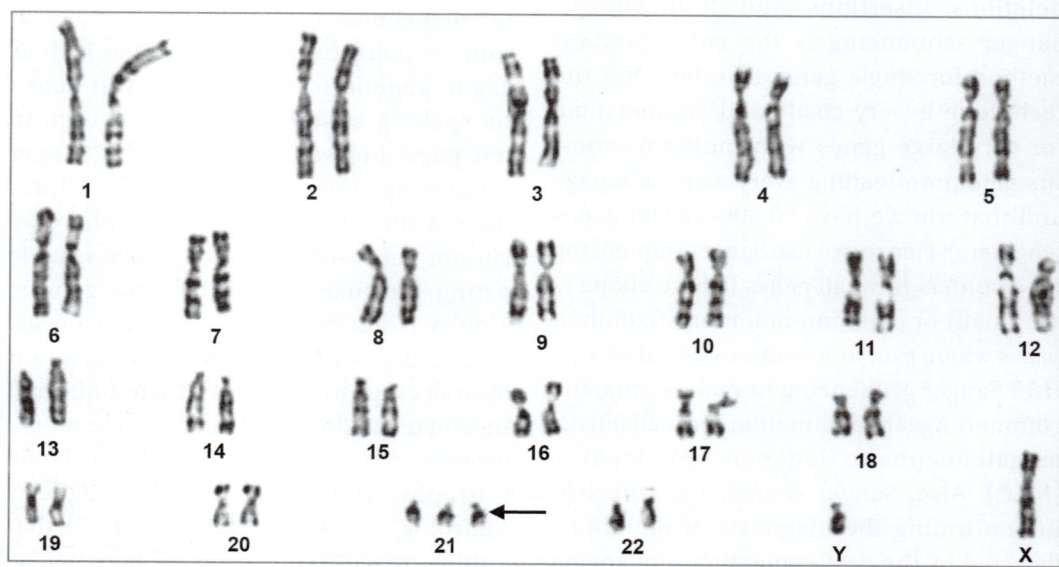

Fig. 1: Karyotype of a child with Down syndrome—46,XY, +21.

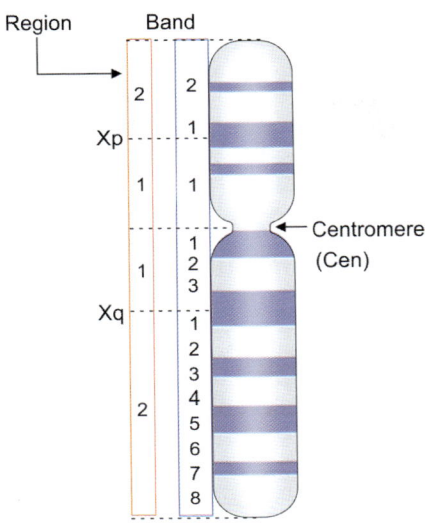

Fig. 2: Chromosome has a short arm (p), long arm (q), region (in red), band (in blue), band, and sub-band.

TABLE 2: Symbols used in karyotype.

Symbol	What does it mean?
46,XX	46 chromosomes, two X chromosome
p	Short arm of chromosome
q	Long arm of chromosome
ter	Terminal
del	Deletion
inv	Inversion
ins	Insertion
dup	Duplication
r	Ring chromosome
i	Isochromosome
t	Translocation

fluorochrome is hybridized with patient sample. The region of this hybridization is visualized using a fluorescent microscope. Its advantage is that it is less time consuming as it can be tested on interphase chromosome and there is no need for cultures as in karyotype. With advent of newer technologies, there is limited utility of FISH in the present era. It is mainly used for determination of gross aneuploidies such as trisomy 13, 18, and 21 in amniotic fluid samples. In addition, there are microdeletion disorders such as Angelman syndrome, Prader–Willi syndrome, William syndrome, and Miller–Dieker syndrome where commercial FISH probes are available.

Multiplex Ligation Probe Amplification

For understanding MLPA, microarray and sequencing, we need to know the concept of CNV and single nucleotide polymorphism (SNP). CNV is a gain or loss in human genome >1 kb in length as compared to the reference genome. This gain or loss may be normal or abnormal. The sequence variations, which are single nucleotide and differ from the reference and not associated with disease, are called single nucleotide polymorphism. For example, GC sequence can be replaced with AT sequence at one specific locus **(Figs. 3A and B)**. This variation can be normally seen in many healthy individuals.

The MLPA probes are targeted at the exons or chromosomal regions, which are responsible for a disease, such as exonic deletion/duplication in Duchenne muscular dystrophy and 16p11.2 deletion/duplication in autism. Each probe is specific for different region of genome. A pair of MLPA probe will hybridize with complementary sequence in the sample DNA. The pair will ligate with each other, amplified by PCR, and analyzed. There are plenty of commercial MLPA probes available for conditions such as Duchenne muscular dystrophy, spinal muscular atrophy **(Fig. 4)** and for common microdeletion syndromes. It takes 24–48 hours for the results. The clinician should ideally have a clinical diagnosis before ordering MLPA (suspected DMD and suspected SMA). However, still at many centers, PCR is being used for molecular diagnosis of DMD.

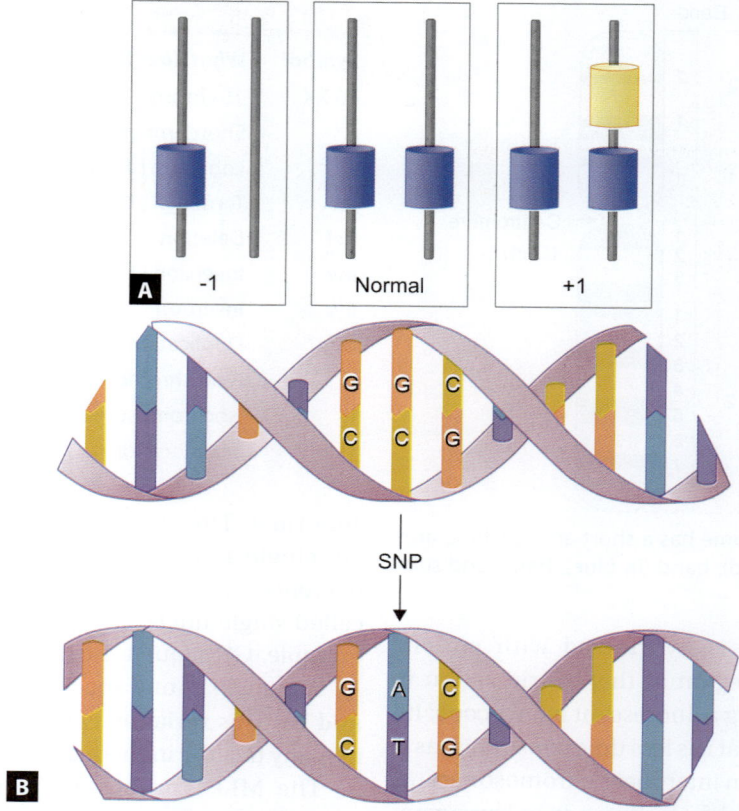

Figs. 3A and B: GC sequence replaced with AT resulting in a sequence with single nucleotide polymorphism (SNP).

Multiplex ligation-dependent probe amplification can detect gross deletions but cannot differentiate between a small deletion and large deletion. For example, in *DMD* gene, if exon 51 is entirely deleted or only a part of it is deleted, MLPA probe for exon 51 will not attach to the sample DNA and will detect it as deleted segment. Also, polymorphisms and point variations near probe binding will alter the results. As it is obvious that MLPA is targeted at a specific locus of the genome and can detect CNVs, hence, it cannot routinely detect mosaicism or anomalies that lie outside the probe regions as compared to the karyotype and cytogenetic microarray that are genomic techniques. Similarly, it cannot routinely detect point mutations, which can be done by sequencing.

Deletions and duplications of the ends of the chromosome (telomere) contribute to around 5% of intellectual disability. MLPA probes for common subtelomeric deletions/duplications can be considered among children with unexplained intellectual disability with normal karyotype. Most common use of MLPA is in the diagnosis of common conditions like spinal muscular atrophy and Duchenne muscular dystrophy. Majority of DMD results from large deletions in the *DMD* gene. There are 79 exons in *DMD*

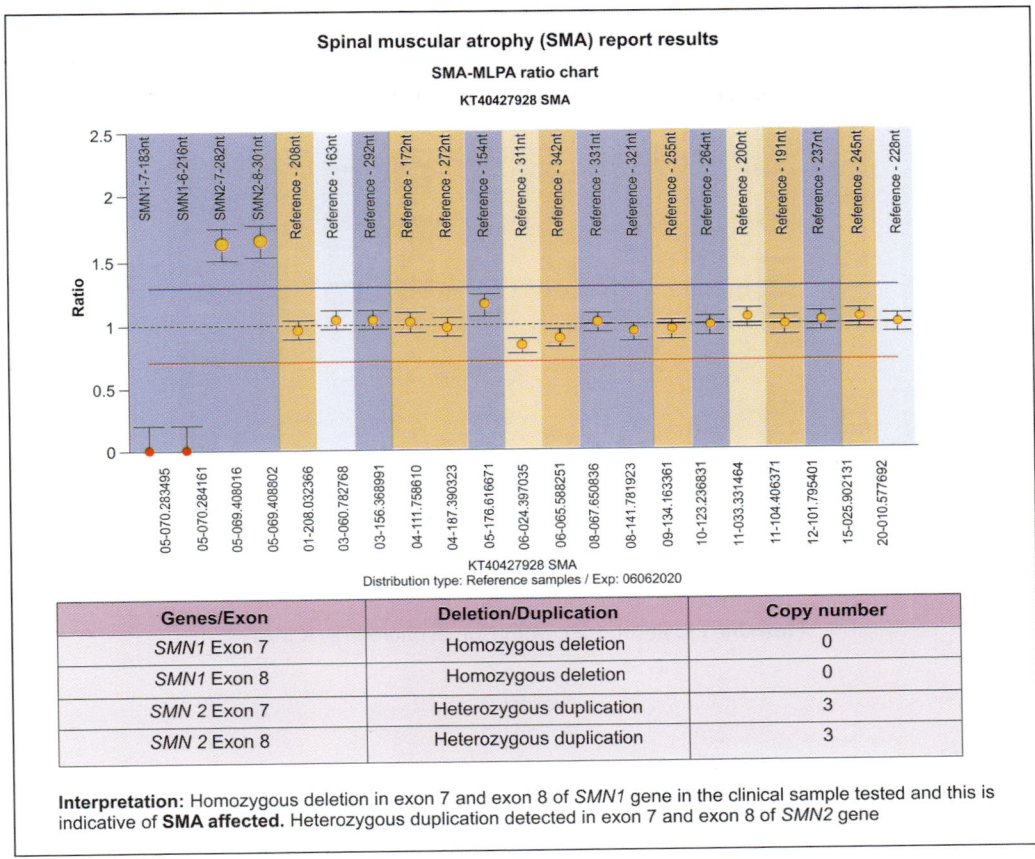

Fig. 4: MLPA report of a patient with spinal muscular atrophy showing homozygous deletion in exon 7 and exon 8 in *SMN1* gene (red dots). (MLPA: multiplex ligation-dependent probe amplification)

gene and most common (hot spot mutations) include exon 45-55 and 2-20. Hence, one could be using 79-exon MLPA to screen for all 79 exons or one could just screen for hot spot regions. A negative MLPA report does not mean that DMD is ruled out. MLPA will not be able to detect point mutation in *DMD* gene, which requires sequencing.

Cytogenetic Microarray (Chromosomal Microarray)

Microarray is a technique to see the chromosome at a high resolution. The earlier and lower resolution ones were comparative genomic hybridization (CGH), which gradually evolved to array CGH and presently most used are the SNP (single nucleotide polymorphism) based arrays. The SNP-based arrays can detect CNVs to a resolution of even 10 kb but if there are no probes in a genomic region that will not be covered. SNP-based arrays will detect mosaicism up to 30%, uniparental disomy, and triploidies. For example, microarray is useful first-line investigation in a child with unexplained GDD with yield of approximately 15%.

Chromosomal microarray covers the entire genome at a very high resolution when compared to karyotype **(Fig. 5)**. CMA is useful

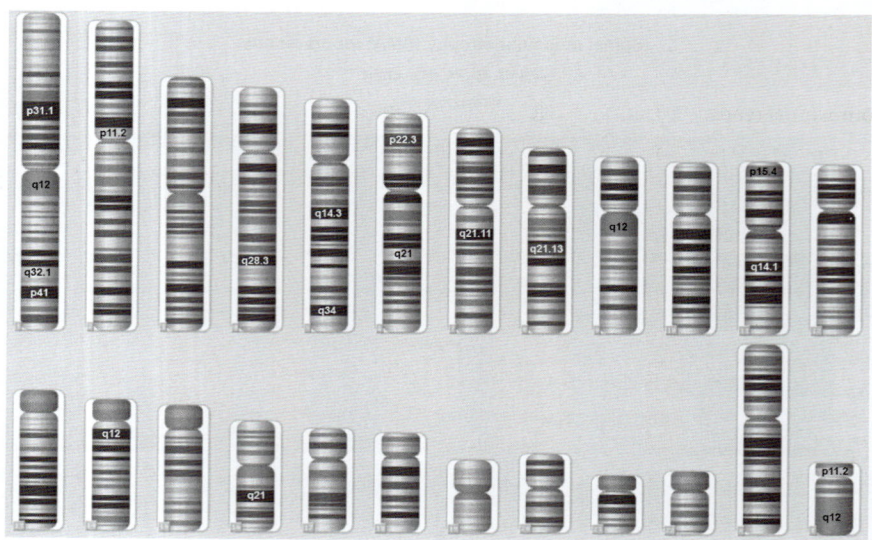

Fig. 5: High-resolution chromosomal microarray—single nucleotide polymorphism (SNP) based.

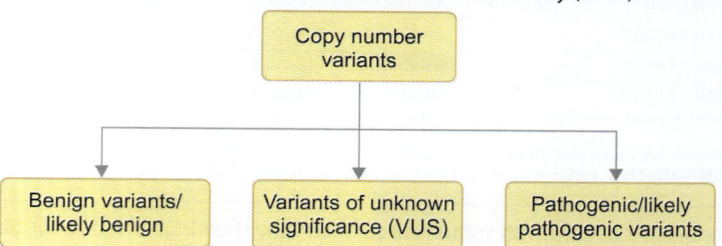

Flowchart 1: Results of chromosomal microarray (CMA).

among children with unexplained GDD, autism spectrum disorder, dysmorphism, or multiple congenital anomalies. CMA platform has miniature chips, which represent each locus of the entire genome. Sample DNA is hybridized to CMA platform and areas of deletions and duplications can be detected. CMA detects CNVs. However, CMA cannot detect balanced translocations and inversions.

Once the results (raw data) of CMA are ready, one can see many copy number variants. It is essential for geneticist to know the clinical phenotype of the patient to interpret these reports **(Flowchart 1)**. This interpretation is a laborious job. Some of these CNVs are detected in healthy normal individuals (benign variants). Some of these CNVs could be associated with certain clinical phenotype as determined by literature (DECIPHER, ISCA, UCSC, and OMIM).

In few cases, CNVs detected in the sample have not been reported in healthy population and there might be insufficient evidence regarding the clinical relevance of these CNVs. Such CNVs are considered as variants of unknown significance (VUS). It is quite possible that the detected CNVs have been reported with some other phenotype, in such a case, it is a good idea to go back and check the phenotype of the patient again (reverse

TABLE 3: Advantages and disadvantages of genetic investigations.

	Karyotype	FISH	MLPA	CMA
Small chromosomal rearrangement*	No	Yes	Yes	Yes
Balanced chromosomal rearrangement	Yes	No	No	No
Mosaicism	Yes	Yes	No	Yes (SNP based)
Low cost	Yes	No	Yes	No
Probe entire genome	Yes	No	No	Yes

*Deletion, duplication, inversion, and translocations are considered as chromosomal rearrangement.
(CMA: chromosomal microarray; FISH: fluorescent in situ hybridization; MLPA: multiplex ligation-dependent probe amplification; SNP: single nucleotide polymorphism)

phenotyping). **Table 3** summarizes the advantages and disadvantages of common genetic investigations.

Targeted Analysis using Next-generation Sequencing (Clinical Exome/Whole-exome/Genome Sequencing)

Polymerase chain reaction (PCR) targets specific DNA region of interest. In PCR, DNA primer anneals to the targeted gene of interest followed by the exponential amplification of targeted gene. PCR output is either qualitative in terms of present or absent or quantitative in terms of quantity such as premutation or mutation as in fragile X testing. Once the product has been amplified by PCR, analysis of actual base pair sequence of specific gene is called *sequencing*. In literal meaning, it means reading the entire nucleotide sequence in that gene. It can detect single nucleotide mutation that can make the gene nonfunctional resulting in a disease. This traditional method called *Sanger sequencing* is the gold standard for genetic diagnosis of single-gene disorders. This method is highly laborious and time consuming, especially if the gene under study is large.

What if we can simultaneously read the nucleotides of all the genes in the genome in a single go along with proofreading the gene multiple times to avoid error. This newer technology where genome (exons, introns, and regulatory elements) can be sequenced to look for errors in nucleotide sequence is called *next-generation sequencing*. If NGS targets a set of genes known to be associated with a specific phenotype, it is called *gene panel testing*, e.g., dystonia panel and ataxia panel. NGS can be used to screen disease causing coding regions (clinical exome sequencing) or all coding regions of the genome (whole-*exome sequencing*). Exons contribute to 1–2% of the whole genome that encodes for proteins but are related to 85% of genetic diseases. If NGS screens the whole genome, both coding and noncoding regions and regulatory regions, then this is called *whole-genome sequencing*.

The NGS-based testing is especially useful among those conditions where clinical diagnosis has not been reached based on clinical examination and various investigations, and we do not have a specific disease phenotype. Exome sequencing might be useful for children with unexplained GDD/ID and other clinical conditions such as microcephaly and syndromic intellectual disability. Since exome/whole-exome/whole-genome sequencing screens for large amount of genome (depending on the tests) and that too multiple times, the test results are voluminous. Many of these detected mutations could be genetic polymorphism that exists in healthy population. You might get incidental mutations (now called secondary findings) which have no clinical correlation, but these mutations could be significant. For example, a clinician might suspect dopa-responsive dystonia and you might not get mutations in any of the dystonia-related gene and rather incidentally pick up *BRCA1* gene mutation known to cause breast cancer. This chance of incidentally picking up genetic mutations must be explained well before ordering the test. There are ACMG (American College of Medical Genetics and Genomics) guidelines formulated to address such issues when secondary findings involve medically actionable variants.

The variants detected in the exome sequencing after application of filters need to be interpreted in the clinical context. Variants are classified into benign, likely benign, variants of uncertain significance, likely pathogenic or pathogenic depending on the clinical correlation **(Flowchart 2)**. When we are not sure whether the detected mutation can cause the phenotype specified by the clinician, then it is classified as VUS. The same mutation classified as VUS can be interpreted by clinician as likely pathogenic, if there is clinical correlation. All pathogenic or likely pathogenic variants always need to be confirmed by Sanger sequencing. Before ordering NGS-based tests, patients should be counseled about the above issues and post-test counseling is a must to deal with issues raised by the NGS tests.

The NGS-based genetic testing is evolving rapidly and it is very important to keep pace with genetic diagnostic techniques, as there are now routinely used NGS-based assays that can determine both the CNV and single-gene variations, bypassing the use of CMA.

The cost of exome sequencing is prohibitive. Hence, the cost, limitation, and utility of exome sequencing need to be explained to parents in advance. Utility of detecting a genetic defect in a child with unexplained intellectual disability might not have any treatment implications, unless you discover a treatable cause, which is quite rare. However, it puts an end to misery of parents as to why it happened to their child, will there be a higher chance of recurrence in their next pregnancy, and can we help them with antenatal diagnosis using chorionic villus sampling (CVS) or amniocentesis to detect affected fetus with same genetic mutation in the future pregnancy.

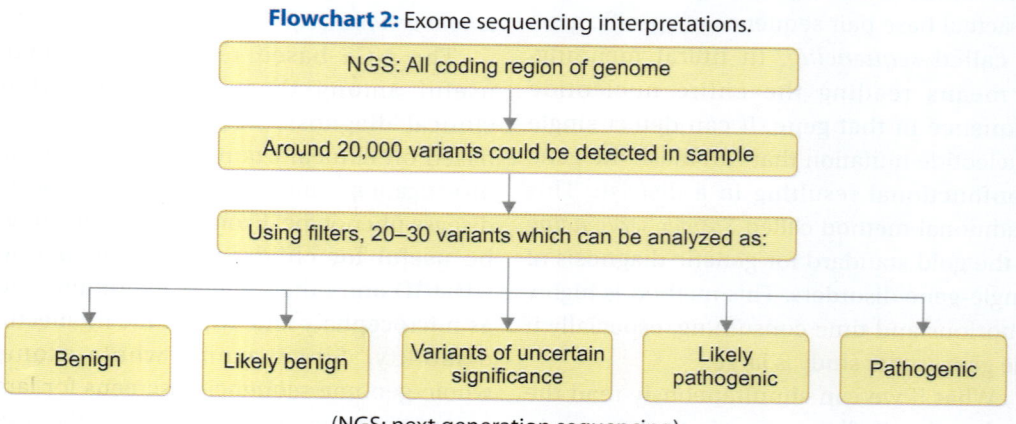

Flowchart 2: Exome sequencing interpretations.

(NGS: next generation sequencing)

CHAPTER 8: Genetic Evaluation in Neurological Diseases

KEY MESSAGES

- Clinician must be aware of the rapid advances in genetics in evaluating patients in pediatric neurology.
- Karyotype is useful for detecting large deletion or duplications but cannot detect microdeletions that can be picked up using CMA, which is literally a magnified karyotype.
- NGS (clinical/whole-exome) sequencing has revolutionized the practice of pediatric neurology and is useful for detecting single gene mutations.
- Molecular diagnostics have been used to confirm or exclude a genetic disease, to provide therapeutic or prognostic purpose, and to prevent uncertainty in diagnosis and bypass burdensome investigations.
- Rapid advances in genetics have been utilized largely to estimate the reproductive risk and enable carrier testing and prenatal testing.

CHAPTER 9

Neural Control of Urinary Bladder

ANATOMY

Urine formation takes place in our two kidneys and reaches the urinary bladder through two respective ureters. The urine collects in the urinary bladder and leaves through urethra. The urinary bladder has detrusor smooth muscle. It is a low-pressure system with capacity of 400–500 mL. There are two sphincters—one internal sphincter and another external sphincter. Internal sphincter is in the neck of the urinary bladder, and external sphincter is in the pelvic wall. External sphincter is under somatic or voluntary control. Total adult bladder capacity is around 750 mL.

Detrusor muscle has β_3 receptor (sympathetic system) and M_3 receptors (parasympathetic system) in its wall; internal sphincter has α_1 receptor (sympathetic system) and external sphincter has nicotinic receptor (somatic system). We have three systems that control the micturition—somatic system, sympathetic system, and parasympathetic system (**Fig. 1**).

- Somatic system arises from sacral spinal segments (S2–S4) through pudendal nerve. This is under our voluntary control. It releases acetylcholine that binds to nicotinic receptors, which contract external sphincter causing retention of urine.
- Parasympathetic system arises from sacral (S2–S4) segment of spinal cord and passes through sacral root and pelvic nerve. It releases acetylcholine that acts on M_3 receptor present in detrusor muscles of urinary bladder causing contraction of bladder. Parasympathetic system through nitric oxide is also known to relax the urethral muscles. Hence, parasympathetic system causes bladder contraction and urethral relaxation, resulting in passage of urine. This system is *not* under our voluntary control.
- Sympathetic system arises from T11–L2 spinal segments through inferior

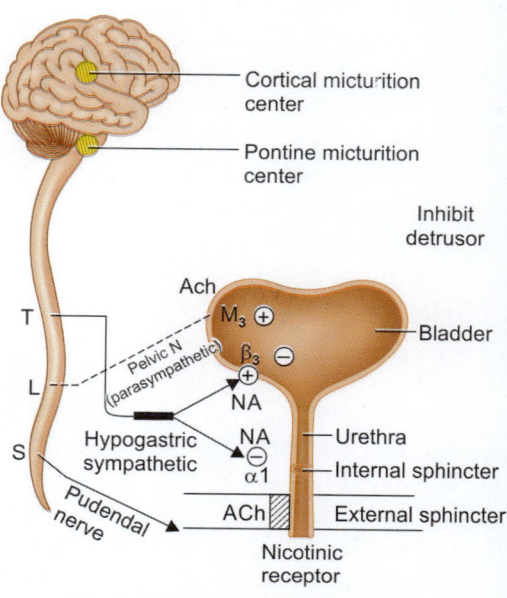

Fig. 1: Neural control of micturition.
(ACh: acetylcholine; NA: noradrenaline)

mesenteric ganglion, and hypogastric nerve.

It releases norepinephrine that acts on β_3 receptors in urinary bladder causing relaxation of bladder and it acts on α_1 receptor in internal sphincter causing its contraction. Hence, sympathetic system causes bladder relaxation and sphincter contraction, resulting in retention of urine. This system is again *not* under our voluntary control.

- There are two main centers in the brain that control the bladder—one is cortical micturition center and another is pontine micturition center (PMC) (Barrington's nucleus).
- Cortical micturition center is in paracentral lobule in frontoparietal cortex that inhibits micturition through PMC, which acts through pudendal nerve and keeps external sphincter closed. Hence, cortex acts to hold the urine until it is socially appropriate to void. We can pass the urine not only when the bladder is full but also when there is minimal urine that is collected as there is voluntary control.
- PMC controls the two opposing systems—parasympathetic (bladder emptying) and sympathetic (bladder filling). When bladder is full, PMC is excitatory to parasympathetic (detrusor contraction) and inhibitory to sympathetic (sphincter relaxation). Whereas, when bladder is empty, PMC is inhibitory to parasympathetic (detrusor relaxation) and excitatory to sympathetic (sphincter contracted, detrusor relaxation).
- Sensory input from cord reaches the periaqueductal gray matter (PAG), which in turn sends signal to hypothalamus, thalamus, prefrontal cortex, and anterior cingulated gyrus. The main job of PAG is to stimulate PMC so that voiding can occur. However, all other brain structures control this impulse of PAG to PMC. Hence, when it is not socially appropriate, PAG is inhibited by prefrontal cortex. This in turn does not stimulate PMC; hence, bladder emptying will not happen till it socially appropriate.
- When the bladder starts filling up to threshold, it asks the cortical center, if it is socially appropriate or not. If appropriate, cortical micturition releases its tonic inhibition on PMC, and similarly, PAG also stimulates PMC to do its job of bladder emptying by stimulating parasympathetic and inhibiting sympathetic impulses. Hence, parasympathetic system is stimulated at sacral level and through Onuf's nucleus, it removes the baseline inhibitory signals to pudendal nerve. This causes external sphincter to relax (pudendal nerve stopped firing) and detrusor to contract (parasympathetic system was stimulated), resulting in passage of urine.

■ **NORMAL BLADDER FUNCTION**

When bladder has just started filling, there is no stretching of the bladder detrusor muscles. Hence, the sensory pelvic nerve will send slow signals in pulse to the spinal cord that keeps hypogastric nerve (sympathetic system) stimulated, which in turn retains the urine. Sensory pelvic nerve also stimulates the pudendal nerve to maintain contraction of external sphincter. Hence, in baseline, sympathetic system is active to retain the urine. Moreover, pontine inhibitory center, also called as pontine storage center, keeps the urethral sphincter muscle contracted. This entire mechanism is called urine storage reflex **(Fig. 2)**.

When the bladder is 100 mL full, first sensation reaches. By 250 mL collection, one

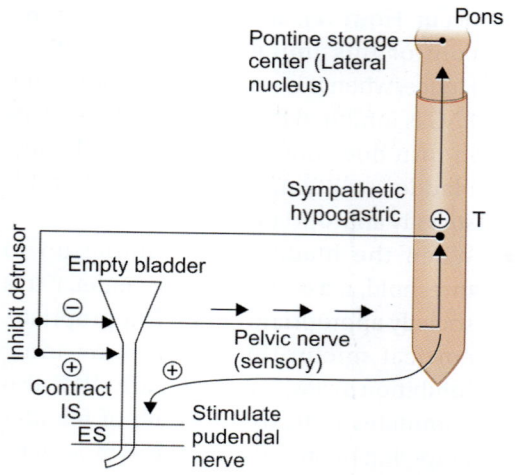

Fig. 2: Mechanism of empty bladder (retention of urine/storage of urine). (ES: external sphincter; IS: internal sphincter)

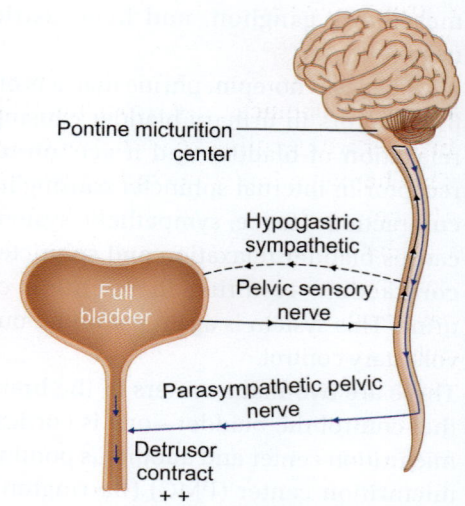

Fig. 3: Bladder emptying voiding reflex.

starts feeling the discomfort, and by 500 mL, it becomes painful, one must take desperate measure to delay the urine. But beyond 650 mL, there is no further cortical control. When the bladder gets full, sensory pelvic nerve sends fast signals to the spinal cord. These fast signals of sensory fibers reach the spinal cord at sacral level. These signals travel up the spinal cord. It asks the cortical micturition center, if it is appropriate to pass urine. If yes, PMC (Barrington nucleus) is stimulated. This in turn stimulates the parasympathetic system and inhibits the sympathetic system and somatic system through pudendal nerve. This action would result in voiding of the urine. As we know, internal sphincter is only under sympathetic control, so it must be suppressed for the urine to pass from the outlet. Once the voiding starts, pelvic afferent nerve will send signals to spinal cord, which in turn will continue to stimulate pelvic parasympathetic nerve to contract the detrusor muscle that results in continued passage of urine **(Fig. 3)**.

> **Key Points**
>
> *Empty bladder:* Sympathetic (hypogastric nerve) is stimulated; parasympathetic (pelvic nerve) is inhibited; pudendal nerve (motor) is stimulated that keeps external sphincter closed.
>
> *Full bladder:* Parasympathetic (pelvic nerve) is stimulated; sympathetic (hypogastric nerve) is inhibited; pudendal nerve is inhibited.

What all can go wrong?
- *When sensory fibers (pelvic nerve) get affected* as in patients with diabetes mellitus, there is no sensation of bladder getting filled (detrusor hyporeflexia). Hence, the bladder will fill and will leak out or overflow automatically. This is called overflow incontinence. Here, there is a failure to store the urine. This bladder is called *autonomous bladder*.
- *When there is cord lesion affecting detrusor output* from S2–S4, but the pudendal nerve is intact, it results in detrusor becoming flaccid and sphincter becoming spastic. When detrusor contracts, outlet must relax for the urine to pass. Similarly, when

detrusor relaxes, outlet must contract. This synergy between detrusor sphincter is essential for the act of micturition. Overactive sphincter and hypocontractile bladder will result in retention of urine. This happens in acute cord pathology. Hence, when a child presents with bladder retention, always think of acute cord pathology apart from local causes of retention.

- When there is a spinal cord lesion above lumbosacral spinal level, there is no control on the bladder reflex (both voluntary and supraspinal control). In acute stage, the bladder becomes flaccid, and there is retention of urine. Slowly, automatic reflex starts developing resulting in bladder to become hyperreflexic (overdrive mode). This is called detrusor overactivity that means detrusor is contracting while the bladder is getting filled. This reflex is inefficient, as it results in simultaneous contraction of detrusor and sphincter resulting in detrusor sphincter dyssynergia. Hence, even a small amount of urine gets collected, it will initiate micturition. Hence, the bladder functions automatically (automatic or spastic or upper motor neuron type bladder). Here, the patient will have sense of urgency to micturate and simultaneously or within few seconds, he/she would pass the urine. This is called urge incontinence. Hence, frequency and urgency are the most common symptoms of detrusor hyperreflexia.

- Cortical lesion can result in uninhibited bladder: In the cortical lesion, baseline suppression of PMC by cortical or subcortical center is lost. Hence, PMC will act independently to empty the bladder. But for lesions above PMC, PMC can coordinate the sympathetic and parasympathetic outflow. Hence, there is no bladder–sphincter dyssynergia. Bladder will become low volume and uninhibited. There is no control on appropriateness of social situation for starting the act of micturition. Hence, the patient passes urine without able to control it when there is an urge **(Figs. 4A and B)**.

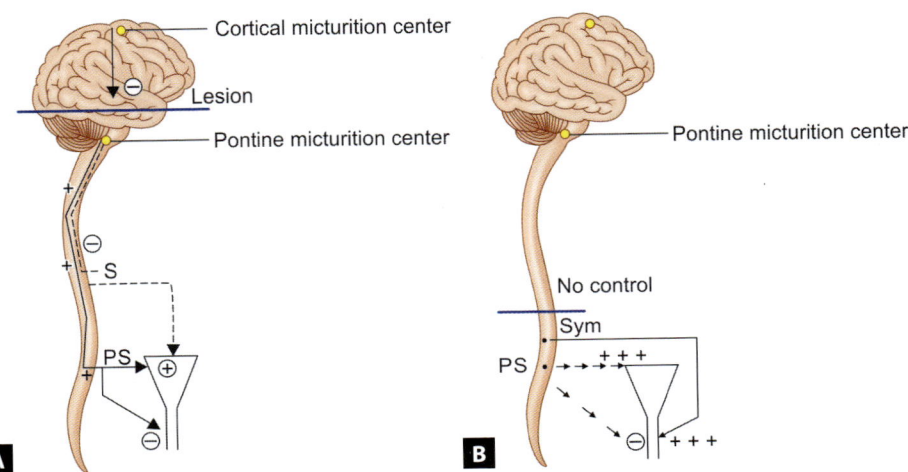

Figs. 4A and B: Patterns of neurogenic bladder: (A) In lesion above pontine micturition center, there is a loss of basal inhibition. Hence, parasympathetic is stimulated and sympathetic is inhibited resulting in voiding without any inhibition (uninhibited bladder); (B) In lesion above T10, there is detrusor overactivity (DTO) so both detrusor and sphincter will be contracted resulting in detrusor sphincter dyssynergia (DSS).

KEY MESSAGES

- Parasympathetic innervation results in voiding through detrusor contraction and urethral relaxation and sympathetic supply results in storage of urine through detrusor relaxation and sphincter contraction.
- PMC controls sympathetic and parasympathetic system coordination with one another. Whereas, cortical center inhibits PMC till it is socially appropriate to void.
- Lesions in cortex result in uninhibited bladder.
- Lesions above T10 level result in retention in acute stage and detrusor overactivity later. Detrusor overactivity results in urge incontinence (inability to void properly).
- Lesion at sacral level results in flaccid bladder resulting in overflow incontinence (patient retain the urine and have constant overflow dribbling).

SECTION 2: Neurological Approach to Diagnosis

10. Seizures, Epilepsy, and Other Paroxysmal Disorders
11. Approach to a Child with Altered Sensorium and Coma
12. Approach to Global Developmental Delay and Intellectual Disability
13. Approach to a Child with Cerebral Palsy
14. Approach to a Child with Developmental Regression
15. Approach to Neuromuscular Weakness
16. Spectrum Disorder and Attention-deficit Hyperactivity Disorder
17. Approach to Diagnosis of Movement Disorders
18. Approach to Diagnosis of Ataxia
19. Approach to Diagnosis of Headache
20. Approach to a Child with Macrocephaly and Microcephaly
21. Approach to Neural Tube Defects
22. Approach to a Child with Vision Loss
23. Approach to a Child with Hearing Loss

CHAPTER 10

Seizures, Epilepsy, and Other Paroxysmal Disorders

■ DEFINITIONS

Seizure

Seizure is a transient alteration in motor function, sensation, or consciousness due to an electrical discharge in brain. Clinical manifestations arising from excessive, hypersynchronous activity of neurons in cerebral cortex are called epileptic seizure. Convulsion refers to motor manifestation of seizure. Hence, what we see is a convulsion and what happens inside the brain is a seizure. Seizure is just an event and not a clinical diagnosis.

Epilepsy

Epilepsy is a clinical diagnosis characterized by recurrent (presence of two or more than two) unprovoked seizures occurring >24 hours apart. All seizures are not epilepsy, you need to have two or more unprovoked seizures to call it an epilepsy. Hence, seizures that are provoked like febrile seizure, a seizure that occurs secondary to hypocalcemia or hypoglycemia or meningitis, will not be called epilepsy. Similarly, the first unprovoked seizure will also not qualify a diagnosis of epilepsy except when the risk of recurrence after the first unprovoked seizure is like that after an epileptic seizure. The definition of epilepsy has been updated by the International League Against Epilepsy (ILAE) in the year 2014.

As per ILAE (2014), epilepsy is a disease of the brain defined by any of the following:
- At least two unprovoked (or reflex) seizures occurring >24 hours apart
- One unprovoked (or reflex) seizure and a probability of further seizures similar to the general recurrence risk (at least 60%) after two unprovoked seizures, occurring over the next 10 years
- Diagnosis of an epilepsy syndrome

Epilepsy is nothing but an enduring predisposition to develop seizures. We know that after one episode of seizure, chances of second seizure are to the tune of 30–40% provided the neuroimaging and electroencephalography reports were normal. If after one episode of seizure, you get an electroencephalogram (EEG) that shows abundant epileptiform discharges from temporal leads or an magnetic resonance imaging (MRI) of brain that shows mesial temporal sclerosis, recurrence risk of a second seizure will be definitely >60%. Therefore, even after the first episode, we can consider this to be epilepsy, considering the recurrence risk. We do not have to wait for the second seizure to label it as epilepsy. This is the meaning of second stem in this definition of epilepsy. The third statement is explained below, if the clinical phenotype along with EEG findings fits into any known electroclinical syndrome, it is obviously epilepsy even if it is only first episode of seizure.

Epilepsy Syndrome

Epilepsy when accompanied by specific patient characteristics and specific EEG abnormality may be considered as an epilepsy syndrome. There are known epilepsy syndromes such as juvenile absence epilepsy, juvenile myoclonic epilepsy, and West syndrome that have a characteristic age of onset, seizure type, and EEG feature. If the clinical seizure type and EEG findings of a child fits into any known epilepsy syndrome, then it qualifies the diagnosis of epilepsy even if it is the first unprovoked seizure.

Example: An adolescent girl presented with three episodes of generalized tonic-clonic seizure in the last 3 months. She also gave history of multiple episodes of early morning jerks in her limbs resulting in dropping of the objects held in her hand. Her EEG revealed 4–6 Hz generalized interictal epileptiform discharges. Presence of generalized seizures and early morning myoclonus with EEG showing generalized discharges in an adolescent fit into a known epileptic syndrome called juvenile myoclonic epilepsy. Similarly, if an infant presents with epileptic spasm with EEG showing hypsarrhythmia, then it qualifies for the diagnosis of West syndrome. Hence, a set of clinical features and certain EEG findings constitute an epilepsy syndrome.

Till now, we have learned that seizure is an abnormal electrical activity in the brain. The motor manifestation of the seizure that we witness is called a convulsion. Seizures can be provoked seizure or unprovoked seizure. If there are two or more than two seizures occurring 24 hours apart, it is called epilepsy. However, if the child has more than one unprovoked seizure within 24 hours' time frame, then it will be considered as first unprovoked seizure rather than true epilepsy.

We need neuroimaging and an EEG for children with epilepsy. If the type of seizure and EEG findings can fit into any known epileptic syndrome, it qualifies the diagnosis of epilepsy syndrome. Now let us understand what the types of seizure are, how can it present clinically (semiology), will it qualify a diagnosis of epilepsy, and if yes, what are the types of epilepsy?

■ SEIZURE

Types

There are broadly two types of seizures: (1) *Generalized seizure* and (2) *focal seizure*. Generalized seizure originates at some point within the brain, but rapidly engage bilaterally distributed network. In contrast, focal seizure originates within networks limited to one hemisphere. The terms such as partial seizure (simple and complex) are no longer used to describe focality. Seizures that begin as focal seizure can evolve to bilateral convulsive seizure, which was earlier described as partial seizure with secondary generalization. ILAE 2017 has revised the classification of seizures **(Flowchart 1)**. It would be good to use ILAE 2017 recommendations to classify the type of seizure. To classify a seizure, we need answers to these three questions:

1. Is it a focal onset, generalized onset, or of unknown onset?
2. Are there motor manifestations or nonmotor manifestations?
3. What is the manifestation (e.g., is it tonic, clonic, atonic or myoclonic)?

Terminologies that have changed in the recent ILAE classification are highlighted in **Box 1** and **Table 1**. It is important to classify the onset of seizure into focal or generalized onset seizure using ILAE 2017 classification. If a child develops clonic jerks of one side of the body, then it is clearly focal seizures.

Flowchart 1: International League Against Epilepsy (ILAE) 2017 classification of seizures.

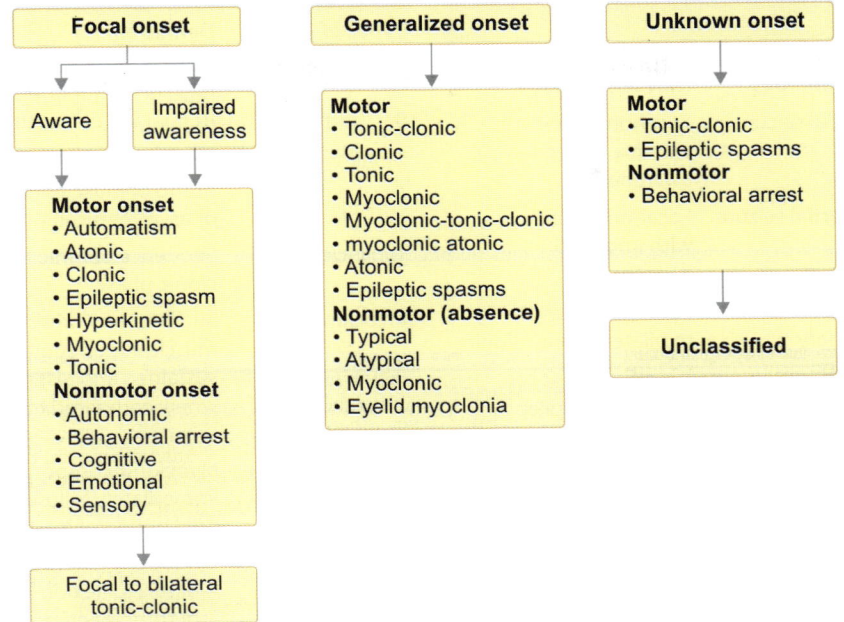

BOX 1: What has changed in recent International League Against Epilepsy (ILAE) 2017 classification?

- Partial seizures are now called focal seizures
- The terms such as simple partial seizure and complex partial seizure are no longer used. We use focal seizure with preserved awareness or focal seizure with impaired awareness
- Partial seizure with secondary generalization is better described as focal seizure evolving to bilateral convulsive seizure
- Seizures can be focal, generalized, unknown onset or unclassified onset. We call it unclassified when the seizure was not witnessed, or it is not clear whether the onset was focal or not
- Seizures like epileptic spasm, and tonic and clonic seizures can be focal as well as generalized
- Etiology can be genetic, structural or unknown etiology instead of idiopathic, symptomatic or cryptogenic
- New seizure types that are now included in the classification include absence with eyelid myoclonia, myoclonic atonic, behavioral arrest, and emotional
- Seizures types that are not used anymore include dyscognitive or psychic seizures type
- The term "benign" as in "benign rolandic epilepsy" is replaced with "self-limiting" or "pharmacoresponsive"
- The term "catastrophic" is no longer used to depict drug-resistant epilepsy as in children with West syndrome and Lennox–Gastaut syndrome

If the child was *aware* during the episode, we call it "focal onset, aware seizure" and if there was impaired awareness during the seizure, we call it "focal onset, impaired awareness". Awareness means knowledge of self and environment. Here, awareness refers to awareness during the seizure. The awareness is ideally described by the child after the seizure ends. The child was aware of what was happening around during that time

TABLE 1: Terminology pertaining to seizure and epilepsy [International League Against Epilepsy (ILAE) classification].

Earlier terminology	New terminology
Simple partial seizure	Focal-onset seizure with preserved awareness
Complex partial seizure	Focal-onset seizure with impaired awareness
Partial seizure with secondary generalization	Focal seizure evolving to bilateral tonic-clonic seizure
Benign epilepsy	Self-limited epilepsy
Catastrophic epilepsy	Pharmacoresistant epilepsy

TABLE 2: Definitions of various types of seizures.

Types of seizure	Definition
Tonic	Sustained contraction of muscle lasting for few seconds to minutes
Clonic	Regular jerking involving a group of muscles (symmetrical or asymmetrical)
Tonic-clonic	Sequence of tonic followed by clonic phase
Myoclonic	Sudden, very brief, involuntary muscle contraction less sustained and less rhythmical when compared to clonic seizure
Myoclonicatonic	Myoclonic component immediately followed by a brief period of loss of tone
Epileptic spasm	• Sudden flexion, extension or mixed flexion-extension of truncal and proximal muscles • They can be as subtle as just grimacing, head nodding, or subtle eye movement. They usually occur in clusters and may be more on awakening from sleep (relation to sleep–wake cycle)
Atonic	Sudden loss or diminution of tone lasting for <2 seconds and not preceded by any myoclonic or tonic component
Absence	Sudden cessation of ongoing activity with blank stare, unresponsiveness with possible brief up rolling of eyeballs
Atypical absence	Gradual onset and not so abrupt offset of absence that lasts for longer than typical absences with or without associated change in muscle tone, not usually witnessed during absence
Behavioral arrest	Arrest of activities, freezing, and immobilization

of seizure even if he does not remember that he had a seizure. For example, at the end of seizure, he may ask the mother as to why she was crying few minutes ago. So, he was able to understand that what was happening around him (mother crying) but he was not aware about his seizure. This will be hence classified as *focal, aware seizure*. It is obviously difficult in infants and young children to clearly say whether the awareness was impaired or preserved.

In the next step, we need to describe whether there were any motor manifestations (*motor onset*) or there were no motor manifestations (*nonmotor onset*). If the onset of seizure is unclear, it is better classified as *unknown onset*. Motor types include tonic, clonic, myoclonic, and atonic seizure; nonmotor types include behavioral arrest and absence (typical and atypical) **(Table 2)**. A few examples are given in the following text.
- If the seizure started like a focal onset but evolved to involve both limbs, it is called *focal to bilateral tonic-clonic seizure*.
- If a child develops sudden onset of forceful turning of face to either of right or left side

CHAPTER 10: Seizures, Epilepsy, and Other Paroxysmal Disorders

with vacant stare and jerks of ipsilateral upper limb with no meaningful response during this episode, we can classify it as *focal onset, impaired awareness, motor onset, and clonic* seizure. Earlier, the same seizure used to be described as complex partial seizure. Note that "awareness or impaired awareness" is applicable in focal-onset seizures and not in generalized-onset seizure.

- A 4-month-old baby presents with multiple episodes of sudden jerks occurring in cluster that occurs when she wakes up from sleep. These episodes are brief and involve all four limbs with neck and head. Using **Flowchart 1**, we can classify them as *generalized onset, motor, epileptic spasms*.
- A 3-year-old child presented with clonic jerks of all four limbs. Parents are not sure how it started, so we do not know whether to call it "generalized onset" or "focal to bilateral tonic-clonic". In such a case, it is better classified as *unknown onset, motor, tonic-clonic*. We may also get a clue once we start investigating the child. Suppose we get right-sided mesial temporal sclerosis on MRI or if we get focal discharges on electro-encephalography, we know it is probably "focal-onset" seizure.

Seizure Semiology

What exactly happened during the seizure event is called semiology. It is based on semiology that we decide whether the seizure was focal-onset seizure or a generalized-onset seizure. There are two concepts in determining the seizure semiology: (1) Lateralization and (2) localization.

Lateralizing Features

Lateralization is to decide whether seizure is originating from right or left side of hemisphere.

- Presence of unilateral dystonic posturing, unilateral forced head turning, unilateral clonic jerks, and postictal hemiparesis point to *contralateral side*.
- Unilateral motor automatism, early head turning, and unilateral eye blinking points to *ipsilateral side*.
- Presence of speech arrest and postictal aphasia points to *dominant lobe involvement*.
- Ictal speech preservation and ictal vomiting points to *nondominant lobe involvement*.

For example, if a child during a seizure turns his head to the right side, has clonic jerks in the right arm with speech arrest, the focus of seizure can be lateralized to left cerebral hemisphere.

Localizing Features

Localization means from which lobe it is arising: Frontal, temporal or occipital lobe **(Box 2)**. Seizure focus is more likely to arise from frontal lobe and temporal lobe.

- *Frontal lobe seizures* are multiple, often daily, nocturnal, abrupt onset, short

BOX 2: Key features of focal epilepsy.

- *Mesial temporal lobe epilepsy:*
  - *Subjective symptoms:* Aura (90%) like epigastric sensation, visual aura, auditory aura
  - *Objective signs:* Motor arrest, staring (dialepsis), automatisms (lip smacking, chewing, licking, and picking up at clothes), head and eye deviation to opposite side, contralateral dystonic posturing, and unilateral eye blinking
- *Neocortical temporal lobe epilepsy:* Motor manifestations are less, early onset of automatism, often begins with staring; automatism is more likely to be auditory or visual, and seizure duration is short
- *Frontal lobe epilepsy:* Brief, nocturnal, abrupt onset, explosive, hypermotor seizures (orbitofrontal), complete recovery, often occurs in clusters, clonic movement (motor cortex), "fencing" posture (supplementary motor cortex), fear or laughter (cingulate gyrus)

duration, hypermotor component, can have bipedal automatism, and can be associated with loud grunt and scream. Frontal lobe seizures have minimal impairment in the postical state.
- *Temporal lobe seizures* are less frequent compared to frontal lobe seizures, have more frequent aura, automatism, and seizures are of longer duration with prominent postictal drowsiness.
- *Occipital lobe seizure* is characterized by visual hallucinations like flashes of color or light in the visual field. This is subjective symptoms which may not described by young children.
- *Parietal lobe seizure* is extremely uncommon. They can present with numbness or tingling sensation in the limbs.

Aura is a term used to describe a warning that a child feels before he develops a seizure. One of the most common auras in children includes rising epigastric sensation. Automatism is a coordinated repetitive motor activity resembling a voluntary movement. This can occur in any part of the body. Lip smacking movement or chewing movement are the most common automatisms. Apart from orofacial automatisms, it can involve limbs including fumbling or tapping movements of hands. **Table 3** summarizes the key points in seizure semiology that point to site the origin.

■ EPILEPSY

Types

Now that we have classified the types of seizure (focal onset, generalized onset or unknown onset), the next step is to see if it qualifies the definition of epilepsy (as discussed before). If it is an epilepsy, what would be the type of epilepsy? Epilepsy is broadly divided into focal epilepsy, generalized epilepsy, combined focal, and generalized epilepsy or unknown type. This will depend on seizure type, whether it was focal onset or generalized onset; it will also depend on any focal abnormality on neuroimaging or focal or generalized abnormality on electroencephalography.

For example, if a child had "unknown onset" of seizure type, his neuroimaging was normal, but EEG revealed left temporal epileptiform discharges, then we would classify the epilepsy as *focal epilepsy*. Here, the seizure type was "unknown onset" and epilepsy type was "focal epilepsy". Probably, the event that was classified as "unknown onset" could have been "focal onset". If the seizure type was "focal onset, impaired

TABLE 3: Seizure semiology and its site of localization.

Clinical manifestation	Localization
Limb automatism	Ipsilateral temporal lobe
Unilateral eye blinking	*Lateralization:* Ipsilateral hemisphere
Postictal nose wiping	Ipsilateral temporal lobe
Rhythmic ictal nonclonic hand movement	Contralateral temporal lobe
Unilateral limb dystonia	Contralateral temporal or frontal lobe
Hyperkinetic seizures	Frontal lobe seizures
Forced head turning	Contralateral frontal lobe
Unilateral clonic movement	Contralateral frontal lobe
Ictal speech arrest	Dominant temporal lobe
Postictal aphasia	Dominant temporal lobe
Dialeptic seizures	Mesial temporal structures

awareness, motor, and clonic" but both neuroimaging and EEG were normal, it would be still classified as "focal epilepsy". Hence, focality in epilepsy is determined by focal seizure type and/or focal abnormality on neuroimaging or EEG.

Etiology

Once a diagnosis of epilepsy is made and type of epilepsy determined, the next step would be to determine the etiology. Etiology is broadly classified into structural, genetic, infectious, metabolic, immune, and unknown causes. Etiology is established based on clinical history, examination, findings on neuroimaging, and other laboratory investigations. For example, if a child has multiple episodes of seizure and his neuroimaging reveals periventricular leukomalacia which is a structural etiology, then it would be called "structural epilepsy". Similarly, epileptic seizures in a child with *SCN1A* mutation would be considered a "genetic epilepsy". If a child has epilepsy and his neuroimaging reveals neurocysticercosis (NCC), it can be called either "infectious etiology" or "structural etiology". Older classification of etiology into idiopathic, symptomatic, and cryptogenic is no longer used.

Once the etiology of epilepsy is established, an attempt at reaching electroclinical syndromic diagnosis must be made. To reiterate, syndromic diagnosis refers to cluster of symptoms such as age at onset, seizure type, and specific EEG findings. As also discussed earlier, an adolescent girl presenting with early morning myoclonus with or without generalized seizure with EEG revealing generalized epileptiform discharges of 4–4.5 Hz, especially on photic stimulation, favors a syndromic diagnosis of juvenile myoclonic epilepsy. In majority of instances, a syndromic diagnosis may not be possible, but efforts should be made to establish it. This will aid in choice of antiepileptic drug and overall prognosis.

■ ELECTROCLINICAL SYNDROME

Electroclinical syndrome is established based on the age at onset, type of seizure, EEG characteristics, response to antiepileptic drug, and outcome. Broadly they can be divided into *self-limited epilepsy* (earlier called benign epilepsy syndrome) and *epileptic encephalopathy* (earlier called catastrophic epilepsy syndrome).

Most common *self-limited epilepsies* include benign myoclonus of infancy, rolandic epilepsy (epilepsy with centrotemporal spikes), childhood or juvenile absence epilepsy, and juvenile myoclonic epilepsy **(Table 4)**. Most common *epileptic encephalopathies* or pharmacoresistant epilepsies include West syndrome, Lennox-Gastaut syndrome, and continuous spike and wave of slow sleep (CSWS) **(Table 5)**.

The term *epileptic encephalopathy* refers to cognitive and behavioral deterioration that occurs as *a direct consequence of frequent seizures* and epileptiform discharge and is not solely due to the underlying cause of the seizures. For example, if a child has global developmental delay secondary to multicystic encephalomalacia, he should be gaining milestones with time. However, if he does not gain any new milestone or loses any attained milestones, one must suspect ongoing epileptic spasms. This means that his cognitive decline is explained by this ongoing epilepsy over and above what multicystic encephalomalacia should have caused.

Epileptic spasm needs to be differentiated from myoclonus. In general, epileptic spasm involves sudden jerk of the body and trunk with resultant flexion (*flexor spasm*)

TABLE 4: Self-limited epileptic seizures and syndromes.

Epilepsy	Clinical features	Electroencephalogram (EEG) pattern
Neonatal onset		
Benign neonatal seizure (fifth day fit)	Unilateral focal clonic seizure on 4th–6th day of life in healthy neonate	Normal or discontinuous EEG background with focal or multifocal abnormalities. Focal, rhythmic theta activity with sharp waves (theta pointu alternans) can be seen in 60% of babies
Benign familial neonatal seizure	Focal clonic seizure with occasional apneic spells on day 2 or day 3 of life, persist longer in otherwise healthy neonate	Normal background or theta pointu alternans
Infantile onset		
Benign myoclonic epilepsy in infancy (BMEI)	Myoclonic jerk for 1–3 seconds in developmentally normal child; onset 4 months to 3 years	Normal EEG background with generalized spike and polyspike discharges
Childhood onset		
Childhood absence epilepsy	Frequent absence seizures in school going child; can be precipitated by hyperventilation	Normal background with 3–4.5 Hz generalized spike wave discharge with frontal dominance
Benign epilepsy with centrotemporal spikes	Seizures during sleep with orofacial motor signs, speech arrest, sialorrhea and unilateral sensory symptoms	Normal sleep background, with sharps/spike waves in centrotemporal region with a horizontal dipole
Early-onset childhood occipital epilepsy (Panayiotopoulos syndrome)	It occurs in sleep with ictal vomiting and autonomic features	Normal EEG background with multifocal and occipital spikes
Late-onset childhood occipital epilepsy (Gastaut syndrome)	Visual hallucinations, colored circular patterns	Runs of rhythmic occipital spikes and sharp waves seen during eye closure called "fixation off" sensitivity. It disappears when eyes are open and fixating at an object "fixation on"
Adolescent		
Juvenile absence epilepsy*	Speech and behavioral arrest without aura. May have automatisms	3–4 Hz spike and wave and polyspike wave discharges
Juvenile myoclonic epilepsy*	Myoclonic jerks in morning, generalized tonic-clonic seizure (GTCS), and absences	4–6 Hz bilateral polyspike wave and spike slow wave discharges; accentuation by photic stimulation
Nocturnal frontal lobe epilepsy	Focal hypermotor seizures during sleep	Runs of bilateral frontal spike, sharp waves

*May require lifelong antiepileptic medications.

TABLE 5: Clinical and EEG features of epileptic encephalopathy.

Age	Clinical phenotype	Interictal EEG features	Background abnormality	Epileptiform abnormalities
Neonatal onset				
Ohtahara syndrome	Tonic spasm	BS in wakefulness and sleep	Bursts of high voltage slow waves of 2–3 seconds followed by suppression of 3–5 seconds	Intermixed multifocal spikes
EME	Erratic fragmentary myoclonus	BS in sleep, may disappear in awake	Burst of 1–3 seconds followed by suppression of 2–10 seconds	Multifocal spikes
Infantile onset				
Migratory focal seizures (previously MPSI)	Multifocal clonic autonomic	Migrating epileptiform discharges	Normal to discontinuous	Migrating or multifocal epileptiform discharges
West syndrome	Epileptic spasms in clusters, after waking up from sleep	Hypsarrhythmia classical or modified	Chaotic, high amplitude, asynchronous slow waves	Multifocal spikes and polyspike
Dravet syndrome	Recurrent febrile and afebrile seizure myoclonic, atypical absence and focal seizures	May be normal initially for 1–2 years	Slow diffuse	Generalized, focal or multifocal discharges
Childhood onset				
MAE (Doose syndrome)	Myoclonic-atonic, absences, tonic-clonic, tonic	Doose rhythm photosensitive	Normal or Doose rhythm (rhythmic parietal theta activity)	Burst of 2–5 Hz generalized spike and polyspike waves
LGS	Tonic seizures, atypical absences, myoclonic seizures	2–2.5 spike wave discharges, PFA	Diffuse slow, absence of sleep markers	2–2.5 spike wave discharges PFA
CSWS	GTCS during sleep, atypical absence, atonic, myoclonic	Frontocentral continuous spike wave	Awake normal *Sleep:* Diffuse slow wave	1.5–2.5 Hz spike wave discharges; activation during sleep; up to 85%
LKS	Seizures in 70% Autistic regression	Temporoparietal spike wave	Awake normal *Sleep:* Diffuse slow wave	Continuous temporoparietal spike wave

(BS: burst suppression; CSWS: continuous spike and wave during sleep; EEG: electroencephalogram; EME: early myoclonic epilepsy; GTCS: generalized tonic-clonic seizure; LGS: Lennox–Gastaut syndrome; LKS: Landau–Kleffner syndrome; MAE: myoclonic astatic epilepsy; MPSI: migrating partial epilepsy of infancy; PFA: paroxysmal fast activity) or extension of the body (*extensor spasm*). They are often associated with autonomic manifestations like crying. In contrast to myoclonus (electric shock like very brief jerk), spasms are more prolonged, they occur on awakening from sleep, and they usually occur in clusters of few jerks together. If a child has epileptic spasm clinically, and EEG shows evidence of hypsarrhythmia with or without developmental delay, we call it an electroclinical syndrome known as West syndrome. Similarly, if child with developmental delay or intellectual disability has multiple types of seizures (nocturnal tonic seizures, atypical absence seizures, head drops) with EEG showing slow spike wave discharges and paroxysmal fast activity, then it is probably Lennox–Gastaut syndrome. Essential features of other epileptic encephalopathies have been summarized in **Table 5**. The terms have been changed in recent 2022 classifications of epilepsy syndromes that begin in neonates and infancy (**Box 3**) and in childhood (**Box 4**) and epilepsy syndromes that begin at any age (**Box 5**). The term idiopathic generalized epilepsies (IGE) include childhood absence epilepsy, juvenile absence epilepsy, juvenile myoclonic epilepsy and epilepsy with GTCS alone.

APPROACH TO DIAGNOSIS IN A CHILD WITH SEIZURES

History-Taking

Majority of diagnosis is based on clinical history alone. We need answers to following questions from the history:
- Is the paroxysmal event a seizure?
- Is it a provoked or an unprovoked seizure?
- If unprovoked, is it a first unprovoked seizure or does it qualify a diagnosis of epilepsy?

> **BOX 3:** International League Against Epilepsy (ILAE) classification (2022) of epilepsy syndrome that begins in neonates and infancy.
>
> - *Self-limited epilepsy:*
>   - Self-limited neonatal epilepsy
>   - Self-limited familial neonatal-infantile epilepsy
>   - Self-limited infantile epilepsy
>   - Genetic epilepsy with febrile seizure plus (GEFS+)
>   - Myoclonic epilepsy in infancy
> - *Developmental and epileptic encephalopathy (DEE):*
>   - Early infantile DEE
>   - Epilepsy in infancy with migrating focal seizures
>   - Infantile epileptic spasm syndrome
>   - Dravet syndrome
> - *Etiology-specific syndromes:*
>   - KCNQ2-DEE
>   - Pyridoxine-dependent DEE
>   - Pyridoxine 5-phosphate deficiency (PNPO)
>   - CDKL-5-DEE
>   - PCDH-19 clustering epilepsy
>   - Glucose transporter-1 deficiency
>   - Sturge–Weber syndrome gelastic seizure with hypothalamic hamartoma

- Is it focal or a generalized epilepsy?
- Does it fit into any syndromic diagnosis of epilepsy?
- What is the most probable etiology?

The main goal of the detailed history is to decide the further investigation and decide for the need of appropriate antiepileptic drug. Priority of the history is to avoid a nonepileptic event being labeled as an epileptic event and to identify and treat the underlying provoking factor.

When to suspect nonepileptic event?
Parents should be asked to narrate the exact sequence of event including what the child was doing prior to the episode, who witnessed the episode, ask the parents to enact as to what they saw in the child. Tonic-clonic movements can also occur at

BOX 4: International League Against Epilepsy (ILAE) classification (2022) epilepsy syndromes with childhood onset.

- *Self-limited focal epilepsies:*
  - Self-limited epilepsy with centrotemporal spikes
  - Self-limited epilepsy with autonomic seizures
  - Childhood occipital visual epilepsy
  - Photosensitive occipital lobe epilepsy
- *Genetic generalized epilepsies:*
  - Childhood absence epilepsy
  - Epilepsy with eyelid myoclonia
  - Epilepsy with myoclonic absence
- *Developmental and epileptic encephalopathy (DEE):*
  - Lennox–Gastaut syndrome
  - DEE-SWAS (spike and wave activation in sleep)
  - EE-SWAS (epileptic encephalopathy-spike and wave activation in sleep)
  - Landau–Kleffner syndrome
  - FIRES (febrile infection-related epilepsy syndrome)
  - HHE (hemiconvulsion hemiplegia epilepsy syndrome)

BOX 5: International League Against Epilepsy (ILAE) classification (2022) epilepsy syndromes with variable age at onset.

- *Focal epilepsy syndromes:*
  - Self-limited
    - Childhood occipital visual epilepsy
    - Photosensitive occipital lobe epilepsy
  - Familial mesial temporal lobe sclerosis
  - Epilepsy with auditory features
- *Generalized epilepsy syndromes:*
  - Juvenile myoclonic epilepsy
  - Juvenile absence epilepsy
  - Epilepsy with GTCS (generalized tonic-clonic seizures) alone
- Epilepsy syndrome with developmental and epileptic encephalopathy (DEE) or with progressive neurological deterioration
  - FIRES (febrile infection-related epilepsy syndrome)
  - Rassmussen syndrome
  - Progressive myoclonic epilepsy

the end of reflex anoxic or breath-holding spells. Hence, we might misdiagnose such nonepileptic events if preceding events such as crying and trivial injury are missed in the history. If parents narrate that in a typically developing toddler, he fell suddenly followed by paleness and he stopped breathing. This sequence clearly suggests a reflex anoxic spell rather than a seizure. Similarly, if a child while playing, became cranky, started crying, then held his breath, became unresponsive, we are probably dealing with breath-holding spells. Majority of children with nonepileptic events are typically developing children (children with normal development). Some of the clinical clues to recognize the common nonepileptic events have been summarized next:

- *Breath-holding spells:* Toddler presenting with sudden onset of paleness, cessation of breathing, perioral duskiness, which may or may not end in tonic-clonic limb movement. This sequence of event can start following a fall, cry, pain or trauma. Hence, it is essential to know what child was doing prior to the onset of paroxysmal event, to avoid misdiagnosis of epilepsy.
- *Sandifer syndrome:* Infant presenting with abnormal tonic posturing of neck, trunk, and limb (opisthotonus) occurring within minutes of feeding and regurgitation of feeds points to possibility of Sandifer syndrome.
- *Benign myoclonus of infancy:* Baby aged 3–15 months presenting with cluster of tonic or myoclonic jerks involving head and trunk with remission within 3 months of onset.
- *Shuddering spells:* Baby aged 3–6 months with paroxysms of behavioral arrest associated with shivering-like movement of head and shoulder as if some cold water was poured on the baby's back is suggestive of shuddering spells.

- *Benign paroxysmal torticollis:* Baby aged 2–8 months with paroxysmal attacks of torticollis associated with pallor, and irritability, favors a possibility of paroxysmal torticollis. This usually remits by 3–5 years of age.
- *Gratification:* Episodes of dystonic posturing, rocking, grunting, facial flushing, and diaphoresis with pressure on perineum that may cease with distraction in a toddler or preschool children is suggestive of gratification.
- *Paroxysmal tonic upward gaze:* Periods of sustained upward tonic conjugate deviation with or without ataxia is suggestive of paroxysmal tonic upward gaze. Oculogyric crises need to be considered among those with such acute episodes following administration of antiemetic medication such as metoclopramide.
- *Spasmus nutans:* Paroxysms of torticollis, nystagmus, and head nodding (no-no movement).
- *Hyperekplexia:* Excessive startle response to unexpected noise or touch resulting in generalized stiffness of body.
- *Paroxysmal dyskinesia:* An adolescent presenting with episodes of abnormal movement consisting of choreoathetoid movement, abnormal twisting movement; multiple such episodes in a day should raise suspicion of paroxysmal dyskinesia rather than seizure.
- *Parasomnias:* These events occur within few minutes to hour of sleep [nonrapid eye movement (NREM) sleep].
- *Syncope:* Prolonged standing in school prayers, skipping breakfast, sudden change of posture after a long interval, unpleasant circumstances could precipitate a syncopal attack. Presence of prodromal symptoms followed by loss of consciousness, pallor, and sweating that are brief with immediate recovery is observed in children with syncope. Rarely, tongue biting, urinary incontinence, and convulsive seizures can occur in syncope.
- *Cardiogenic syncope:* Paroxysmal episode of loss of consciousness with or without motor manifestation that occur following an exercise, point to prolonged *QT syndrome* or cardiogenic syncope.
- *Psychogenic paroxysmal nonepileptic events:* Paroxysmal events that occur following psychological stressor (school maladjustment, peer bullying, parental quarrels, and separation anxiety) could hint toward psychogenic paroxysmal nonepileptic events. These paroxysmal events usually occur in stressful situations or when other people are watching him/her. They usually do not occur when the child is alone. They are bizarre nonstereotypic motor movement, no resultant injury, presence of resisted eyelid opening (he shuts his eyes tight when we try to open it during that paroxysm), avoidance or guarding behavior, no effect of antiepileptic drug, and not accompanied by electrophysiological changes.
- *Dystonia:* History of drug ingestion (metoclopramide or prochlorperazine) prior to the episode could point to possibility of dystonic reaction (oculogyric crises).

Is it a provoked seizure or an unprovoked seizure?

It is essential to differentiate a provoked seizure from unprovoked seizure. Unprovoked seizure would be considered when the seizure cannot be explained by an immediate and obvious provoking cause. Definition of unprovoked seizure would be a seizure or a cluster of seizures occurring within 24 hours in a

TABLE 6: Definitions of terms related to febrile seizures.

Seizure type	Definition
Simple febrile seizures (SFS)	SFS are generalized, last <15 minutes, and have one episode in 24 hours
Complex febrile seizure (CFS)	CFS can be focal, prolonged (duration >15 minutes), or more than one episode in 24 hours
Simple febrile seizure plus (SFS+)	SFS+ are generalized seizure that last for <15 minutes but have more than one episode in 24 hours. SFS+ behaves like SFS rather than CFS and the overall prognosis is same as SFS
Febrile seizure plus (FS+)	FS+ refers to febrile seizure that begins either after 6 years or persists beyond 6 years of age with or without afebrile seizure/s
Febrile status epilepticus (FSE)	FSE refers to single seizure or series of seizure, with no interim recovery, lasting for >30 minutes, and otherwise meeting the definition of febrile seizure

TABLE 7: Risk of recurrence and risk of future epilepsy among children with febrile seizure.

Risk of recurrence	Risk of future epilepsy
Five risk factors include: 1. Age at onset <15 months 2. Epilepsy in first-degree relative 3. Febrile seizure in first-degree relative 4. Frequent febrile illness 5. Low temperature at onset of febrile illness	Four risk factors: 1. Family history of epilepsy 2. Abnormal neurological or developmental examination 3. Fever seizure interval (interval between onset of fever and onset of seizure; shorter the duration, higher the risk) 4. Complex febrile seizure including focal febrile seizure and febrile status epilepticus
Percentage risk of recurrence: • *10%:* No risk factor • *25–50%:* 1–2 risk factors • *50–100%:* >3 risk factors	*Percentage risk of epilepsy:* • *0.5%:* If there was no history of any febrile seizure • *1.5%:* If there is history of simple febrile seizure • *4%:* If there is a history of complex febrile seizure

person older than 1 month of age, occurring in the absence of precipitating factors.

Provoking factors include head trauma, fever, prolonged fasting (documented hypoglycemia), meningitis, and documented hypocalcemia or history of diarrhea (dyselectrolytemia). By convention, provoked seizures are not considered an epilepsy as treatment of underlying factor will treat the seizure. Hence, once you treat hypoglycemia, seizures get controlled; you do not need anticonvulsants in such cases. One of the most common provoked seizures in children is febrile seizure. Febrile seizures are common in the age group of 6 months to 5 years **(Table 6)**. There are two major concerns once a child develops febrile seizure: what is the chance that he/she will have another episode and what is the chance that he/she will develop future epilepsy requiring long-term antiepileptic drugs **(Table 7)**. Key investigations in febrile seizures are summarized in **Box 6**.

BOX 6: How to investigate a child with febrile seizure?

Indications of lumbar puncture in the first episode of simple febrile seizure:
- Presence of meningeal signs
- Infant 6–12 months when not vaccinated for *Haemophilus influenzae* type b (Hib) or pneumococcal or immunization status not known
- Optional if pretreated with antibiotic

Electroencephalogram (EEG) and magnetic resonance imaging (MRI) brain in febrile seizure: No role in simple febrile seizure; role of EEG and MRI is restricted to focal febrile seizure and febrile status epilepticus

Indications of EEG:
- Abnormal development
- Family history of epilepsy
- >1 complex feature

Indications for intermittent prophylaxis (using clobazam):
- >3 seizures in 6 months
- >4 seizures in 12 months
- Seizure lasting >15 minutes
- Seizure that require abortive medication like midazolam

Indications for continuous prophylaxis (using sodium valproate):
- Febrile status epilepticus
- Complex febrile seizure

Examination

Rapid assessment of airway, breathing, and circulation is the priority in examination in a child presenting to emergency room with acute seizure. General physical examination must focus to look for any evidence of neurocutaneous stigmata. Some of the neurocutaneous markers include port wine stain (Sturge–Weber syndrome), ash leaf macule, shagreen patch, adenoma sebaceum (tuberous sclerosis), hypopigmented lesions along the lines of Blaschko (hypomelanosis of Ito), and café-au-lait macules (neurofibromatosis). Presence of injury marks on forehead could indicate drop attacks or myoclonic jerks.

Higher mental function must focus on cognition, learning, behavior, communication, social interaction, sleep, and memory. Children with epilepsy often have associated learning difficulties, behavioral problems, sleep problems, and memory disturbances. Children with recent onset of altered sensorium, cranial nerve deficits, and motor deficits need neurological evaluation for underlying etiology.

How to provide clinical diagnosis?

Clinical diagnosis is made as per following five subheadings:

1. *Type of seizure:* Focal (aware or impaired awareness) or generalized (motor onset or nonmotor onset)
2. *Type of epilepsy:* Focal, generalized, combined focal and generalized, and unknown
3. *Etiology of seizure/epilepsy:* Structural, genetic, infectious, metabolic, immune or unknown
4. *Syndromic epilepsy diagnosis (if any):* Self-limiting or pharmacoresistant epilepsy syndromes
5. *Comorbidities:* Intellectual disability, vision or hearing impairment, motor impairment [in terms of Gross Motor Function Classification System (GMFCS)]

Example: A 7-year-old boy presented with version of head and eyes to right side with unresponsiveness that lasted for 3 minutes followed by postictal drowsiness for 1 hour. He was complaining of vague abdominal pain before onset of this episode. He had multiple episodes of febrile seizure between 1 and 4 years of age. He was brought to emergency room where he was loaded with phenytoin. MRI brain revealed left-sided mesial temporal sclerosis. EEG showed frequent interictal epileptiform discharges from left temporal leads.

Analysis: Presence of version to the right side lateralizes to left hemisphere. Similarly, presence of aura (epigastric sensation) and prolonged period of unresponsiveness localizes to temporal lobe. Hence, the seizure semiology points to left temporal lobe. History of frequent febrile seizures in the past also points to possible development of mesial temporal sclerosis. This being a structural abnormality, the etiology of this focal seizure is structural. This child had first unprovoked seizure, rest all were provoked event. Will we call it epilepsy? Yes. MRI shows mesial temporal sclerosis which increases the chances of recurrence. So, you do not have to wait for a second seizure to call it epilepsy as discussed earlier. In this child, there were no other comorbidities. This child does not fit into any known epilepsy syndrome; hence, there is no possible syndromic diagnosis.

Diagnosis:
- *Seizure classification:* Focal seizure with impaired awareness, nonmotor, and behavioral arrest
- *Type of epilepsy:* Focal epilepsy
- *Etiology:* Structural etiology
- *Epilepsy syndrome:* None
- *Comorbidity:* No significant comorbidity

Investigations for Seizures

All children with acute seizure presenting to emergency room should be subjected to blood glucose level, serum electrolytes, and blood calcium. Among those with fever, workup for underlying cause of fever needs to be determined. In children with suspected toxic or drug-induced etiology, blood levels of suspected drug must be ordered. In children who present with fever and seizure, indications of lumbar puncture include those with meningeal signs or where the history and examination suggest an intracranial infection.

Neuroimaging

Readers are advised to read the **Chapter 5** on basics of neuroimaging. Neuroimaging is indicated for evaluating a child with epilepsy, especially among those with convulsive seizures, focal seizures, cluster of seizures or focal neurological deficit. There are two options, CT head and MRI brain. CT head is easy and quick to perform and is cheap, but has the risk of radiation exposure. MRI brain has a better yield, although it takes longer time to perform and requires sedation. Contrast-enhanced computed tomography (CECT) is helpful in identifying etiologies such as NCC, tuberculoma, meningitis (meningeal enhancement), ventricular size, and vascular infarct. Among those with history of head trauma or where intracranial bleed is suspected, noncontrast computed tomography (NCCT) will be indicated. Abnormalities such as periventricular leukomalacia, cortical malformation, mesial temporal sclerosis, hippocampal malrotation are better delineated on MRI brain. MRI brain (contrast) would be indicated in nonemergent, nontraumatic cases with seizures and among those with developmental delay, and intellectual disability. In children with refractory seizures and those with suspected temporal lobe epilepsy, MRI brain with dedicated epilepsy protocol would be useful. These dedicated epilepsy protocols look for finer details of hippocampal volumetric on MRI brain and diagnose mesial temporal sclerosis **(Fig. 1)**. Restrict the use of CT to only patients with trauma as we know that bones are better visualized in CT brain as compared to MRI brain. It is important to note that epilepsy syndromes like juvenile absence epilepsy or juvenile myoclonic epilepsy often do not warrant a neuroimaging.

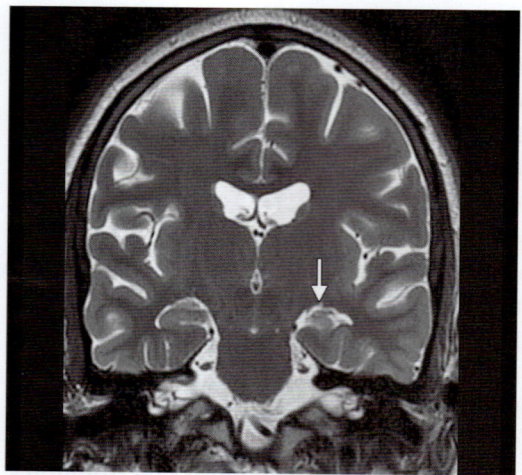

Fig. 1: Magnetic resonance imaging T2 coronal image showing left-sided hippocampal atrophy and mesial temporal sclerosis (arrow).

Electroencephalogram

Kindly read the basics of electroencephalogram (EEG) from **Chapter 6**. EEG must be considered among those with unprovoked seizure where neuroimaging is normal. Should we get both MRI brain and EEG simultaneously or should we get it done sequentially? If sequential, should we perform MRI first or EEG first? In endemic zone for NCC as in north India, MRI brain is preferred first before considering EEG. This contrasts with American and European guidelines, where EEG is preferred as the first-line investigation among those presenting with unprovoked seizure. Focal slowing on EEG could suggest underlying structural focal pathology.

An EEG is useful in diagnosis of the event, identification of a specific syndrome, and for prediction of long-term outcome/recurrence. EEG abnormalities are considered the best predictors of recurrence in children who were neurologically normal. It is estimated that recurrence risk was significantly less among those with normal EEG (25% of 165 children) when compared to those with abnormal EEG (54% of 103 children). Ideally, EEG must be performed within 4 weeks of the episode. However, in centers with large burden of patients, this short duration is often not feasible.

Other investigations in epilepsy include interictal positron emission tomography (PET) scan and ictal single-photon emission computerized tomography (SPECT) scan. If there are multiple episodes of focal seizure semiology with focal EEG findings but MRI is normal, then an interictal PET scan or ictal SPECT scan would be useful for localizing the site or focus of seizures. Many such patients are good candidates for epilepsy surgery, especially when conventional antiepileptic medications are not working well.

■ CASE VIGNETTES

Case 1

A 10-year-old boy presented with first episode of twitching of right angle of mouth with frothing and lack of awareness during the episode that lasted for 20 minutes followed by drowsiness for next 30 minutes. He is school going, studying in 5th standard. There is no family history of seizure, epilepsy. There was no history of head trauma or febrile illness.

Analysis:
- *Seizure type:* Focal motor seizure with impaired awareness
- *Provoked or unprovoked:* Probably unprovoked seizure
- *Is it an epilepsy:* It is the first unprovoked seizure
- *Will you get MRI brain or CECT:* Would prefer MRI brain with a focus on mesial temporal structures (mesial temporal lobe sclerosis)
- *Is there a role of EEG:* EEG will be useful provided common lesions such as NCC or tuberculoma have been ruled out to predict the chances of recurrence. In areas not endemic for NCC, EEG is the first option. If MRI reveals NCC, treat the NCC. There is no point in getting both

MRI and EEG done simultaneously in such case. Get an EEG before tapering the antiepileptic drugs. If MRI is normal, get a good sleep deprived EEG done to look for focal epileptiform abnormalities.

Case 2

A 2-year-old boy presented with history of multiple episodes of generalized seizure following a fall from the roof of the house. He is hemodynamically stable. There are no neurological deficits.

Analysis:
- *Is it a seizure?* Probably yes.
- *Is it provoked or unprovoked seizure?* It is clearly a provoked seizure, following head trauma.
- *Is it epilepsy?* It is difficult to predict at this point of time.
- *Which is the investigation of choice:* Would prefer NCCT scan with bone window to look for fractures.
- *Is there a role of EEG?* It might not be helpful at this point of time; it may be useful before deciding to taper antiepileptic drugs.

Case 3

A 6-month-old boy presented with multiple episodes of epileptic spasms for last 1 month. It involves a jerk involving all the four limbs.

He had not attained any developmental milestones. He had history of perinatal asphyxia.

Analysis:
- *What is the seizure type?* Generalized onset and epileptic spasm
- *Provoked or unprovoked:* Unprovoked seizure
- *Is it an epilepsy?* Yes
- *Does it qualify a syndromic diagnosis?* Probably yes, especially if the EEG can demonstrate hypsarrhythmia or its variant.
- *What is the investigation of choice?* EEG should be done on priority to look for evidence of hypsarrhythmia. MRI brain is required for establishing the underlying etiology.

Case 4

A 10-year-old girl presented with episodes of sudden head drop followed by brief period of unresponsiveness that lasts for few seconds. She is otherwise normal, attending her school.

Analysis
- *What is seizure type?* Generalized onset, motor onset, and myoclonic absence
- *Is it provoked or unprovoked?* Unprovoked
- *Is it epilepsy?* Yes, multiple such episodes in a day
- *Does it qualify a syndromic diagnosis?* Probably yes, if EEG findings are suggestive of generalized epileptiform discharges, then it could support electroclinical syndrome of "epilepsy with myoclonic absence".
- *Investigation:* Yield of abnormality on MRI brain is very low. EEG will be a useful investigation for this child.

KEY MESSAGES

- Identify the paroxysmal event; could it be a seizure or nonepileptic event? Focus on the complete description of the event before concluding that it is a true seizure.
- All seizures are not epilepsy; presence of more than two unprovoked seizure would qualify a diagnosis of epilepsy.
- Seizures are classified as focal onset, generalized onset or unknown onset. Epilepsy is classified as focal epilepsy, generalized epilepsy, and mixed epilepsy.
- Etiology of epilepsy is categorized into structural, genetic, infectious, metabolic, immune or unknown causes.
- Epilepsy syndrome could be self-limited epilepsies or pharmacoresistant epilepsy (epileptic encephalopathy).

CHAPTER 11

Approach to a Child with Altered Sensorium and Coma

■ INTRODUCTION

Encephalopathy refers to a global dysfunction of mental status. It is essential to differentiate it from *encephalitis*, which refers to inflammation of brain parenchyma. Most children with encephalitis will thus present with encephalopathy, but not all children with encephalopathy have encephalitis as the underlying cause. Causes of encephalopathy can be broadly categorized as infective, parainfectious, autoimmune, traumatic, metabolic, toxic, and malignant **(Table 1)**.

Initial Assessment and Stabilization

Steps in initial management include stabilization of airway, breathing, and maintaining circulation. It is essential to treat hypoglycemia (blood sugar <50 mg/dL) and dyselectrolytemia, if any. Seizures need to be controlled with appropriate antiepileptic medication, and measures should be instituted to decrease raised intracranial pressure (ICP) **(Table 2)**. Once these initial steps are addressed, the patient needs to be evaluated to establish the cause of altered sensorium by detailed history, examination, and investigations.

■ CLINICAL PRESENTATION

Presenting Complaints

Clinical presentation can be highly variable depending on the etiology and age of presentation. Children with acute encephalopathy often present in an acute emergency setting with one or more of the following complaints for a duration of <7 days:
- Altered consciousness or altered sensorium
- Multiple episodes of convulsion
- Multiple episodes of vomiting and severe headache (older children)
- Excessive irritability and repeated episodes of vomiting (infants)

History of Presenting Illness

The following points need to be covered in the history of presenting illness among children who present with acute encephalopathy.

Elaboration of Presenting Complaints

- *Fever:* Grade of fever, documented temperature; any relief with medication must be elicited. Chronology of fever with the development of acute encephalopathy is a useful link to etiology. Presence of ongoing fever with encephalopathy points to an infective pathology like meningoencephalitis. History of febrile illness, diarrheal illness, or vaccination in the recent past in a child with acute encephalopathy points to parainfectious etiology like acute disseminated encephalomyelitis (ADEM). In the absence of fever, infective causes are fairly ruled out.
- *Altered sensorium:* The focus of history would be to determine the extent or depth

TABLE 1: Causes of encephalopathy in infants and children.

Broad etiology	Causes
Infective	• Meningitis/meningoencephalitis • Brain abscess (secondary to CSOM/mastoiditis)
Parainfectious/autoimmune	• ADEM • Autoimmune encephalitis (NMDA and VGKC) • Hashimoto encephalitis
Traumatic (head trauma)	Traumatic intracranial bleed (subarachnoid, subdural, and intraparenchymal)
Intracranial bleed (nontraumatic)	• Rupture of AV malformation and cavernous malformation • Bleeding diathesis (thrombocytopenia/coagulopathy)
Seizures	Postictal event or nonconvulsive status epilepticus
Metabolic	• Hypoglycemia • Dyselectrolytemia (hypo-/hypernatremia) • Hepatic encephalopathy • Uremic encephalopathy • Metabolic acidosis (lactic acidosis in mitochondrial cytopathies) • Hyperammonemia • Hypoxic ischemic encephalopathy (poststatus epilepticus, postcardiac arrest, prolonged mechanical ventilation, postdrowning) • Hypertensive encephalopathy • Toxic causes (carbon monoxide, heavy metals, and drugs)
Vascular	• Cerebral venous sinus thrombosis • Arterial ischemic stroke
Malignancy	• Primary malignancy with sudden hemorrhage • Secondary metastasis

(ADEM: acute disseminated encephalomyelitis; AV: arteriovenous; CSOM: chronic suppurative otitis media; NMDA: N-methyl D-aspartate receptor; VGKC: voltage-gated potassium channel)

TABLE 2: Basic steps in management of a patient with coma.

Goal	Principle
Establishing airway: Intubation and mechanical ventilation	*Indication:* Glasgow Coma Scale (GCS) ≤ 8, impaired airway reflexes, signs of raised ICP, SpO$_2$ <92% despite high flow oxygen, fluid refractory shock
Establish IV cannula and maintain circulation	Management of shock as per standard guidelines [fluid challenge 20 mL/kg (may be repeated) followed by inotropic support]
Hypoglycemia (<50 mg/dL)	IV dextrose (5 mL/kg)
Seizure	Lorazepam (0.1 mg/kg) followed by phenytoin (15–20 mg/kg loading dose at a maximum rate of 1 mg/kg/min)
Raised ICP: Abnormal pupil, decerebration, bradycardia, hypertension, abnormal respiratory pattern, and papilledema	Mannitol or 3% hypertonic saline, moderate hyperventilation, and head end elevation to 30°
Fever	Antipyretic drugs

(ICP: intracranial pressure; IV: intravenous; SpO$_2$: oxygen saturation of arterial blood)

of impaired consciousness. We remember that sensorium has two components of wakefulness (preserved sleep–wake cycle) and awareness [interest in surrounding, interest in toys, ability to recognize and obey parental commands, indicating for food (hunger), and wet pants (passage of urine/stool)]. Absence of wakefulness and awareness would indicate coma. Does the child give any meaningful or suboptimal response to commands from the parents (minimally conscious child)? For example, a child cries every time mother talks to him instead of responding the way he used to do before illness (response is suboptimal but reproducible, qualifying the depth of impaired consciousness to be minimally conscious state).

- *Seizure:* Episode of abnormal movement in the form of jerky movement of limbs (clonic), tight posturing followed by jerky movement of limbs (tonic-clonic seizure), forced turning of face/eyes to one side (focal seizure), twitching of the mouth (focal), and repeated blinking of the eyes. Presence or absence of unresponsiveness during the paroxysmal event must be elicited.
- *Headache:* Severe continuous and diffuse headache disturbing sleep and performance of day-to-day activities is suggestive of headache secondary to raised ICP. The headache is often associated with vomiting and the child may have temporary relief of headache with vomiting. Infants with raised ICP may have excessive irritability, headbanging, and refusal to feed with repeated vomiting on an attempt to feed.
- *Vomiting:* Many children with raised ICP at the onset of illness can describe the sudden onset of violent vomiting without any nausea that forces the vomitus to fall in the distance from where the child is standing (projectile vomiting). Infants may vomit every feed.

History to Ascertain the Extent of Involvement

- *History of altered sensorium:* Lack of alertness (sleep–wake cycle preserved or absent) and lack of awareness (inability to indicate for bladder/bowel/hunger needs, not recognizing parents, and lack of any meaningful response to verbal/physical stimuli). When the sleep–wake cycles are preserved, parents know that now the child is awake and now he/she is sleeping. If this cycle is absent, it indicates a lack of wakefulness. By awareness, we mean the ability to understand and respond to external environmental cues.
- *History of cranial nerve (CN) involvement:* They can have associated malalignment of eyes (3rd, 4th, and 6th CN), drooping of eyelids (3rd CN), deviation of angle of mouth, drooling of saliva (7th CN), nasal regurgitation of feeds, or alteration in voice and difficulty in swallowing (9th and 10th CN).
- *History of motor involvement:* Other motor symptoms must be enquired including tightness (may indicate spasticity) or abnormal twisting postures (indicates dystonia which needs to be confirmed on the examination) or flail-ness of limbs (indicates hypotonia on examination), and paucity of movement of any half of the body (indicates hemiparesis)
- History of *neck stiffness* (indicates meningeal irritation)

Etiological History

The following etiological history needs to be elucidated:

- History of preceding convulsions (postictal state of altered sensorium would

- recover within few minutes to hours or if the child develops hypoxic brain injury secondary to status epilepticus, then the recovery may take longer and may leave behind neurological sequelae)
- History of rash (measles, rickettsia, meningococcemia, and dengue)
- Small reddish spots (petechiae) or bluish patches in the skin all over the body (meningococcemia)
- History of preceding diarrhea (enteroviral meningoencephalitis and cerebral cortical venous sinus thrombosis)
- History of prior vaccination and febrile illness (ADEM)
- History of ear discharge [brain abscess secondary to chronic suppurative otitis media (CSOM)]
- History of bleeding from any other site (bleeding diathesis with an intracranial bleed as in infants with vitamin K deficiency)
- History of excessive sweating, behavioral disturbances, and alteration in sleep–wake cycle [autoimmune encephalitis including N-methyl D-aspartate receptor (NMDAR) encephalitis]
- History of bony pains, swelling or mass in the abdomen, and unexplained weight loss (paraneoplastic neurological manifestation secondary to malignancy)
- History of rash, joint pain, and arthralgia (systemic vasculitis like systemic lupus erythematosus)
- History of jaundice (hepatic encephalopathy)
- History of polyuria, polydipsia, and inability to gain weight (uremic encephalopathy)
- History of onset of altered sensorium following an overnight fast (hypoglycemia)
- History of profuse diarrhea and prior fluid administration (dyselectrolytemia like hypo-/hypernatremia)
- History of eating raw litchi in empty stomach (acute toxic encephalopathy with litchi consumption)
- Past history of head trauma (subdural hemorrhage can present with acute encephalopathy)
- Past history of similar encephalopathy (toxic causes or inborn errors of metabolism)
- History of consanguinity, recurrent abortions, sibling loss, affected siblings, affected family members, and abnormal urinary odor (inborn error of metabolism)
- Any prior medical illness like cyanotic congenital heart disease (CHD) (venous sinus thrombosis or brain abscess), chronic renal failure (posterior reversible leukoencephalopathy), and nephrotic syndrome (venous sinus thrombosis or posterior reversible leukoencephalopathy)
- History of drug intake (sedative drugs) or possible toxin exposure (organic solvents, heavy metal exposure, cyanide, and carbon monoxide). *Note:* Sleeping in a closed room in winter months with a heater might expose the family to high levels of carbon monoxide. History of aspirin intake has been linked to development of Reye syndrome.
- History of prior epilepsy [children with nonconvulsive status epilepticus (NCSE) might present with acute onset of encephalopathy; any child whose sensorium does not recover following convulsive seizure for a sufficiently prolonged period must be considered for NCSE].

EXAMINATION

Vital Signs

Vital signs were evaluated as a part of the initial assessment. The presence of tachycardia with poor pulse volume would indicate septic shock. The presence of bradycardia and hypertension could point to the feature of raised ICP. Presence of hypertension alone could point to the possibility of posterior reversible encephalopathy syndrome (PRES) (also known as reversible posterior leukoencephalopathy) and hypertensive encephalopathy.

General Physical Examination

- Presence of anemia (intracranial bleeding and cerebral malaria)
- Presence of jaundice (hepatic encephalopathy)
- Presence of central cyanosis and clubbing (cyanotic CHD with either cerebral venous sinus thrombosis or brain abscess)
- Presence of rash (measles encephalitis, meningococcemia, dengue fever, and rickettsial fever)
- Presence of petechiae or ecchymotic patches (dengue hemorrhagic fever, rickettsial infection, and meningococcemia)
- *Signs of trauma:* Look for head contusion, concussion or any other injury marks in the scalp

Assessment of Sensorium

Consciousness has two components: Awareness and wakefulness. Wakefulness refers to the preservation of sleep–wake cycle, whereas awareness is assessed in terms of eye opening, motor response, and verbal response. Alteration of sensorium can be classified as conscious, minimally conscious state, coma, and vegetative state **(Table 3)**.

Sensorium is assessed bedside using Glasgow Coma Scale (GCS) **(Table 4)**. GCS was developed to assess the level of neurological injury in head injury patients. It has three components: Eye opening (score 1–4), motor response (score of 1–6), and verbal response (score of 1–5). The minimum GCS score is 3 and the maximum score is 15. As per GCS, brain injury was classified as severe (GCS ≤ 8), moderate (GCS 9–12), and mild (GCS > 13). Considering difficulty in interpreting verbal scores among intubated patients, we use the letter "T" to denote GCS score of an intubated patient. Hence, GCS in an intubated patient can range from a minimum of 3 scores to a maximum of 11 scores (4 for eye opening, 6 for motor response, and 1 minimum for verbal score). Spontaneous eye opening indicates arousal response (intact brainstem) and not intact awareness. Eye opening to speech must be tested before giving painful stimulus as it is essential to determine the best or highest level of response. A verbal response is difficult to comment on among intubated and aphasic patients. Similarly, the verbal component of GCS is challenging to assess among preverbal children below 3 years of age, although pediatric GCS somewhat takes care of this fallacy. The motor response is difficult to comment among patients on neuromuscular-blocking drugs or those with spinal cord pathology.

TABLE 3: Interpretation of state of consciousness.

State of consciousness	Conscious	Minimal conscious state	Coma	Vegetative state
Self-awareness	Present	Limited	Absent	Absent
Perception of pain	Yes	Yes	No	No
Sleep–wake cycle	Preserved	Preserved	Lost	Preserved
Motor function	Purposeful	Severe limitation	No movement	No movement
Respiratory function	Normal	Variably depressed	Variably depressed	Normal

TABLE 4: Glasgow Coma Scale (GCS).*

Scores	Eye opening	Scores	Motor response (pediatric GCS)	Scores	Verbal response (pediatric GCS)
4	Spontaneous	6	Obey command (spontaneous movement)	5	Oriented (coos and babbles which is age appropriate)
3	Eye opening to speech	5	Localizes to pain (withdraws to touch)	4	Confused response (irritable and cries)
2	Eye opening to pain	4	Withdraws to pain	3	Inappropriate words (cries to pain)
1	No eye opening	3	Abnormal flexion response	2	Incomprehensible sounds (moans to pain)
		2	Abnormal extension response	1	No verbal response
		1	No motor response		

*Minimum score is 3 and maximum score is 15.

Other scales used for assessment of sensorium in an emergency setting include:
- Test responsiveness, obeys, localizes, or less (TROLL):
  - Obeys command
  - Localizes to pain
  - Withdrawal to pain or less
- Alert verbal pain unresponsiveness (AVPU)
  - Alert
  - Responds to verbal stimuli
  - Responds to painful stimuli
  - Unresponsive to all stimuli
- Alert, confused, drowsy, unresponsive (ACDU)
  - Alert
  - Confused
  - Drowsy
  - Unresponsive
- Full outline of unresponsiveness (FOUR) scores **(Fig. 1)**

Assessment of Eye Movement

Oculocephalic Reflex

Eyelids must be held open to observe for spontaneous eye movement; conjugate movement of eyes indicates an intact ocular motor system. Among those in whom cervical trauma has been ruled out, eye movement must be tested by oculocephalic reflex (doll's eye response). Among patients with coma with the intact brainstem, eyes move in a counter direction to direction of movement of the head, i.e., if the head is moved to the right extreme, eyes move to left and at the extreme when the head is held, eyes move to mid position. This reflex must be tested in both a horizontal and vertical gaze. In an awake patient, voluntary control of gaze overcomes reflex eye movement. Hence, there is little utility of the doll's eye response in a conscious or minimally conscious state. It is essential to remember that preserved doll's eye response indicates an intact brainstem pathway, especially the pathway from the vestibular nucleus lower pons (pontine tegmentum). It is also important to note that ocular motor pathways are very close to the reticular activating system that maintains consciousness.

Vestibular–ocular Reflex

Among those with cervical trauma and those with a poor response on oculocephalic

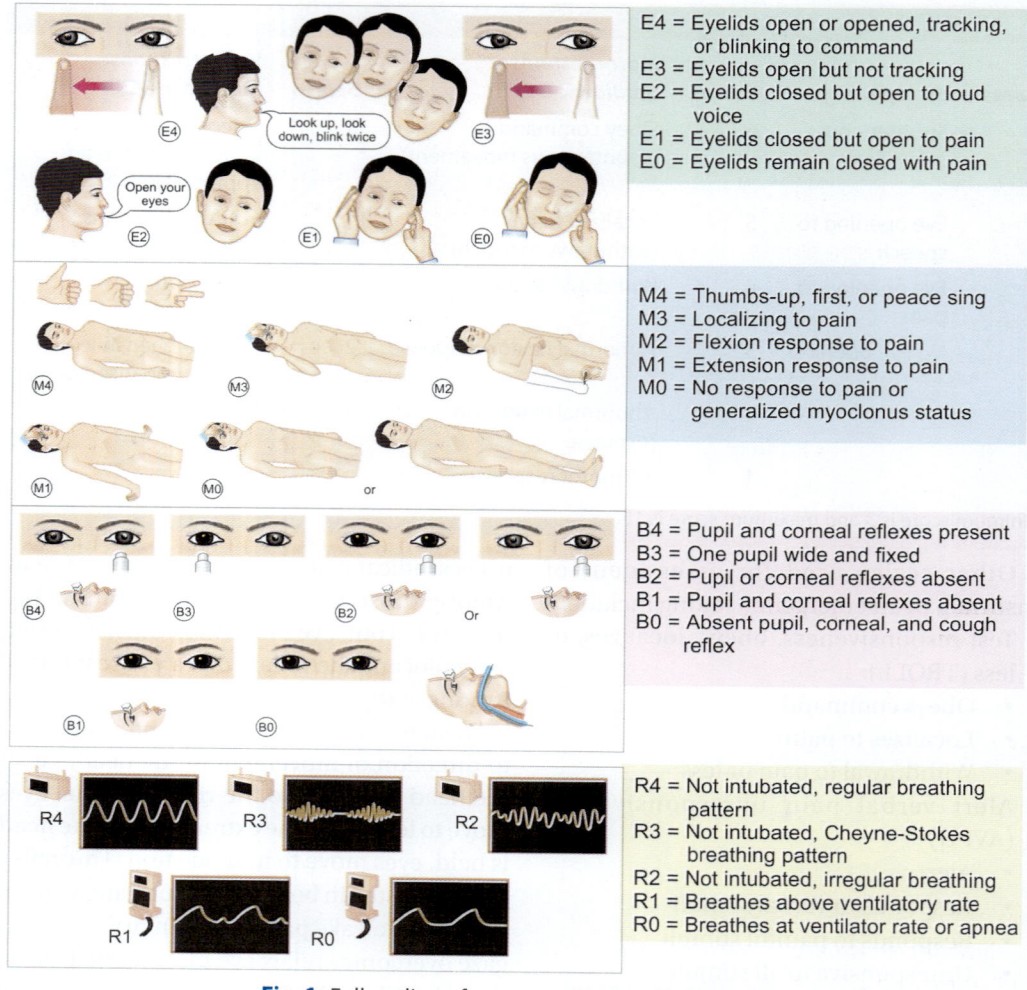

Fig. 1: Full outline of unresponsiveness (FOUR) score.

reflex, the caloric vestibular–ocular response needs to be tested. The head end is raised to 30°; ice water is infused into the ear canal at 10 mL/min for 5 minutes. In an awake patient, cold water irrigation results in the slow drift toward the side of irrigation with compensatory rapid nystagmus to the midline in the opposite direction (cold, opposite; warm, same; refers to fast compensatory direction). In a comatose patient, cold water irrigation results in tonic deviation toward the same side. The absence of caloric response indicates brainstem dysfunction or bilateral vestibular dysfunction (aminoglycoside and phenytoin).

Interpretation of Eye Movement Findings in a Comatose Patient

The frontal eye field governs the saccadic eye movement in the horizontal gaze. The frontal eye field stimulates contralateral paramedian pontine reticular formation (PPRF), which in turn stimulates ipsilateral 6th nerve causing

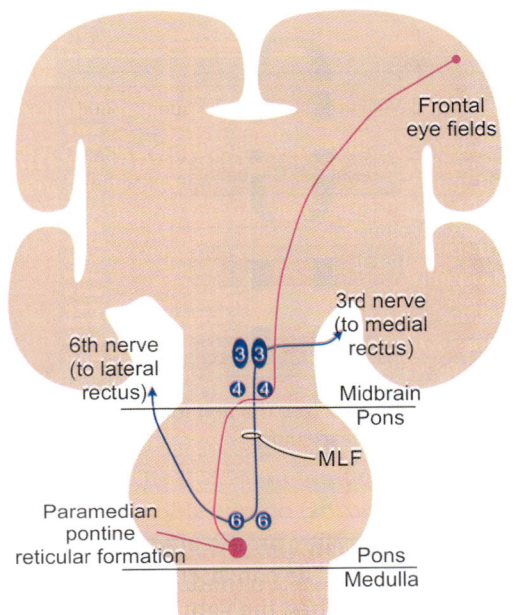

Fig. 2: Supratentorial control of extraocular eye movements. (MLF: medial longitudinal fasciculus)

abduction and contralateral 3rd nerve [through medial longitudinal fasciculus (MLF)] causing adduction **(Fig. 2)**. Hence, left frontal eye field will result in the abduction of the right eye and adduction of the left eye causing conjugate gaze toward the right. In a comatose patient, when the head is turned to right normally, the eyes will deviate toward the left in a conjugate manner, and similarly, when the head is turned to left, there will be conjugate eye deviation toward the right. This indicates normal brainstem function, including MLF and PPRF. Read **Chapter 1** on clinical neuroanatomy for understanding the basis of abnormalities in the eye movement.

The following abnormalities in eye movement can be noticed:

- *Tonic deviation to one side:* When eyes are tonically deviated to one side, it indicates a contralateral irritative cortical lesion or ipsilateral destructive cortical lesion. Hence in a comatose child, if eyes are tonically deviated toward the left side, it could be an irritative focus on the right cortex, destructive focus on the left cortex, or destructive lesion of the left side of pons. The irritative focus will tonically activate the frontal eye field, forcing the eyes to look in opposite direction, whereas a destructive lesion in one side will decrease stimulation from that side, forcing the other frontal eye field to deviate the eyes to the same side. The focus of seizure is an example of irritative lesion. Brain abscess or gliosis are examples of destructive lesions.
- *Abnormalities on oculocephalic reflex (doll's eye reflex):* When we move the head of the doll to one side, her eyes move in the opposite direction. A similar response in a comatose patient would indicate intact brainstem. In such a case, if we move the head to the left side, we expect the eyes to deviate to the right. If on moving the head to the left side, the left eye turn right, but the right eye does not turn right, it indicates right-sided 6th nerve or lateral rectus palsy **(Fig. 3)**. We remember that MLF interconnects one-sided 6th CN nucleus to contralateral 3rd CN nucleus so that eyes can move together (conjugate eye movement). If we move the eye of a comatose patient to the right side, then both eyes turn left. But when we move the eye to the left, the left eye does not move, and right eye abducts with endpoint nystagmus, it indicates right-sided MLF lesion. If there is a right MLF lesion, right PPRF will stimulate the right 6th nerve but cannot stimulate the left 3rd nerve. This results in a failure of the adduction of the left eye. If both eyes fail to adduct, it will indicate a bilateral MLF lesion.

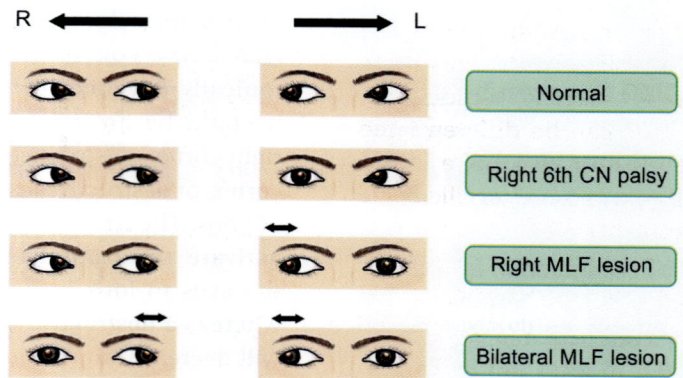

Fig. 3: Ocular movement in comatose patients on oculocephalic reflex (see the text for explanation). (CN: cranial nerve; MLF: medial longitudinal fasciculus)

Assessment of Pupillary Reflex

Assessment of pupillary size and reaction to light gives an important clue to neuroanatomical localization in a comatose patient. It is very important to remember that pupillary response is not affected in metabolic coma. Hence, presence or absence of pupillary response helps in differentiating structural coma from metabolic coma. Pupillary response is determined by sympathetic innervations from C8-T2 sympathetic chain causing pupillary dilation and parasympathetic innervations from the Edinger–Westphal nucleus causing pupillary constriction. In addition to pupillary response, ciliospinal reflex must be used to test integrity of lower brainstem to spinal cord pathway. In this reflex, pinching neck skin will result in ipsilateral pupillary dilatation. Following pupillary abnormalities can be observed among comatose patients:

- *Normal reflex:* When the light is shown on one eye, both pupils constrict to direct and consensual light reflex. When the light is shifted from one side to the other side, that pupil constricts to direct light reflex and the other eye to consensual light reflex.
- *Relative afferent pupillary defect:* When there is damage to the retina or optic disc (*optic neuritis*) on one side, there will be no direct reflex on the affected side, but the affected side constricts on consensual light reflex when the light is shown on the opposite side. Hence, when the light is swung from normal to abnormal side, the pupil constricts on the normal side with consensual constriction of the pupil in the affected side. But when the light reaches the affected side, consensual constriction starts to dilate, and since direct light reflex will be absent on that side, the affected eye shows dilation of the pupil (paradoxical). This phenomenon is called relative afferent pupillary defect (RAPD).
- *Unilateral fixed dilated pupil:* It is considered the most ominous sign, which indicates uncal lobe herniation unless proven otherwise. (Rule out mydriatic use in the affected eye.) Other causes of unilateral fixed dilated pupil include rupture of posterior communicating artery aneurysm, which compresses on 3rd CN.
- *Unilateral small reactive pupil with associated ptosis and anhidrosis represent Horner syndrome.* The presence of Horner syndrome in a comatose patient with arterial ischemic stroke often points to arterial dissection at the carotid level.

- Bilateral large or mid-dilated fixed pupil often results from damage to the oculomotor nucleus at midbrain tegmentum. This can be differentiated from the fixed dilated pupil of a brain-dead patient by the presence of ciliospinal reflex in the former.
- Pinpoint pupil results from extensive damage to the sympathetic pathway, as seen in an extensive pontine tegmental injury like pontine hemorrhage.
- Small reactive pupil can be seen in a diencephalic lesion or in metabolic causes of coma.

Assessment of Motor Response to Stimuli

Decorticate posturing refers to flexion of upper limbs (at elbow, wrist, and fingers) and extension and internal rotation of lower limbs. This results from extensive dysfunction of forebrain till rostral midbrain. Any lesion below rostral midbrain results in decerebrate posturing where there is hyperextension of both upper and lower limbs with opisthotonic posturing. In contrast, lesions of forebrain and diencephalon often result in hemiparesis with the opposite side showing few meaningful localizing signs.

Assessment of Respiratory Pattern

Table 5 outlines the type of respiratory pattern observed among comatose patients.

This can provide a clue to the site of the lesion.

ANALYSIS OF HISTORY AND EXAMINATION

Review of history and examination can be made under the following heads:
- *State of consciousness/depth of coma:* Coma, vegetative state, and minimally conscious state.

TABLE 5: Types of abnormal respiration and its neurological localization.

Type of respiration	Site of lesion
Cheyne–Stokes breathing	Metabolic coma, diencephalic lesion, and forebrain lesion
Central neurogenic hyperventilation	Metabolic encephalopathy
Apneustic breathing	Bilateral pontine lesion
Cluster or ataxic breathing	Pontomedullary junction

- Are there any signs of raised ICP or features of herniation?
- *Possible extent of involvement and neuro-anatomical localization:* Extensive cortical lesion, unilateral cortical lesion, diencephalic lesion, brainstem involvement (midbrain, pons, and medulla involvement), or multifocal involvement
- *Possible etiology:* Infective, parainfectious, vascular, metabolic, or traumatic **(Table 1)**

■ CASE VIGNETTES

Case 1

A 3-month-old boy presented with a history of a flurry of multifocal seizures, progressive paleness of body, and altered sensorium for the last 2 days. On examination, heart rate (HR)—72 beats/min, respiratory rate (RR)—24 breaths/min, and blood pressure (BP)—110/70 mm Hg (>95th centile). Severe pallor was present. Anterior fontanel was bulging tense. The child was in a minimally conscious state with motor hypertonia with brisk deep tendon reflex (DTR) and extensor plantar response. Pupils were small and reactive. There was no evident CN palsy.

Analysis

- *State of consciousness:* Minimally conscious state

- *Features of raised ICP:* Present (hypertonia, brisk reflex, and bulging fontanel)
- *Neuroanatomical site:* Cortical lesion (seizure, altered sensorium, features of raised ICP, and no CN palsy)
- *Possible etiology:* Vascular etiology like hemorrhagic stroke or venous strokes are more likely considering the acute onset of encephalopathy with features of raised ICP. In absence of fever, and any febrile illness in the recent past, infective or parainfectious etiology is less likely. Screening ultrasonography can be performed to confirm the diagnosis of intracranial bleed. This intracranial bleed can result from vitamin K deficiency.

Case 2

A 14-month-old boy diagnosed with tetralogy of Fallot at the age of 9 months was on propranolol. He presented with a history of seizure followed by altered sensorium. He was comatose with GCS = 6. His pupils were fixed and dilated. The oculocephalic reflex was absent. He had decerebrate posturing with hyperventilation. He was intubated electively and mechanically ventilated.

Analysis

- *State/depth of consciousness:* Coma
- *Features of raised ICP:* Present
- *Neuroanatomical site:* Multifocal (cortical in view of seizures, encephalopathy; brainstem lesion below rostral midbrain in view of absent oculocephalic reflex, fixed dilated pupil, and decerebrate posturing). This could be secondary to central herniation.
- *Possible etiology:*
  - Cerebral venous sinus thrombosis (in view of underlying cyanotic CHD)
  - Arterial ischemic stroke could result in features of raised ICP and central herniation in children with cyanotic CHD. Brain abscess is less likely in view of the absence of fever.

Neuroimaging, preferably magnetic resonance imaging (MRI) brain with magnetic resonance (MR) venography, is essential to look for venous sinus thrombosis. In view of raised ICP, it would be prudent to defer lumbar puncture till neuroimaging is performed.

Case 3

An 8-year-old boy presented with multiple episodes of seizures, high-grade fever, and altered sensorium for 2 days. The child was developmentally normal and was going to school before the onset of illness. There was no history to suggest any CN involvement and no history of any motor deficit or any abnormal movement. There was no meningeal sign. There was no hepatosplenomegaly. Currently, he is in altered sensorium (minimally conscious state).

Analysis

- *State or depth of consciousness:* Minimally conscious state
- Are there any features of raised ICP? Probably no
- What is the extent of lesion? It is involving the sensorium but probably sparing the CNs, motor functions, sensory functions, or meningeal irritation. The most probable neuroanatomical site of lesion is gray matter (cortex).
- *Etiology:* In the presence of ongoing fever, infective etiology needs to be kept. We are probably dealing with acute febrile encephalopathy with no clinical features of raised ICP. The clinical differentials would be encephalitis (bacterial or viral) and cerebral malaria (absence of splenomegaly and anemia are point against).

Case 4

A 12-year-old girl presented with altered behavior, excessive shouting, and altered sensorium for duration of 10 days. There was no clear preceding febrile illness or vaccination. She developed an episode of seizure on the 10th day of illness. She was brought to casualty convulsing. Once seizures were aborted, she remained in a minimally conscious state. There was no evidence of any CN palsy, no motor deficit, and no meningeal signs. The systemic examination was unremarkable.

Analysis

- *State of consciousness:* We are probably dealing with acute to subacute (history of 10 days) neurological illness with seizures and encephalopathy. The child is in a minimally conscious state.
- There are no clear signs of raised ICP.
- *Extent of lesion and neuroanatomical site:* In this case, again CNs, motor functions, sensory functions, and signs of meningeal irritation are spared. The possible neuroanatomical site is the cerebral cortex (gray matter).
- *Etiology:* In the absence of ongoing fever, infective pathology looks less likely when compared to the possibility of parainfectious pathology. Clinical possibilities of ADEM and autoimmune encephalitis, therefore, need to be entertained in priority. Structural pathology cannot be ruled out by the sheer absence of clinical signs of raised ICP. In this child, the neuroimaging was normal. This fairly rules out demyelination, vascular, traumatic, and neoplastic etiologies. Considering the predominance of neuropsychiatric manifestations, subacute encephalopathy, possibility of NMDAR encephalitis (NMDARE) was

kept. Cerebrospinal fluid (CSF) study was normal in cytology, protein, and sugars. CSF was positive for the NMDA receptor antibody.

■ INVESTIGATION

Initial Workup

All children presenting with encephalopathy must be screened for blood sugar (to detect hypoglycemia), serum sodium (to look for hypo-/hypernatremia), serum calcium, hemoglobin level (to assess the degree of anemia), total leukocyte count (indicator of infection), and platelet count (to look for thrombocytopenia). Blood gas analysis is useful to detect metabolic acidosis (mitochondrial disorder) and respiratory alkalosis (hyperventilation). Among those with suspected coagulopathy, additional samples for prothrombin time can be obtained. Among those with clinical evidence of jaundice or clinical suspicion of hepatic encephalopathy, serum bilirubin level, and serum aminotransferase [serum glutamic pyruvic transaminase (SGPT)] levels may be obtained. Blood urea and serum creatinine levels are useful among those with suspected uremic encephalopathy.

Computed Tomography Brain

Neuroimaging is the first investigation required to determine the etiology of encephalopathy. Computed tomography (CT) scan brain is often readily available in an emergency setting and is less time-consuming. However, there is a remarkable risk of radiation associated with performing CT scans for children. Among children presenting with coma, the following clinical entities can be picked up on CT scan:

- Noncontrast CT brain is useful to detect hemorrhagic stroke, dense arterial

ischemic stroke, cord sign in cerebral venous sinus thrombosis, and hypoxic-ischemic changes following prolonged asphyxia.
- Contrast CT brain is useful to detect meningeal enhancement **(Fig. 4)**, brain abscess, and intracranial space-occupying lesions like neurocysticercosis, tuberculoma, and malignancy.

It is essential to make a hypothesis regarding your clinical possibility and accordingly order the neuroimaging. Getting noncontrast CT scan followed by contrast CT scan would improve the yield of diagnosis, but it also means two times the radiation exposure. Common radiological findings on CT brain among children presenting with coma are summarized in **Table 6**.

Clinical diagnosis and suspicion are extremely important before radiological findings are interpreted. For example, in a child presenting with acute febrile encephalopathy, detecting arachnoid cyst on CT scan has no clinical relevance and is often an incidental finding rather than the primary etiology. In addition, the number of clinical conditions like autoimmune encephalitis, metabolic encephalopathy, epileptic encephalopathy, and meningitis may have normal neuroimaging findings. However, the yield of abnormal neuroimaging improves with MRI brain compared to the CT brain. Hence, in nonemergent situations with stable hemodynamic parameters, MRI brain is preferable to CT brain among children with coma.

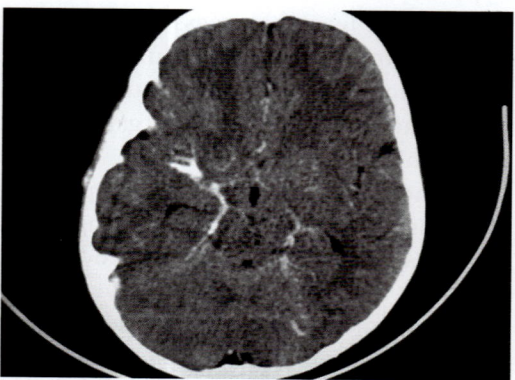

Fig. 4: Contrast-enhanced computed tomography (CECT) brain showing basal cistern enhancement with effacement of sulci and gyri which could be consistent with diagnosis of tubercular meningitis.

TABLE 6: Common CT scan findings among children presenting with coma.

Clinical condition resulting in coma	Radiological findings on CT scan
Meningitis (bacterial)	Normal or meningeal (basal and/or pachymeningeal) enhancement on CECT brain
Meningitis (tubercular)	Basal exudates, tuberculoma, vascular stroke in middle cerebral artery (MCA) territory, meningeal enhancement, and hydrocephalus
Brain abscess	Ring enhancing lesion with central hypodensity and peripheral enhancement of wall
Hypoxic ischemia secondary to prolonged asphyxia	Diffuse hypodensity involving entire cerebral hemisphere with sparing of cerebellum (white cerebellar sign)
Arterial ischemic stroke	Hypodensity along the vascular arterial distribution
Cerebral venous sinus thrombosis	Dense cord sign on NCCT and rim enhancement on CECT brain

(CECT: contrast-enhanced computed tomography; CT: computed tomography; NCCT: noncontrast computed tomography)

Magnetic Resonance Imaging Brain

Magnetic resonance imaging brain is useful to decipher the etiology of encephalopathy in children, especially if CT head is normal or inconclusive **(Table 7)**. MRI brain is superior to CT brain in detecting ischemia (diffusion restriction can be detected early on MRI brain when CT can be normal) **(Figs. 5 and 6)**. Demyelinating conditions like ADEM are best appreciated on MRI brain; presence of asymmetric and patchy white matter hyperintensities with diffusion restriction are highly suggestive of ADEM **(Fig. 7)**. MRI brain can also point toward an underlying metabolic disorder like mitochondrial disorder **(Fig. 8)**, which can present with acute alteration of sensorium. The presence of a history of prolonged ventilation, status epilepticus, or need for resuscitation following cardiac arrest would indicate a possibility of hypoxic injury. It is appreciated by loss of gray matter–white matter differentiation and gross cerebral edema. In prolonged hypoxia, watershed infarcts are appreciated **(Fig. 9)**.

TABLE 7: Magnetic resonance imaging findings and its clinical correlate in children with acute febrile encephalopathy.

Clinical entity	Clinical presentation	Radiological features
Japanese encephalitis	Febrile encephalopathy with predominant extrapyramidal manifestations (hypokinetic or hyperkinetic)	Bilateral symmetrical signal changes in thalamus (87%), midbrain (substantia nigra) (28–45%), and basal ganglia (40–50%)
Herpes encephalitis	Febrile encephalopathy with predominant behavioral or neuropsychiatric features with or without focal signs	Signal hyperintensity in medial temporal lobe, cingulate gyrus, and orbital surface of frontal lobe with hemorrhagic transformation
Enterovirus 71	Febrile encephalopathy with multiple cranial nerve palsy and other brainstem signs including ataxic breathing, loss of oculocephalic, corneal reflex (brainstem encephalitis)	Signal hyperintensity in dorsal pons, medulla, midbrain, and dentate nucleus of cerebellum
West Nile virus	Febrile encephalopathy with pyramidal and/or extrapyramidal features	Signal hyperintensity in basal ganglia, thalamus, and brainstem (pons)
Nipah virus	Acute febrile encephalopathy	Multiple white matter signal changes on T2
Rotavirus	Encephalopathy following diarrheal infection	Transient corpus callosum (splenium) lesion
Acute measles encephalitis	Febrile encephalopathy with measly rash	Cortical edema, symmetrical hyperintensity in caudate, and putamen
Lyme disease	Febrile encephalopathy with erythema migrans on the skin in background of recent travel to endemic zone/tick bite	Bilateral white matter signal hyperintensity, meningeal or cranial nerve enhancement
Leptospirosis	Acute encephalopathy in setting of hepatic and renal compromise	Normal, cerebral edema or arterial ischemic stroke

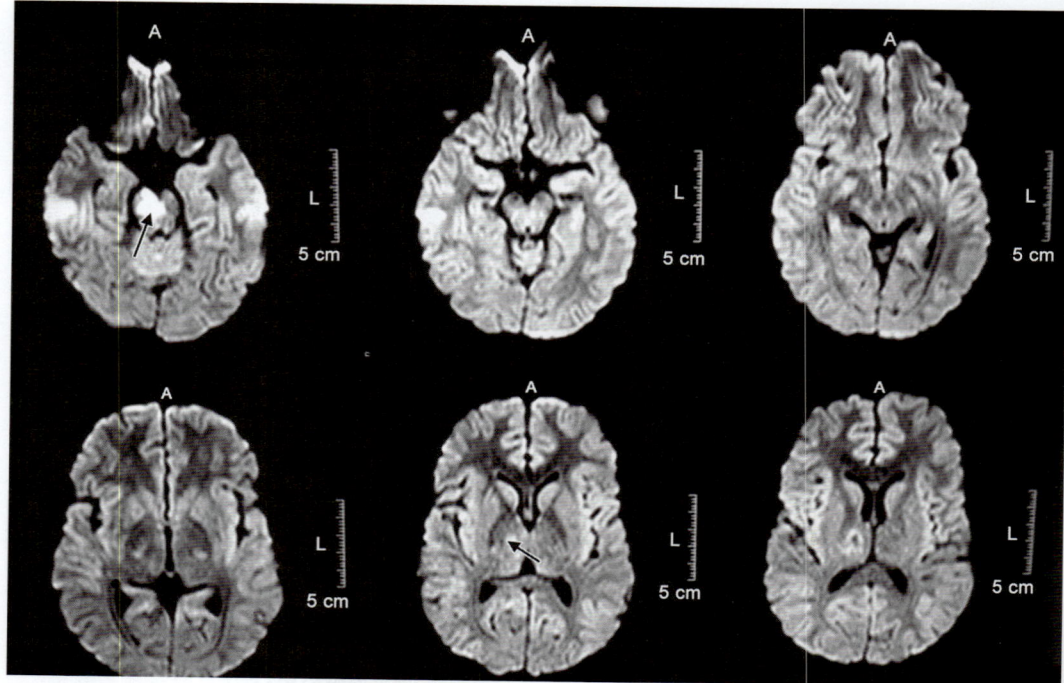

Fig. 5: Magnetic resonance imaging brain diffusion-weighted images reveal diffusion restriction in the right-sided thalamus and midbrain suggestive of right posterior circulation stroke.

It is again reemphasized that neuroimaging findings need to be interpreted in the clinical context. The radiologist must be provided with clinical details and consulted one to one for your clinical impression. For example, in a child with febrile encephalopathy, bilateral symmetrical signal abnormalities in thalamus would point to Japanese encephalitis (JE), whereas it may point to deep venous sinus thrombosis in a child with acute encephalopathy following dehydration. Similarly, if a child presents with seizures and transient encephalopathy with MRI showing occipital hyperintensities that resolve within a few days, it suggests posterior reversible leukoencephalopathy (PRES) **(Fig. 10)**.

Electroencephalography

Electroencephalogram (EEG) is indicated among children presenting with seizure or unexplained encephalopathy to rule out NCSE. NCSE is suspected among children with known epilepsy presenting to a casualty with unexplained features of encephalopathy. In addition, the presence of focal slowing **(Fig. 11)** is an indicator of underlying structural etiology, and diffuse, generalized slowing, or background attenuation is also an indicator of depth of coma. Periodic lateralized epileptiform discharges **(Fig. 12)** can be observed in focal structural lesions as well as in focal cerebritis like herpes encephalitis and focal arterial ischemic stroke.

Metabolic Screening

Metabolic screening for inborn errors of metabolism (organic acidemia, urea cycle disorders, and aminoacidopathies) can be performed among those with suspected metabolic coma. The following clinical

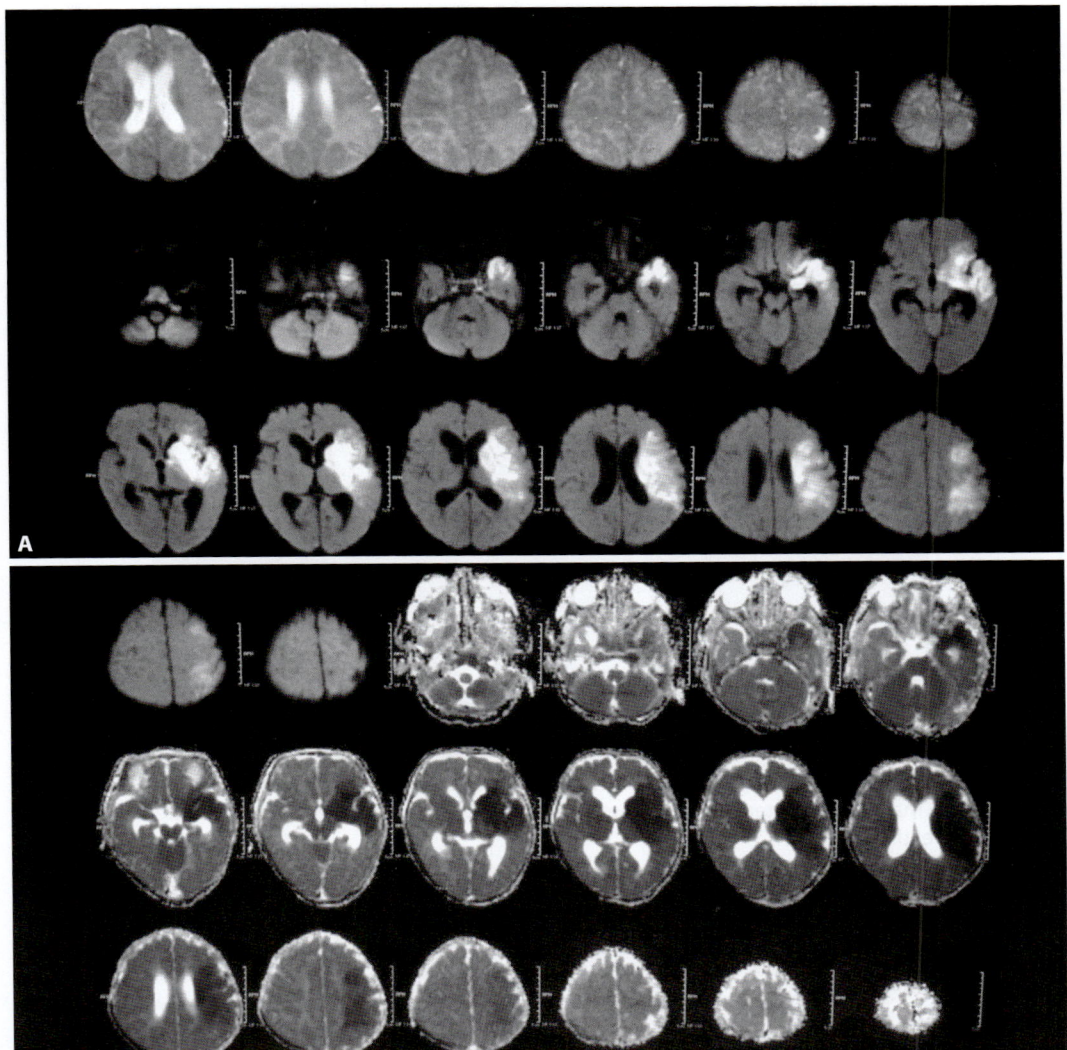

Figs. 6A and B: Magnetic resonance imaging brain [(A) diffusion-weighted imaging (DWI) and (B) apparent diffusion coefficient (ADC) map] revealing diffusion restriction across left middle cerebral artery (MCA) suggestive of left MCA stroke.

features point to neurometabolic etiology: Consanguinity, recurrent abortions/stillbirths, family history of affected siblings, abnormal urinary odor, unexplained metabolic acidosis/hyperlactatemia/hyperammonemia, global developmental delay, and recurrent encephalopathy. Clinical worsening with febrile illness or trivial stress often points to underlying mitochondrial leukoencephalopathy. MRI brain is a useful adjunct in categorizing the type of neurometabolic disorder so that appropriate workup can be planned. Among those with a suspected neurometabolic

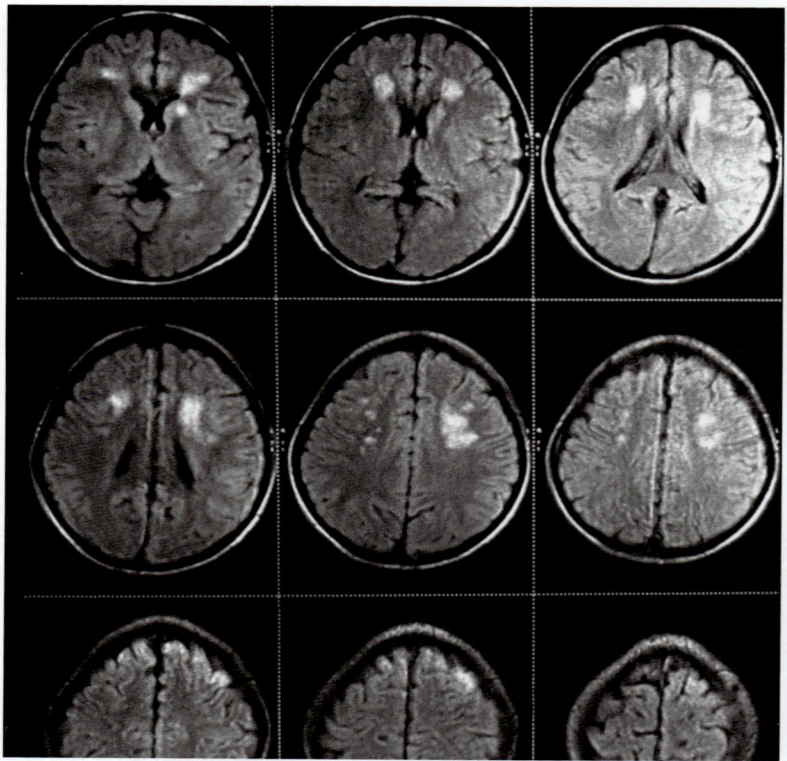

Fig. 7: Magnetic resonance imaging T2 fluid-attenuated inversion recovery (FLAIR) axial images revealing discrete white matter hyperintensities that are bilateral and asymmetric suggestive of acute disseminated encephalomyelitis (ADEM).

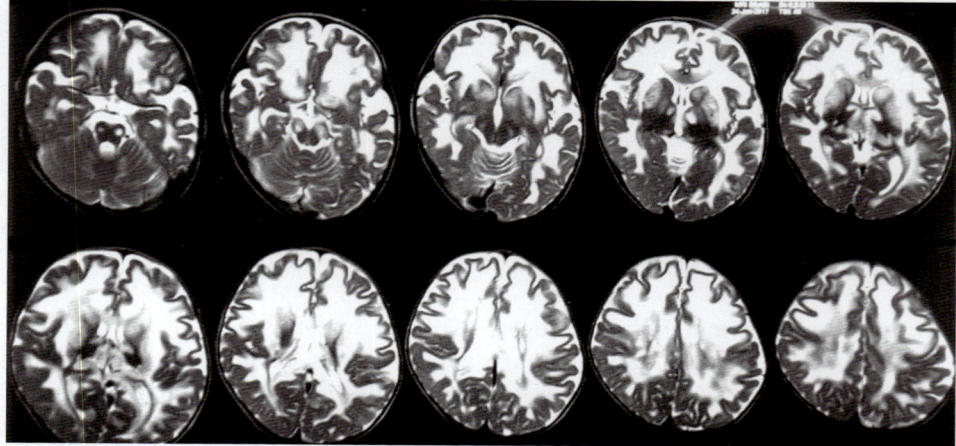

Fig. 8: Magnetic resonance imaging brain T2-weighted images reveal multicystic involvement of deep and periventricular white matter with involvement of midbrain corticospinal tracts, caudate, and putamen in a child with mitochondrial disorder.

disorder, screening with blood glucose, electrolytes, lactate, ammonia, anion gap (blood gas analysis), and ketone (urine) can be performed (mnemonic GELAAK). Amino acid profile, free carnitine, acylcarnitine levels, and free fatty acid can be estimated by tandem mass spectrometry and confirmed by urinary gas chromatography.

Metabolic disorders that can present with acute encephalopathy include methylmalonic aciduria, propionic aciduria, maple syrup urine disease, multiple carboxylase deficiency, isovaleric aciduria, and glutarylcoenzyme A dehydrogenase deficiency.

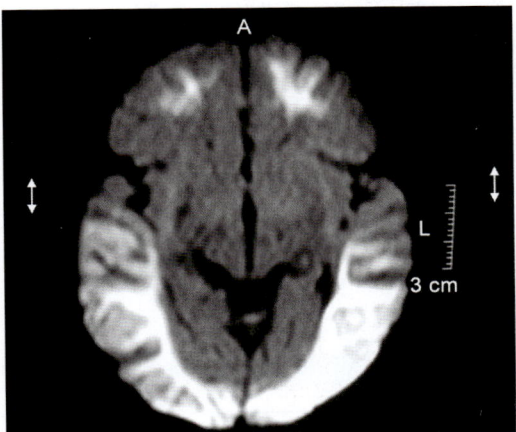

Fig. 9: Magnetic resonance imaging brain (diffusion-weighted imaging) reveals bilateral watershed infarcts which suggest prolonged hypoxic damage.

Autoimmune Workup

Children presenting with new onset of psychiatric manifestation, movement disorder, autonomic disturbances, seizures, and cognitive problems followed by encephalopathy must be evaluated for autoimmune encephalitis, especially NMDARE

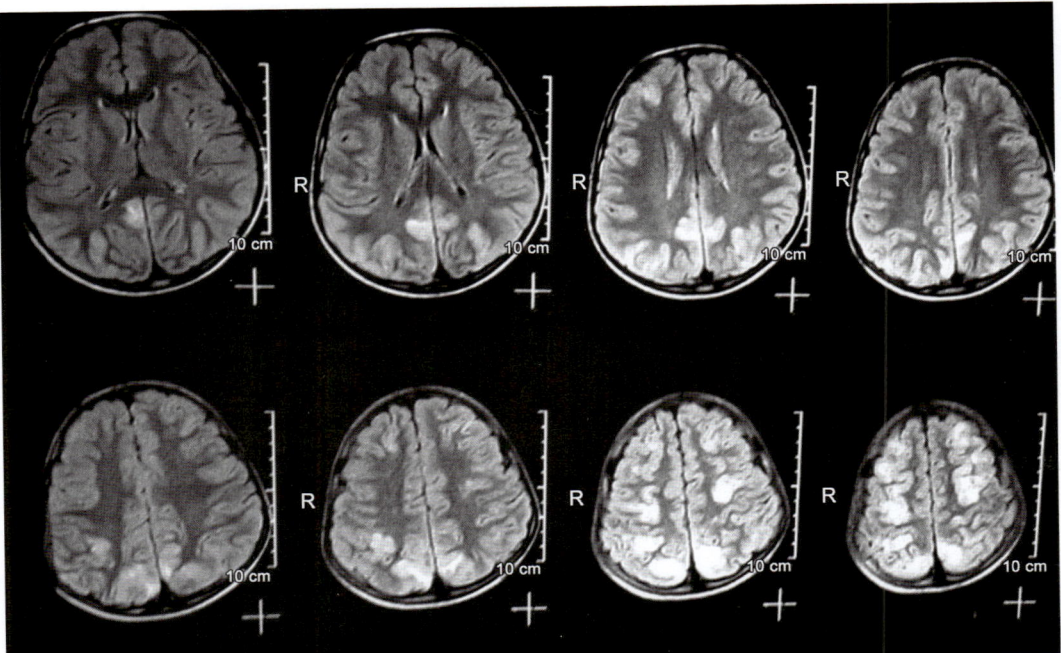

Fig. 10: Magnetic resonance imaging brain (T2/FLAIR images) revealing bilateral parieto-occipital gray matter hyperintensities suggestive of posterior reversible leukoencephalopathy (PRES).

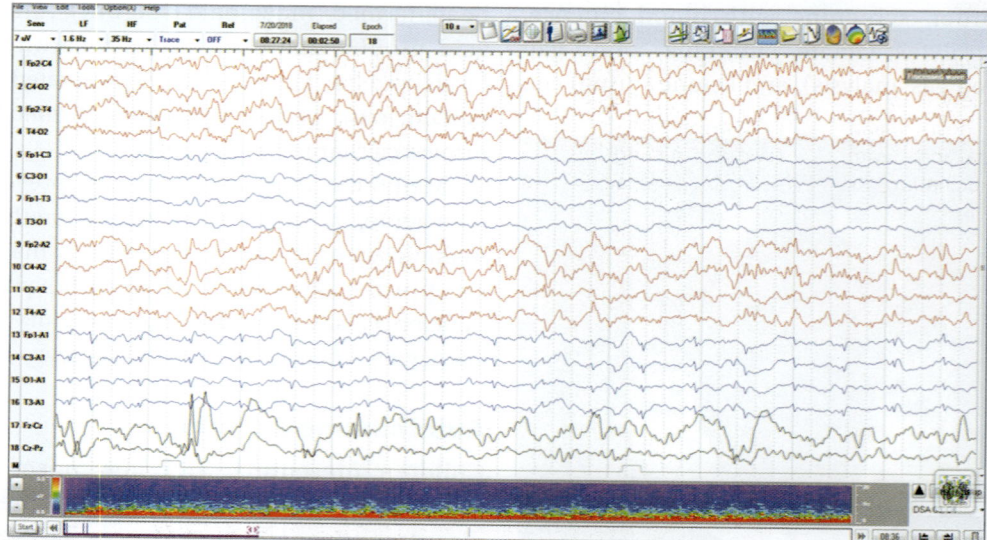

Fig. 11: Electroencephalography showing slowing of left hemispheric leads which indicates a possible left hemispheric structural pathology.

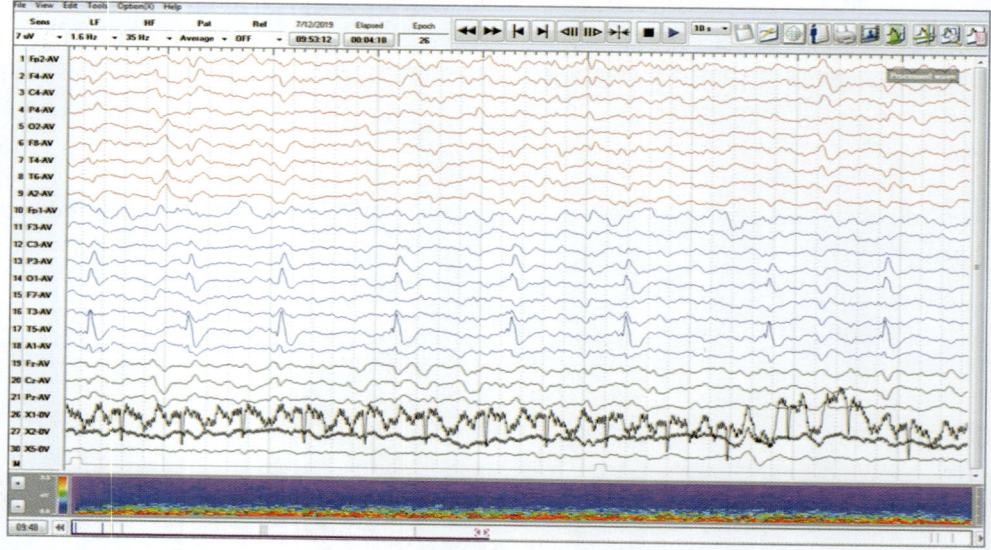

Fig. 12: Electroencephalography showing periodic sharp waves in left temporal leads suggestive of periodic lateralized epileptiform discharges.

(Table 8). Those with positive NMDA receptor antibody must be screened for underlying tumor, especially ovarian tumors among girls. The thyroid function test and thyroid antibody [antithyroid peroxidase (anti-TPO) antibody] must be screened among those with suspected autoimmune encephalitis. Children with suspected central nervous

TABLE 8: Key features of NMDA receptor encephalitis.

Psychiatric features	Movement disorder	Cognitive problems	Autonomic instability
Anxiety, fear, psychosis, mania, visual and auditory hallucination, and insomnia	Orofacial dyskinesia (45%) (chewing, tongue thrusting, lip smacking, and facial grimacing)	Short-term memory loss, reduced verbal output, echolalia, echopraxia, mutism, altered consciousness (variable), signs of raised ICP uncommon, masked by psychiatric manifestation	Tachycardia, hypertension, hyperthermia (86%), and hypersalivation urinary incontinence
Social withdrawal and stereotypical behavior are common	Choreoathetosis and dystonia		
Behavioral changes: Tantrums, irritability, hyperactivity, and aggressive	Complex stereotypies (pelvic thrusting, pseudopiano playing movement)		

(ICP: intracranial pressure; NMDA: N-methyl D-aspartate)

system (CNS) vasculitis must be screened for antinuclear antibody (ANA), antineutrophil cytoplasmic antibody (ANCA), and erythrocyte sedimentation rate (ESR). Rheumatology consultation must be sought for workup of children with suspected CNS vasculitis.

Role of Angiography and Venography

Magnetic resonance angiography (MRA) is useful among children with arterial ischemic stroke and those with suspected CNS vasculitis. MRA is useful in detecting arteriopathy, including moyamoya disease (MMD). Children with MMD often present with seizures, encephalopathy, and bilateral ischemic stroke with MRA showing evidence of extensive collaterals secondary to stenosis at the level of distal internal carotid artery, proximal middle cerebral artery, and anterior cerebral artery (puff of smoke appearance). Conventional angiography (digital subtraction angiography) is often required among those with suspected arterial aneurysms, arteriovenous malformation, arterial dissection, and CNS vasculitis.

Magnetic resonance venography is required among those with suspected venous sinus thrombosis. One must remember that venous strokes secondary to cerebral venous sinus thrombosis more often present with encephalopathy and seizures as compared to an arterial ischemic stroke, which presents with focal deficits like hemiplegia, CN palsy, and aphasia. Noncontrast CT scan reveal dense transverse sinus with "dense clot sign". When the venous sinus is patent, CT will show sinus to be dark (hypodense), but it becomes hyperdense (bright) when a clot is formed. This is called a dense clot sign. When we give intravenous contrast (which looks bright on a CT scan), it reaches the venous sinuses leaving the central area of the clot that looks dark (looks like an empty delta). Hence, contrast CT scan reveals a triangular area of enhancement called "empty delta sign". Venous sinus thrombosis often results in loss of flow voids on MRI. Venous infarcts

Flowchart 1: Clinical approach to a child with encephalopathy.

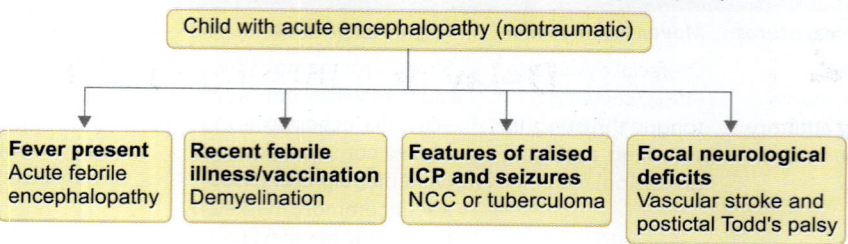

(ICP: intracranial pressure; NCC: neurocysticercosis)

secondary to venous sinus thrombosis often undergo a hemorrhagic transformation.

Further coagulation workup and cardiac evaluation are required among those with confirmed arterial ischemic or venous strokes.

A broad approach to a child with nontraumatic coma has been outlined in **Flowchart 1**.

KEY MESSAGES

- Assessment of a comatose child must include assessment of consciousness, pupil size, and reactivity, eye movement, respiratory pattern, and presence of brainstem reflexes.
- Presence of focal neurological deficit like hemiparesis or CN palsy in a comatose child would indicate a possible structural etiology.
- Neuroimaging must precede lumbar puncture in the evaluation of children with nontraumatic encephalopathy considering the imminent risk of herniation among those with raised ICP.
- One must consider a possibility of autoimmune encephalitis among adolescent girls presenting with subacute encephalopathy with neuropsychiatric manifestations and extrapyramidal symptoms.
- Neuroimaging (MRI brain) provides an essential clue to the underlying etiology of comatose children.

CHAPTER 12: Approach to Global Developmental Delay and Intellectual Disability

DEFINITIONS

Global developmental delay (GDD) refers to significant (more than 2 standard deviations) delay in two or more of the following domains—motor (gross/fine), language/communication, social, cognitive, and activities of daily living. If there is a significant difference between developmental rates of two domains, it would be considered *developmental dissociation*. For example, if there is a significant motor delay when compared to cognition, it would be considered developmental dissociation. In general, the term GDD is used for children <5 years of age. The term intellectual disability is used beyond 5 years of age.

Intellectual disability (ID) is defined as significant limitation in intellectual function and adaptive behavior expressed in terms of conceptual, social, and practical adaptive skills with onset <18 years of age. The Diagnostic and Statistical Manual of Mental Disorders, 5th edition (DSM-5) criteria are considered gold standard for diagnosis of ID **(Box 1)**. These deficits are in comparison to age, gender, and socioculturally matched peers. The International Classification of Diseases, 11th Revision (ICD-11) uses the term intellectual developmental disorder for ID. The term mental retardation (MR) is no longer used and is replaced with ID. Hence, a child who was labeled as GDD could possibly evolve to ID as the age advances. We often use the term GDD/ID, as they refer to spectrum of the same problem.

APPROACH TO DIAGNOSIS

Clinical Diagnosis

Intellectual disability is a nonprogressive disorder, although fluctuations are known to occur. The severity of ID may vary depending on the underlying etiology and ongoing therapies. Many children with GDD/ID will have few autistic symptoms. However, majority of them do not qualify the diagnosis of autism spectrum disorder (ASD) as per DSM-5 criteria. DSM-5 criteria allow comorbid diagnosis such as ID with ASD, ID with attention deficit hyperactivity disorder (ADHD). Traditionally, IQ scores alone

---

BOX 1: DSM-5 criteria for intellectual disability.

- Deficit in intellectual functions such as reasoning, problem-solving, planning, abstract thinking, judgment, academic learning, and learning from experience
- Deficit in adaptive functioning in one or more of activities of daily living such as communication, social participation, and independent living across multiple environment such as home, school, work, or community
- Onset of intellectual and adaptive deficit during the developmental period

(DSM-5: Diagnostic and Statistical Manual of Mental Disorders, 5th edition)

were used for categorization of ID **(Box 2)**. Culturally appropriate and psychometrically sound tools need to be used for determination of intellectual functioning.

There is a transition from traditional IQ scores to impairment of adaptive functioning in assessing the severity of ID (DSM-5). IQ scores are less reliable in lower end of IQ range. IQ scores are also affected by associated hearing deficit, visual problems, epilepsy, disorders of communication, language, and motor or sensory function disorders. ID (DSM-5) includes both deficit in intellectual functioning and adaptive functioning. Adaptive functioning is assessed in terms of conceptual (academic), social, and practical domain during the developmental period **(Box 3)**. Conceptual domain includes assessment of memory, language, reading, and writing; social domain includes awareness of other's feelings, friendship, and interpersonal communication skill; practical domain includes personal care and job responsibility.

Etiology of Intellectual Disability

Intellectual disability can result from genetic cause or acquired cause. Genetic cause can be broadly divided into chromosomal disorders, single-gene disorder, or metabolic disorder **(Table 1)**. The most common genetic cause of ID is Down syndrome followed by fragile X syndrome. In India, acquired causes such as perinatal asphyxia and prematurity predominate.

History

Focus of clinical history among children with ID is to determine the underlying etiology. Key points in the history include the following:
- *Antenatal history:* Fever, rash, and swellings in the neck [congenital rubella infection and other TORCH (toxoplasmosis, others—syphilis, hepatitis B, rubella, cytomegalovirus, herpes simplex) infection], drug intake (warfarin, valparin, phenytoin, and other teratogenic drugs), and risk factors for intrauterine growth restriction (IUGR) (pre-eclampsia, anemia, and gestational diabetes)
- *Natal history:* Prematurity, low birthweight, APGAR scores, neonatal encephalopathy, neonatal seizure, neonatal meningitis, intracranial bleed, kernicterus/neonatal jaundice, and need for mechanical ventilation/inotropic support
- *Postnatal history:* Postnatal insult in terms of head trauma, meningitis, and intracranial bleed needs to be determined.
- *Associated comorbidity:* Hearing, vision, seizure, feeding difficulties, behavior problem, motor deficit (spasticity/dystonia), sensory deficit, autistic features, features of hyperactivity, and sleep disturbances
- Family history with three-generation pedigree charts is essential, affected

---

BOX 2: Severity of intellectual disability.

Intelligence quotient (IQ) score:
- *IQ < 70:* Intellectual disability (ID)
- *IQ 50–69:* Mild ID
- *IQ 35–49:* Moderate ID
- *IQ 20–34:* Severe ID
- *IQ < 20:* Profound ID

BOX 3: Intellectual and adaptive functioning.

Intellectual functioning:
- Reasoning
- Problem-solving
- Planning
- Abstract thinking
- Judgment
- Academic learning
- Learning from experience

Adaptive functioning:
- Communication
- Social participation
- Independent living across home, school, work, and community

CHAPTER 12: Approach to Global Developmental Delay and Intellectual Disability

TABLE 1: Common etiology of intellectual disability.

Category	Etiology
Chromosomal disorders	Down syndrome, Prader–Willi syndrome, and William syndrome
Single-gene disorder (syndromic)	Fragile X syndrome, Rubinstein–Taybi syndrome, Coffin–Lowry syndrome
Single-gene disorder (nonsyndromic)	OPHN1, FMR2, SLC6A8, and SHANK-3
Metabolic	Phenylketonuria, galactosemia, Smith–Lemli–Opitz syndrome, and mutation in thyroid hormone transporter
Acquired	Fetal alcohol syndrome, maternal phenylketonuria, maternal iodine deficiency, maternal drug intake, TORCH infection, HIV infection, perinatal insult (hypoxic-ischemic encephalopathy, kernicterus, prematurity, neonatal meningitis, and intracranial hemorrhage), postnatal insult (meningitis and head trauma), and chronic lead exposure

[HIV: human immunodeficiency virus; TORCH: toxoplasmosis, others (syphilis, hepatitis B), rubella, cytomegalovirus, herpes simplex]

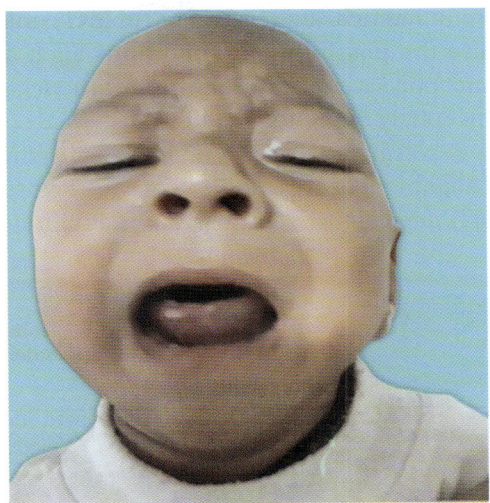

Fig. 1: Primary microcephaly.

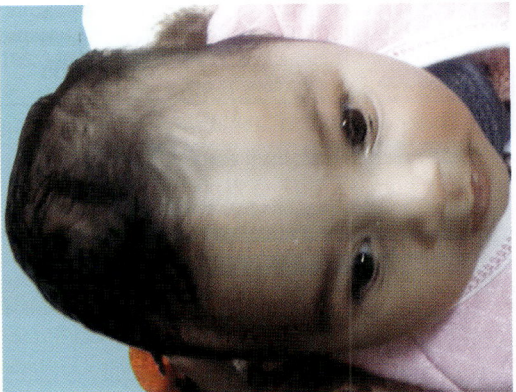

Fig. 2: Overriding of sutures (craniosynostosis) in a child with global developmental delay.

family members with ID, history of consanguinity, and history of repeated abortions/pregnancy loss.

Examination

The focus of examination is to determine the possible etiology of ID. The most crucial information is head circumference at birth. Microcephaly at birth implies antenatal insult or congenital anomaly of skull **(Fig. 1)** and brain like primary craniosynostosis **(Fig. 2)**. Children with various microdeletion syndromes and chromosomal disorders have microcephaly. If the head circumference at birth was within the normal limit and subsequently he developed microcephaly, it is most likely secondary to natal or postnatal insult such as birth asphyxia, prematurity, and neonatal meningitis **(Fig. 3)**. In tropical countries, majority of patients with ID and microcephaly are secondary to perinatal insult. In a child with ID, head circumference >2 SD (macrocephaly) could raise the possibility of conditions such as mucopolysaccharidosis or those with megalencephaly like Sotos syndrome.

Assessment of facial dysmorphism in terms of alignment of eyes, position of ears (low-set ears), depressed nasal bridge, flat philtrum, any cleft lip or cleft palate must be noted (**Fig. 4**). In presence of dysmorphism, classification into any known syndromic cause must be attempted (**Table 2**). Obvious syndromes such as Down syndrome (**Fig. 5**), fragile X syndrome (**Fig. 6**), and William syndrome (**Fig. 7**) can be recognized by most of the pediatricians.

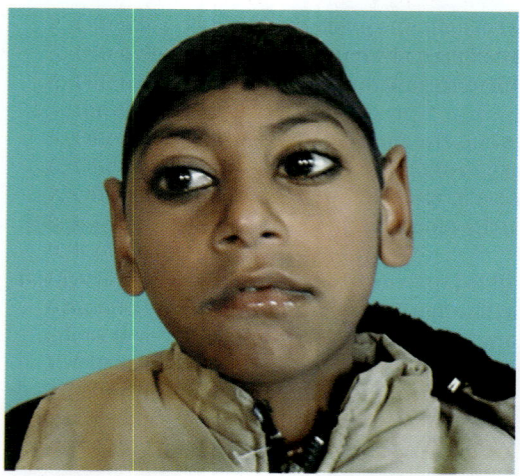

Fig. 3: A child with intellectual disability and microcephaly sequelae to perinatal asphyxia.

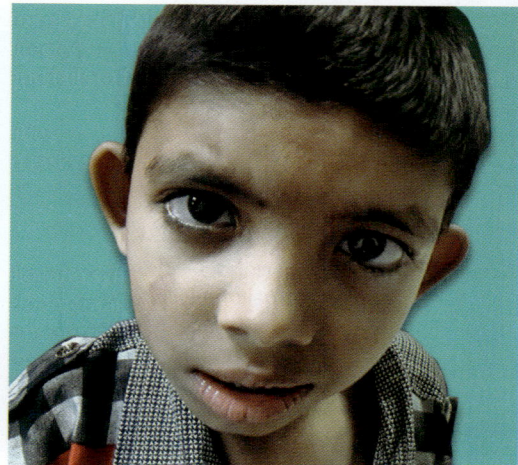

Fig. 4: A child with intellectual disability and facial dysmorphism (depressed nasal bridge and prominent ears).

TABLE 2: Syndromic causes of intellectual disability (ID).

Syndrome	Clinical features
Fragile X syndrome	ID, hyperactivity, broad forehead, elongated facies, prominent ears, high-arched palate, hyperextensible joints, and enlarged testis
William syndrome	Happy puppet, tetanic spasm, good verbal skills, hyper social behavior, hyperacusis, puffy eyes, and depressed nasal bridge, mid facial hypoplasia and thick lips
Fetal alcohol syndrome	Epicanthic folds, small palpebral fissure, thin upper lip, and smooth philtrum
Cornelia de Lange syndrome	Low hairline, synophrys (joined eyebrows of both eyes), low set ears, anteverted nares, long thin philtrum, limb abnormalities, sensorineural hearing loss, short stature, and aggressive and self-injurious behavior
Cri-du-chat syndrome	Round flat facies, hypertelorism, depressed nasal bridge, micrognathia, poorly formed ears, simian crease, dexterity, and inquisitiveness
Rubinstein–Taybi syndrome	ID, self-soothing behavior, microcephaly, prominent forehead, hypertelorism, beaked nose, micrognathia, grimacing smile, broad thumb, great toes with angulation, posterior rotation of ears, pulmonary stenosis, hyperextensible joints, and hypoplastic kidneys

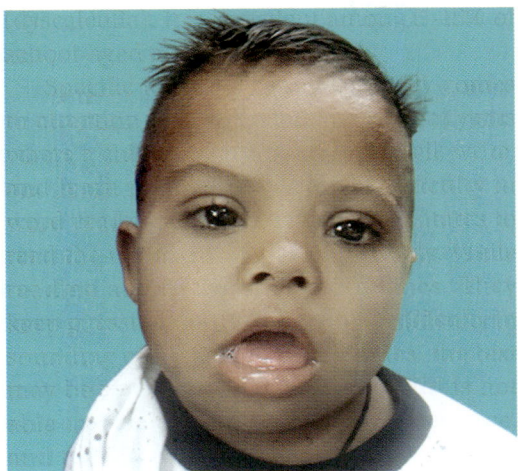

Fig. 5: Down syndrome.

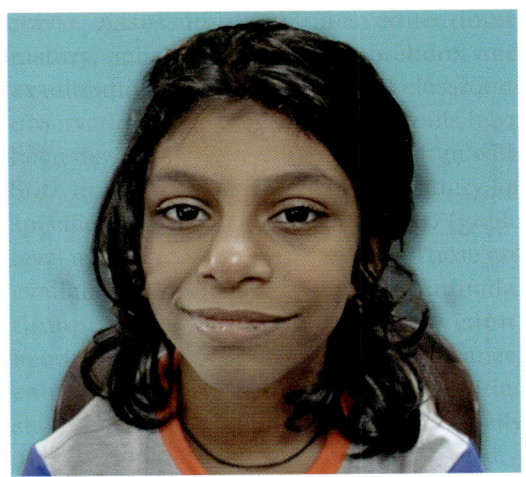

Fig. 7: Patient with William syndrome (note the midface hypoplasia and thick lips).
Courtesy: Professor Neerja Gupta, AIIMS, Delhi.

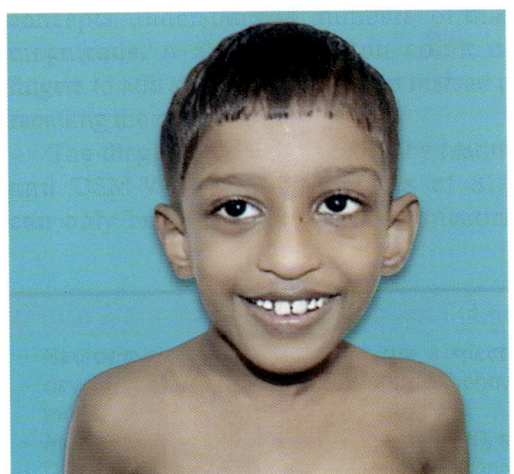

Fig. 6: Patient with fragile X syndrome (note the elongated face and prominent ears).
Courtesy: Professor Neerja Gupta, AIIMS, Delhi.

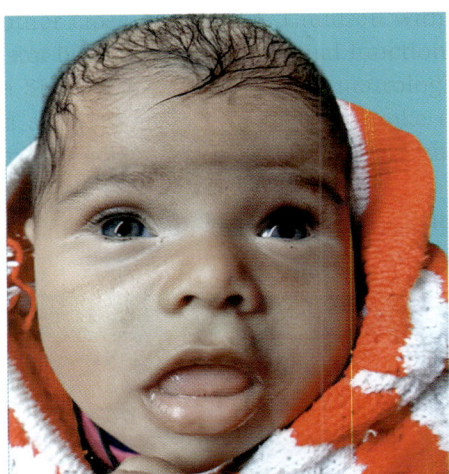

Fig. 8: Congenital hypothyroidism (note the open mouth with protruded tongue).

Treatable disorders such as congenital hypothyroidism must never be missed **(Fig. 8)**. Consultation with a geneticist would be useful among children with ID and facial dysmorphism. There are few free mobile apps such as Face2Gene, which can help a clinician to reach a possible diagnosis. It is a good idea to download this app from Play Store and use it for evaluation of children with dysmorphism. It might not clinch the diagnosis, but still will be useful to narrow the differentials.

Examination of skin is essential to look for neurocutaneous markers **(Table 3)** among all children with ID. Neurocutaneous syndromes such as neurofibromatosis, Sturge–Weber syndrome, and tuberous sclerosis can present with ID alone. One must look for ash-leaf macule **(Fig. 9A)**, Shagreen patch **(Fig. 9B)**, facial angiofibroma **(Fig. 10)**, port-wine stain **(Fig. 11)**, and café-au-lait macule **(Fig. 12)**. Similarly, presence of ichthyosis could suggest a possibility of Sjögren–Larsson syndrome and inverted nipples with fat pads would indicate possibility of congenital disorders of glycosylation (CDG) **(Fig. 13)**. Multiple injury marks over forehead or other parts of body in a child with ID will indicate possible myoclonic jerks in the child **(Fig. 14)**.

Ophthalmic evaluation is mandatory among all children with ID. Presence of ocular signs such as cataract, retinitis pigmentosa, conjunctival telangiectasia **(Fig. 15)** and corneal clouding could point to underlying etiology of ID **(Table 4)**. Importance of clinical signs in evaluation of patients with ID is summarized in **Table 5**.

Detailed neurological examination is mandatory among children with ID. Higher mental function including cognition needs to be assessed. Cranial nerve examination must focus on visual impairment, hearing impairment, and squint. Presence of motor deficits such as spasticity, dystonia, and dyskinesia warrants associated diagnosis of cerebral palsy. Majority of children with ID do not have any motor deficits. The two terms

TABLE 3: Key features of neurocutaneous syndromes presenting with intellectual disability.

Syndrome	Key features
Neurofibromatosis	Café-au-lait macules, axillary freckling, neurofibroma, Lisch nodules in iris, optic glioma, and sphenoid wing dysplasia
Sturge–Weber syndrome	Port-wine stain, ocular abnormality (glaucoma, choroidal angioma, and heterochromia iridis), seizures, and developmental delay
Tuberous sclerosis	Facial angiofibroma, ash-leaf macule, shagreen patch, seizures, intellectual disability, behavioral problems, and magnetic resonance imaging (MRI) brain shows subependymal nodule
Incontinentia pigmenti	Bullous rash evolving to verrucous plaque to hyperpigmented swirling pattern along the lines of Blaschko

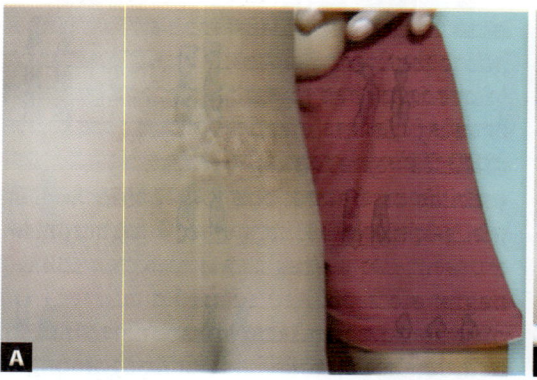 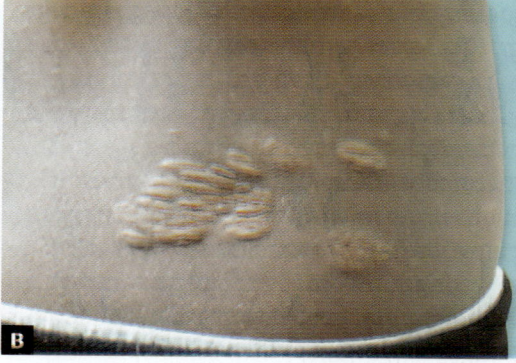

Figs. 9A and B: (A) Ash-leaf macule and (B) Shagreen patch in two children with tuberous sclerosis.

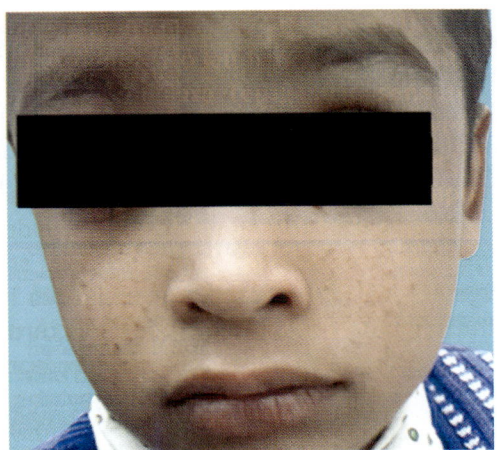

Fig. 10: Facial angiofibroma in a child with tuberous sclerosis.

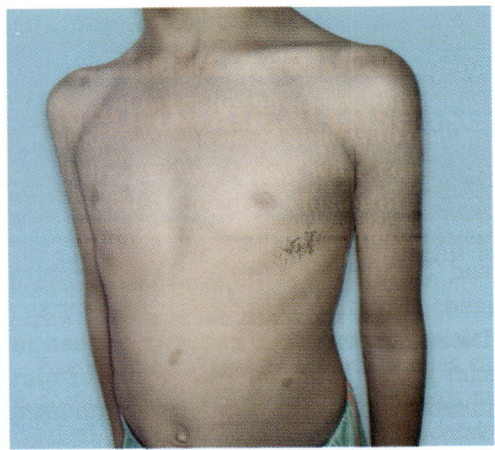

Fig. 12: Multiple café-au-lait macules in a child with neurofibromatosis.

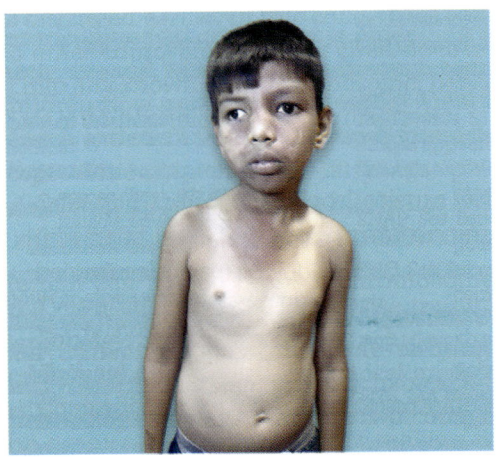

Fig. 11: Port-wine stain in a child with Sturge–Weber syndrome.

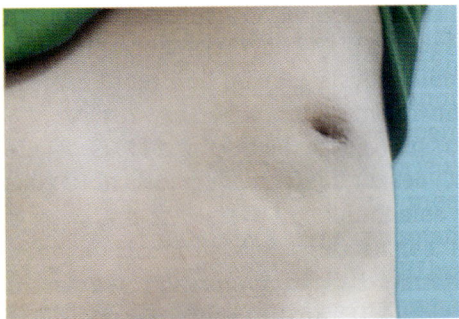

Fig. 13: Inverted nipple and subcutaneous fat pads in a child with congenital disorder of glycosylation.

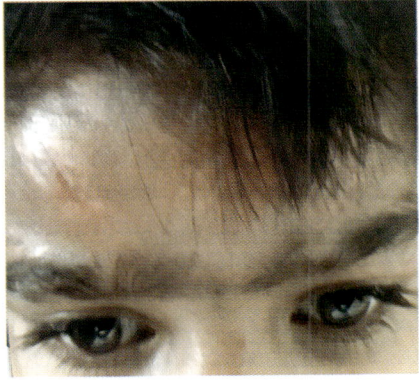

Fig. 14: A child with intellectual disability having multiple injury marks over the forehead secondary to myoclonic seizures.

"intellectual disability" and "cerebral palsy" are distinct. Cerebral palsy is a disorder of movement and posture. All children with ID do not have motor deficit (cerebral palsy) and all children with cerebral palsy do not necessarily have ID. Children with spastic quadriplegic cerebral palsy often have lower cognitive and adaptive scores when compared to those with diplegic or hemiplegic cerebral palsy.

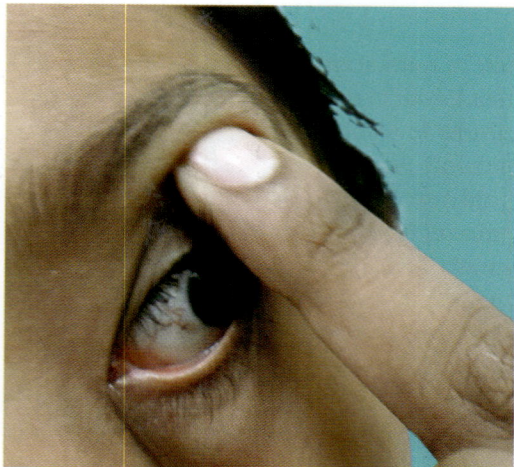

Fig. 15: Ocular telangiectasia in a child with ataxia telangiectasia.

Analysis and Clinical Differentials

Final analysis can be summarized in the following manner:
- Is it a GDD or developmental dissociation?
- Does it qualify the diagnosis of ID (based on definition of ID)?
- Is it a static or a progressive illness? (Progressive disorders are not classified under ID. If things are worsening with time, it is more likely to be a progressive neurodegenerative disease. ID is a static disorder and cognition often improves with time.)
- Is there a neurological deficit or any focal neurological sign (like hemiparesis, paraparesis, and cranial nerve deficits)?
- *Are there any comorbidities*—vision impairment, hearing impairment, behavioral abnormalities, seizures, spasticity, dystonia/dyskinesia, or contractures?
- Is there a microcephaly, macrocephaly, or normocephaly?
- *Are there any extraneural signs*—changes or clinical clues in the skin, hair, facial dysmorphism, changes in the eyes, hepatosplenomegaly?

TABLE 4: Ocular signs in intellectual disability.

Ocular sign	Common conditions
Cherry red spot	• Gangliosidosis (GM1) • Tay–Sachs disease/Sandhoff disease (GM2) • Niemann–Pick disease (NPD) type A • Gaucher disease
Cataract	• Cockayne syndrome • Galactosemia • Lowe syndrome • Congenital rubella syndrome • Marinesco–Sjögren syndrome
Chorioretinitis	TORCH (toxoplasmosis, others—syphilis, hepatitis B, rubella, cytomegalovirus, herpes simplex) infection
Dislocated lens	• Homocystinuria • Sulfite oxidase deficiency
Glaucoma	• Rubinstein–Taybi syndrome • Sturge–Weber syndrome
Nystagmus	Joubert syndrome
Retinitis pigmentosa	• Cockayne syndrome • Ataxia telangiectasia • Hallervorden–Spatz disease (pantothenate kinase-associated neurodegeneration—PKAN) • Mitochondrial (Kearns–Sayre syndrome) disorder • Neuronal ceroid lipofuscinosis (NCL)
Vertical supranuclear gaze palsy	Niemann–Pick disease type C

- Is there a family history of similar illness?
- What is the most probable etiology (chromosomal, syndromic single gene, nonsyndromic single-gene, metabolic, or acquired)?

Note: It is essential to differentiate GDD from developmental dissociation. We have two broad categories of presentation—the first one is GDD evolving to ID. It is usually secondary to some antenatal, natal, or postnatal insult. This group forms many children with ID and includes all children with ID and cerebral palsy. Second group of children with ID includes those who usually have subtle or no motor delay but with speech and cognitive delay from beginning (*developmental dissociation*). This group of children usually has no antenatal, natal, or postnatal insult. Majority of them have genetic basis for their ID such as chromosomal disorder (e.g., Down syndrome and Cri-Du-Chat syndrome), syndromic (e.g., fragile X syndrome), or nonsyndromic single-gene disorder (e.g., *STXBP-1* gene and *SHANK-3* gene mutation).

■ CASE VIGNETTES

Case 1

A 3-year-old child with delay in all spheres and autistic features has preserved vision, hearing, no seizures, and no motor deficit. There is evidence of facial dysmorphism. Her head circumference was normal. She had an uneventful antenatal, natal, and postnatal period.

TABLE 5: Clinical signs in children with intellectual disability.

Clinical sign	Possible differentials
Hepatosplenomegaly	Gaucher disease, glycogen storage disease, mucopolysaccharidosis, and Niemann–Pick disease
Hair abnormality	• *Fine hair:* Homocystinuria • *Friable:* Menkes, argininosuccinic acid deficiency • *Premature gray:* Ataxia telangiectasia • *White hair:* Methionine metabolism
Hearing loss	Mitochondrial (Kearns–Sayre syndrome, MELAS, and MERRF), Refsum disease
Hyperacusis	Tay–Sachs disease, GM1 gangliosidosis, and Krabbe disease
Café-au-lait macule	Neurofibromatosis, ataxia telangiectasia, and Bloom syndrome
Excessive Mongolian spot	GM1 gangliosidosis
Depigmented nevi	Tuberous sclerosis
Eczema	Phenylketonuria
Malar flush	Homocystinuria
Photosensitivity	Hartnup disease
Synophrys	Cretinism and Cornelia De Lange syndrome
Nystagmus	Joubert syndrome
Fat pad distribution	Congenital disorders of glycosylation (CDG)

Analysis	Present case
Is it a global developmental delay or developmental dissociation?	It is a global developmental delay with autistic features
Does it qualify the diagnosis of intellectual disability?	Child is 3 years of age; we usually use ID beyond 5 years of age
Is it a static or a progressive encephalopathy?	As things are probably improving with time, it is likely to be a static encephalopathy
Is there a neurological deficit?	None
What are the comorbidities?	None
Any extraneural signs	Facial dysmorphism
Microcephaly/macrocephaly or normocephaly	Normocephaly
Is there a family history?	There is no family history
Etiology	Most likely is syndromic single-gene disorder (genetic etiology) or chromosomal disorder

Note: Presence of facial dysmorphism with intellectual disability often warrants an opinion from a geneticist, if it can fit into any known syndromes.

Case 2

A 10-month-old baby presented with nonattainment of milestones, clinical signs of hypotonia, and presence of hepatosplenomegaly. There were excessive Mongolian spots. There was no frank evident dysmorphism. His vision and hearing were preserved. He had no seizures. His head circumference corresponds to +2 SD (macrocephaly). Fundus examination revealed cherry red spot. He had uneventful neonatal and postnatal period. He was born to nonconsanguineous married couple with history of recurrent abortions.

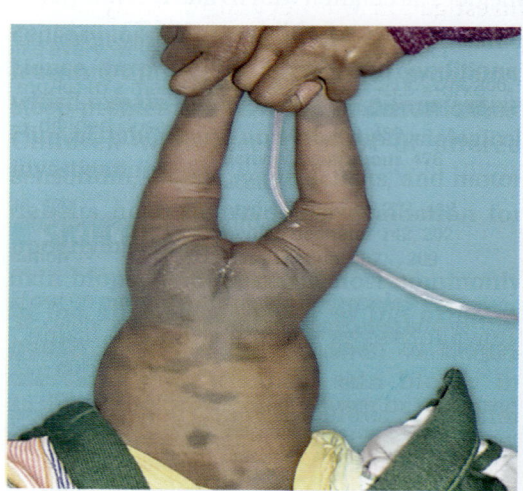

Analysis	Present case
Is it a global developmental delay or developmental dissociation?	There is nonattainment of any milestones, it can be considered as global developmental delay
Does it qualify the diagnosis of intellectual disability?	Child is 10 months old; we usually use ID beyond 5 years of age
Is it a static or a progressive encephalopathy?	As things are the same, it is difficult to interpret whether it will be a static or progressive encephalopathy. Time will likely determine the course of illness
Is there a neurological deficit?	Hypotonia
What are the comorbidities?	None
Any extraneural signs	Hepatosplenomegaly, excessive Mongolian spots, and cherry red spot on fundus
Microcephaly/ macrocephaly or normocephaly	Macrocephaly
Is there a family history?	No affected member, but there was history of recurrent abortions
Etiology	Most likely cause is metabolic. Considering 10 months age, cherry red spots, hepatosplenomegaly, macrocephaly, hypotonia, global developmental delay possibility of lysosomal storage disease such as GM1 gangliosidosis

INVESTIGATIONS FOR INTELLECTUAL DISABILITY

Investigation will depend on analysis and possible underlying etiology determined by history and examination **(Table 6)**. Cytogenetics includes high-resolution G-banding karyotype, fluorescent in situ hybridization (FISH), multiplex ligation (MLPA), array comparative genomic hybridization (CGH), next-generation sequencing, whole-exome sequencing, and whole-genome sequencing. Among children with ID, karyotype is abnormal in 4%, array CGH in 7.8%, subtelomeric FISH in 6.6%, and fragile X mutation study in 2.6%. Screening for inborn errors of metabolism (IEMs) has yield in 0.2–4.6% and congenital disorders of glycosylation (CDG) screening in 1.4%. Third tier investigations for ID include serum uric acid, urine organic acid, plasma amino acid, testing for CDG, VLCFA (very low chain fatty acid), 7-dehydrocholesterol, and urine MPS testing (to screen for mucopolysaccharidosis).

Common clinical scenarios and their investigation plan are as follows:
- In a child with ID, if there was a clear history of perinatal insult or postnatal insult and child is otherwise improving with time, then neuroimaging becomes the investigation of choice. This would document the nature and extent of insult.
- If the child with ID has signs of dysmorphism, then it would be prudent to identify any recognizable syndrome and investigation can be planned accordingly. For example, if features clearly suggest

TABLE 6: Indications of investigation in children with intellectual disability (ID).

Investigation	Indication
MRI (magnetic resonance imaging) brain	Children with global developmental delay progressing into ID, with or without presence of microcephaly and history of perinatal insult. Yield of detecting abnormality ranges from 40 to 70%
MR spectroscopy	Unexplained ID with autistic features to look for creatine deficiency
Karyotype	ID with dysmorphism or any recognizable chromosomal disorder like Down syndrome or as a first step in evaluation of unexplained ID
FISH (fluorescent in situ hybridization)	ID with dysmorphism in the form of recognizable microdeletion syndrome like Cri du chat syndrome
MLPA (multiplex ligation probe analysis)	Unexplained ID with no recognizable syndrome to look for common microdeletions/microduplication
Array CGH (comparative genomic hybridization)	First-line investigation for all children with nonsyndromic ID
MECP2 (Methyl CpG binding protein 2)	Females with moderate-to-severe ID
FMR1 testing (fragile X testing)	All nonsyndromic males with ID
Metabolic testing [tandem mass spectrometry, urine gas chromatography mass spectrometry (GCMS), homocysteine, arterial lactate, and ammonia]	Children with ID, history of consanguinity, recurrent abortions, sibling loss, multiorgan involvement, regression of attained milestones, and clinical or radiological clue to underlying metabolic cause

Down syndrome, karyotype should be performed and if features suggest Prader–Willi syndrome, genetic testing for Prader–Willi syndrome can be ordered directly.
- If the child has ID and based on the phenotype suspicion of William syndrome and Miller–Dieker syndrome is kept and the laboratory has FISH probes for diagnosis of these conditions, then FISH can be ordered.
- If the child with ID has features of dysmorphism but no recognizable syndrome, or if the child with ID has no dysmorphism, then karyotype can be a first-line screening investigation followed by MLPA for common microdeletion syndromes. However, if cost is not prohibitive, then array CGH is the investigation of choice.
- If a boy with unexplained severe ID with normal or large head has normal karyotype, fragile X testing must be

Flowchart 1: Treatable intellectual disability endeavor protocol to identify the treatable causes of intellectual disability (ID).

1st tier: In all patients with unexplained ID, nontargeted screening identify 54 (60%) treatable IEMs

Blood:
- Plasma amino acids
- Total homocysteine
- Acylcarnitine profile
- Copper, ceruloplasmin

Urine:
- Organic acids
- Purines and pyrimidines
- Creatine metabolites
- Oligosaccharides
- Glycosaminoglycans

2nd tier: Targeted metabolic workup to identify 35 (40%) treatable IEMs requiring 'specific testing'

- According to patient's symptomatology and clinician's expertise
- Utilization of textbooks and digital resources (webapp: www.treatable-id.org)
- Consider the following biochemical/gene tests:
  - Whole blood manganese
  - Plasma cholestanol
  - *Plasma 7-dehydroxy-cholesterol*: Cholesterol ratio
  - Plasma pipecolic acid and urine α-aminoadipic semialdehyde
  - Plasma vary long chain fatty acids
  - Plasma vitamin B_{12} and folate
  - Serum and CSF lactate: Pyruvate ratio
  - *Enzyme activities (leukocytes)*: Arylsulfatase A, biotinidase, glucocerebrosidase, fatty aldehyde dehydrogenase
  - Urine deoxypyridinoline
  - CSF amino acids
  - CSF neurotransmitters
  - *CSF*: Plasma glucose ratio
  - CoQ measurement fibroblasts
  - *Molecular analyses*: CA5A, NPC1, NPC2, SC4MOL, SLC18A2, SLC19A3, SLC30A10, SLC52A2, SLC52A3, PDHA1, DLAT, PDHX, SPR, TH genes

(CoQ: Coenzyme Q; CSF: cerebrospinal fluid; IEMs: inborn errors of metabolism)

performed with or without fragile X phenotype.
- If there is family history of affected males with ID, fragile X testing is warranted. Panel testing for X-linked ID using next-generation sequencing (exome sequencing) is warranted, if fragile X testing is negative.
- If a child is born to consanguineous parents, with mother having a history of recurrent abortions, affected siblings or other family members, and has clinical or radiological features to suggest a metabolic disorder, then metabolic testing is warranted.

Among children with unexplained ID, normal karyotype, and array CGH, clinical exome sequencing may be advised.

Role of electroencephalography (EEG) is restricted to those with seizures. Among children with ID, recent onset of behavioral disturbances and sleep disturbances should be evaluated to rule out continuous spike wave of slow sleep (CSWS).

There is a wide list of around 81 treatable disorders of ID, which although uncommon must not be missed. In the last 2 years, there has been a paradigm shift in investigating a child with ID with shift of focus in establishing a diagnosis to identifying and treating treatable disorders. In this endeavor, TIDE (treatable intellectual disability endeavor) protocol was formulated by Clara van Karneback **(Flowchart 1)**. There are two tiers of investigations. It is considered that the first-tier investigations could pick around 60% of these treatable disorders. TIDE protocol is also available as a mobile app, called *"treatable ID"*, which is free app and extremely useful to those who cannot remember all 81 disorders. It provides provision to feed the neurological symptoms and arrive at possible differentials and plan the investigation accordingly. Hence, TIDE protocol (at least the first-tier investigations) must be used in conjunction to the standard genetic investigations discussed above.

KEY MESSAGES

- Intellectual disability refers to a significant limitation in both intellectual function and adaptive behavior, and severity is not solely dependent on IQ scores.
- In a child with ID and dysmorphism, an attempt to fit into any known genetic syndrome should be made. If not possible, one may consider karyotype or microarray and fragile X (males) and MECP2 in females.
- Consider neuroimaging among all children with ID with head size abnormality, neurocutaneous markers, and associated epilepsy.
- Unexplained ID/GDD should be investigated with microarray, fragile X testing, and first-tier testing for IEM.
- Use TIDE (treatable intellectual disability endeavor) protocol in conjunction with the standard American Academy of Pediatrics (AAP) recommendations for evaluating a child with GDD/ID.

CHAPTER 13

Approach to a Child with Cerebral Palsy

INTRODUCTION

Cerebral palsy (CP) is a permanent disorder of movement and posture that appears during infancy or early childhood, resulting in activity limitation that occurs due to a nonprogressive damage to developing brain. Although, CP is considered nonprogressive, clinical manifestations may change over time. CP is a static neuromotor impairment, which may be accompanied by several impairments/comorbidities **(Fig. 1)** CP could be secondary to insult in antenatal, natal, or postnatal period **(Box 1)**.

MOTOR IMPAIRMENT

Motor impairment in children with CP is attributable to the following:

- *Spasticity:* Inability to relax the muscle resulting in unnecessary contractions during the movement
- *Weakness:* The muscles are weak and are unable to generate force to perform the movement.
- *Loss of selectivity:* There is loss of selective control of relaxation of antagonist muscle when agonist contracts. This results in simultaneous contraction of agonist and antagonist resulting in dystonic movement instead of desired voluntary movement **(Fig. 2)**.
- *Loss of balance* and loss of cortical sensation of movement may be present in CP.
- Primitive reflexes must disappear for advanced postural reflexes to appear. Persistence of primitive reflex and delayed appearance of advanced postural reflex for balance and equilibrium are observed in children with CP. Hence, motor impairment in CP is complex and is not merely attributable to spasticity alone. It is further complicated by development

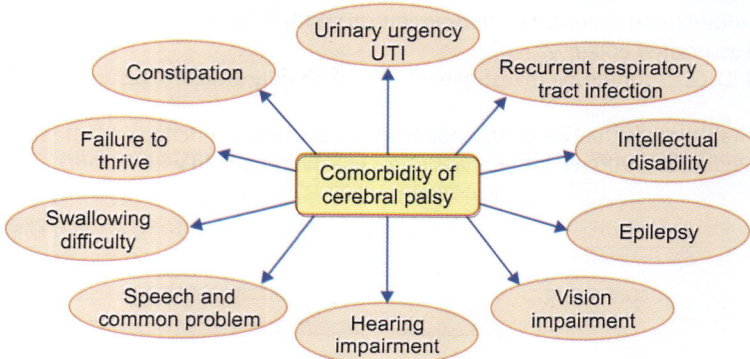

Fig. 1: Comorbidities of cerebral palsy. (UTI: Urinary tract infection)

of contractures and deformities with resultant secondary adaptive mechanism to compensate for contractures. The common muscles affected by contracture (**Flowchart 1**) and various deformities (**Flowchart 2**) in CP are depicted.

> **BOX 1:** Etiology of cerebral palsy.
>
> *Prenatal:*
> - TORCH infection
> - Maternal preeclampsia
> - Maternal diabetes mellitus
> - Maternal drug/smoking
>
> *Perinatal:*
> - PROM
> - Hypoxic ischemic
> - Prematurity
> - Low birthweight
> - Prolonged labor
>
> *Postnatal:*
> - Meningitis
> - Encephalitis
> - Kernicterus
> - Trauma
> - Hypoglycemic seizures

(TORCH: toxoplasmosis, others (syphilis, hepatitis B), rubella, cytomegalovirus, herpes simplex; PROM: premature rupture of membranes)

■ TYPES OF CEREBRAL PALSY

Broadly, there are three types of CP: Spastic CP, dyskinetic CP, and mixed CP. Other uncommon types include ataxic CP, and hypotonic CP. Based on topographic involvement, spastic CP is divided into quadriplegic, (all 4 limbs UL > LL) hemiplegic (one side UL > LL), and diplegic (LL > UL). (**Fig. 3**) Dyskinetic CP could be choreoathetoid CP *or* dystonic CP. From therapist point of view, the cerebral palsy could be unilateral (monoplegia or hemiplegia) or bilateral cerebral palsy. **Table 1** summarizes the key difference between various types of cerebral palsy.

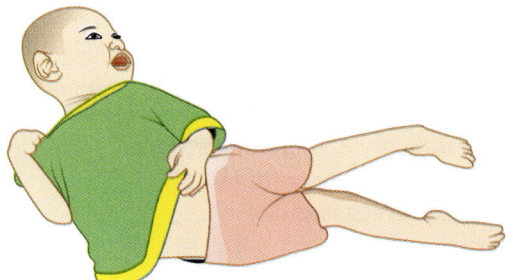

Fig. 2: Dystonic posturing in a child with cerebral palsy.

Flowchart 1: Contractures in cerebral palsy.

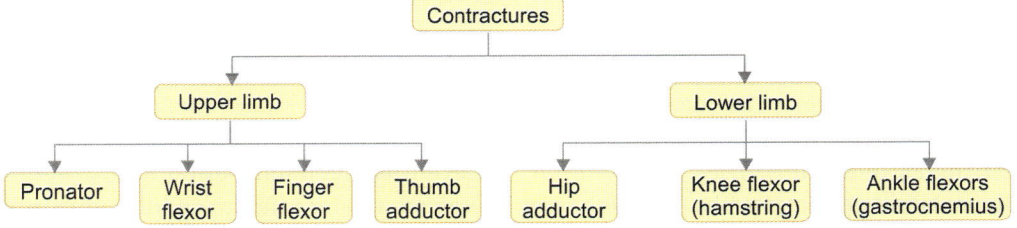

Flowchart 2: Deformities in cerebral palsy.

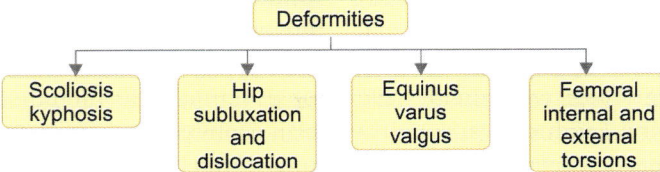

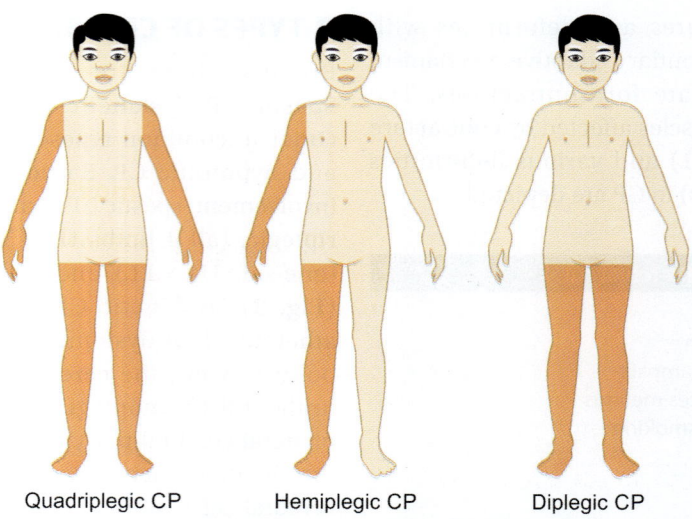

Fig. 3: Types of cerebral palsy (CP).

TABLE 1: Key differences between types of cerebral palsy (CP).

	Quadriplegic CP	Diplegic CP	Hemiplegic CP
Limb involvement	UL > LL	LL >> UL	One side UL > LL
Intellectual disability	++	–	–/+
Seizures	++	–	–/+
Feeding difficulty	++	–	–
MRI finding	Multicystic encephalomalacia	Periventricular leukomalacia	Focal cerebral infarct

(LL: lower limb; UL: upper limb)

Children with spastic quadriplegic CP are usually nonambulatory. They have associated seizure, intellectual disability, and spasticity involving all four limbs. They mostly result from profound perinatal asphyxia with resultant multicystic encephalomalacia. Children with spastic diplegia are result of prematurity with magnetic resonance imaging (MRI) features of periventricular leukomalacia. Diplegic children have difficulty in changing nappies, scissoring of legs when held, have commando crawling (adductor spasticity) and toe walking (spasticity of gastrocnemius) **(Fig. 4)**. Various gait problems in diplegic children are summarized in **Figure 5**. Most children with hemiplegic CP will have uneventful neonatal period and would be detected in later infancy/childhood. It often results from focal cerebral infarction during the perinatal period **(Fig. 6)**. Dyskinetic CP would be classified based on predominant movement disorder into choreathetoid CP and dystonic CP. Two most common insults for dyskinetic CP include kernicterus and term asphyxia. One must screen for contractures through clinical evaluation **(Fig. 7)**.

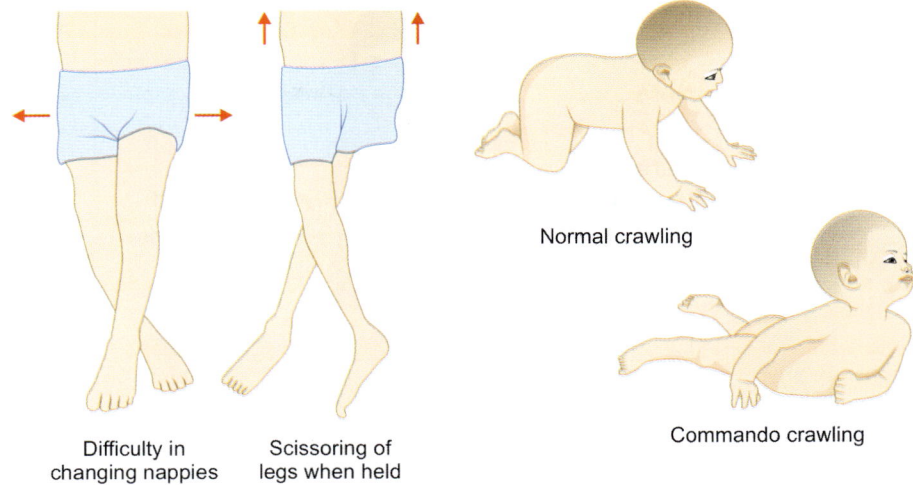

Fig. 4: Clinical features of spastic diplegia.

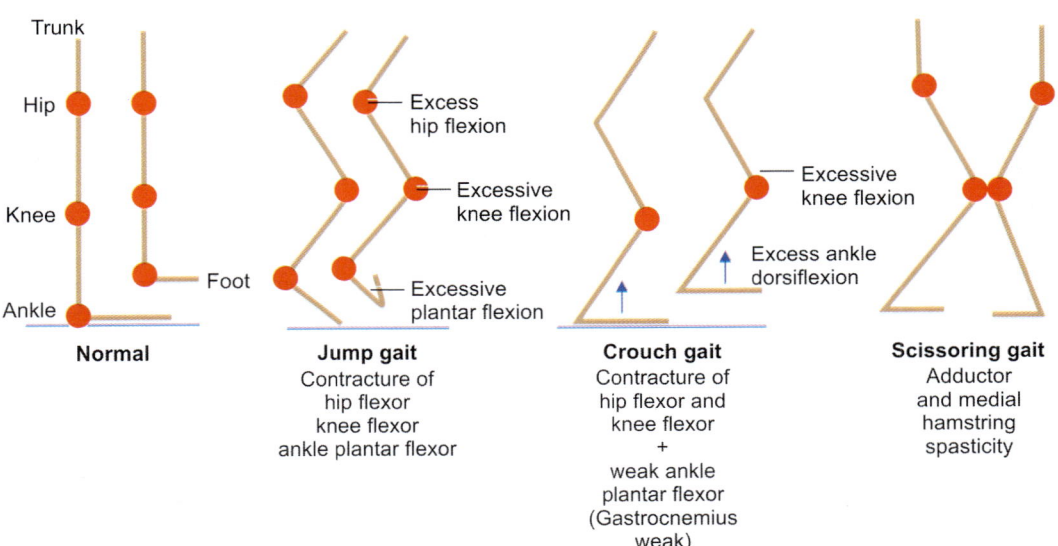

Fig. 5: Various gait problems in diplegic CP. (CP: cerebral palsy)

■ SEVERITY OF IMPAIRMENT

Severity of impairment in motor function is assessed by Gross Motor Function Classification System (GMFCS), which evaluates the gross motor function. The impairment in fine motor function is assessed and classified using Manual ability classification system (MACS). The impairment in day-to-day communication function classification system (CFCS) and ability to eat/eating drinking ability classification system (EDACS) can also be

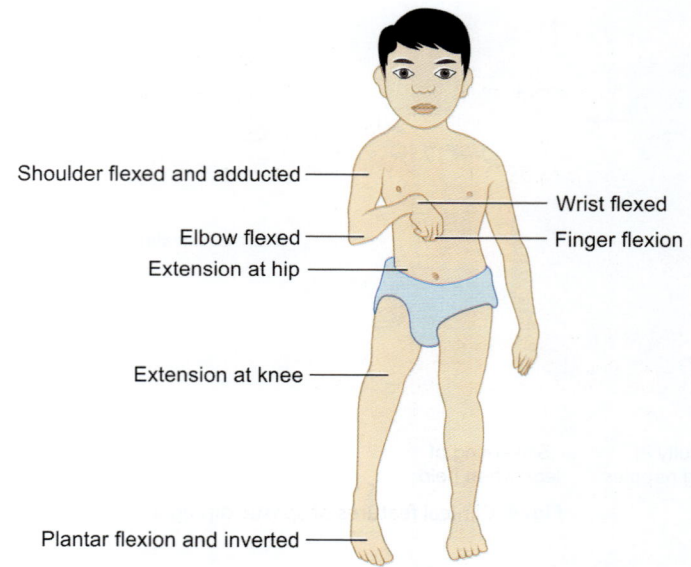

Fig. 6: Description of right hemiplegic posture.

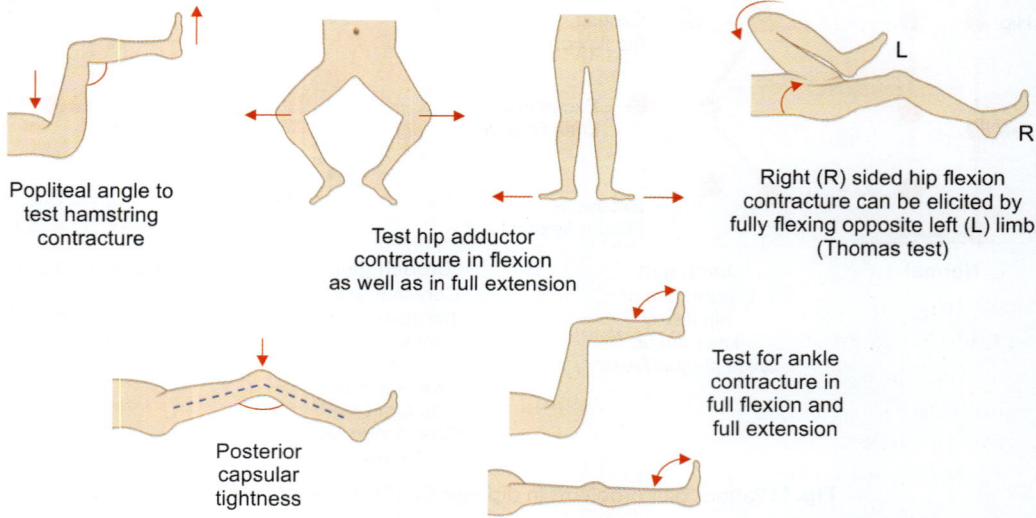

Fig. 7: Screening for contractures in CP. (CP: cerebral palsy)

graded and classified. GMFLS and MACS are discussed on chapter on case of cerebral palsy **(Chapter 24)**. A broad clinical approach to a child with cerebral palsy is summarized in **Figure 8**.

INVESTIGATING A CHILD WITH CEREBRAL PALSY

Diagnosis of cerebral palsy is clinical; investigation have limited role in evaluating a child with cerebral palsy.

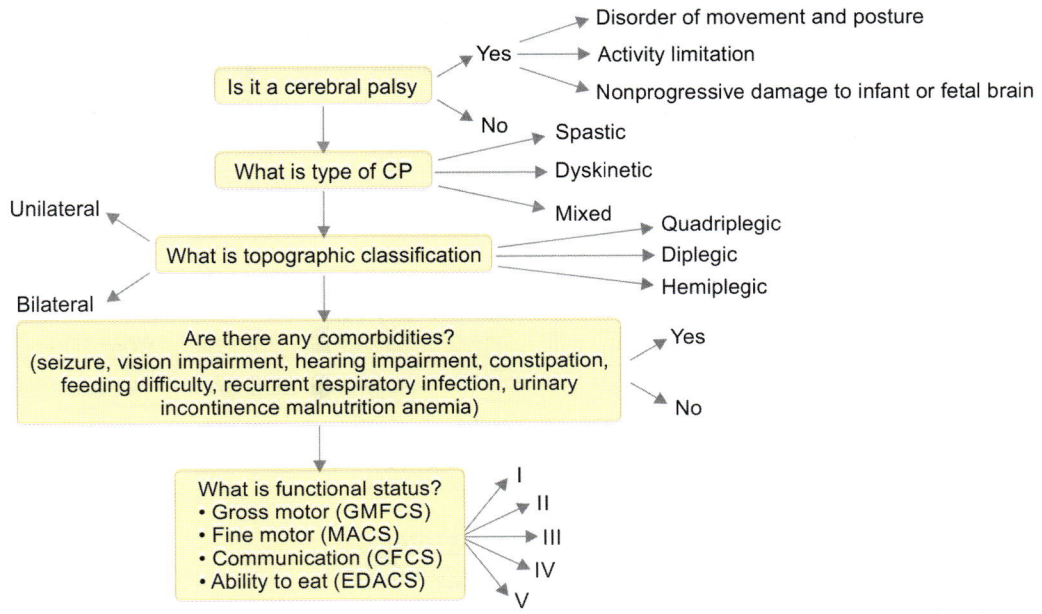

Fig. 8: Broad clinical approach to a child with cerebral palsy. (CFCS: communication function classification system; EDACS: eat/eating drinking ability classification system GMFCS: gross motor function classification system; MACS: manual ability classification system)

- *MRI Brain:* MRI brain is often recommended to confirm and support the clinical diagnosis of CP. Lack of history of neonatal insult in a child with CP is a definitive indication for neuroimaging to establish the etiology. The common findings in MRI brain are depicted **Table 2**. We must remember that 10–20% of children with CP may have normal MRI findings. However, high index of suspicion for CP mimics like dopa-responsive dystonia, and other neurotransmitter disorders must be considered if neuroimaging is normal **(Table 3)**. **Figure 9** enumerates the differential of CP mimics of dyskinetic CP.
- *Compute tomography (CT) Head:* It is usually not recommended for evaluation of child with CP, except for identifying periventricular calcifications in congenital cytomegalovirus (CMV) infection.
- *Electroencephalography* (EEG) must be considered only among those with associated epilepsy.
- *Hip surveillance:* Hip dysplasia is common in CP and increases with increasing severity of GMFCS. Apart from clinical surveillance, anteroposterior (AP) pelvis radiographs are recommended to measure migration percentage to quantify the degree of hip displacement.
- *Gastroesophageal reflux disease (GERD) scan:* Gastroesophageal Reflux (GER) scan is useful among children with CP (GMFCS 4/5) with feeding difficulty, repeated respiratory tract infection, and failure to thrive.
- *Visual evoked potential (VEP) scan:* VEP will be useful among those with vision impairment and normal ophthalmological evaluation (normal fundus).

TABLE 2: Magnetic resonance imaging (MRI) findings in various types of cerebral palsy (CP).

Type of CP	MRI findings
Spastic diplegia CP	Periventricular leukomalacia
Spastic hemiplegic CP	Focal/ischemic necrosis
Dyskinetic CP and mixed CP	Bilateral globus pallidus hyperintensity (kernicterus) hyperintensity involving ventrolateral thalamus (term asphyxia)

TABLE 3: Cerebral palsy (CP) mimics of spastic diplegia.

Clinical features	What to think of?
Spastic paraparesis, hairy patch over back, scoliosis patchy sensory loss, bladder/bowel incontinence	Spinal dysraphism
Spastic paraparesis, positive family history of gait difficulty, with urinary urgency and decreased vibration sense	Hereditary spastic paraparesis (HSP)
Spasticity with history of regression of motor or cognitive milestone with suggestive MRI findings (clinical features and age at onset will vary)	Leukodystrophy
Spastic paraparesis, with regression of cognitive skills with failure to thrive	Arginase deficiency
Spastic paraparesis with congenital ichthyosis and cognitive delay	Sjögren-Larsson's syndrome
Spastic paraparesis with optic atrophy	Late-onset biotinidase deficiency
Spastic paraparesis with development delay, autism, microcephaly	Cerebral folate deficiency
Spastic diplegia with normal MRI brain	Atlantoaxial dislocation

(MRI: magnetic resonance imaging)

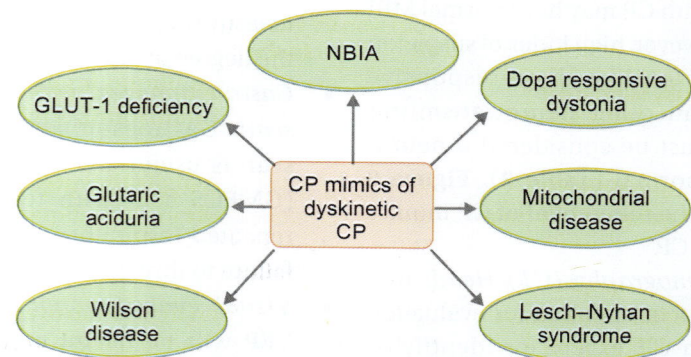

Fig. 9: CP mimics of dyskinetic CP. (CP: cerebral palsy; NBIA: neurodegeneration with brain iron accumulation; GLUT: glucose transporter)

- *BERA (brainstem-evoked response audiometry)* response would be required among those with hearing impairment.

Management of cerebral palsy has been discussed in **Chapter 38** (management of developmental disorders)

KEY MESSAGES

- Cerebral palsy is a disorder of movement and posture resulting from nonprogressive damage to developing brain.
- Motor impairment in children with cerebral palsy results from combination of increased tone, weakness, loss of selectivity, and loss of balance.
- Cerebral palsy can be divided into spastic CP, dyskinetic CP, and mixed cerebral palsy. Topographically, it can be divided into quadriplegic, hemiplegic, and diplegic cerebral palsy.
- Spasticity selectively involves hip adductors, knee flexors and ankle plantar flexors in lower limb; elbow flexors, wrist flexors, pronators, and shoulder adductors in upper limb
- Comorbidities in children with cerebral palsy include epilepsy, behavioral problems, sleep disturbances, feeding difficulty, recurrent respiratory tract infection, constipation, and urinary tract infection.

CHAPTER 14

Approach to a Child with Developmental Regression

■ INTRODUCTION

Progressive encephalopathy refers to disorders with gradual loss of cognitive function. It could result from genetic or acquired causes (toxic, infectious, inflammatory, or neoplastic). Few examples of acquired causes include subacute sclerosing panencephalitis (SSPE), human immunodeficiency virus (HIV) infection, and multiple sclerosis. Genetic causes of progressive encephalopathy include neurometabolic disorder and neurodegenerative disorders (NDDs).

■ NEUROMETABOLIC DISORDERS

Neurometabolic disorders refer to disorders where the progressive encephalopathy is attributable to a specific defect in the metabolic pathway. These can be broadly divided into three groups—intoxication disorders, energy deficiency disorders, or storage disorders. They can present in three forms—acute presentation (neonates and late infancy), recurrent or intermittent, and chronic progressive presentation.

■ NEURODEGENERATIVE DISORDERS

- NDDs are genetic disorders that result in progressive encephalopathy. This heterogeneous group can present with progressive loss of motor, amino acid (phenylketonuria and maple syrup urine disease), sugar (galactosemia), and ammonia (urea cycle disorder).
- *Energy deficiency disorders* can present with a congenital malformation or cerebral dysgenesis. Examples include mitochondrial disorders, fatty acid oxidation disorders, and defects in glycogen synthesis. They are also called large molecule disorders.
- *Organelle disorders* include the accumulation of incompletely metabolized tissues in various cellular organelles. Examples include mucopolysaccharidosis, lysosomal storage disease, and oligosaccharidosis. **Table 1** summarizes the clinical features of these three broad groups of neurometabolic disorders.
- *Intoxication disorder* occurs secondary to a defect in metabolic pathway resulting in accumulation of proximal metabolite. They are also called small molecule disorders. Symptoms begin in infancy or childhood with no apparent embryonic toxicity. There can be an accumulation of cognitive or perceptual function. There is a marked overlap between neurometabolic disorders and NDDs, as many so-called NDDs have a metabolic basis. For example, metachromatic leukodystrophy results from the deficiency of arylsulfatase enzyme.

TABLE 1: Classification of neurometabolic disorders.

Classification	Presentation	Disease
Disorders of intoxication	• Acute decompensation with stress or increased metabolic demand • There will be a period of symptom-free interval • It usually does not interfere with fetal development • They can present at any age. Acute management is crucial	• Organic acidemia (MMA and IVA) • Aminoaciduria (MSUD and PKU) • Urea cycle disorder • Sugar intolerance (galactosemia and HFI) • Metal disorders (Wilson and Menkes)
Disorder of energy failure	• Majority of them have failure to thrive • Illness is often precipitated by stress-like fever, surgery • May have a fluctuating clinical course (mitochondrial) • They often have multisystemic involvement (mitochondrial) • Few mitochondrial and PPP defects can affect fetal development: Dysmorphism and dysplasia	• Mitochondrial disorders (more severe) • Cytoplasmic defects (less severe presentation)
Organelle disorder	• Coarse facies, hepatosplenomegaly, corneal opacity, PME phenotype, CR spots on fundus, and gaze palsy (LSD) • Congenital anomalies, hypotonia, abnormal fat pads, and abnormal coagulation (CDG) • Retinopathy, sensorineural hearing loss, brain malformation, and dysmorphism (peroxisomal disorder) • GDD and multiple congenital anomalies (cholesterol biosynthesis)	• Lysosomal storage disorders • Peroxisomal disorders • Disorders of intracellular trafficking (α-antitrypsin deficiency) • CDG deficiency • Cholesterol biosynthetic defect

(CDG: congenital disorders of glycosylation; CR: cherry red; GDD: global developmental delay; HFI: hereditary fructose intolerance; IVA: isovaleric acidemia; LSD: lysosomal storage disorder; MMA: methylmalonic acidemia; MSUD: maple syrup urine disease; PKU: phenylketonuria; PME: progressive myoclonic epilepsy; PPP: pentose phosphate pathway)

Approach to Neurodegenerative Disorders

Neurodegenerative disorders can be approached by their main clinical presentation, age at onset, and neuroimaging findings. A broad clinical approach to NDD includes consideration for the following key points:
- Is it a neurodegenerative disease?
- What is the age of onset?
- Is it acute, intermittent, or chronic?
- What is the clinical presentation?
- Is it a gray matter or white matter disease?
- Does it also involve the peripheral nervous system?
- Are there any extraneurological features?

Is it a Neurodegenerative Disorder?

Regression of attained milestones is *not* synonymous with NDDs. There can be various causes of regression of milestones in a child with static encephalopathy like cerebral palsy. These include increasing spasticity, new-onset movement disorders, new-onset seizures or spasm, progressive hydrocephalus, or parental misperception of attained milestones. It is a good idea to look at old photographs or videos of the baby when parents perceive that the baby was fine. Questions like "As the time is progressing, do you think the things are worsening or improving?" often help to differentiate static encephalopathy from progressive encephalopathy. If clinical features are overall improving with time, but tightness has worsened, we know that it is pseudoregression in a static encephalopathy owing to increasing spasticity rather than a true neurodegenerative disease.

What is the Age at Onset?

Based on the age at onset, the NDD can be classified into those that begin in the neonatal period, infancy, or childhood **(Table 2)**. Considering that the majority of these NDD will have overlapping clinical features, knowledge of age at the onset will help exclude or include few differentials. In a 6-month-old baby with progressive cognitive decline and myoclonus, we will not think of SSPE despite that being the most common cause of progressive myoclonic epilepsy (PME) in an Indian setup. We would rather think of neuronal ceroid lipofuscinosis (NCL).

Is it Acute, Intermittent, or Chronic?

Neurodegenerative disorders can present in acute, intermittent, or chronic patterns. Disorders including urea cycle disorder, organic acidemia, and maple syrup urine disease can present acutely whereas mucopolysaccharidosis, lysosomal storage disease, and NCL present with chronic progressive encephalopathy.

TABLE 2: Classification of neurodegenerative disorder based on the age at onset.

Age at onset	Examples
Neonatal onset (<1 month)	• Neonatal adrenoleukodystrophy • GM1 gangliosidosis • Glycogen storage disorder type I • Mucolipidosis
Early infantile (1–6 months)	• Infantile neuronal ceroid lipofuscinosis (NCL) • Pompe disease • Maple syrup urine disease • Galactosemia
Late infantile (6–12 months)	• Tay–Sachs disease • Krabbe disease • Niemann–Pick disease type A • Canavan disease • Lesch–Nyhan disease • Mitochondrial disorder • Infantile neuroaxonal dystrophy
Early childhood (1–5 years)	• Metachromatic leukodystrophy • Niemann–Pick disease type C • Mucopolysaccharidosis
Late childhood (5–15 years)	• Juvenile NCL • Adrenoleukodystrophy • Subacute sclerosing panencephalitis • Sanfilippo syndrome • Juvenile metachromatic leukodystrophy (MLD) • Gaucher type III

What is the Clinical Presentation?

Recognition of clinical phenotype is important in reaching the exact etiology. The common clinical presentation includes cognitive decline, seizures, difficulty in vision, evolving spasticity, extrapyramidal

TABLE 3: Clinical presentation of common neurodegenerative disorders in children.

Predominant clinical presentation	Neurodegenerative disorders (age >2 years)	Neurodegenerative disorders (age <2 years)
Cerebellar ataxia	• Friedreich ataxia • Spinocerebellar ataxia • Ataxia telangiectasia • Abetalipoproteinemia	• Ataxia telangiectasia • Mitochondrial disorders
Dystonia	• Segawa disease (dopa-responsive dystonia) • Pantothenate kinase-associated neurodegeneration (PKAN) • Wilson disease • Huntington chorea	• Lesch–Nyhan disease • Glutaric aciduria type I
Spasticity	• Metachromatic leukodystrophy • Adrenoleukodystrophy	• Krabbe disease • Mitochondrial disorder
Progressive myoclonic epilepsy	• Subacute sclerosing panencephalitis (SSPE) • Lafora body disease	• Neuronal ceroid lipofuscinosis (NCL) • Myoclonic epilepsy with ragged red fiber (MERRF)
Coarse facies	Mucopolysaccharidosis (MPS)	• Mucopolysaccharidosis • Mucolipidosis • GM1 gangliosidosis
Hepatosplenomegaly	MPS	• Gaucher disease • Niemann–Pick disease • MPS • GM1 gangliosidosis
Macrocephaly	Megalencephalic leukoencephalopathy with subcortical cyst (Van der Knaap disease)	• Canavan disease • Alexander disease • Tay–Sachs disease

symptoms (choreoathetosis and dystonia), ataxia, and motor weakness. Based on the age at onset and predominant clinical presentation, a broad group of the NDD can be often recognized. **Table 3** outlines the symptomatology of common NDDs.

Is it a Gray Matter or White Matter Degeneration?

Traditionally, NDDs were classified into the gray matter and white matter degenerative brain disorders (DBDs). With the advent of genetics, it is realized that there is a marked overlap of clinical features in gray matter and white matter DBD. This distinction of gray matter and white matter DBD is blurring. However, traditional teaching still can be used to narrow our differential diagnosis **(Table 4)**.

By convention, gray matter disorders present with psychomotor regression, cognitive decline, seizures, and/or extrapyramidal manifestations. Fundus examination can reveal pigmentary retinopathy (NCL) or cherry-red spot (Tay–Sachs disease). In contrast, white matter disorders present with spasticity and/or peripheral neuropathy and optic atrophy. This cannot be a rule

TABLE 4: Differentiating white and gray matter degenerative brain disorders (DBDs).

	White matter DBD	Gray matter DBD
Age at onset	Mostly late	Early
Head size	May have macrocephaly	Usually microcephaly
Seizures	Late and rare	Early and common
Cognitive impairment	Affected late	Common
Peripheral neuropathy	Demyelination	Axonal
Spasticity	Early and severe	Late
Cerebellar signs	Early and prominent	Late

for differentiating white matter and gray matter DBD. End stage of most white matter DBD, including adrenoleukodystrophy and metachromatic leukodystrophy, will have cognitive decline. Similarly, upper motor neuron signs including spasticity can be seen in gray matter DBD like NCL and mitochondrial disorders.

Does it also Involve Peripheral Nervous System?

Among children presenting with predominant motor regression, it is often imperative to differentiate central nervous system (CNS) versus peripheral nervous system (PNS) as the site of the lesion. By convention, those with hypotonia, hyporeflexia or areflexia, and mute or flexor plantar response are presumed to be secondary to lower motor neuron (LMN) pathology. There are few conditions where peripheral neuropathy is associated with CNS pathology. For example, demyelinating peripheral neuropathy is common among children with Krabbe disease, adrenoleukodystrophy, and metachromatic leukodystrophy. Axonal polyneuropathy is observed among those with abetalipoproteinemia, pyruvate dehydrogenase deficiency, and cerebrotendinous xanthomatosis. Infantile neuroaxonal dystrophy (INAD) can present with hypotonia and hyporeflexia, often mimicking myopathic process.

What are the Extraneural Clinical Manifestations?

Systemic findings in eyes, hair, face, skin, hearing loss, and hepatosplenomegaly offer clinical clues to underlying etiology **(Table 5)**. Head circumference may also give a hint at the underlying etiology: microcephaly in Krabbe disease, NCL, and macrocephaly in Tay–Sachs disease, gangliosidosis, Alexander disease, and Canavan disease.

Is there a Family History?

A family history of similar illness gives a hint toward the mode of inheritance. The majority of neurometabolic disorder and NDDs have an autosomal recessive inheritance. A family history of affected siblings, recurrent abortions, and consanguinity points toward an autosomal recessive disorder. Disorders such as Lesch–Nyhan syndrome and adrenoleukodystrophy can have an X-linked mode of inheritance. Mitochondrial disorders can have autosomal or mitochondrial inheritance depending on the involvement of nuclear or cytoplasmic genes.

TABLE 5: Extraneural signs in neurodegenerative diseases.

Extraneural organ	Clinical finding	Neurodegenerative disease
Hair	Friable tufted hair	Menkes disease and argininosuccinate lyase deficiency
	Premature gray	Ataxia telangiectasia
Ear	Deafness	• Mucopolysaccharidosis (MPS) • Mitochondrial disorders [myoclonic epilepsy with ragged red fiber (MERRF)]
	Hyperacusis (excessive startle)	Tay–Sachs disease
Skin	Rash	Biotinidase deficiency
	Café-au-lait macules	Ataxia telangiectasia
Hepatosplenomegaly		Mucopolysaccharidosis, Gaucher, Niemann–Pick disease, and glycogen storage disorder
Fundus	Pigmentary changes	• Ataxia telangiectasia • Pantothenate kinase-associated neurodegeneration (PKAN) • Mitochondrial disorders • Neuronal ceroid lipofuscinosis (NCL)
	Optic atrophy	Krabbe disease
	Cherry-red spot	• GM1 gangliosidosis • Niemann–Pick disease (NPD) type A • Tay–Sachs disease
Eye	Cataract	Galactosemia
	Telangiectasia	Ataxia–telangiectasia

◼ LEUKODYSTROPHY

Leukoencephalopathy encompasses all disorders that affect exclusively or predominantly white matter.

Leukodystrophy refers to genetically determined leukoencephalopathy. Based on the radiological pattern of white matter involvement, it can be classified as focal, periventricular, diffuse cerebral, and multifocal **(Table 6)**.

Table 7 summarizes the key differences between *dysmyelinating, demyelinating,* and *hypomyelinating* leukodystrophy.

If there is no myelin formation, it would be considered hypomyelinating. If the myelin that is formed is abnormal, it would be dysmyelinating. If the myelin was formed normally and later due to some insult, it gets destroyed; this is called demyelinating. Mature, healthy myelin will look bright (hyperintense) on T1 and dark (hypointense) on T2. Abnormal myelin (dysmyelination) or destructed myelin (demyelinating) will look bright on T2 and dark on T1. Hypomyelinating leukodystrophy will look bright on T2 and isointense on T1. On MRI brain, it is difficult to differentiate dysmyelinating from demyelinating pathology, as both will look T2 hyperintense and T1 hypointense.

Hypomyelinating Leukodystrophy

One of the most practical ways to diagnose hypomyelinating leukodystrophy is to look for structures that get myelinated at birth like the posterior limb of internal capsule (PLIC). Structures that are myelinated at

TABLE 6: Patterns of leukodystrophy.

Focal	Periventricular	Diffuse cerebral	Multifocal
• Alexander (Frontal) • CTX (Cerebellum) • Alexander (Cerebellum) • Leigh (Brainstem) • LBSL (Brainstem) • ALD (Occipital)	• MLD • Krabbe • Sjögren–Larsson syndrome • LBSL • NCL	• MLC • VWMD • Mitochondrial • Merosin-negative CMD	• PML • MS/NMO • Mitochondrial • Galactosemia • Brucellosis

(ALD: adrenoleukodystrophy; CMD: congenital muscular dystrophy; CTX: cerebrotendinous xanthomatosis; LBSL: leukoencephalopathy with brainstem and spinal cord with elevated lactate; MLC: megalencephalic leukodystrophy with subcortical cyst; MLD: metachromatic leukodystrophy; MS: multiple sclerosis; NCL: neuronal ceroid lipofuscinosis; NMO: neuromyelitis optica; PML: progressive multifocal leukoencephalopathy; VWMD: vanishing white matter disease)

TABLE 7: Key differences between types of white matter abnormalities.

Abnormality of white matter	What does it mean?
Dysmyelinating	Formation of abnormal myelin; distribution is symmetrical and confluent
Demyelinating	Destruction of normal myelin; majority of them are patchy, asymmetrical, and multifocal
Hypomyelinating	Reduction in the amount of myelin
Delayed myelination	When there is a delay in maturation

birth include PLIC, dorsal brainstem, and perirolandic gyrus. If PLIC is myelinated (T1 hyperintense and T2 hypointense), then it is very unlikely to be a hypomyelinating leukodystrophy. Myelination can be delayed in many syndromes such as Down syndrome and acquired causes such as hypoxic–ischemic encephalopathy. Diagnosis of delayed myelination is made on serial scans performed at a minimum interval of 6 months. If the myelination is progressing on serial scans, then it is probably delayed myelination, but if there is no myelination from the beginning with no further myelination on the serial scan, it is probably hypomyelinating leukodystrophy. Majority of myelination proceeds after birth. It proceeds from posterior to anterior and central to the periphery. Majority of myelination is completed by 18–24 months.

Identifying the Etiology

It is essential to have a good knowledge of pattern involvement in leukodystrophy to identify the underlying etiology **(Flowchart 1)**. Periventricular white matter is involved in metachromatic leukodystrophy, Krabbe disease; subcortical white matter is involved in Canavan disease and megalencephalic leukoencephalopathy with subcortical cyst (MLC); frontal white matter is involved in Alexander disease; occipital white matter in adrenoleukodystrophy; corticospinal tract involved in Krabbe disease and Leigh disease; and cerebellar involvement in Krabbe disease and mitochondrial disorders. Key clinical features of common leukodystrophies are summarized in **Table 8**. MRI images of common leukodystrophies, including metachromatic leukodystrophy, adrenoleukodystrophy, megalencephalic leukoencephalopathy with a subcortical cyst, Alexander disease, and Pelizaeus–Merzbacher disease, are shown in **Figures 1 to 5**.

Flowchart 1: Classification of leukodystrophy based on imaging findings.

```
                          Leukodystrophy
    ┌──────────────────┬──────────┬──────────────────┐
Demyelinating    Hypomyelinating   Spongiform         Cystic
• ALD            • PMD             • Canavan disease  • VWM disease
• MLD            • 4H syndrome     • MLC              • Alexander disease
• Krabbe disease
```

(4H: hypomyelination, hypogonadotropic, hypogonadism, and hypodontia; ALD: adrenoleukodystrophy; MLC: megalencephalic leukoencephalopathy with subcortical cyst; MLD: metachromatic leukodystrophy; PMD: Pelizaeus–Merzbacher disease; VWM: vanishing white matter)

TABLE 8: Key clinical and radiological features of commonly encountered leukodystrophy.

Leukodystrophy	Clinical phenotype	Radiological phenotype
Pelizaeus–Merzbacher disease (*PLP1* gene)	Infancy, nystagmus, axial hypotonia, motor delay > cognitive delay	T2 hyperintense (homogeneous); T1 normal with normal basal ganglia (BG), cerebellum (Cbl), brainstem (BS)
Megalencephalic leukoencephalopathy with subcortical cyst (MLC)	Infancy, macrocephaly, subtle developmental delay, common in Agarwal community	Diffuse white matter involvement T2 hyperintense, T1 hypointense with anterior temporal lobe cyst, sparing of BG, Cbl, and BS
Adrenoleukodystrophy (ALD)	School-going children, hyperactivity, behavioral issues, spasticity, and visual loss	Posterior (parieto-occipital) white matter involvement T2 hyperintense, T1 hypointense, and contrast uptake
Metachromatic leukodystrophy (MLD)	Onset 2–5 years of age, spasticity, and preserved cognition	Periventricular white matter involvement with a tigroid appearance
Vanishing white matter disease	Neuroregression following trivial trauma or febrile illness, and ataxia	Diffuse white matter involvement with cystic changes
Neuronal ceroid lipofuscinosis	Age at onset (infantile, later infantile, and juvenile), developmental delay, ataxia, visual loss, pigmentary retinopathy, microcephaly, and myoclonic epilepsy	Cerebellar atrophy and periventricular signal changes
Alexander disease	Infancy, macrocephaly is the only constant finding, others include acute presentation with features of raised ICP	Bilateral symmetrical frontal predominant white matter involvement
Canavan disease	Infancy onset, hypotonia, macro-cephaly, and developmental delay	Subcortical white matter involvement with involvement of globus pallidus, N-acetyl aspartate (NAA) peak on magnetic resonance spectrometry
Krabbe disease	Infancy onset, excessive irritability, microcephaly, exaggerated startle, and spasticity	Periventricular, posterior limb of internal capsule, corpus callosum, and cerebellar involvement with hyperdense thalamus

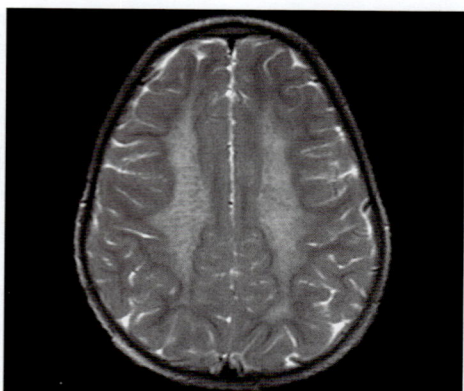

Fig. 1: T2-weighted magnetic resonance imaging (MRI) showing periventricular white matter signal changes with tigroid pattern with sparing of basal ganglia and cerebellum (not shown) suggestive of metachromatic leukodystrophy.

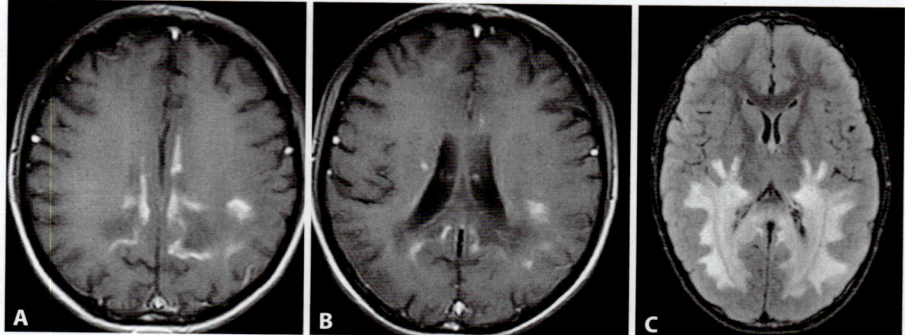

Figs. 2A to C: (A and B) T1-weighted images (contrast); (C) T2 FLAIR image showing posterior predominant (occipital) white matter signal changes with contrast enhancement in a child with adrenoleukodystrophy (ALD).

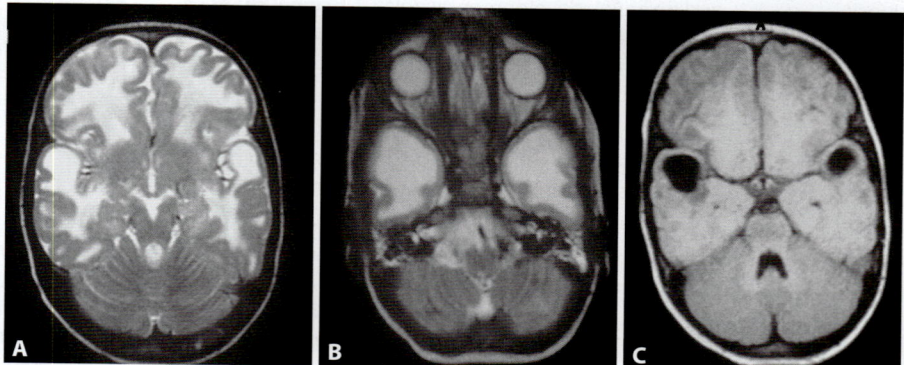

Figs. 3A to C: T2-weighted MRI brain sequences (A and B) showing T2 hyperintense and T1 hypointense (C) diffuse white matter involvement (both periventricular and subcortical) with sparing of basal ganglia, brainstem, and cerebellum in a child who has subtle motor delay with macrocephaly. MRI was done following a trivial fall from bed. These findings are suggestive of megalencephalic leukoencephalopathy with subcortical cyst (MLC).

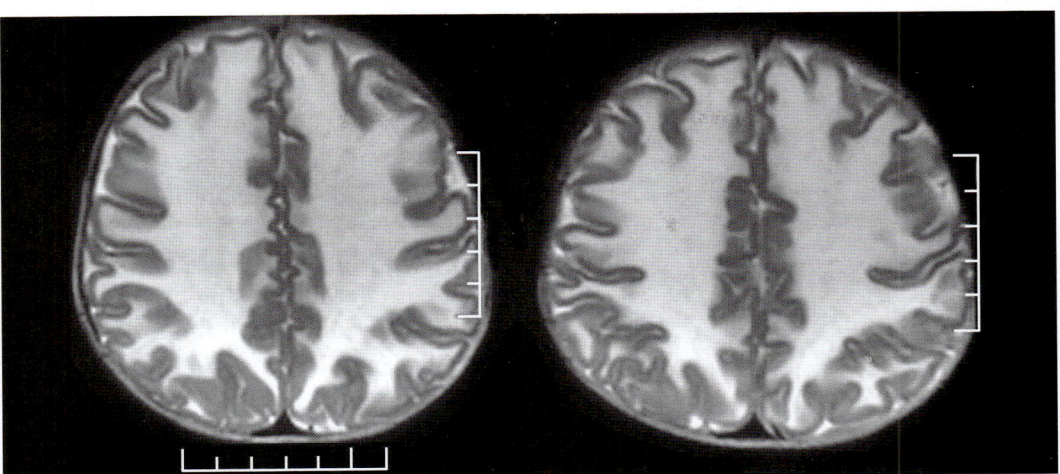

Fig. 4: T2-weighted magnetic resonance imaging (MRI) brain showing dense white matter signal changes in a child with developmental delay and macrocephaly suggestive of Alexander disease.
Courtesy: Dr Rachana Dubey Gupta, Indore, Madhya Pradesh, India.

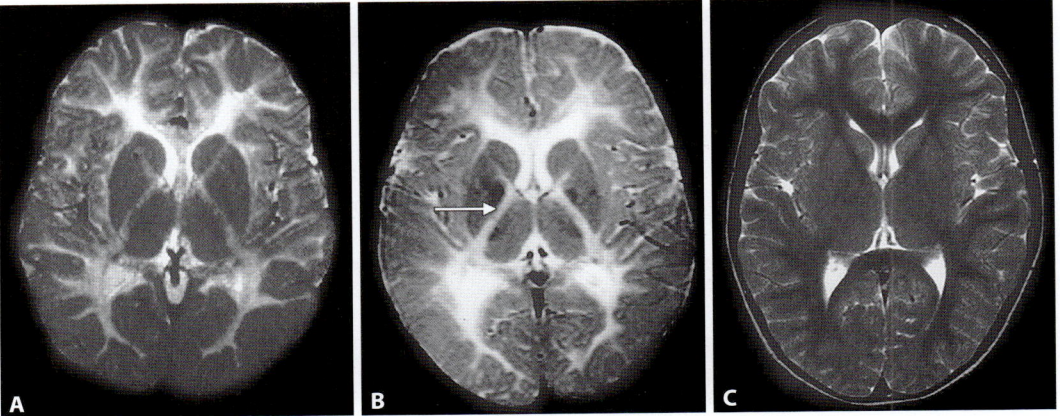

Figs. 5A to C: T2-weighted magnetic resonance imaging (MRI) brain showing T2 hyperintensity with T1 isointense diffuse white matter involvement in a child with hypotonia, nystagmus, hyporeflexia suggestive of clinical diagnosis of Pelizaeus–Merzbacher disease (PMD). Look at the unmyelinated posterior limb of internal capsule (PLIC) (arrow).

■ CASE VIGNETTES

Case 1

An 8-year-old boy presented with complaints of repeated episodes of fall while walking, with a progressive decline in basic understanding for the last 3 months. Before the onset of illness, he was studying in 3rd grade and was average in academic activity. Examination reveals myoclonic jerks involving trunk and limbs. There are no signs of spasticity or extrapyramidal features. There was no dysmorphism or any signs of organomegaly. Fundus showed pigmentary changes.

Analysis

Analysis	Index case
Is it a neurodegenerative disease?	Yes, as things are worsening with time
What is the age at onset?	It started at 8 years of age
Is it acute, intermittent, or chronic?	It has an insidious onset and is a slowly progressive disease
What is the clinical presentation?	There are myoclonus and progressive cognitive decline
Is it a gray matter or white matter disease?	Considering the lack of spasticity, the presence of seizures (myoclonic), and cognitive decline, it appears to be gray matter DBD
Is it CNS or PNS?	There appears to be no involvement of PNS
Are there any extraneural features?	There was no dysmorphism, organomegaly. The fundus examination revealed pigmentary changes

We are dealing with an 8-year-old first affected child with progressive cognitive decline and myoclonus. It is likely to be a gray matter DBD with PME. Differentials will include SSPE, NCL, Unverricht–Lundborg disease, Lafora body disease, juvenile Gaucher disease, juvenile GM2, mitochondrial disorders (MERRF), and sialidosis **(Table 9)**. Now consider the following:

- Absence of splenomegaly rules out Gaucher and Niemann–Pick disease.
- Absence of pyramidal or extrapyramidal signs (rule out NCL and Lafora disease)
- Normal hearing makes the diagnosis of MERRF unlikely.
- No cherry-red spot on fundus rules out sialidosis.
- Presence of cognitive decline in the present case makes a diagnosis of Unverricht–Lundborg disease to be unlikely.
- Rapid cognitive decline within 3 months of onset could point toward Lafora body disease.
- Presence of PME phenotype with pigmentary retinopathy could point to NCL or SSPE.

TABLE 9: Key features of conditions presenting with progressive myoclonic epilepsy.

Progressive myoclonic epilepsy (PME)	Key features
Unverricht–Lundborg disease	Cognition is preserved till late, often myoclonus involves face, and it is stimulus sensitive
Lafora body disease	Usually rapidly progressive cognitive decline, with occipital seizures and visual hallucinations with presence of pyramidal signs
Neuronal ceroid lipofuscinosis (NCL)	Rapidly progressive cognitive decline, pyramidal and extrapyramidal signs, visual loss, and pigmentary retinal changes
Juvenile Gaucher disease	Gaze palsies, abnormal eye movement, cerebellar ataxia, pyramidal and extrapyramidal signs, early dementia, and presence of hepatosplenomegaly
Mitochondrial [myoclonic epilepsy with ragged red fiber (MERRF)]	Optic atrophy, muscle weakness, and sensorineural hearing loss
Sialidosis	Facial myoclonus, visual deficit, cherry-red spot, and painful neuropathy

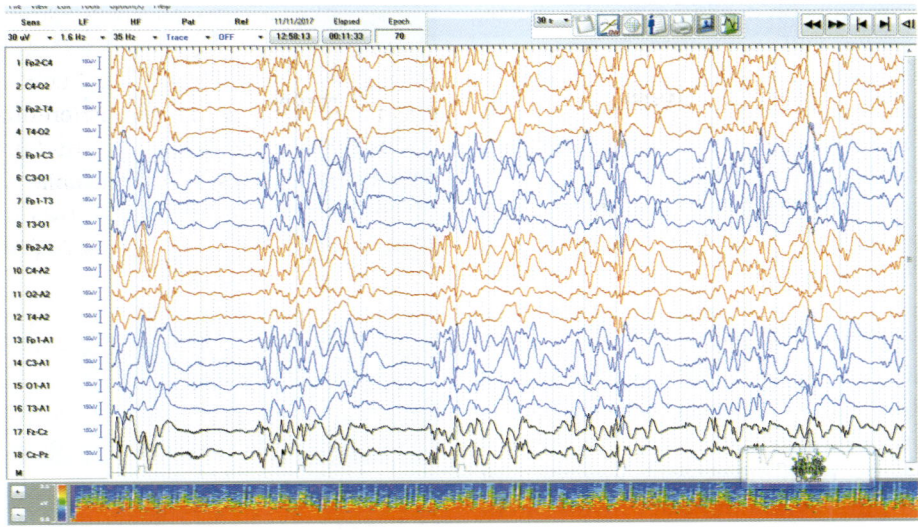

Fig. 6: Electroencephalography showing generalized epileptiform discharges in pseudoperiodic interval.

Hence, three close differentials in the present case would be SSPE, NCL, and Lafora body disease. Investigations were planned accordingly.

- MRI brain was normal in the case. The absence of cerebellar atrophy makes NCL less likely.
- Electroencephalogram (EEG) revealed generalized interictal epileptiform discharges in pseudoperiodic intervals **(Fig. 6)**, favoring a clinical diagnosis of SSPE.
- Lumbar puncture was performed, and CSF was examined for antimeasles antibodies. A high titer confirmed the diagnosis of SSPE.

Case 2

A 3-year-old boy presented with progressive difficulty in walking and repeated falls for the last 6 months. There is no history of seizures. He has preserved cognition, vision, and hearing. There are signs of spasticity with absent deep tendon reflexes (DTRs) on examination. The fundus examination was normal. Head circumference is age appropriate. There are no signs of anemia or any other signs of malnutrition.

Analysis

Analysis	Index case
Is it a neurodegenerative disease?	Probably yes, as things are worsening with time
What is the age at the onset?	It started at 2.5 years of age
Is it acute, intermittent, or chronic?	It has an insidious onset and is a slowly progressive chronic disease
What is the clinical presentation?	Motor regression and spasticity
Is it a gray matter or white matter disease?	Presence of spasticity, favors white matter DBD
Is it CNS or PNS?	Involvement of PNS is possible considering areflexia despite presence of spasticity
Are there any extraneural features?	There was no dysmorphism or organomegaly. Normal fundus. No extraneural markers

We are probably dealing with a child having white matter DBD with onset at 2.5 years of age. Differentials could include metachromatic leukodystrophy, Krabbe disease, mitochondrial disorders, Canavan disease, and Alexander disease. Now, consider the following:
- Most children with Krabbe disease will have microcephaly and would have an earlier onset.
- Children with mitochondrial disorders usually have a failure to thrive and can have multisystemic involvement and extrapyramidal involvement. Considering normal anthropometric parameters, absence of multisystemic involvement, and pure pyramidal tract involvement, mitochondrial disorders will be lower down in the differential.
- Canavan disease and Alexander disease usually have macrocephaly.
- This narrows down our differential diagnosis to metachromatic leukodystrophy (MLD), Krabbe disease, and mitochondrial disorder in that sequence. Absent reflexes with PNS involvement are observed in MLD. Neuroimaging revealed white matter hyperintensity involving periventricular white matter and centrum semiovale. The pattern suggested metachromatic leukodystrophy **(Fig. 7)**.

Case 3

A 9-year-old boy presented with progressively increasing difficulty in speech, difficulty in walking, and abnormal twisting movement of hands and feet for the last 6 months. There is no history of seizures. The child is almost bedridden now. He has generalized dystonia, difficult to elicit reflexes, and variable tone. Eye examination reveals normal fundus. There is evidence of extrapyramidal dysarthria. Cognition is relatively preserved. Vision and hearing are normal.

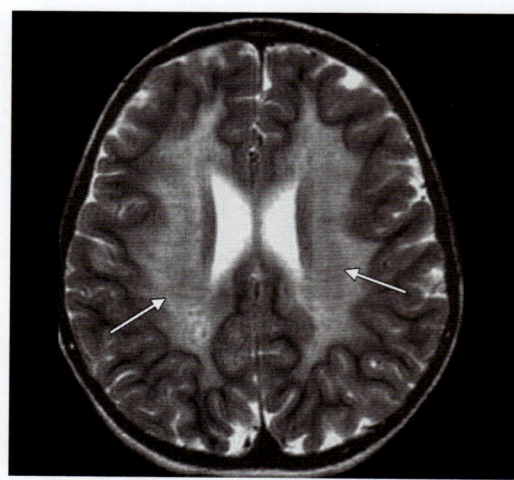

Fig. 7: Magnetic resonance imaging (MRI) brain T2 images revealed T2 hyperintense and T1 hypointense white matter signal changes showing tigroid appearance suggestive of metachromatic leukodystrophy.

Analysis

Analysis	Index case
Is it a neurodegenerative disease?	Probably yes, as things are worsening with time
What is the age at the onset?	It started at 8.5 years of age
Is it acute, intermittent, or chronic?	It has an insidious onset; slowly progressive chronic disease
What is the clinical presentation?	Generalized dystonia with preserved cognition (pure extrapyramidal syndrome)
Is it a gray matter or white matter disease?	Pure extrapyramidal syndrome points to basal ganglia involvement (gray matter DBD)
Is it CNS or PNS?	Despite difficult to elicit reflexes during dystonia, there is no clinical evidence to suggest PNS involvement
Are there any extraneural features?	There was no dysmorphism and organomegaly. Normal fundus. No extraneural markers

In this 9-year-old boy with progressive generalized dystonia with preserved vision and hearing, possible differentials would include Wilson disease, dopa-responsive dystonia, pantothenate kinase-associated neurodegeneration (PKAN), Huntington disease, and juvenile NCL **(Table 10)**.

Considering preserved cognition and absence of seizures, the possibility of juvenile Huntington, mitochondrial disorder, and juvenile NCL becomes less likely. Normal fundus with lack of pigmentary changes again points against NCL. A progressive pure extrapyramidal syndrome is thus suggestive of Wilson disease, PKAN, or dopa-responsive dystonia. These conditions are listed in **Table 11**. Investigations need to be planned accordingly. In this child, eye examination

TABLE 10: Differential diagnosis of progressive dystonia with preserved cognition, vision, and hearing.

Differential diagnosis	Classical features	Features in this case
Wilson disease	Age 7–10 years, faciolingual rigidity, generalized dystonia, behavioral problems, and Kayser–Fleischer ring on slit-lamp examination	• Extrapyramidal dysarthria • Generalized dystonia • Age onset 7.5 years • Need to look for Kayser–Fleischer ring
Dopa-responsive dystonia	Dystonia begins with one limb, gradually involves all four limbs, diurnal variation, remarkable response to levodopa	• Generalized dystonia • No diurnal variation • Insidious onset in all limbs
PKAN (Hallervorden–Spatz disease)	Age at onset 3–5 years; generalized dystonia; oromandibular dyskinesia; night blindness, preserved cognition till late stage	Generalized dystonia, oromandibular dystonia, preserved cognition; late onset
Huntington chorea	Rigidity, dysarthria, cognitive decline, seizures, ataxia, disorders of ocular movement, and chorea	Absence of seizures/cognitive decline
Juvenile neuronal ceroid lipofuscinosis (NCL)	Parkinsonian rigidity, seizures, visual failure, retinitis pigmentosa, cognitive decline	Preserved cognition, no seizures, and normal fundus

TABLE 11: Comprehensive list of conditions with predominant extrapyramidal syndrome.

Genetic conditions	Neurometabolic disorders
• Primary dystonia (*DYT* gene mutation: 1-12) • Pantothenate kinase-associated neurodegeneration (PKAN) • Spinocerebellar ataxia (SCA)-3 • Huntington disease • Neuronal ceroid lipofuscinosis • Neuroacanthocytosis • Aceruloplasminemia • Hypoprebetalipoproteinemia, acanthocytosis, retinitis pigmentosa, pallidal degeneration (HARP) syndrome	• Wilson disease • Glutaric aciduria • Tay–Sachs disease • GM1 gangliosidosis • Niemann–Pick disease type C • Metachromatic leukodystrophy • Lesch–Nyhan syndrome • Mitochondrial disorders • Methylmalonic aciduria • Homocystinuria • Tyrosinemia

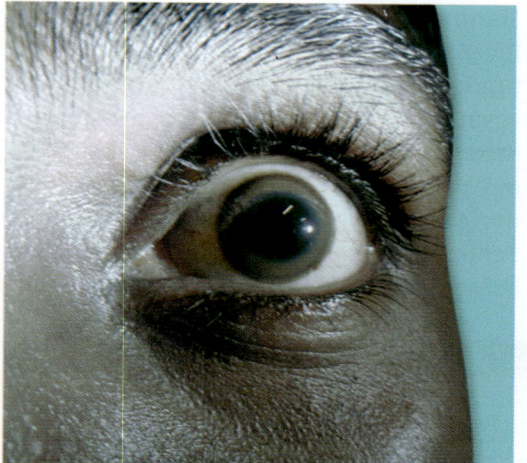

Fig. 8: Kayser–Fleischer ring in a child with Wilson disease.

revealed Kayser–Fleischer (KF) ring **(Fig. 8)**, pointing to Wilson disease.

Case 4

A 9-year-old boy presented with repeated falls and wobbly gait for the last 2–3 years. Examination revealed ataxic gait, nystagmus, slow saccades, dysarthria, areflexia, optic atrophy, and signs of cerebellar involvement. Auscultation of heart revealed a systolic murmur. His foot shows pes cavus deformity. MRI brain reveals cerebellar atrophy. There was no significant family history.

Analysis

Analysis	Index case
Is it a neurodegenerative disease?	Probably yes, as things are worsening with time
What is the age at the onset?	It started at 7 years of age
Is it acute, intermittent, or chronic?	It has an insidious onset and slowly progressive chronic disease

Contd...

Contd...

What is the clinical presentation?	Chronic progressive cerebellar ataxia
Is it gray matter or white matter disease?	Pure cerebellar involvement
Is it CNS or PNS?	There is pes cavus deformity, areflexia which often points to associated PNS involvement
Are there any extraneural features?	There was no dysmorphism or organomegaly. Normal fundus. CVS examination reveals systolic murmur

This 9-year-old boy has chronic progressive cerebellar ataxia with preserved cognition and pes cavus (evidence of peripheral neuropathy). Possible differentials are described below with their key features:

- *Friedreich ataxia (FA):* Onset before 10 years of age, autosomal recessive disorder, gait ataxia, dysarthria, absent DTR, dorsal column signs, kyphoscoliosis, pes cavus, and hypertrophic cardiomyopathy
- *Ataxia with vitamin E deficiency:* Features are same as FA except for no cardiomyopathy, no peripheral neuropathy, and slow progressive.
- *Refsum disease:* Sensorineural hearing loss, retinal degeneration, chronic sensory polyneuropathy, and ichthyosis.
- *Spinocerebellar ataxia (SCA):* Cerebellar ataxia, progressive course, variable involvement of extrapyramidal symptoms, deafness, dorsal column signs, and peripheral neuropathy depending on the type of SCA
- *Cerebrotendinous xanthomatosis*
- *Others:* Early onset ataxia including ataxia telangiectasia, ataxia with oculomotor

apraxia, and mitochondrial disorders look less likely considering the late onset of the disease

In this case, serum vitamin E levels and nerve conduction study might narrow our differentials. If the nerve conduction study reveals evidence of neuropathy and serum vitamin E level is normal, it will raise the possibility of FA. Genetic testing for FA would be useful in such a case. If, at the end of the examination, we still have wide differentials, then it would be better to go for ataxia genetic panel rather than testing for FA alone.

Case 5

A 3-day-old neonate presents with unexplained encephalopathy and refractory seizures that failed to respond to conventional antiepileptic drugs as well as pyridoxine. The baby had an uneventful antenatal period. He was born full-term by normal delivery, and birth history was unremarkable and had a birth weight of 3.2 kg. The pupils were sluggishly reacting. Investigations revealed two readings of hypoglycemia. The rest of the investigations were unremarkable, including normal ultrasonography of the brain.

Analysis

Analysis	Index case
Is it a neurodegenerative disease?	Cannot comment considering an acute presentation
What is the age at onset?	Neonatal period after 24 hours
Is it acute, intermittent, or chronic?	Acute onset
What is clinical presentation?	Unexplained encephalopathy
	Contd...

Contd...

Is it gray matter or white matter disease?	Cannot comment in such a small baby
Is it CNS or PNS?	No evidence to suggest a PNS involvement, although difficult to comment
Are there any extraneural features?	There was no dysmorphism or organomegaly

Considering acute presentation of a neonate with an uneventful neonatal period who presented with unexplained acute encephalopathy with refractory seizures and hypoglycemia strongly favors the possibility of neurometabolic disorders. Various such disorders in neonates are shown in **Figure 9**.

Neurometabolic disorders can also present in infancy and early childhood **(Figs. 10A and B)**.

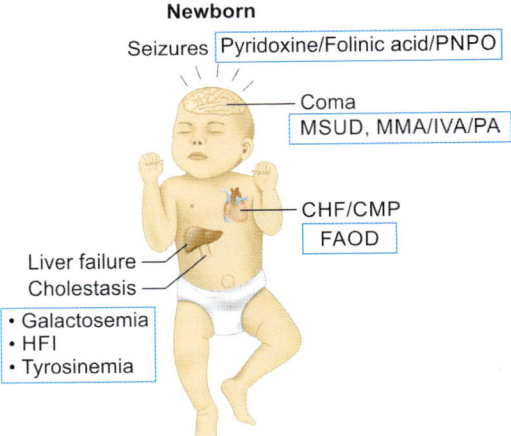

Fig. 9: Neurometabolic disorders of neonate and their clinical presentations. (FAOD: fatty acid oxidation disorder; HFI: hereditary fructose intolerance; IVA: isovaleric acidemia; MMA: methylmalonic acidemia; MSUD: maple syrup urine disease; PA: propionic acidemia; PNPO: pyridoxine 5′-phosphate oxidase deficiency)

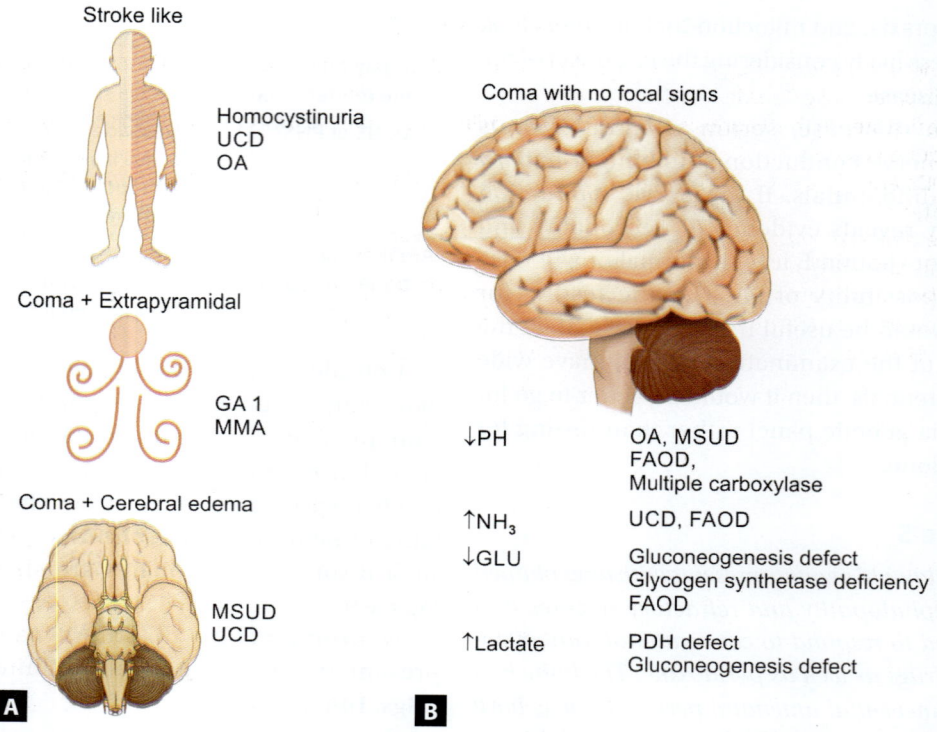

Figs. 10A and B: Neurometabolic disorders that present with acute neurological features in infancy and early childhood. (FAOD: fatty acid oxidation disorder; GA1: glutaric aciduria; MMA: methylmalonic acidemia; MSUD: maple syrup urine disease; NH_3: ammonia; OA: organic acidemia; PDH: pyruvate dehydrogenase deficiency; UCD: urea cycle disorder)

Case 6

A 10-month-old boy presented with regression of attained milestone of ability to hold the neck and social smile in the last 45 days. There was a global developmental delay from the beginning. There was a history of perinatal asphyxia requiring mechanical ventilation. He now remains irritable and cranky. On probing further, he has also developed epileptic spasms, multiple episodes that occur in a cluster, and happen on awakening from the sleep. Examination revealed microcephaly, evolving spasticity of all four limbs. His EEG revealed hypsarrhythmia.

Analysis

The regression of milestones, in this case, is attributable to the development of epileptic spasms. Once the epileptic spasms are treated effectively, the child may regain his baseline milestone. This group of conditions where cognitive decline is attributable to ongoing epileptic activity is called epileptic encephalopathy. This case provides an example of pseudoregression owing to epilepsy. Hence, the regression of milestones does *not* always mean neurodegenerative disease.

CHAPTER 14: Approach to a Child with Developmental Regression

KEY MESSAGES

- Genetic causes of progressive encephalopathy presenting with cognitive decline could result in neurometabolic disorder or NDDs.
- The first step in the diagnosis of NDDs includes ruling out pseudoregression and to look for any possible acquired cause.
- NDDs are a heterogeneous group of conditions with variable age at onset, clinical, and radiological pattern.
- The clinical pattern of NDDs would include extrapyramidal syndrome, cerebellar syndrome, pyramidal syndrome, PME, and cognitive decline.
- *Rule of three:* Neurometabolic disorders are divided into three groups—small molecule, large molecule, and organelle disorders. They can have three presentations—acute neonatal presentation or late-onset acute presentation, recurrent/intermittent, and chronic progressive clinical presentation.

CHAPTER 15

Approach to Neuromuscular Weakness

INTRODUCTION

Weakness refers to lack of muscle strength, whereas hypotonia refers to loss of muscle tone. A hypotonic baby may be weak and floppy with limited movement of the limbs or may be strong with preserved antigravity movement. The former results from a lesion in the motor unit (peripheral hypotonia) and the latter results from a lesion in the central nervous system (central hypotonia) **(Table 1)**. Neuromuscular (NM) weakness refers to weakness resulting from a lesion in the motor unit. A motor unit consists of anterior horn cell, nerve root, peripheral nerve, NM junction, and muscles. The muscle weakness can also result from upper motor neuron lesions, but these conditions are *not* considered under NM weakness. Now let us understand how to localize the site of lesion in a child with NM weakness. NM diseases can be classified depending on the site of lesion into *neuronopathies* (anterior horn cell involvement), *neuropathies* (peripheral nerve involvement), *NM transmission disorders* (myasthenic syndromes), or *myopathies* (muscle diseases).

NEUROANATOMICAL LOCALIZATION

Neuronopathy

Neuronopathy refers to anterior horn cell involvement that results in severe muscle atrophy, areflexia, and tongue fasciculation. Spinal muscular atrophy (SMA) is a classic example of neuronopathy. SMA manifests with marked weakness and hypotonia of limbs with limited antigravity movement, global areflexia [all deep tendon reflexes (DTRs) are absent], and tongue fasciculation. Other diseases that affect anterior horn cell include poliomyelitis, Pompe disease, and motor neuron disease.

Neuropathy

Clinical presentation of children with early-onset neuropathy (e.g., congenital hypomyelinating neuropathy) includes floppy infant, distal muscle weakness, sensory loss, atrophy of muscles (pes cavus deformity of foot), and hyporeflexia or areflexia. By convention, sensory

TABLE 1: Differentiating central from peripheral hypotonia.

Central hypotonia	Peripheral hypotonia
Hypotonia > weakness	Weakness > hypotonia
Preserved antigravity movement	Decreased or absent antigravity movement
DTRs are normal or brisk	DTRs are sluggish or absent
Associated cognitive delay, dysmorphism, and seizures	Cognition is preserved (floppy and alert)

(DTRs: deep tendon reflexes)

involvement with areflexia is a strong pointer toward peripheral nerve involvement. Other conditions that can present as floppy infant secondary to involvement of peripheral nerve include hereditary motor sensory neuropathy (HMSN), hereditary sensory autonomic neuropathy (HSAN), and giant axonal neuropathy.

Neuromuscular Transmission Disorder

Children with disorders of NM transmission often have extraocular muscle weakness, ptosis, hypotonia, and preserved DTRs. Common disorders that affect NM transmission include myasthenia gravis, congenital myasthenia, and botulism. Presence of diurnal variation (improvement with rest or during morning hours and worsening with time or by evening hours), fluctuating illness, and worsening with febrile illness are common in disorders of NM junction.

Myopathy

Children with myopathy often present with proximal weakness and hypotonia with or without facial weakness. Weakness is predominantly proximal with variable DTRs depending on the bulk of muscle. One of the characteristic features of myopathy is weakness out of proportion to the degree of muscle atrophy. In myopathy, muscle does not look that atrophic till terminal stages, but weakness is quite significant. This contrasts with neuropathy where atrophy is proportional to weakness.

To summarize, three clinical signs, which help in localization of the site of lesion in NM weakness, include muscle power, tone, and DTRs. The site of localization could be anterior horn cell, nerve root/fiber, NM junction, muscle, or central nervous system **(Box 1)**.

> **BOX 1:** Site of lesion in neuromuscular disorders.
> - *Central:* Hypotonia, normal strength, normal or exaggerated deep tendon reflex (DTR), extensor plantar response, seizure ±, dysmorphism ±
> - *Anterior horn cell:* Hypotonia, generalized weakness, absent DTR, fasciculation present, and mute or flexor plantar response
> - *Nerve:* Hypotonia, distal weakness, absent DTR, and sensory involvement ±
> - *Neuromuscular:* Ptosis, proximal girdle weakness, normal DTR, and flexor plantar response
> - *Muscle:* Proximal girdle weakness, normal or diminished DTR, and flexor plantar response

The following points help us to determine the site of lesion:

- Severe muscle weakness with atrophy, hypotonia, and areflexia with fasciculation points to anterior *horn cell pathology*.
- Distal muscle weakness, distal muscle atrophy, and hypotonia, with hyporeflexia or areflexia, point to *neuropathy*.
- Muscle weakness, variable tone, and preserved DTR, in the presence of extraocular muscle involvement (ptosis/extraocular weakness), point to *NM pathology*.
- Muscle weakness (proximal), hypotonia, normal or diminished DTR, and flexor plantar response point to *myopathic pathology*.

CLINICAL APPROACH TO NEUROMUSCULAR WEAKNESS

Mode of Onset

The mode of onset can be acute or insidious. We often consider the weakness to be of insidious onset when parents cannot recall the exact age at onset. Although there is no clear cutoff to define the duration of illness to be acute, subacute, or chronic, often we consider the symptoms to be acute when the duration of symptom is <14 days (2 weeks), subacute when between 2 and 4 weeks, and chronic when >4 weeks. Acute and subacute weakness of the muscle (acute flaccid paralysis) and its clinical differentials have been discussed in **Chapter 28**. This chapter primarily deals with insidious onset and chronic duration illness with NM weakness.

Age at Onset

Most of chronic NM diseases often start from the birth although the symptoms might be noticed when the child has delay in attainment of motor milestones. SMA, congenital myopathy, congenital muscular dystrophy (CMD), congenital myotonic dystrophy, and metabolic myopathy often begin in early infancy. Few disorders such as SMA type 0, congenital myotonic dystrophy, CMD, few types of congenital myopathy, metabolic myopathy (Pompe disease), and congenital myasthenic syndromes may present at birth. Few disorders can have antenatal onset in the form of decreased fetal movement, polyhydramnios, and floppiness at birth.

By convention, we consider congenital weakness to be the one where weakness starts from beginning. However, few congenital disorders such as SMA type 3, few variants of congenital myopathy, and CMD may manifest in late childhood. Similarly, children with muscular dystrophy often present late in the childhood. Conditions such as chronic inflammatory demyelinating neuropathy (CIDP), myasthenia gravis, and dermatomyositis often have a new onset of acquired weakness. Hence, age alone cannot differentiate congenital from acquired causes. Common clinical presentation of NM weakness includes floppy infant and muscular dystrophy. Floppy babies often present with motor delay and children with dystrophy present with proximal hip-girdle weakness in the form of difficulty in getting up from the floor or recurrent falls. Common presenting complaints of pediatric NM weakness are depicted in **Table 2**.

Patterns of Weakness

Ascertain the pattern of muscle weakness:
- Proximal weakness, distal weakness, and both proximal and distal weakness

TABLE 2: Presenting complaints of children with floppy infant and muscular dystrophy.

Floppy infant	Muscular dystrophy
Inability to hold the neck till now	Difficulty in getting up from floor, climbing stairs, getting downstairs, and raising from low-lying stool
Paucity of movement of all the four limbs noticed since birth	Repeated falls while walking with twisting of legs since he started walking
Looseness or flailness of limbs	Thin muscle mass over the limbs or large calves noticed since 3–4 years of age
Infant being floppy since birth	Episode of breathlessness, perspiration, or swelling over the feet (cardiac)
Repeated episodes of cough, fever, and fast breathing	Pain in muscles, exercise intolerance, and easy fatigability
Feeding difficulty or choking while feeding	Muscle cramps and passage of dark-colored urine following strenuous exercise

CHAPTER 15: Approach to Neuromuscular Weakness

TABLE 3: Pattern of weakness among various neuromuscular conditions in children.

Pattern of weakness	Differential diagnosis
Progressive proximal limb-girdle weakness	• Muscular dystrophy (Bethlem myopathy, dystrophinopathies, and FSHD) • Inflammatory myopathy (dermatomyositis and polymyositis) • Juvenile spinal muscular atrophy • Metabolic myopathy (acid maltase deficiency, carnitine deficiency, debrancher enzyme deficiency, and mitochondrial myopathy) • Endocrine myopathy
Progressive distal limb weakness	• *Congenital myopathy:* Nemaline rod, central core, and centronuclear myopathy • Muscular dystrophy (EDMD and FSHD) • Neuropathy (CMT, giant axonal neuropathy, drug induced, and systemic vasculitis) • Distal myopathy (myotonic dystrophy)
Scapuloperoneal weakness	• Scapuloperoneal dystrophy • Emery–Dreifuss muscular dystrophy • LGMD 1B (laminopathy) • LGMD 2A (calpainopathy) • LGMD 2C-F (sarcoglycanopathy) • LGMD 2I (FKRP)
Ptosis	Myasthenia gravis, centronuclear and nemaline rod myopathy, and myotonic dystrophy
Ptosis and ophthalmoplegia	Progressive external ophthalmoplegia, oculopharyngeal muscular dystrophy, myasthenia gravis, and Lambert–Eaton syndrome
Prominent neck extensor weakness	• Dermatomyositis • Polymyositis • FSHD • Myotonic dystrophy types 1 and 2

(CMT: Charcot–Marie–Tooth disease; EDMD: Emery–Dreifuss muscular dystrophy; FSHD: facioscapulohumeral dystrophy)

- Upper limb, lower limb, trunk, and neck flexor/extensor weakness
- Facial involvement
- Bulbar involvement
- Extraocular muscle involvement

Pattern of muscle weakness will give clue regarding the possible underlying cause **(Table 3)**.

Lower Limb Weakness

Presenting complaints of frequent falls, tripping over floor, stamping or high steppage gait, and difficulty in walking are suggestive of *distal lower limb weakness*. Difficulty in getting up from floor, walking up and down stairs, rising from low-lying chair, and waddling gait are suggestive of *proximal lower limb weakness*. This is often elicited clinically when the child is asked to get up from sitting position on floor. A child with proximal hip-girdle weakness will adopt the following sequence to rise to standing position (Gower sign). It is described below.

Gower sign:
- He puts hand on floor and stretches his leg behind and wide apart.
- He keeps the toe on the ground and pushing backward, gets knee straight so

that weight of trunk is born by hands and feet.
- He places one hand on the knee and pushes down to support hip extension, so that he can raise to upright position.

Gower sign is an indicator of hip-girdle weakness and can be seen in Duchenne muscular dystrophy (DMD), limb-girdle muscular dystrophy (LGMD), and juvenile SMA.

Upper Limb Weakness

The proximal upper limb weakness could present with inability to lift the arm to pick up object from shelf, inability to lift arm to comb his/her hair, and inability to lift heavy objects. *Distal upper limb weakness* manifests with inability to hold the objects, clumsiness in holding the objects, difficulty in buttoning and unbuttoning his/her shirt, and poor handwriting.

Other Muscle Weakness

Weakness could also manifest with inability to lift head off the bed (*neck flexor weakness*), inability to sit up from lying-down position or inability to turn prone to supine and back (*truncal weakness*), drooping of eyelids (*ptosis*), diplopia (*extraocular muscle weakness*), and difficulty in deglutition or nasal regurgitation of feeds (*bulbar weakness*). Dull facial expression, wasting of temporalis muscle, failure to close the eyes completely, inability to purse the lips, and inability to suck from a straw or blow balloons are markers toward *facial weakness*. Presence of slurred speech with difficulty in pronouncing words d, n, l, and t points to *tongue muscle weakness*.

It is important to differentiate NM weakness from gait alteration resulting from ataxia, spasticity, dystonia, choreoathetosis, or other movement disorder. Presence of swaying while standing (truncal ataxia) along with other cerebellar symptoms such as past pointing and jerky eye movements often points to cerebellar ataxia. Presence of abnormal twisting postures of upper and lower limbs (dystonia) and presence of dance-like choreiform flowing movement or distal writhing movement of hands (athetoid movement) often point to an underlying movement disorder rather than NM weakness.

Static versus Progressive Weakness

It is crucial to differentiate a static weakness from progressive weakness. By convention, dystrophic pathology has progressive worsening of weakness. Majority of children with muscular dystrophy such as DMD have progressive worsening of weakness, as the time progresses. In contrast, children with other NM conditions such as congenital myopathy and congenital myotonic dystrophy usually improve with time except when they develop new contractures or develop recurrent respiratory tract infections. It is imperative to understand that normal childhood motor development often masks the progressive nature of weakness. This is often perceived by parents as subjective improvement or stabilization despite a dystrophic pathology. Similarly, outdoor play activities often result in marginal improvement in weakness. This can again be perceived as gain in NM power to perform better.

Intermittent or Episodic Weakness

Children with NM disorders such as mitochondrial myopathy and myasthenia often have waxing and waning nature of weakness. The weakness may worsen with febrile illness. There will be bad days where a child is completely bedridden when he/she has fever and then recovers to a premorbid functional state a few days after the febrile illness subsides. Inflammatory myopathy such as dermatomyositis may also have waxing and waning characteristic of weakness. History of diurnal variation with weakness worsening by evening hours but improves after taking rest or better in the early morning hours points toward myasthenia and other NM junction abnormalities.

Episodic weakness manifests with recurrent episodes of sudden onset of NM weakness that resolves within few days. Episodic weakness or periodic paralysis and myotonia are considered channelopathies.

- *Sodium channelopathy* (hyperkalemic periodic paralysis and paramyotonia congenita)
- *Chloride channelopathy:* Myotonia congenita (Thomsen and Becker disease)
- *Calcium channelopathy:* Hypokalemic periodic paralysis
- *Others:* Schwartz–Jampel syndrome, Anderson syndrome, and Brody disease.

Presence of Precipitating Cause

Muscle pain is often a nonspecific complaint in typically developing children. If the muscle pain is associated with a new onset of NM weakness, it often points to inflammatory pathology. This includes Guillain–Barré syndrome, infective or tropical pyomyositis, or dermatomyositis. Presence of severe muscle cramps, weakness, or myoglobinuria following exercise is a complaint specific to metabolic myopathy (fatty acid oxidation defect, lipid storage defect, and mitochondrial disorder). Weakness that develops following heavy carbohydrate meal is observed in adolescents with hypokalemic periodic paralysis. Weakness that worsens with fasting often points to fatty acid oxidation defects. Worsening of muscle stiffness with cold is seen in paramyotonia congenita.

Other Organ System Involvement

Ocular involvement in the form of ptosis and extraocular muscle weakness is observed in disorders of NM transmission such as myasthenia gravis. Ocular involvement is also seen in congenital myasthenic syndrome, CMD, and certain subtypes of congenital myopathy. Cardiac involvement occurs in children with DMD, Becker muscular dystrophy (BMD), myotonic dystrophy, Pompe disease, LGMD type 1B, and carnitine deficiency. Early respiratory compromise may occur in SMA, congenital myopathy, DMD, Pompe disease, and carnitine deficiency. Hepatic involvement may occur in Pompe disease, mitochondrial disorder, and carnitine deficiency. Multisystemic involvement with failure to thrive, short stature, sensorineural hearing loss, cardiac conduction defects, and hepatic involvement often points to mitochondrial cytopathy.

Look for Complications

Contractures, deformities, gastroesophageal reflux disease, recurrent chest infection, failure to thrive, and obesity (nonambulatory patients) are some of common complications observed in children with NM disorder. Comorbid cognitive deficits are seen in children with DMD and certain forms of syndromic CMD.

Family History

A three-generation pedigree is essential to look for the inheritance pattern. History of any affected family member who uses wheelchair, has skeletal deformity, or has any functional limitations must be elicited. NM disorders can have autosomal dominant, autosomal recessive, or X-linked inheritance **(Table 4)**.

TABLE 4: Inheritance pattern in neuromuscular disorders.	
Autosomal dominant	FSHD, LGMD, and myotonic dystrophy
Autosomal recessive	LGMD and metabolic myopathy
Maternal transmission	Mitochondrial myopathy
X-linked recessive	Duchenne, Becker, and EDMD

(EDMD: Emery–Dreifuss muscular dystrophy; FSHD: facioscapulohumeral dystrophy; LGMD: limb-girdle muscular dystrophy)

Broad Category of Disease Phenotype

Once the mode of onset, age at onset, and pattern of weakness are determined, the next step is to categorize into a broad group of NM disorder.
- *Differential diagnosis of a floppy infant with peripheral hypotonia:*
  - SMA (anterior horn cell)
  - Congenital myopathy (muscle)
  - CMD (muscle)
  - Congenital myotonic dystrophy (muscle)
  - Congenital myasthenic syndrome (NM transmission junction)
  - Metabolic myopathy (glycogen, lipid, and storage) (muscle)
  - Mitochondrial myopathy (muscle)
  - Hereditary motor sensory polyneuropathy (peripheral nerve)
- *Differential diagnosis of a child with proximal hip-girdle weakness and Gower sign:*
  - DMD/BMD
  - LGMD
  - Juvenile SMA (type 3)
  - Inflammatory myopathy dermatomyositis and polymyositis
  - Metabolic myopathy (Pompe disease and carnitine deficiency)
  - Endocrinal myopathy (hypothyroid)

FOCUSED EXAMINATION

Anthropometry
- Overweight/obesity can be seen once children with DMD reach a nonambulatory stage.
- Failure to thrive can be seen in children with NM weakness. They have recurrent chest infection and feeding difficulties.

General Physical Examination
- Presence of facial dysmorphism is a pointer to syndromic CMD.
- Tented upper lip with wide open mouth is suggestive of congenital myotonic dystrophy.
- Presence of flat facial expression, high-arched palate, and bitemporal hallowing is suggestive of myopathic facies (congenital myopathy and congenital myasthenia).
- Presence of hyperlaxity of joints, velvety feel of skin, and hypertrophic scar points to Ullrich CMD.
- Look for fixed contractures, deformities, hip dislocation, scoliosis, and lordosis.
- Look for pectus excavatum and other chest deformities.
- Joint contractures as a feature of arthrogryposis need to be documented, if present.
- Do not miss signs of vitamin D deficiency (rickets) in a hypotonic baby—frontal bossing, rachitic rosary, Harrison sulcus, and wrist widening.
- *Eyes:* Cataract (myotonic dystrophy) and ptosis/ophthalmoplegia (myasthenia gravis, congenital myasthenic syndrome).

Systemic Examination
- *Hepatomegaly:* Presence of hepatomegaly in a floppy baby often raises the possibility of Pompe disease, mitochondrial myopathy, and glycogen storage disorders.

- *Cardiac involvement:* Presence of signs of congestive heart failure (tachycardia, tachypnea, and hepatomegaly) in a floppy baby points to metabolic etiology (Pompe disease, fatty acid oxidation defect, and glycogen storage defects).
- *Respiratory failure* is a presenting complaint of many NM disorders including SMA (type 1), congenital myopathy, and CMD.

Neurological Evaluation

- *Functional assessment of muscle weakness* can be done by assessment of gait and posture. Formal muscle power testing of individual muscles is often difficult among children. It is suggested to perform an overall functional assessment by asking the patient to stand with feet closed, standing and walking on heels and toes, run, jump, rising from low chair or squatting posture without using arms, and rising from supine to sitting without arm. These maneuvers will give an overall pattern of muscle weakness. It will also elicit subtle neurological weakness, which otherwise might be missed with routine neurological examination. Look for gait (ambulatory) and posture (nonambulatory):
  - Waddling gait and lordotic posture are suggestive of proximal hip-girdle weakness observed among children with muscular dystrophy.
  - Stamping gait (or weakness of foot dorsiflexor) is common in peripheral neuropathy.
  - Toe walking is an indicator of muscular dystrophy, spinal dysraphism, spastic diplegia, or a normal variant.
- *Look for DTR:* Hypotonia with areflexia is a pointer toward involvement of motor unit (neuronopathy, myopathy, neuropathy, and NM disorders), whereas hypotonia with brisk reflexes is a pointer toward CNS etiology. Preserved ankle DTR in a hypotonic baby often points to a central cause.

Other Features

- *Look for clinical features in face:* Lack of facial expression (FSHD), ptosis (myasthenia gravis), ophthalmoplegia (Kearns–Sayre syndrome), myotonia of eyelid (myotonia congenita), and protuberant auricles (DMD)
- *Presence of tongue fasciculation* and fine tremulous movement of outstretched hand (polyminimyoclonus) is suggestive of neuronopathy such as SMA.
- *Clinical features in upper limb and trunk:* Neck flexor weakness (DMD), paraspinal contractures (rigid spine syndrome), winged scapula (FSHD), and contractures of elbow (Emery–Dreifuss muscular dystrophy)
- *Clinical features in lower limb:* Inverted champagne bottle (peroneal muscular atrophy), hypertrophy of calf (DMD), and pes cavus (Friedreich ataxia)
- *Examine the mother for evidence of myotonia:* Ask the mother to close the fist and then open it suddenly. A myotonic patient will have delayed time to open the fist.
- *Look for wasting of muscles* including sternocleidomastoid muscle, trapezius muscle, winging of scapula, and atrophy of intrinsic muscles of hands. Wasting of quadriceps muscle, anterior compartment of legs, tapering of legs distally, tightness of heel cords, pes cavus, pes planus, and presence of foot drop point to peripheral nerve involvement.
- *Look for exaggerated lumbar lordosis* is indicative of hip-girdle weakness observed in patients with DMD, LGMD, and juvenile SMA.

BOX 2: Steps in clinical evaluation of neuromuscular care.

- Age of child and gender of child
- Mode of onset
- Age at onset
- Static versus progressive
- Pattern of weakness
- Functional status and complications
- Family history
- Any known precipitating cause
- Any signs of multiorgan dysfunction
- Key findings in neurological examination
- Neuroanatomical site of localization
- Possible differentials with points in favor and against

■ MAKING THE DIAGNOSIS

In order to summarize the clinical evaluation of NM case, use the scheme given in **Box 2**.

When to think of congenital myopathy?
- Onset in infancy or childhood with variable clinical presentation ranging from severe manifestations at birth to mild limb-girdle pattern of weakness manifesting in late childhood
- Nonprogressive muscle weakness with hypotonia with hyporeflexia
- Poor muscle bulk is often a feature of congenital myopathy
- Facial involvement (high-arched palate, elongated facies, and dolichocephalic head) is common [nemaline rod myopathy (NM), centronuclear myopathy (CNM), MTM1 (myotubularin), RYR1 (ryanodine receptor), and DNM2 (dynamin)].
- Extraocular involvement (ophthalmoplegia and ptosis) is uncommon [CNM (MTM1, RYR1, and DNM2)].
- Bulbar weakness and severe respiratory weakness at birth are uncommon [NM, CNM (MTM1), severe RYR1].
- Rarely hip dislocation or other orthopedic deformity (RYR1)
- Rare presentation also includes marked axial involvement, early-onset scoliosis, and rigid spine [SEPN1 (selenoprotein) and RYR1].
- Clinical features have marked overlap with congenital myotonic dystrophy, congenital myasthenic syndrome, and CMD.

When to think of congenital muscular dystrophy?
- It can present at birth or early infancy with hypotonia and weakness. Few children present later in childhood with motor delay or contractures.
- Weakness is relatively static or slowly progressive (in contrast to another dystrophy such as DMD, which is rapidly progressive).
- Involvement of upper limb is more as compared to lower limb weakness (merosin-negative CMD and dystroglycanopathy).
- Most of these children achieve sitting, but independent ambulation is unlikely except patients with partial merosin deficiency.
- Cognition is relatively preserved except for syndromic CMD such as POMT1-related CMD.
- Ocular abnormalities such as persistent primary vitreous, microphthalmia, and myopia may be seen in few patients (dystroglycanopathy).
- Distal joint laxity, early contractures of proximal joints, velvety skin, protrusion of calcaneum, and hypertrophic scars can be seen among Ullrich CMD.
- Rare presentations include rigid spine and early respiratory involvement (SEPN1-related CMD).

When to think of congenital myasthenic syndrome?
- Early onset of weakness and hypotonia (onset <2 years) with few presenting in

neonatal period with early respiratory involvement [choline acetyltransferase (CHAT) deficiency and acetylcholinesterase deficiency]
- Weakness predominantly involving facial muscles, extraocular muscles (ophthalmoplegia and ptosis), and/or bulbar and respiratory muscle
- Episodic worsening with intercurrent illness (fever and exertion)
- Skeletal deformities are uncommon (acetylcholine receptor resistance and fast channel CMS)

When to think of congenital myotonic dystrophy?
- Neonatal-onset generalized weakness and hypotonia
- Respiratory failure, feeding difficulties, and clubfoot deformities are common clinical features.
- History of polyhydramnios and decreased fetal movement may be elicited.
- Facial involvement is classical with open mouth and tented upper lip.
- Intellectual disability, autism spectrum disorder, and learning difficulties are not uncommon among children with congenital myotonic dystrophy.
- Mothers of these children might have clinical evidence of myotonia (grip myotonia and percussion myotonia), cataract, ptosis, and slender stature/wasting (clinical myotonia is *not* evident in a neonate with congenital myotonic dystrophy)

■ CASE VIGNETTES

Case 1

A 3.5-year-old girl presented with delay in attainment of motor milestones.

History

She has difficulty in getting up from the bed (neck flexor weakness), standing up from sitting position (proximal hip-girdle weakness), and difficulty in lifting arms (proximal shoulder-girdle weakness) with poor grip (distal hand weakness). She can walk few steps independently (functional status). There is no diurnal variation in weakness (*observed in myasthenia*) and no worsening with trivial febrile illness (*seen in myasthenia and mitochondrial myopathy*).

There is no history of muscle pain (*seen in inflammatory myopathy*). There is no history of breathing difficulty, excessive perspiration, and swelling over feet (*to look for cardiac involvement*). There is no history of passage of red-colored urine after prolonged play activity (*seen in McArdle disease and other metabolic myopathy*). She is intelligent, studying in preschool, and doing well in studies (*preserved cognition*). There is no family member affected with history of weakness, thinning of muscles, or prolonged time in relaxing when making a fist (*ruling out myotonic dystrophy*). The antenatal period of the mother did not reveal any history of polyhydramnios or decreased fetal movement. She was born by normal delivery and had an uneventful neonatal period with no history of prolonged labor. Her early neonatal and infantile period did not witness adverse feeding problems or recurrent respiratory illness. Her hearing and vision are normal.

Examination

Physical examination revealed normal anthropometric variables (*failure to thrive is seen in mitochondrial myopathy*). Facial weakness was present (*favors congenital myopathy, congenital myasthenia, and congenital myotonic dystrophy*). There was marked generalized hypotonia. There is marked thinning of muscles with no focal atrophy or hypertrophy (*ruling out dystrophinopathies*). There were no fasciculations in tongue (*rules out anterior horn cell involvement*). All DTRs were sluggish. There was sparing of extraocular muscles with no evidence of ptosis (*rules out myasthenia and certain variants of congenital myopathy*). There was no respiratory involvement or any obvious chest deformity. There was no hepatomegaly (*for Pompe disease*). There was no distal laxity or evidence of hypertrophic scars/keloids/prominent calcaneum (*for Ullrich CMD*). There was dynamic contracture of both Achilles tendon.

Step 1: Determining neuroanatomical site. Considering proximal and distal weakness, hyporeflexia, hypotonia, facial weakness, contractures, absence of tongue fasciculations with absence of diurnal variation, and sparing of extraocular muscles, the *possible neuroanatomical site of lesion is muscle.*

Step 2: Points in favor and against the possible differential diagnoses **(Table 5)**

Step 3: Rearrange the clinical differentials based on points in favor. I would keep following differentials (in the order of priority) based on clinical evaluation:
- Congenital myopathy (nemaline rod or centronuclear myopathy)
- CMD (merosin negative)
- Congenital myasthenic syndrome
- *Others:* Congenital myotonic dystrophy, SMA, mitochondrial myopathy, and Pompe disease.

Step 4: Plan investigations according to clinical differential diagnoses:
- *Total creatine phosphokinase (CPK) level:* If CPK levels are elevated, it indicates dystrophic muscle pathology, then obviously CMD will be a strong possibility.
- *Electromyography (EMG):* One may decide to omit this step, as it is obvious that we are dealing with myopathic pathology. But, however, if tongue fasciculation

TABLE 5: Points in favor and against the possible differential diagnoses.

Disease entity	Points in favor	Points against
Congenital myopathy	Weakness and hypotonia; facial involvement; loss of muscle bulk; presence of contracture	
Congenital myotonic dystrophy	Weakness and hypotonia	Facies not typical of congenital myotonic dystrophy; late age at onset; achieved ambulation; mother healthy with no evidence of myotonia; early muscle atrophy
Congenital myasthenic syndrome	Weakness and hypotonia; facial weakness	No ptosis, no ophthalmoplegia; no diurnal variations; late age at onset
Congenital muscular dystrophy	Weakness and hypotonia	No skin changes: no ocular involvement, cognition being preserved (for syndromic CMD)
Spinal muscular atrophy type 2	Weakness and hypotonia; muscle wasting	No tongue fasciculations
Mitochondrial myopathy	Weakness and hypotonia	No worsening with febrile illness, normal anthropometry; no systemic involvement
Metabolic myopathy (Pompe disease)	Weakness and hypotonia	Late age at onset, no hepatomegaly, no cardiac symptoms

was not very convincing and one is not sure whether the neuronopathic process could be a differential, we can go ahead with EMG to differentiate myopathic versus neuropathic EMG pattern. EMG of mother will be useful to rule out myotonia as congenital myotonic dystrophy is a differential.

- Genetic testing: Most of genetic testing is phenotype driven. For example, if there is weakness, hypotonia in setting of joint laxity, proximal contractures, and skin changes, we are dealing with Ullrich CMD; hence, the genetic testing can be driven toward the same. However, in the case discussed above, the clinical features/phenotype is inconclusive and broad, and it would be advisable to look for clinical exome sequencing for congenital myopathy and CMD. Gene panels are available commercially, but cost is prohibitive. Phenotype-driven genetic testing for single-gene disorders is always better and cost-effective approach.
- Role of muscle biopsy: In this era of genetic testing, the role of muscle biopsy is limited. Biopsy can serve as a guide for targeted genetic testing rather than looking for the spectrum of muscular disorders. In this case, if the muscle biopsy is suggestive of nemaline rod myopathy (congenital myopathy), genetic analysis for targeted genes such as *TPM3, ACTA1, NEB, KBTBD,* and *KLHL40* could be performed.

Case 2

A 10-year-old boy presents with difficulty in getting up from floor, difficulty in using Indian style of toilet, and repeated falls while walking which have been noticed for the last 3 years. Weakness has been slowly increasing over the last 3 years. He has developed fixed contractures in both feet with thinning of muscles of legs.

There is no history of muscle cramps or stiffness or red-colored urine following exercise (*metabolic myopathy*). There is no history of pain in muscles or skin rash (*to rule out dermatomyositis*). There is no episodic fluctuation with fever or stress (*mitochondrial myopathy*). There is no specific relation with fasting (*glycogen storage disorder*). There is no history suggestive of dizziness, difficulty in breathing on lying down, syncope, or chest pain (*to rule out cardiac involvement*). There is no history of breathing difficulty or sleep disturbances (*to rule out respiratory involvement*).

He is in 5th class, average in studies, and no evident behavioral disturbances. Antenatal and neonatal periods were uneventful. He had attained age-appropriate motor milestones although parents cannot really recollect the exact age. There are two siblings with one elder sister who is doing fine. There are no affected family members on three-generation pedigree charting.

Examination findings suggest proximal limb weakness involving lower limb > upper limb with sparing of facial, bulbar, and respiratory muscles. DTRs are sluggish but preserved. There is no clinical evidence of cardiac or respiratory involvement. Cognition is intact. The current functional ability of independent ambulation is up to 10 meters. There is selective atrophy of distal muscles of leg with bilateral Achilles tendon contracture. There is scapular winging.

Step 1: Determine Neuroanatomical Site of Lesion

Considering proximal hip and shoulder-girdle weakness with preserved ankle DTR with no fixed diurnal variation, the most likely site of lesion is muscle. But distal atrophy and sluggish DTR also make us think of peripheral nerve as a possible site of lesion (but neuropathies by convention have distal weakness rather than proximal weakness).

It is not a bad idea to think broad and entertain neuropathic causes as well in this child.

Step 2: Points that Favor and Against Following Clinical Differentials

Step 2 is given in **Table 6**.

Step 3: Rearrange Clinical Differentials Based on Strength of Points in Favor

I would keep the following differentials in this child:
- Calpainopathy (LGMD)
- Becker muscular dystrophy
- SMA type III

- *Others:* Limb-girdle myasthenia, late-onset Pompe disease, Charcot–Marie–Tooth disease, and DMD (outlier)

Step 4: Plan Investigations Accordingly

- *Total CPK level:* If CPK level in this index case was 8,000 IU/L, which is raised, my clinical differentials of calpainopathy and BMD are retained. Late-onset Pompe disease can also have elevated CPK but not to the tune of 8,000 IU/L. SMA is probably out.
- *Muscle biopsy versus genetic testing:* Muscle biopsy is an option where the facility for immunoblot is available. In the absence of availability of immunoblot, histopathology alone describing dystrophic changes might

TABLE 6: Points that favor and against following clinical differentials.

Disease entity	Points in favor	Points against
Duchenne muscular dystrophy	Proximal hip-girdle weakness	Age at onset late; no focal atrophy/hypertrophy, no family history, and foot muscle atrophy
Becker muscular dystrophy	Proximal hip-girdle weakness; age at onset	No focal atrophy/hypertrophy, no family history, foot muscle atrophy
Limb-girdle muscular dystrophy (calpainopathy)	Proximal hip-girdle weakness, foot atrophy, tendoachilles contractures, age at onset, ambulatory till now (slowly progressive)	None
Limb-girdle myasthenia	Proximal hip-girdle weakness	No diurnal variation, atrophy, and tendoachilles (TA) contractures
Spinal muscular atrophy type 3	Proximal hip-girdle weakness, distal atrophy, and contracture	No tongue fasciculations, deep tendon reflex (DTR) elicitable, and normal motor milestones
Pompe disease (late onset)	Proximal hip-girdle weakness	Atrophy, contracture, no hepatomegaly, and no cardiac involvement
Charcot–Marie–tooth disease	Atrophy of leg muscles	DTR elicitable and proximal hip-girdle weakness

not be very useful. Considering biopsy as invasive investigation, one may prefer genetic analysis. Since clinical and laboratory phenotypes strongly suggest calpainopathy, one can prefer targeted *CAPN3* gene mutation study. If negative, we have two options—plan genetic panel for muscular dystrophy or else biopsy-driven genetic analysis. Genetic analysis of suspected DMD/BMD will include testing for deletion or duplication by multiplex ligation-dependent probe amplification (MLPA) and if negative, sequencing of the entire *DMD* gene can be performed.

■ SPECIFIC CONDITIONS

When to think of limb-girdle muscular dystrophy?

- Proximal hip-girdle weakness more involved as compared to shoulder-girdle weakness
- Hip extensor, knee flexor, and hip adductors are severely involved in calpainopathy and sarcoglycanopathy as compared to hip abductor and quadriceps group involvement in DMD. Since hip abductors are spared in sarcoglycanopathy, children while getting up from floor splay their thigh abducted (hip abduction sign).
- Calf hypertrophy [sarcoglycanopathy and LGMD type 1 (Fukutin)] or calf atrophy (calpainopathy) can be seen in LGMD.
- Early Achilles tendon contractures (calpainopathy)
- Prominent scapular winging (calpainopathy and sarcoglycanopathy)
- Rarely sudden onset of muscle pain and weakness with hyperCKemia can be seen (dysferlinopathy).
- Selective atrophy with biceps atrophy and deltoid hypertrophy (dysferlinopathy) can be seen.
- Elbow contractures and neck flexor weakness are prominent in LGMD type 1B.
- Onset usually childhood or adolescence but less than 20 years
- Sparing of facial, ocular, respiration, and bulbar muscles is common
- Cardiac involvement (dilated cardiomyopathy) and respiratory involvement are uncommon (sarcoglycanopathy, lamin A/C, and LGMD type 1). Cardiac conduction defects can be seen in LGMD type 1B (laminopathy).

When to think of Becker muscular dystrophy?

- Age at onset being 10–20 years (50% by 10 years and 90% by 20 years)
- Pelvic-girdle weakness and thigh muscle weakness with presence of calf hypertrophy
- Relative sparing of tibialis anterior, peroneal group of muscles, neck flexor, and intrinsic muscles of hand
- Contractures and scoliosis are less common when compared to children with DMD.
- Cognition is relatively preserved with cardiac involvement being uncommon when compared to DMD.
- Most of them remain ambulatory beyond 16 years of age.

When to think of Charcot–Marie–Tooth (CMT) disease?

- Presence of foot deformities (pes cavus and hammer toe) with distal weakness, atrophy, and areflexia with sensory loss (CMT1A)
- Nerve hypertrophy, ataxia, and upper limb tremor can be seen in CMT1A.
- *Age at onset:* Late childhood or early adolescent period (onset in second decade in CMT type 2A; early onset and severe manifestations in CMT3 and CMT4)
- Rarely sensory predominant forms can present with self-mutilation ulcers (CMT2B).

ROLE OF INVESTIGATION IN NEUROMUSCULAR DISEASE

Serum Creatine Phosphokinase Level

Serum CPK levels are a sensitive marker for NM disorders in children. The serum CPK level must be interpreted in clinical context and not in isolation. Markedly elevated CPK levels >10,000 IU/L are seen in inflammatory myopathy, dermatomyositis, and dysferlinopathy (LGMD). CPK levels are elevated 5,000–10,000 IU/L in DMD and sarcoglycanopathy. CPK levels in range of 2,500–5,000 IU/L are seen in calpainopathy (LGMD2A), caveolinopathy (LGMD1C), and Fukutin-related LGMD (LGMD2I). CPK levels are marginally elevated in CMD and Pompe disease. However, CPK levels are often normal in SMA, congenital myopathy, congenital myotonic dystrophy, and congenital myasthenia syndrome. Often, CPK levels are nearly normal in majority of causes of floppy baby. One should be careful that CPK levels can be elevated following EMG; hence, CPK levels must be done prior to EMG.

Nerve Conduction Study

Investigations must be planned only after clinical differentials have been analyzed. Nerve conduction study will be useful for evaluation of neuropathies, especially CMT disease. It can broadly categorize the type of CMT into axonal (CMT2) or demyelinating (CMT1, CMT3, CMT4). Nerve conduction study will have limited role in evaluation of floppy infant, unless congenital hypomyelinating neuropathy or early-onset CMT (CMT4) is kept in clinical differentials, and more common causes have been ruled out by conventional genetic analysis. Compound muscle action potential (CMAP) may be decreased in muscle atrophy. It is also useful in characterizing HSAN that presents with self-mutilating ulcers and sensory loss over the distal extremities. Readers are suggested to go through **Chapter 6** on basics of neurophysiology.

Electromyography

Electromyography (spontaneous activity) reveals evidence of fibrillations/positive sharp waves in a myopathic process. In a neuropathic process, spontaneous activity reveals fasciculations or myokymia. Myotonic EMG discharges may be seen in myotonic dystrophy and congenital myotonia. EMG findings in myopathic pathology include short duration, low amplitude, and polyphasic motor unit action potential (MUAP) with early recruitment. In contrast, high-amplitude, long-duration MUAPs with poor recruitment could indicate neuropathy or neuronopathy.

Muscle Biopsy Findings

Muscle biopsy in children is performed under local anesthesia and sedation. Open biopsy from vastus lateralis is preferred. One must avoid muscles where EMG has been performed for biopsy. Muscle biopsy examination includes histological examination (to detect inflammation, myofiber necrosis, perimysium, and endothelial connective tissue proliferation), histochemical staining (modified Gomori trichrome stain for collagen and mitochondria, ATPase stain to differentiate type I from type II fibers, NADH-TR oxidative enzyme stain, succinate dehydrogenase stain for mitochondria, and periodic acid–Schiff reaction), and immunocytochemical staining (for dystrophinopathies, dystroglycanopathy, and merosin staining). Electron microscopy is useful in mitochondrial myopathy (paracrystalline inclusion, stacked, and whorled cristae). Few molecular genetic analyses are performed on muscle biopsy tissue, especially mitochondrial genetic analysis.

Dystrophic change in muscle biopsy includes necrotic myofibers, regenerating myofibers, increased endomysial connective tissue, variation in fiber size, fiber splitting, and increased internal nucleation. Denervation atrophy, fiber-type grouping, group atrophy, and reinnervation atrophy with angulated fibers are evident in SMA. Children with dermatomyositis will demonstrate perivascular inflammation. Mitochondrial myopathy may demonstrate ragged red fiber on Gomori trichrome stain. PAS-positive subsarcolemmal granules are classical of McArdle disease.

Genetic Analysis

Indications for genetic analysis are to establish the diagnosis, predict the prognosis, and predict the risk of recurrence in next pregnancy and risk of asymptomatic disease in family members. Providing genetic diagnosis for a child is crucial to end the ordeal of parents seeking final diagnosis for their child. Molecular genetic testing plays a vital role in diagnosis of NM disorders. Targeted gene analysis by MLPA or polymerase chain reaction (PCR) is preferred for phenotype-driven analysis (*DMD* gene testing for DMD; *SMN* gene testing for SMA; CTG triplet analysis for congenital myotonic dystrophy). In clinical conditions where the phenotype of the patient does not fit clearly into any known NM disorder, there are two options for further genetic testing: Gene panel or clinical exome analysis. Gene panel testing for congenital myopathy and muscular dystrophy is available commercially. Clinical exome sequencing will sequence known disease genes and would analyze further if a mutation is not identified. Recurrence risk for future pregnancy will depend on mutation in index case. If mutation is de novo or spontaneous, then parents are unlikely to harbor the mutation; hence, the chances of recurrence are <1%. Prenatal testing for targeted gene using chorionic villus sampling at 10–12 weeks or amniocentesis beyond 16 weeks is useful to guide parents for continuation of pregnancy. Other viable options for parents desiring a healthy baby include donor sperm, donor egg, adoption, or preimplantation genetic diagnosis (PGD). PGD is a method by which only embryos without the familial mutation are transferred into uterus.

Neuromuscular Imaging

Ultrasonography of superficial skeletal muscle is easy and noninvasive imaging with no radiation risk. Information that be conveyed by a trained sonographer will include atrophy, hypertrophy, and changes in muscle architecture (dystrophic changes). Sensitivity of detecting dystrophic changes in muscle ranges from 25 to 60% among patients with muscular dystrophy. MRI muscle is increasingly used among children with a suspected inherited NM disorder. Dystrophic changes with fatty degeneration can be detected in short tau inversion recovery (STIR) sequences. Depending on the group of muscles affected on MRI, clinical differentials can be narrowed **(Table 7)**. Similarly, inflammatory changes such as muscle edema in patients with suspected dermatomyositis or inflammatory myopathy can be detected in T2-imaging sequences.

TABLE 7: Muscle involvement in MRI muscle.

Disease	Group of muscle involvement
Calpainopathy	Gluteus posterior compartment, leg posterior compartment
Dysferlinopathy	Adductor magnus and posterior compartment of leg
Sarcoglycanopathy	Anterior compartment of thigh
FKRP (LGMD2I)	Biceps femoris, gastrocnemius, and soleus
LGMD2J	Tibialis anterior

KEY MESSAGES

- Hypotonia with preserved reflexes and preserved antigravity movement suggests central cause; hypotonia with marked muscle weakness, hyporeflexia, or areflexia points to motor unit dysfunction.
- Pattern of weakness (proximal or distal weakness) and extent of weakness (upper limb, lower limb, trunk, neck muscle, ocular, bulbar and extraocular muscle, ptosis) give an important clue to a possible underlying disease.
- There is limited role of electromyography (EMG) and muscle biopsy in diagnosis of NM disorders in children in the current era of rapid advances in genetics.
- Clinical exome sequencing and targeted gene panel testing have revolutionized the diagnosis of NM disorders.
- There is an emerging interest in NM imaging including MRI muscle as a supplementary guide to diagnosis.

16. Spectrum Disorder and Attention-deficit Hyperactivity Disorder

■ AUTISM SPECTRUM DISORDER

Introduction

Autism is a neurodevelopmental disorder characterized by impairment in social communication along with the presence of a restricted, repetitive pattern of behavior, interest, and activities. Leo Kanner was the first to publish his seminal paper in the year 1943, entitled "autistic disturbance of affective contact". He described a series of 11 children who were highly intelligent but had a "powerful desire of aloneness", "anxiously obsessive desire for the preservation of same", delayed echolalia, and oversensitivity to few stimuli.

Autism was earlier classified under childhood schizophrenia. Later in the year 1980, "infantile autism" was classified separately under Diagnostic and Statistical Manual of Mental Disorder, 3rd edition (DSM-III). The current diagnostic criteria for autism spectrum disorder (ASD) based on DSM-V club all pervasive developmental disorders (Asperger syndrome, Rett syndrome, and pervasive developmental disorder—not otherwise specified) into a single umbrella diagnosis of "ASD".

Diagnosis

The approach to diagnosis has been summarized in **Flowchart 1**. Clinical diagnosis of ASD is often based on criteria described in DSM-V (**Box 1**). DSM-V includes two domain levels—(1) impairment in social interaction and social communication (three items) and (2) restrictive, repetitive patterns of behavior, activity, and interest (four items). Diagnosis of ASD requires all three of three items in the first domain and at least two of four items in the second domain. In addition, these symptoms must be present in the early childhood. In many occasions when the symptoms are mild, they manifest only when the child grows up and is not able to cope up to the expectations of his age or in other words, symptoms manifest when social demands exceed limited capacity. These symptoms must cause significant impairment in social and/or occupational functioning.

DSM-V classifies autism severity into three levels—*level 1*: requiring support, *level 2*: requiring substantial support, and *level 3*: requiring very substantial support. These levels are decided on the extent of deficit in social communication, restrictive interest, and repetitive behavior. There is considerable overlap of symptoms between ASD and other conditions including global developmental delay (GDD), intellectual disability (ID), and attention-deficit hyperactivity disorder (ADHD). For example, inattention and impaired social interaction can be present in both ASD and ADHD. These symptoms are called overlapping symptoms.

Flowchart 1: Outlining approach to diagnosis of children with autism spectrum disorder (ASD).

Red flag signs
Infancy: No joyful expressions, no sharing of sounds, no babbling, and no waving or pointing
>1 year: No words by 16 months; no phrases by 24 months; and lack of social interaction

↓

Screening for ASD: M-CHAT, SCQ

↓

At risk for autism

↓

Comprehensive evaluation of ASD
- *Diagnostic evaluation of ASD:* DSM-V or ICD-10 criteria, diagnostic tools like ADI-R, ADOS, CARS, INDT-ASD, and ISAA tool can be used
- Evaluation of cognition, speech, behavior using appropriate psychological tool
- *Comorbidities:* Sleep, gastrointestinal, psychiatric, behavioral, sensory, and neurological (seizures and tics)

↓

Diagnosis of ASD

(ADI-R: autism diagnostic interview revised; ADOS: Autism Diagnostic Observation Schedule; ASD: autism spectrum disorder; CARS: Childhood Autism Rating Scale; DSM-V: Diagnostic and Statistical Manual of Mental Disorders-V; ICD: International Classification of Diseases; INDT-ASD: INCLEN diagnostic tool for autism spectrum disorder; ISAA: Indian Scale for Assessment of Autism; M-CHAT: modified checklist for autism; SCQ: social communication questionnaire)

When an individual is affected with two distinct disorders but occurring together, then this is called *comorbidity*. Comorbid conditions include psychiatric conditions, behavioral disturbance, sensory disturbance, neurological disturbance, and gastrointestinal and sleep-related issues **(Table 1)**. Conditions that are commonly associated with ASD include ADHD, anxiety, depression, and conduct disorder. *Diagnostic overshadowing* occurs when the salient features of one disorder, for example, ID, overshadow the consideration of another disorder, say ASD. In such a case, when symptoms of ASD can be explained solely by ID, then diagnosis of ASD alone is not made. DSM-V allows comorbid diagnosis. Hence, one can make a diagnosis of ASD-ID, ASD-ADHD, ASD-GDD, and so on. There are various metabolic disorders, single-gene disorders, and chromosomal disorders known to be associated with ASD **(Box 2)**.

Clinical Features

- *Impairment of social interaction and communication:*
    - *Reduced sharing of interest:* Lack of showing or bringing objects of interest to other people (e.g., if he sees a beautiful toy, he will get excited but will not bring it and share his liking with his parents or others).

BOX 1: DSM-V diagnostic criteria for autism spectrum disorder.

A. Persistent deficits in social communication and social interaction across multiple contexts as manifested by the following (three of three criteria):
   1. *Deficits in social–emotional reciprocity:* Ranging from abnormal social approach, failure of normal back to forth conversation, to reduced sharing of interests, emotions or affect, failure to initiate or respond to social interaction
   2. Deficits in nonverbal communicative behavior used for social interaction ranging from poorly integrated verbal and nonverbal communication; abnormal eye contact and body language; deficits in understanding and use of gestures; to total lack of facial expression and nonverbal communication
   3. *Deficits in developing and maintaining relationships:* Ranging from difficulties adjusting behavior to suit social contexts; difficulties in sharing, imaginative play, in making friends, and absence of interest in others
B. Restricted, repetitive patterns of behavior, interests, or activities as manifested by at least two of four following symptoms:
   1. Stereotyped or repetitive motor movements, use of objects or speech
   2. Insistence on sameness, inflexible adherence to routines, or ritualized patterns of verbal or nonverbal behavior
   3. Highly restricted and fixated interests that are abnormal in intensity or focus
   4. Hyper- or hyporeactivity to sensory input or unusual interest in sensory aspects of environment
C. Symptoms must be present in early childhood (but may not manifest until social demands exceed limited capacities)
D. The symptoms cause clinically significant impairment in social, occupational, or other important areas of functioning
E. These disturbances are not better explained by GDD or intellectual disability

(DSM-V: Diagnostic and Statistical Manual of Mental Disorders-V; GDD: global developmental delay)

TABLE 1: Comorbid conditions of autism spectrum disorder.

Broad category	Comorbid condition
Psychiatric	• Anxiety (43–84%) • Depression (2–30%) • Obsessive–compulsive disorder (37%) • Oppositional defiant disorder (7%) • Behavioral problems
Behavioral	• Disruptive • Irritable • Aggressive behavior (8–32%) • Self-injurious behavior (34%)
Sensory disturbances	• Tactile (80–90%) • Auditory sensitivity (5–47%)
Neurological	• Seizures and epilepsy (5–49%) • Tics (8–10%)
Gastrointestinal	• GERD (8–59%) • Constipation (8–59%)
Sleep disturbances	Sleep disruptions (52–73%)

(GERD: gastroesophageal reflux disease)

> **BOX 2:** Diseases associated with autism spectrum disorder.
>
> - *Metabolic disorders:*
>   - Phenylketonuria
>   - Adenosylsuccinate lyase deficiency (disorder of purine metabolism)
>   - Adenosine deaminase deficiency
>   - Succinic semialdehyde dehydrogenase (SSADH) deficiency
>   - Disorder of creatine transport and metabolism (arginine glycine aminotransferase deficiency and guanidine acetate methyltransferase deficiency)
>   - Cerebral folate deficiency
>   - Smith–Lemli–Opitz syndrome
>   - Mitochondrial disorders
> - *Chromosomal disorders:*
>   - Dup 7q11.23
>   - Dup or Del 16p 11.2
>   - Del 17q 12
>   - Del or Dup 15q13
>   - Del 22q 13
> - *Monogenic disorders:*
>   - Neurofibromatosis
>   - Tuberous sclerosis
>   - Fragile X syndrome

(Del: deletion; Dup: duplication)

- *Reduced sharing of emotions/affect:* Failure to share enjoyment, excitement, or achievements with others (e.g., child might get excited to see a cat, but will not call parents to show his excitement), lack of response to praise, lack of response to physical affection such as kissing and hugging, and lack of response when greeted with a social smile.
- Preference to play alone and getting irritated when other kids try to play with him. Hence, there is lack of joint play (e.g., when he goes to park, he often does not mingle with other kids, often plays alone, keeps running in the park or pushing other kids, cannot understand the rules of the game, cannot sustain a joint play).
- *Abnormal social approach:* For example, he might initiate social interaction with some intrusive abnormal touching or licking.
- *Lack of back and forth conversation:* Child does not initiate a conversation unless to fulfill his desires, he does not add anything significant for conversation to continue, he will not clarify what he means to say, most of the talks are one sided.

■ *Deficit in nonverbal communicative behavior used for social interaction:*
- Lack of mature pointing to bring attention to the object of his/her interest [e.g., if he wants a biscuit box kept above the fridge, then he will hold the hands of parents to take them (hand leading) to fridge rather than pointing out with his index finger that he needs that biscuit box]. Lack of understanding appropriate gestures such as head nodding and waving
- *Lack of social use of eye contact:* He often has no eye contact or ill-sustained eye contact during social interaction. Similarly, he might not face the person who is speaking to him (lack of appropriate body posture)
- Lack of social affect like inappropriate or lack of facial expression, inability, or limitation in conveying his emotions through words, expressions, gestures, or tone of voice
- Lack of coordinated verbal and nonverbal communication (coordinating eye contact with gestures and words)

■ *Deficits in developing and maintaining relationship appropriate to the developmental level:*
- Difficulty in making friends, lack of developing preferences in friends, lack of joint play (beyond 24 months)

- Prefers to play alone, avoids groups of children, limited interest in others, does not play with children of his age (prefers younger or older children)
- Lack of imaginative play with peers (imitative role plays like doctor–patient and teacher–student)
- *Abnormal behavior out of social context:* He cannot understand if he is being bullied or teased; he cannot understand if the other person is not interested in an activity; he is often unaware of social context and might express emotions or speak at inappropriate place or time; he might not understand the emotional impact of his behavior.

■ Stereotyped or repetitive speech, motor movement, or use of object:
  - Stereotyped speech:
    ◆ Jargon speech beyond developmental age of 24 months
      – Idiosyncratic or neologistic words that a child uses to communicate
      – Infantile squeals, guttural sounds, and repetitive humming can be observed in nonverbal children.
      – Immediate echolalia where the child repeats the words asked, so when asked, "what is your name", he will answer "what's your name" rather than answering his name
      – Delayed echolalia refers to repetition of words or phrases that he heard few minutes to hours back.
      – Lack of usage of "I" in speech. He would rather say "Rohan wants milk" instead of "I want milk".
      – He may replace "I" for "you".
  - *Stereotyped motor movement or use of object:*
    – Repetitive hand flapping and clapping movement
    – Excessive spinning and repetitive foot tapping
    – Toe walking
    – Unusual facial grimacing and teeth grinding
    – *Unusual use of object:* Lining up of toys, repetitive closing and opening of doors, and repetitively turning light on and off.

■ *Excessive adherence to routines, ritualized pattern of verbal and nonverbal behavior, excessive resistance to change, and rigid thinking:*
  - Insistence on rigidly following specific routines and getting irritated when disturbed. For example, taking one particular route to home, taking dinner in some specific patterns
  - Verbal rituals like saying one thing in a specific way, nonverbal rituals, or compulsions like turning three times before entering a room
  - Rigid thinking with inability to understand humor or sarcasm; inability to understand implied meaning or second meaning of some statement

■ *Highly restricted or fixated interests that are abnormal in intensity or focus:*
  - Narrow range of interest on few objects, topics, or activities
  - Excessive focus on nonfunctional parts of object such as wheels of car
  - Preoccupation with few colors and timetables
  - Preoccupied with unusual objects such as strings or rubber band

■ *Hypo- or hyperreactivity to sensory stimuli or unusual interest in sensory surroundings:*
  - Intolerance or excessive tolerance to pain.

- Preoccupation with texture or touch (he might like touching his mother's hairs or father's printed design in his t-shirt) or he may be averse with some touch like averse to toenail cutting, hair cutting, brushing teeth, etc.
- Unusual visual exploration like looking through corner of eye, holding objects in an unusual angle and looking at it, and unusual fascination with moving objects like fan, wheels of toy, and opening and closing of door.
- Unusual smelling of food before eating and licking his hands (smell and taste)
- Covers his ears repeatedly on unusual loud sounds like whistle of pressure cooker in kitchen.

Screening for Autism Spectrum Disorder

The average age at diagnosis for ASD is 4 years. There is a growing interest in early identification and intervention for children with ASD. The American Academy of Pediatrics (AAP) recommends general developmental screening at 9, 18, and 30 months with specific screening for ASD at 18 and 24 months. Screening tool (age of administration) for autism includes modified checklist for autism in toddlers, revised with follow-up (M-CHAT R/F) (16–30 months), early screening for autistic trait (ESAT) (14–15 months), infant toddler checklist (ITC) (6–24 months), social communication questionnaire (SCQ) (more than 4 years), social responsiveness scale (SRS) (>2½ years), and Gilliam Autism Rating Scale (GARS) (3–22 years).

Most commonly used screening tools for ASD include M-CHAT-R/F for children below 3 years of age and SCQ for children above 3 years. Majority of screeners are parent self-administered or parent interview based, except for an interactive tool such as screening test for autism in toddlers and young children (STAT).

Comprehensive Evaluation of Autism: Diagnosis

Definitive diagnosis of ASD is based on DSM-V criteria or ICD-10 criteria. Differential diagnosis and comorbidities of ASD must be considered before reaching a final diagnosis. Comprehensive evaluation also includes assessment of cognition, communication, motor skills, and functional adaptive skills. Autism-specific diagnostic tool needs to be used in conjunction with tools for cognitive, behavioral, motor, and functional skills. For example, assessment of intelligence (Wechsler Intelligence Scale or Vineland Social Maturity Scale) is required among children with ASD and ID. Similarly, comorbid diagnosis of ADHD in children with ASD would require an ADHD-specific diagnostic tool like Conner's Rating Scale.

Diagnosis of autism can be reached using diagnostic tools with high specificity and at least moderate sensitivity. The diagnostic tools could be parental interview based or observation based. Interview-based diagnostic tools include Autism Diagnostic Interview-Revised (ADI-R), parent interview for autism, GARS, and pervasive developmental disorder screening test. Observation-based diagnostic tools include Childhood Autism Rating Scale (CARS), Autism Diagnostic Observation Schedule (ADOS), INCLEN Diagnostic Tool for ASD (INDT-ASD), and Indian Scale for Assessment of Autism (ISAA). ADOS and ADI-R have largest evidence in diagnosis of ASD.

Differential Diagnosis and Diagnostic Overlap

The most common differential diagnosis of ASD includes ID, ADHD, and social communication disorder. Children with isolated impairment of social interaction and communication without restrictive repetitive behavior are often labeled under social communication disorder. Clinical features of ASD and ID tend to overlap, leading to ambiguity of comorbid diagnosis of ASD and ID versus ID alone explaining the autistic features. It has been observed that restricted interest or repetitive behavior best differentiates ASD and ID. When impairment in social communication and interaction corresponds to the developmental level of his nonverbal skills like fine motor skills or nonverbal problem-solving skill, then it is more likely to be ID alone. In contrast, there will be discrepancy in both among children with ASD and ID.

DSM-V allows comorbid diagnosis of ID, ADHD, and other genetic diagnoses unlike DSM-IV. Hence, diagnosis of ASD with ID is possible under DSM-V. Specifiers in DSM-V diagnosis of ASD include intellectual impairment and language impairment. DSM-V gives liberty to the clinician to allow comorbid diagnosis of ASD and ADHD. Majority of individuals with ASD have ADHD symptomatology, and it is considered that 15–25% of ADHD children have features suggestive of ASD. Diagnosis of this comorbidity is faced with a large number of diagnostic and therapeutic challenges. It is considered that comorbid diagnosis of ASD and ADHD has more impairment in executive as well as adaptive functioning when compared to either of them being alone.

When not to Think of Autism?

- When there is isolated impairment of social interaction, isolated impairment of communication, or absence of restrictive repetitive stereotyped behavior (social communication disorder)
- When there is a significant cognitive impairment in a child with few autistic features. ASD is often a comorbidity of ID.
- When the child was typically developing and now has developed autistic features (new onset of autistic features). When these new-onset autistic features are associated with autonomic involvement (like excessive sweating), extrapyramidal involvement (like choreoathetosis), cognitive decline, or seizures, a possibility of autoimmune N-methyl-D-aspartate (NMDA) receptor encephalitis needs to be kept.
- Autistic regression beyond 3 years of age is unusual for ASD, which may have regression at around 1½–2 years of age. Mothers will often complain that the child had attained few meaningful words that he lost subsequently. When such regression occurs beyond 3 years of age, possibility of continuous spike-waves during slow-wave sleep (CSWS) and Landau–Kleffner syndrome (LKS) should be considered **(Table 2)**. Children with LKS will have verbal auditory agnosia, i.e., they will not respond to auditory stimulus despite normal hearing physiology. They often consult multiple ENT physicians for hearing assessment. Children with CSWS often present with seizures and global regression along with autistic features. Among these children, electroencephalogram (EEG) record obtained in the sleep might reveal activation of epileptiform discharges called electrical status epilepticus of sleep (ESES).

Recommendations for Investigating a Child with Autism Spectrum Disorder

The American Academy of Pediatrics, American College of Medical Genetics (ACMG), and American Academy of Neurology (AAN) have published their

TABLE 2: Key differences between Landau–Kleffner syndrome, continuous spike-waves during slow-wave sleep (CSWS), and autistic regression.

Landau–Kleffner syndrome	CSWS	Autistic regression
Onset 2–8 years (peak 4–5 years)	Onset 4–8 years	Usually 18–24 months (before 3 years)
Normal language and cognitive development prior to the onset	Up to one-third have preexisting developmental delay	Speech delay from beginning or after attainment of 4–5 meaningful words
Verbal auditory agnosia is common	Majority will have seizures; one-third will have abnormal MRI findings	Majority will have normal MRI; seizures and significant cognitive impairment are uncommon
EEG spike localization: Temporal	*EEG spike localization:* Frontal	Normal EEG

(EEG: electroencephalogram)

recommendations for investigating a child with ASD. Recommendations include the following:

- Metabolic investigation needs to be done only if the symptoms are suggestive of one of the outlined syndromes **(Box 2)**. Metabolic etiology is considered in the presence of consanguinity, recurrent sibling loss, unexplained lethargy, early onset seizures, and abnormal urinary odor.
- High-resolution karyotyping and fragile X study are recommended among males with ASD, especially in the presence of ID or if there is a family history of ID or dysmorphic features.
- MRI brain is not required routinely but may be indicated in children with tuberous sclerosis and epilepsy.
- EEG should be done only if there is a history of seizure or suspicion of subclinical seizure. Children with ASD may have regression of speech in 1–2 years, but unusually late onset of speech regression could raise a possibility of LKS that warrants a sleep EEG.
- *MECP2* gene study may be considered among ASD females with regression.
- Microarray is required among those with cognitive impairment/ID.
- Phosphatase and tensin homolog (*PTEN*) mutation is recommended, if head circumference is >2 standard deviation (SD) above the mean.
- There is no role of celiac serology, allergy testing, vitamin levels, thyroid profile, or mitochondrial screening with lactate and pyruvate among children with ASD.

ATTENTION-DEFICIT HYPERACTIVITY DISORDER

Introduction

Attention-deficit hyperactivity disorder is a common neurodevelopmental disorder in children. It mainly affects the executive brain functioning. ADHD affects approximately 5.9–7.1% of children under 18 years, worldwide. It is characterized by inattention, hyperactivity, and impulsivity. Different terminologies such as "brain-injured child syndrome", "hyperkinetic impulse disorder", or "hyperactive child syndrome" have been used for ADHD. In 1968, DSM-II adopted it as "hyperkinetic reaction of childhood" under childhood disorders. For the first time in 1980, the term "attention deficit disorder" (ADD) was used in DSM-III. It was later renamed as "attention deficit hyperactivity disorder" in DSM-III-TR, signifying the incorporation of all three (hyperactivity, inattentiveness, and impulsivity) core symptoms in the manual.

Extensive work in ADHD research suggested that hyperactivity and impulsivity form a single behavioral domain. As a result, DSM-IV identified two distinct domains of inattention and hyperactivity–impulsivity with a specific set of symptoms for each domain. For the first time, a subtype with hyperactive impulsive behavior without inattention was also discussed in DSM-IV. In the year 2013, DSM-V was published with broadening the age group for clinical diagnosis of ADHD. DSM-V describes three basic forms of ADHD—(1) predominantly inattentive, (2) predominantly hyperactive/impulsive, and (3) combined.

Clinical Features

Symptoms of ADHD can present as early as 3–6 years of age. They can continue into adolescence and adulthood. The three core symptoms of ADHD are inattention, hyperactivity, and impulsivity which interfere with functioning and development of child. Diagnostic criteria of ADHD are as per DSM-V (**Box 3**). Some inattention is normal in child but in ADHD, they are more severe, occur more often, and hamper social functioning. The symptoms of ADHD have been enumerated in the following examples.

Inattention

Fictitious character *master X* lacks persistence, wanders off tasks that require sustained mental effort, overlooks or misses details, and works inaccurately. He is unable to concentrate on activities like a long lecture, lengthy readings, and looking at picture books. School teachers often complain that his mind seems elsewhere and is distracted easily with even little distractions such as vendors, traffic, or animal sounds. At home, he often starts a task like homework but quickly loses interest and is unable to complete it. He is very disorganized, messy, and has difficulty in managing sequential tasks that often require time management. *Master X*'s parents complain that he loses things like books and pencils at school. It is very difficult to get *master X* ready for school and he often forgets to bathe or brush or dress him completely. During his adolescence, he may develop problems completing forms, writing long reports, and meeting deadlines at work.

Hyperactivity and Impulsivity

Master X is fidgety in class and keeps tapping fingers. He squirms, moves his hands and feet, and keeps twisting his body while sitting on his bench. He is unable to remain seated in his or her place for long. He runs around excessively at school and even when he is at home. While playing games, like chess, he often quarrels and is unable to sit quietly. Parents often tell that he is very talkative, interrupts others' conversations, and answers even before the question is complete. He cannot wait for his turn and he does not like to wait in queues. The child is very intrusive and interrupts games and other activities, which leads to frequent quarrels. He has limited friends and often fights with them over trivial issues.

Evolution of Symptoms

Symptoms of ADHD vary with age. Parents may notice subtle features like very high motor activity. This may well be a part of normal behavior of a child <4 years of age. Hyperactivity and impulsiveness are more prominent during the preschool age of 3–5 years. When the child starts to go to school, inattention is noticed more often. In adolescents and adults, hyperactivity seems to lessen and may remain only as restlessness.

Evaluation and Diagnosis

Approach to the diagnosis of ADHD has been summarized below. Evaluation involves focused history, examination, and plan investigations if essential.

History

- The presenting complaints are often pertaining to core symptoms (inattention, hyperactivity–impulsivity) based on DSM-V.
- Consider inputs from parents/teachers, coaches, and guardians.
- *Age of onset:* Symptoms are often recognized at school by teachers and parents seek advice based on suggestions from the schoolteachers.
- Duration of core symptoms needs to be determined (minimum 6 months).
- Document the parent–child interaction in office settings (symptoms must be present in the home as well as in your clinic).
- Developmental history with developmental milestones, especially language milestones. Majority of children with isolated ADHD attain age-appropriate milestones. Presence of developmental delay and/or cognitive delay must point toward ADHD being comorbidity for ID rather than isolated ADHD.
  - Family history of ADHD or other neurological comorbidities must be enquired.
  - Medical history for drugs such as anticonvulsants, antihypertensive, ephedrine pseudoephedrine, MAO inhibitors; conditions such as hypertension, hepatic diseases, glaucoma, heart disease (these medications can have interactions with ADHD medications), head trauma, and CNS infections (can be a contributing factor).
- Other comorbidities that exist with ADHD including seizures, vision problems, hearing problems, and motor disability such as spasticity or dystonia must be demonstrated.
- Degree of the functional impairment in daily functioning in terms of family interactions, school performance, family dysfunction (e.g., drug abuse, chronic illness, financial problems), social skills, substance abuse, psychosocial, and family stressors. It is essential to determine the degree of impairment in daily functioning to decide on the need of medication.

Examination

- Growth (anthropometric) parameters including head circumference. Presence of macrocephaly along with typical facies may favor possibility of fragile X syndrome.
- Vision and hearing assessment
- Presence of dysmorphic features may point toward syndromic association such as William syndrome or fragile X syndrome
- Neurocutaneous markers must be searched to look for evidence of tuberous sclerosis or neurofibromatosis.
- Comprehensive psychological assessment includes screening for core symptoms of ADHD, assessment of cognition (intelligence), and assessment of behavior. Various rating scales for parents and teachers have been formulated to screen the child. These include ADHD Comprehensive Teacher Rating Scale, 2nd edition, Vanderbilt ADHD Teacher Rating Scale, Conner's Parent and

Teacher Rating Scales-Revised (CPRS-R and CTRS-R), Swanson, and Nolan and Pelham IV Questionnaire.
- Complete neurological examination including mental status (affect, cognition, speech, and thought patterns).

Diagnostic Criteria

Diagnosis of ADHD is a clinical diagnosis based on DSM-V criteria **(Box 3)**. Many European countries use ICD-10 for diagnosis of ADHD. A total of 6 out of 9 criteria in inattention domain and hyperactivity–impulsivity domain for a minimum duration of 6 months are required for clinical diagnosis of ADHD. It is mandatory that these symptoms must be present in at least two different settings like home and school. ADHD has been classified into mild, moderate, and severe depending on the degree of impairments in social or occupational functioning. It is possible that all requisite number of criteria could not be fulfilled in the last 6 months, as the child is in *partial remission*. DSM-V classifies based on the criteria into three types:

1. *Combined presentation:* If both criterion A (inattention) and criterion B (hyperactivity–impulsivity) are met
2. *Predominantly inattentive presentation:* If criterion A (inattention) is met but criterion B (hyperactivity–impulsivity) is not met
3. *Predominantly hyperactive/impulsive presentation:* If criterion B (hyperactivity–impulsivity) is met and criterion A (inattention) is not met.

Differential Diagnosis

There is considerable overlap of symptoms between ADHD and other conditions including GDD, ID, and ASD. For example, inattention and impaired social interaction can be present in both ADHD and ASD. These symptoms are called *overlapping symptoms*. Motor stereotypes in stereotypic movement disorder and autism can often be confused with fidgetiness of ADHD. The social dysfunction and peer rejection of ADHD must be differentiated from isolation and difficulty in social interaction in autism.

Conditions that are commonly associated with ADHD include ID and ASD. Oppositional defiant disorder is the most common comorbid condition that occurs in about 42% and 25% of children with combined and predominantly inattentive types of ADHD, respectively. It is characterized by antisocial behavior such as stubbornness, aggression, frequent temper tantrums, and stealing. About 25% of combined-type ADHD have co-occurrence of conduct disorder.

The most common differential diagnoses of ADHD are oppositional defiant disorder, intermittent explosive disorder, anxiety and depressive disorder, substance abuse, and personality disorder. Children with oppositional defiant disorder often resist doing schoolwork due to their defiant behavior. This must be differentiated from the inability of engaging in mentally demanding tasks in a child with ADHD. Secondary oppositional behavior may also develop in some children with ADHD and may make differentiating these two disorders more difficult.

Inattention, restlessness, and inability to focus are also seen in specific learning disorder (SLD), anxiety, and depressive disorders. In ADHD, these symptoms are present all the time unlike in depression where they present during depressive episodes. They are often associated with worry and rumination in anxiety disorders and help to differentiate it from ADHD. Inattention in learning disabilities is due to limited abilities and frustration. In contrast to ADHD, it is only limited to academic work.

> **BOX 3:** Diagnostic and Statistical Manual of Mental Disorder (DSM)-V diagnostic criteria for attention-deficit hyperactivity disorder.
>
> Persistent pattern of inattention and/or hyperactivity–impulsivity that interferes with functioning or development, as characterized by (A) and/or (B):
>
> A. *Inattention:* Six (or more) of the following symptoms have persisted for at least 6 months to a degree that is inconsistent with developmental level. For older adolescents and adults (age 17 years and older), at least five symptoms are required:
>   1. Often fails to give close attention to details or makes careless mistakes in schoolwork, at work, or during other activities
>   2. Often has difficulty sustaining attention in tasks or play activities
>   3. Often does not seem to listen when spoken to directly
>   4. Often does not follow through the instructions and fails to finish schoolwork, chores, or duties in the workplace
>   5. Often has difficulty in organizing tasks and activities
>   6. Often avoids, dislikes, or is reluctant to engage in tasks that require sustained mental effort
>   7. Often loses things necessary for tasks or activities
>   8. Is often easily distracted by extraneous stimuli?
>   9. Is often forgetful in daily activities?
> B. *Hyperactivity and impulsivity:* Six (or more) of the following symptoms have persisted for at least 6 months to a degree that is inconsistent with developmental level; for older adolescents and adults (age 17 years and older), at least five symptoms are required:
>   1. Often fidgets with or taps hands or feet or squirms in seat
>   2. Often leaves seat in situations when remaining seated is expected
>   3. Often runs about or climbs in situations where it is inappropriate
>   4. Often unable to play or engage in leisure activities quietly
>   5. Is often "on the go," acting as if "driven by a motor"?
>   6. Often talks excessively
>   7. Often blurts out an answer before a question has been completed
>   8. Often has difficulty waiting for his or her turn
>   9. Often interrupts or intrudes on others
> C. Several inattentive or hyperactive–impulsive symptoms were present prior to age 12 years
> D. Several inattentive or hyperactive–impulsive symptoms are present in two or more settings (e.g., at home, school, or work)
> E. There is clear evidence that the symptoms interfere with or reduce the quality of social, academic, or occupational functioning
> F. The symptoms do not occur exclusively during the course of schizophrenia or another psychotic disorder and are not better explained by other mental disorders (e.g., mood disorder, anxiety disorder, dissociative disorder, personality disorder, substance intoxication, or withdrawal)

Impulsivity is a symptom common to both ADHD and intermittent explosive disorder but presence of aggression points toward the latter. Personality disorders present with aggressive and narcissistic behavior, which is perceived as socially intrusive and inappropriate. Hence, narcissistic personality can be confused with ADHD.

■ SPECIFIC LEARNING DISORDERS

Specific learning disorder is another neurodevelopmental disorder, which affects the learning of academic skills by the child. It does not affect the intelligence and has been described in DSM-V as an umbrella term for reading (dyslexia), writing (dysgraphia), and mathematics expression disorders (dyscalculia). It is prevalent among 5–15% of school-aged children.

Specific learning disorder usually comes to attention during elementary school years where a child is required to read, spell, write, and learn math. He or she has difficulty in word reading wherein the child hesitates to read the word or it is read incorrectly. While reading aloud, the child skips lines. They keep guessing the word and have difficulty in sounding out the word. Sometimes, the text may be read accurately but the child is not able to understand the meaning, sequence, and the deeper meaning of what was read. Multiple grammatical and punctuation errors are often seen. Teachers and parent complain of untidy and illegible handwriting. There is difficulty in application of mathematical concepts, understanding numbers, or their magnitude. A child will often count on fingers to add single digit numbers instead of recalling the math fact.

The diagnosis of SLD is made by history and DSM-V criteria. Diagnosis of SLD can only be made after formal education starts. Assessment includes educational history, school documents (notebook and examination papers) review, and classroom observations by teachers. Various tools have been devised for assessment of children with SLD. In Indian setting, NIMHANS battery for specific learning disability and GLAD (grade level assessment device) are used. These are available in English, Hindi, and Kannada. Comprehensive assessment of vision, hearing, intelligence, academic performance, communicative status, and motor abilities should be done. The diagnosis must specify all domains and subskills that are impaired.

Specific learning disorder can often be confused with low performance in academics due to varied causes such as lack of opportunities or poor instructions. ID is another close differential. Children with ID do not have normal intellectual functioning like SLD. Many children with neurological and sensory disorders such as stroke and hearing impairment can present with similar symptoms and so these must be ruled out before a diagnosis of learning disorder is made.

KEY MESSAGES

- Neurodevelopmental disorders are a spectrum of heterogeneous conditions that disrupt the developmental, cognitive, emotional, behavioral, psychosocial, and adaptive functioning of an individual.
- Most diagnosed disorders are ASD, ADHD, ID, and SLD.
- DSM provides a common language for all clinicians, researchers, and psychologists to diagnose these neurodevelopmental disorders.
- Autism is a neurodevelopmental disorder characterized by an impairment in social interaction and communication along with the presence of restricted, repetitive pattern of behavior, interest, and activities.
- ADHD is characterized by an impairment of attention, hyperactivity, and impulsivity, while SLD affects an individual's ability to perceive and process the information required to develop academic skills.

CHAPTER 17

Approach to Diagnosis of Movement Disorders

INTRODUCTION

An essential prerequisite for smooth coordination of movement includes normal muscle power along with normal inputs from eyes, cerebellum, posterior column, and vestibular system. *Movement disorders are characterized by abnormal involuntary movement or impaired performance of voluntary movement, not resulting from neuromuscular weakness or abnormality of tone.* Identifying the movement disorder is essential to plan an appropriate workup and design a management plan accordingly.

Characterization of movement disorder in children is often challenging; and, in many instances, it becomes difficult to differentiate it from other events such as seizures. A detailed description of the movement as described by parents often needs to be supplemented with a video recording of the event to precisely understand the nature of movement and characterize it accordingly. The approach should focus on the description of movement rather than identifying the type of movement. It is essential to realize that children often have mixed type of movement disorder rather than pure forms of chorea, athetosis, or dystonia.

JONATHAN MINK APPROACH TO MOVEMENT DISORDER

Step 1: Is the Pattern of Movements Normal (Developmental Variations) or Abnormal for Age?

An abnormal movement could be normal at one state and abnormal at a different state. For example, myoclonus would be normal at the onset of sleep (benign sleep myoclonus). It would be abnormal when it occurs in an awake state. Few movement disorders are considered normal for that developmental age. For example, benign neonatal sleep myoclonus, and jitteriness in a newborn is normal. These movement disorders are considered as developmental variations. Shuddering spells, paroxysmal torticollis, Sandifer syndrome, and spasmus nutans are few developmental variations observed in infancy. They are often mistaken as seizures. The first step in the analysis of movement disorder is to recognize the pattern of these normal developmental movement disorders. Following are some of the clinical clues to recognize them:

- When a typically developing infant presents with multiple episodes of paroxysm of behavioral arrest with

shivering-like movement of head and trunk (mistaken for episodes of tremulous movement) as if someone has poured cold water over his/her back, then we must think of *shuddering spells*.
- Children with *gratification* have dystonic posturing of lower limbs with rocking, grinding, and pressure-like movement on the perineum. These movements are often associated with flushing and diaphoresis.
- Excessive startle response to unusual sounds with generalized stiffening of the body in early infancy often points to *hyperekplexia* (often mistaken for myoclonus).
- Paroxysmal episodes of torticollis with pallor and irritability could favor *benign paroxysmal torticollis* (often mistaken for dystonia of neck muscles).
- A combination of torticollis, nystagmus, and head nodding is seen in *spasmus nutans*.
- Abnormal extensor posturing of the neck, trunk, and limbs occurring immediately after feeds (mistaken for generalized dystonia) could point to the possibility of *Sandifer syndrome*.

Step 2: Are there Excessive Movements (Hyperkinetic), or Is There a Paucity of Movement (Hypokinetic)?

Broadly, movement disorders can be categorized into hyperkinetic and hypokinetic movement disorders **(Box 1)**. By convention, hyperkinetic movement disorders are more common than hypokinetic movement disorders in children. In many instances, the exact characterization of the hyperkinetic movement disorder could not be made. The term "dyskinesia" is often used to describe such uncharacterizable hyperkinetic movement disorder.

> **BOX 1:** Broad classification of movement disorders.
>
> *Hyperkinetic movement disorder*
> - Chorea
> - Athetosis
> - Ballismus
> - Dystonia
> - Tremors
> - Tics
> - Stereotypies
>
> *Hypokinetic movement disorder:*
> - Bradykinesia/Parkinsonian movement disorder (akinetic rigid syndrome)

Step 3: Which Part of the Body is Involved [Face, Neck, Upper Limb, and Lower Limb (Proximal or Distal)]?

Abnormal movement can involve the face, upper limb, lower limb, trunk, and neck muscles in isolation or in combination. By convention, focal involvement is uncommon in children. Most of the movement disorders are generalized. For example, generalized dystonia is far more common in children, whereas focal dystonia, like blepharospasm or laryngeal dystonia is more common in adults. If there is a limb involvement, the description must include if it is proximal or distal predominant movement.
- Athetoid movements are distal predominant movement, whereas choreiform movements are proximal.
- *Tics* are more evident in the face and neck muscles.
- *Tremors* are often observed on outstretched hands (positional tremor), or while approaching an object (intentional tremors) or at rest (resting tremors).
- *Stereotypies* often manifest in hands and appear like "handwashing movement" or "hand wringing movement."

Step 4: Description of the Movement

The next step is the characterization of the movement disorder. Description of movement disorder includes the right choice of words. For example, *chorea* is a bizarre, flowing movement; *athetosis* is a distal writhing movement; *dystonia* is an abnormal twisting movement with fixed postures; *myoclonus* is electric shock-like movement; *ballismus* is high-amplitude choreiform movement; *stereotypies* are patterned movement; and *tremors* are rhythmic oscillating movement around a fixed axis **(Table 1)**.

It is often challenging to characterize the type of abnormal movement into chorea, athetosis, dystonia, or mixture of them. Hence, it is a description of this abnormal movement in the above format that helps in understanding the movement disorder rather than naming the type of movement disorder. Few clinical markers that can help in identifying the type of movement disorder are depicted in **Table 2**. Many of the movement disorders mimic each other. Paroxysmal movement disorder can mimic seizure; myoclonus can mimic dystonia;

TABLE 1: Description of movement disorders in children.

Movement disorder	Description (keywords are marked in italics)
Athetosis	• *Slow, distal, writhing, continuous,* and involuntary movements • They are commonly associated with chorea (choreoathetosis)
Ballismus	• *Involuntary, high-amplitude,* and *flinging* movements that typically occur proximally • It is an uncommon movement disorder encountered in pediatric practice
Chorea	• Involuntary, *semipurposive, bizarre,* and *chaotic* movement • It is continual and irregular hyperkinetic disorder • Movements occur unpredictably and randomly with variable rate and direction that *flows* from one body part to other • It can involve upper limb and/or lower limb; can involve both proximal and distal muscles • Motor impersistence in chorea is demonstrated by milkmaid grip, supinator sign, darting tongue, and spooning of hands
Dystonia	• Dystonia is a syndrome of sustained muscle contractions, frequently causing *abnormal twisting* and repetitive movements, or *abnormal postures* • It is caused by simultaneous contraction of agonist and antagonist • It is triggered by attempted voluntary movement and subsides with rest/sleep • It cannot be suppressed voluntarily • Touching one part of body may relieve the dystonic spasm (sensory tricks or *geste antagoniste*) • It can be focal dystonia (e.g., writer's cramp and cervical dystonia), or generalized dystonia
Myoclonus	• Quick, very brief, involuntary, and nonsuppressible *shock-like movements* of one or more muscles • It can, at times, be elicited by sensory stimulus (reflex myoclonus) or movement (action myoclonus) • It can be positive (sudden contraction) or negative (sudden and brief interruption of contraction in active postural muscles) • It can be focal, multifocal, segmental, or generalized
Parkinsonism	Presence of two or more of the cardinal features of Parkinson's disease: tremor at rest, *bradykinesia, rigidity,* and postural instability

Contd...

Contd...

Movement disorder	Description (keywords are marked in italics)
Stereotypies	• Involuntary, *patterned, coordinated*, repetitive, nonreflexive movements that occur in the same fashion with each repetition • It is exacerbated with excitement, stress, or fatigue • It may stop once the child is distracted • These movements are relatively stable over a period and do not change over time • Stereotypic movements include hand flapping, and finger wiggling movements. They are common in an intellectually disabled child, and those with autism spectrum disorder including Rett syndrome
Tics	• Sudden, *rapid, abrupt*, repetitive, and nonrhythmic movement • Movement can involve the head, neck, or upper body (simple or complex motor tics) such as eye blinking, grimacing, jerking of the neck, and shoulder elevation • It can involve voice (vocal tics) such as sniffing, throat clearing, and coughing. It often is a combination of motor and vocal tics • It is preceded by an uncomfortable feeling or *urge* that is relieved by carrying out the movement • It can be *suppressed voluntarily* for a brief period • It often involves the head and upper body • It can occur multiple times a day • It has a waxing and waning course over a period of time
Tremors	• *Oscillating* and *rhythmic* movements about a fixed point, axis, or plane that occur when antagonist muscles contract alternately • It can be rest tremor (occurs at rest), intention tremor (occurs while approaching an object), or action tremor (occurs during maintained posture or movement) • Tremors can involve upper limb, head, lower limb, and voice

TABLE 2: Clinical markers for identification of movement disorder.

Characteristics	Movement disorder
Movement that is evident at rest	Chorea, athetosis, and myoclonus
Movement that is more evident with action	Dystonia (abnormal twisting posture) and chorea (semipurposive)
Movement that is evident with certain posture (like outstretched hands)	Tremors
Movement that subsides with sleep	Most of movement disorders subside with sleep
Presence of premonitory urge, voluntarily suppressible for brief period, and exacerbation with emotional stress	Tics

and high-amplitude ballismus can mimic myoclonus **(Table 3)**.

■ *Relation to sleep:* The majority of movement disorders including chorea, athetosis, and dystonia subside in sleep. Myoclonus of neurodegenerative diseases might persist during sleep. In contrast, benign neonatal sleep myoclonus occurs only during sleep.

■ *Relation to emotional state:* Choreoathetoid movement and dystonia often increase with emotional challenge and stress.

TABLE 3: Few close differentials of movement disorders.

Movement disorder	What does it mimic like?	Clinical pointers
Low-amplitude chorea	Fidgety appearance	Presence of milk maid grip, darting tongue, and spooning of hands point to chorea
Rhythmic myoclonus	Tremor	Tremor often oscillates around an axis that may worsen with certain posture/action unlike myoclonus that often has characteristic of shock-like contraction
Stereotypies	Complex tics	Stereotypies remain the same over time; tics tend to fluctuate with time and also change from one type to another
Paroxysmal dystonia	Seizures	Dystonia is abnormal twisting posture of body that subsides with sleep, occurs through the day unlike seizures that although may be multiple episodes they tend to have definitive onset and offset and may be associated with impairment of consciousness

- *Awareness of movement:* Children with choreoathetoid movements are often aware of their movement and, to hide it, they perform some purposive movements like trying to comb the hair or touch the cheek. These movements are hence called quasipurposive movements.
- *Does the child have a premonitory urge and can he/she suppress the movement?* Children with tic disorder often can control the movement for a few seconds but have severe urge to perform it again and again.
- *Relation to rest, action, or specific posture:* The majority of hyperkinetic movement disorders, including choreoathetosis and dystonia, occurs at rest and increases on an attempt to perform specific action. Tremors can occur at rest (resting tremors of Parkinsonism), action (intentional tremors of the cerebellum), or posture (wing beating tremors of Wilson disease).

Step 5: Is the Movement Paroxysmal, Continual, or Continuous?

It could be paroxysmal (sudden onset for a brief period which may recur), continual (repeated again and again), or continuous (without stop). Majority of movement disorders are continual or continuous. Paroxysmal movement disorders include developmental movement disorder such as shuddering spells and gratification. Paroxysmal dyskinesia is a group of conditions characterized by recurrent episodes of dystonia, chorea, athetosis, ballismus, or a combination of them with complete recovery and normal neurological examination in-between the episodes **(Table 4)**. These episodes are often mistaken as seizures, and children are often on multiple antiepileptic drugs before the condition is diagnosed.

Step 6: Is it Static or Progressive?

Progression in movement disorder is an important clue to the possibility of underlying neurodegenerative disorder. If the child had a one-time insult (e.g., perinatal asphyxia, kernicterus, trauma, intracranial hemorrhage, and meningoencephalitis) followed by the onset of movement disorder that is otherwise improving with the progress of time, it would suggest a static insult. Progressive diseases can be relentlessly progressive as in subacute sclerosing panencephalitis (SSPE) or might

TABLE 4: Paroxysmal movement disorders.

Paroxysmal movement disorder	Clinical description
Paroxysmal kinesigenic dyskinesia (PKD)	Children aged 5–15 years with attacks of dystonia with choreiform movement lasting for few seconds, often precipitated by sudden movement, occurring multiple times in a day in an otherwise typically developing school-going child; *PRRT2* gene mutation; PKD responds well to carbamazepine. Other treatment options include phenytoin, levetiracetam, and phenobarbitone
Paroxysmal nonkinesigenic dyskinesia (PNKD)	Episodes of hyperkinetic movement (dystonia and/or chorea) lasting for minutes to hours, starting with one limb spreading to all, remain conscious during the episode, onset in early infancy or childhood, *PNKD* gene mutation; drugs that may be useful include clonazepam, haloperidol, and acetazolamide
Paroxysmal exercise-induced dyskinesia (PED)	Attacks of hyperkinetic movement within minutes to hours of exercise, lasting for few minutes; *SCL2A1/GCH* and *Parkin* gene mutations are implicated
Episodic ataxia type 1	Episodes of ataxia lasting for seconds to minute often triggered by exercise, fever, stress with an onset in early childhood; *KCNA1* gene mutation; favorable response to acetazolamide
Episodic ataxia type 2	Episodes of ataxia, migraine lasting for minutes to days with interictal nystagmus; favorable response to acetazolamide; *CACNA1A* gene mutation

have fluctuations with clinical worsening on trivial infection or stress (mitochondrial disorders). Few movement disorders could change over time (started with one movement and evolved to other movement types). For example, dystonia that started from one limb at the beginning that ultimately progressed to all four limbs with diurnal variation (worsening in evening hours) might point towards dopa-responsive dystonia. Children with ataxia–telangiectasia can manifest with choreoathetosis that resolves before ataxia and becomes a prominent manifestation.

Step 7: Is Development Normal, and are there Findings on the Examination to Suggest Focal Neurologic Deficit?

The presence of developmental delay in a child with movement disorder often points to underlying static insult during the perinatal period such as kernicterus and perinatal asphyxia. This often results in dyskinetic cerebral palsy, which could be a choreoathetoid or dystonic or mixed type of cerebral palsy. The onset of paroxysmal movement disorder in early infancy in an otherwise typically developing child indicates developmental movement disorder.

The presence of focal neurological deficit, including hemiparesis and cranial nerve palsy in an acute setting with a movement disorder, especially hemichorea, would point to structural or vascular pathology in the contralateral side of the brain.

Step 8: What could be Probable Etiology?

Etiology can be broadly divided into infective, parainfectious (demyelinating/

autoimmune), structural, vascular, metabolic, traumatic, neoplastic, drug/toxin-induced, nutritional, and genetic causes. Most of the movement disorders could be attributable to one or more of the above categories.

- *Infective:* The presence of ongoing fever favors infective etiology. Encephalitis with the involvement of basal ganglia and thalamus (like Japanese encephalitis) can result in choreoathetoid and dystonic movement. Children with subacute sclerosing panencephalitis can present with myoclonus and cognitive decline.
- *Parainfectious:* History of recent febrile illness or vaccination prior to onset of neurological symptom points toward parainfectious/demyelinating like acute disseminated encephalitis (ADEM) that may present with new onset of movement disorder. Similarly, the subacute onset of autonomic manifestations, movement disorders, with or without a cognitive decline in an older child, could raise a possibility of autoimmune (like NMDA receptor encephalitis). Children with encephalitis lethargica (von economo disease) can manifest with a hypokinetic movement disorder. Sydenham chorea follows weeks to months after group A *Streptococcal* infection.
- *Structural etiology:* Children with structural causes such as cerebral palsy, stroke, trauma, and encephalitis often have a static course with gradual improvement in symptoms. The most common cause of dyskinesia in children is dyskinetic cerebral palsy sequelae to kernicterus or perinatal asphyxia. History of the perinatal event, history of head trauma, history of encephalitis, or stroke-like illness could provide hint among children with a static or nonprogressive course of illness.
- *Vascular etiology:* Arterial ischemic stroke can manifest with new onset of movement disorder. Most of vascular (arterial) etiologies have a focal neurological deficit (hemiparesis, cranial nerve palsy, oculomotor involvement, and speech involvement) in addition to movement disorder, which often is asymmetric. Asymmetry in movement disorder could point to either structural or vascular pathology on the contralateral side. Central nervous system (CNS) vasculitis such as systemic lupus erythematosus and anticardiolipin/antiphospholipid antibody syndrome can present with new onset of chorea (history of rash, fever, joint pain, and photosensitivity).
- *Traumatic:* History of trivial trauma in infancy followed by the onset of hemidystonia and hemiparesis could favor the diagnosis of mineralizing angiopathy of childhood. Similarly, head trauma-induced basal ganglia stroke or bleed could often manifest with asymmetric movement disorders.
- *Metabolic:* There is a wide list of metabolic disorders that manifest with movement disorders such as chorea, dystonia, and myoclonus **(Table 5)**. Children with storage disorders may have associated developmental delay with or without coarse facies and organomegaly. Fundus evaluation may show a cherry-red spot (Niemann–Pick disease) or pigmentary retinal changes (neuronal ceroid lipofuscinosis). Children with white matter degenerative brain disease (leukodystrophy) may manifest with neuroregression with variable combination of spasticity, dystonia, and/or choreoathetoid movement. Hereditary or genetic causes may have an affected family member. Genetic causes can

TABLE 5: Examples of neurometabolic disorders that present with movement disorder.

Neurometabolic disorder	Examples
Storage disorders	GM1 gangliosidosis and Niemann–Pick disease type C
Organic acidemia	Methylmalonic acidemia (MMA), propionic acidemia (PA), nonketotic hyperglycinemia (NKH), mitochondrial disorders (Leigh syndrome), and glutaric aciduria type 1
Leukodystrophies	Metachromatic leukodystrophy and Pelizaeus–Merzbacher disease
Others	Lesch–Nyhan syndrome and Wilson disease

TABLE 6: Genetic conditions presenting with mixed movement disorder.

Disease	Classical clinical feature
Wilson disease	Age 7–10 years, fasciolingual–pharyngeal rigidity, wing-beating tremors (20–50%), mask-like facies, dyskinesia of limbs (10–60%), psychiatric manifestation, loss of emotional control, presence of Kayser–Fleischer ring, serum ceruloplasmin (<20 mg/dL), 24-hour urinary copper > 100 g/day; *ATP7B* gene mutation; chelation with D-penicillamine, trientine, and zinc acetate
Aceruloplasminemia	Slowly progressive late-onset dystonia, chorea, dysarthria with low ceruloplasmin, decreased serum iron, and raised serum ferritin
Childhood-onset Huntington disease	Early onset presents with features of dystonia, seizures, and cognitive decline; later onset presents with Parkinsonian rigidity, dysarthria, cognitive decline, seizures, and slow saccades; MRI brain shows atrophy of caudate; genetically confirmed triplet repeats (CAG repeats)
Neuroacanthosis	Late onset > 10 years, orofasciolingual and pharyngeal dyskinesia, rigidity, tic-like manifestation, blood acanthocytosis, MRI showing caudate atrophy

present with various movement disorders, including mixed movement disorders **(Table 6)**, chorea **(Table 7)**, dystonia **(Table 8)**, or myoclonus **(Table 9)**. While describing myoclonus, it would be useful to understand its site of origin—cortical, subcortical, spinal, or peripheral myoclonus **(Box 2)**. Classical clinical features of some of the common genetic diseases manifesting with a movement disorder are outlined in **Tables 6 to 9**. Although there is an exhaustive list of causes of dystonia and chorea, we are restricting to common genetic disorders.

- *Toxic/drug-induced/endocrinal causes:* Sedatives, neuroleptics, calcium channel blocker, stimulants (amphetamine and cocaine), few antiepileptic drugs (valproate, phenytoin, and carbamazepine), and antiemetics have been implicated in drug-induced movement disorders including chorea, dystonia, tremors, and Parkinsonian features. Similarly, arsenic, lead, and cyanide poisoning can induce tremors. Endocrinal causes include hyperthyroidism-induced chorea and tremor; hypoparathyroidism can result in hypocalcemia with resultant tremors.

TABLE 7: Genetic diseases presenting with movement disorders (chorea).

Movement disorder	Genetic disease	Clinical features
Choreoathetoid movement	Ataxia telangiectasia (*ATM* gene mutation)	Early-onset cerebellar ataxia, choreoathetoid movement, impaired oculomotor saccades, recurrent sinopulmonary infection, increased radiosensitivity, decreased levels of IgG2 and IgA, and elevated α-fetoprotein
	Ataxia with oculomotor apraxia (AOA type 1) (*APTX* gene mutation)	Early onset of chorea, ataxia, and oculomotor apraxia (impaired ocular saccades) may have hypoalbuminemia.
	Ataxia with oculomotor apraxia type 2 (AOA type 2) (*SETX* gene mutation)	Ataxia, oculomotor apraxia, peripheral neuropathy, and occasional chorea/dystonia
	Benign hereditary chorea (BHC)	Motor delay with hypotonia, early onset of nonprogressive chorea, autosomal-dominant inheritance, normal cognition, absence of epilepsy, may have associated learning disabilities and ADHD

(ADHD: attention deficit hyperactivity disorder)

TABLE 8: Genetic diseases presenting with movement disorders (dystonia).

Genetic disease	Clinical features
Pantothenate kinase-associated neurodegeneration (PKAN)	Onset 3–10 years of age with dystonia starting in the leg, progressing to involve the entire body, choreoathetosis, ballismus, dysarthria, bradykinesia with MRI brain clinching the diagnosis with typical "eye of tiger sign"; common in few communities (Agarwal)
Dopa-responsive dystonia (DYT-5) mutation in *GTP cyclohydrolase 1* gene	Onset at around 6 years of age, dystonia starting from one limb progressing to other limb associated with Parkinsonian features, with a diurnal variation that worsens by evening hours, dramatic improvement with the trial of L-dopa
Dystonia myoclonus syndrome (DYT-11) (mutation in epsilon sarcoglycan protein)	Myoclonus can involve neck, trunk, arms, along with focal dystonia in the form of torticollis and arm dystonia; is often associated with behavioral issues; treatment includes benzodiazepines, valproate, and trihexyphenidyl
DYT-1 dystonia	Dystonia that starts in one limb progressing to generalized dystonia with age at onset being 10 years, variation in progression, does not respond to L-dopa

(GTP: guanosine triphosphate)

Step 9: Summary, Differential Diagnosis, and Planning Investigation

Summarize under following subheadings:
- Age and gender
- Consanguinity and family history
- Prior development
- Age at onset
- Is it normal or abnormal?
- Is it hyperkinetic or hypokinetic?
- What parts of body are involved?
- What is the type and description of movement disorder (does it subside

TABLE 9: Genetic diseases presenting with movement disorder (progressive myoclonus epilepsy).

Genetic disease	Classical clinical features
DRPLA (dentato-rubropallido-luysial atrophy)	Late onset >10 years; features of cerebellar ataxia, cognitive decline, choreoathetoid movement with myoclonus; MRI brain showing pontocerebellar ataxia
Myoclonic epilepsy with ragged red fiber (MERRF)	Progressive myoclonic epilepsy in a child with short stature, deafness, peripheral neuropathy, raised CSF lactate; maternal inheritance
Lafora disease	Presence of visual hallucination, occipital seizures, and rapid course of progressive myoclonic epilepsy; MRI brain showing cerebellar atrophy; skin biopsy showing Lafora bodies (PAS+ve cytoplasmic inclusion)
Unverricht disease	Disabling myoclonus; stimulus sensitive myoclonus; other seizure types; onset 6–16 years; relatively preserved cognition and slowly progressive disease in a child with PME phenotype; giant SSEP (somatosensory evoked potentials); EEG showing slow background with generalized spike wave discharges
Sialidosis	Progressive visual loss with fundus showing cherry-red spot in a child with progressive myoclonic epilepsy with cerebellar ataxia; MRI brain showing cortical and cerebellar atrophy
Subacute sclerosing panencephalitis	PME in a child with or without past history of measles, fundus showing perimacular chorioretinitis, EEG showing periodic complexes of generalized spike and polyspike wave complexes; nonspecific asymmetric white matter changes on MRI; CSF antimeasles antibody positive; drug treatment—isoprinosine, and interferon-α

(CSF: cerebrospinal fluid; EEG: electroencephalography; PAS: periodic acid–Schiff; PME: progressive myoclonus epilepsy)

BOX 2: Classification of myoclonus.

Myoclonus can be localized to cortical, brainstem, spinal, or segmental myoclonus:
- *Cortical myoclonus:* Involves upper limb/face, action myoclonus, focal, affect speech, and gait
- *Subcortical (brainstem) myoclonus:* Generalized, stimulus sensitive (auditory), e.g., hyperekplexia
- *Spinal myoclonus:* Involves few contiguous spinal segments; no relation to sleep/action/stimulus
- *Peripheral myoclonus:* Mostly involves a segment supplied by root, nerve, or plexus lesion

BOX 3: Example depicting how to present a movement disorder.

A 2-year-old boy presented with abnormal (*normal or abnormal*) body movement involving all the four limbs (*parts of the body involved*) in the form of twisting postures (*nature of abnormal movement*) of upper limb, especially when trying to approach an object and fixed postures in lower limb when made to lie down supine. These movements are nearly continuous (*paroxysmal, continuous, or continual*) and increase when he cries or gets emotionally charged (*change with emotion*) and subside totally when he sleeps (*change with sleep*). There are no associated flowing (*choreiform*) or distal writhing (*athetoid*) movements or any electric shock like jerks (*myoclonic*). These movements probably suggest generalized dystonia

with sleep; does it increase with stress or emotions?
- What is the most probable etiology?

Box 3 provides an example of how to describe a movement disorder.

CASE VIGNETTES

Case 1

A 3-year-old boy, born to nonconsanguineously married couple with no significant family history, presented with global developmental delay and abnormal movement since 8–9 months of age. These movements were hyperkinetic, consisting of abnormal twisting postures of both upper limb and lower limb that increases on crying or getting excited. It subsides in sleep, and during the wakeful state, it is present continuously. The baby was born by vaginal delivery and cried immediately at birth. He developed neonatal jaundice on day 2 of life, requiring exchange transfusion.

Analysis

Considering the static course, the possibility of dyskinetic cerebral palsy secondary to bilirubin-induced neurological dysfunction can be considered. MRI brain to look for globus pallidus involvement could clinch the diagnosis of kernicterus. Had there been no history of jaundice with MRI brain showing bilateral globus pallidus involvement, neurometabolic causes including mitochondrial disorders, and organic acidemia (methylmalonic acidemia) needs to be considered. The following text summarizes the steps of analysis in arriving at the diagnosis of generalized dystonia secondary to kernicterus.

Description of movement	Case
Is it normal or abnormal movement?	Abnormal movement disorder
Is it hyperkinetic or hypokinetic?	It is hyperkinetic movement
Parts of body involved	Abnormal twisting postures involve upper limb, lower limb with arching of back, and neck, suggestive of generalized dystonia
Paroxysmal/continual/continuous	It is nearly continuous for the entire day
Change over time	Almost the same since beginning, marginal improvement with age

Contd...

Contd...

Rest/action/specific posture	It subsides with rest and exacerbated when the child attempts to reach an object
Response to emotional stress/stimuli	Yes. These movements increase when child is being handled like changing his clothes, being taken in lap, and while crying
Does it subside with sleep?	Yes. These movements subside with sleep
Awareness of movement, voluntary suppression, and premonitory urge	Difficult to assess in children with developmental delay and intellectual disability

Case 2

A 10-year-old girl, student of class 5, presents with abnormal flowing movements of the upper limbs and lower limbs for 3 weeks. These movements were preceded by a history of sore throat 40 days back.

Analysis

The following text narrates the steps of analysis in arriving at the diagnosis of choreoathetoid movement. New onset of abnormal involuntary, bizarre, continuous, quasipurposive flowing movement involving all four limbs that increases with stress and subsides with sleep in the background history of the sore throat could point to parainfectious etiology. Among parainfectious causes, Sydenham chorea, basal ganglia encephalitis, autoimmune basal ganglia disease, and paraneoplastic involvement of basal ganglia can be kept as differential diagnoses. In an Indian setup, Sydenham chorea is the most prevalent cause of new-onset chorea. Hence, the first investigation to be considered is antistreptolysin (ASO) antibody levels. If ASO titers are elevated, further evaluation for rheumatic chorea can be considered, which includes erythrocyte sedimentation rate/C-reactive protein (ESR/CRP) (to look for rheumatic activity), electrocardiography (ECG) (to look for PR interval), and echocardiography (to look for underlying rheumatic heart disease). If ASO titers were negative, MRI brain to look for structural causes and further autoimmune, paraneoplastic workup needs to be planned.

Description of movement	Case
Is it normal or abnormal movement?	These movements cannot be considered normal for this age
Is it hyperkinetic or hypokinetic?	It is hyperkinetic movement
Parts of body involved	They are bizarre, chaotic, continuous movement involving upper limb, neck, trunk flowing from one part to another part of the body
Paroxysmal/continual/continuous	It is nearly continuous through the day
Change over time	It was worst at the beginning; it gradually improves with time
Rest/action/specific posture	It decreases but does not subside with rest and exacerbated when she attempts to perform any activity
Response to emotional stress/stimuli	Yes. These movements increase while she is closely watched or observed. It also increases when she gets emotional or stressful
Does it subside with sleep?	Yes. These movements subside with sleep
Awareness of movement, voluntary suppression, and premonitory urge	She is aware of movement and tries to hide these movements as if performing some action (semipurposive). There is a premonitory urge. She cannot suppress these movements

Case 3

A 6-year-old boy presented with an abnormal twisting posture of the body for the last 18 months. In addition, he has difficulty in speech (dysarthria) and eating (dysphagia). He can understand, comprehend, and respond by appropriate gestures. He has constant drooling of saliva. He was ambulatory till 6 months back, and gradually twisting postures have worsened to make him bedridden now. These movements are rather continuous, worsen with emotion, stress, and while trying to perform some action, and it totally subsides during sleep. Prior to the onset of illness, he was going to playschool and performing well when compared to his peers. There was no fever, seizure, encephalopathy, head trauma at the onset of illness (to rule out static insult). There was no history of drug intake (to rule out drug-induced movement disorder). His examination revealed normocephaly, with no neurocutaneous markers. Fundus revealed pigmentary retinopathy. There were no Kayser–Fleischer (KF) rings on the slit-lamp examination. There was evidence of severe generalized dystonia involving both upper and lower limbs with extensor posturing of trunk, resulting in arching of the back.

Analysis

This appears to be a neurodegenerative disease with extrapyramidal manifestation with pigmentary retinopathy with age at onset being 4.5 years with no family history. It appears to be genetic or neurometabolic disease considering the progressive course. MRI brain needs to be obtained to look for "eye of tiger sign" in PKAN (pantothenate kinase-associated neurodegeneration), "leukodystrophy" as in metachromatic leukodystrophy, bulky basal ganglia with hypomyelination in GM2 gangliosidosis. Normal MRI favors the diagnosis of primary/

genetic dystonia that includes DYT-1 and DYT-5. Fundus revealing pigmentary retinopathy favors the diagnosis of PKAN and NCL.

Case 4

An 8-year-old girl presented with complaints of sudden jerks while walking with aggressive and disruptive behavior for the last 2 months. These jerks were paroxysmal, non-rhythmic in nature involving the neck, trunk, upper, and lower limb. It occurs both in rest and action. There is no relation to auditory stimuli. It occurs throughout the day as well as in sleep. It is not aggravated with emotional stress. There is no preceding urge, no associated abnormal flowing movement, twisting posture, or distal writhing movement. There is a progressive decline in cognition, and abnormal hyperactive, aggressive, and disruptive behavior noticed for 2 months. There are no focal neurological signs. Fundus evaluation is normal.

Analysis

This case study points to progressive neurodegenerative disease with myoclonus with cognitive decline (progressive myoclonic epilepsy) and behavioral problems for 2 months. Considering the epidemiological context, SSPE remains the first possibility. Electroencephalography (EEG) would reveal periodic discharges, and further confirmation can be done by cerebrospinal fluid (CSF) antimeasles antibody. If EEG did not reveal characteristic periodic discharges, MRI brain needs to be planned to look for other possibilities such as neuronal ceroid lipofuscinosis (cerebellar atrophy), myoclonic epilepsy with ragged red fiber (MERRF) (basal ganglia involvement), Unverricht–Lundborg disease, and Lafora body disease.

Case 5

A 13-year-old boy presented with an abnormal rhythmic jerky movement of head and eyelid that persists the whole day for last 2.5 years. He says he can control those movements for a little while but has an urge to perform them. The mother notices that he behaves a little oddly, keeps checking his bag and purse for some missing object. He has become very stubborn, argues, and fights with his sibling. His school grades have started dropping, and his mother faces a lot of complaints during the parent–teacher meetings. There are no affected family members. Neurological examination is unremarkable.

Analysis

This is a child with chronic tic disorder with predominant motor tics. The presence of behavior problems favors the possibility of Tourette syndrome (genetic cause).

Case 6

A 10-year-old girl presented with tremulous movements of outstretched hands for the duration of the last 2 years. These tremors are more evident while approaching and handling any object. These movements never occur during rest. Her school performance has been good. There is no abnormal behavior. Both father and grandfather have similar tremors while handling fine objects. Grandfather is now unable to hold objects and has lost his handwriting. There is no history of drug intake. There is no history of excessive sweating or heat intolerance to suggest hyperthyroidism. Examination reveals postural tremors.

Analysis

Coarse postural tremors (nonprogressive) with intact cognition and strong autosomal-dominant inheritance favor the diagnosis of benign essential tremors. We do not expect any changes in imaging; hence, probably there is no need for MRI brain. In the absence of any significant family history in an adolescent with new onset of bizarre uncharacterizable movement disorder, keep a possibility of psychogenic movement disorder.

Functional (psychogenic) movement disorder can include multiple bizarre, reproducible movements such as abnormal gait, violent flinging movements, and other complex movements that could not be characterized into any known type of movement disorder. It often occurs in the awake state, in the presence of other family members, no resultant injuries, and has the background of stressful family or school environment. This is a diagnosis of exclusion and needs to be kept in mind, especially in adolescent females with stressful family situations such as broken family, frequent fights and quarrels, and stressful academic expectations.

KEY MESSAGES

- Movement disorder can be hyperkinetic or hypokinetic movement disorder.
- Hyperkinetic movement disorder includes chorea (dancing/flowing movement), dystonia (abnormal twisting postures), athetosis (distal writhing movement), myoclonus (shock-like movement), tics (suppressible and involuntary movement with premonitory urge), and tremors (rhythmic oscillatory movement).
- Type of movement disorder can be characterized by body part involved, its relationship with rest/action/posture/sleep/emotion/stress, presence of urge, suppressibility of movement, prior developmental level, and family history of movement disorder.
- Emphasize on the description of movement disorder rather than arriving at classifying the movement disorder into chorea, athetosis, dystonia, and myoclonus, as majority of the movement disorders are mixed.
- Home video records are a very useful adjunct to the analysis of the symptoms.

CHAPTER 18

Approach to Diagnosis of Ataxia

INTRODUCTION

Ataxia is defined as a disturbance in fine control of posture and movement or inability to perform a smooth, coordinated, and voluntary motor act. It may involve the movement of the limb (limb ataxia) or trunk (truncal ataxia). Limb ataxia results in difficulty in performing a task, whereas truncal ataxia results in titubation while sitting. Ataxic disorders can also involve motor speech system and eye movement. The ataxia most commonly presents with an abnormal gait, which is often wide-based and lurching. Many parents describe their child's walking is like that of a drunk person. Young ataxic children often refuse to walk and get cranky when made to stand unsupported.

It can result from dysfunction of the cerebellum (cerebellar ataxia), its major inputs from the frontal lobe, posterior columns of the spinal cord (sensory ataxia), or from vestibular involvement (vestibular ataxia) **(Table 1)**. Based on the onset and progression of ataxia, it can be divided into *acute* (hours to days), *subacute* (week to months), or *chronic* (months to years). The most common causes of acute ataxia in children are acute cerebellar ataxia and drug-induced ataxia. Friedreich ataxia is the most common hereditary form of chronic or progressive ataxia.

What is not considered as ataxia?

Gait instability can also result from motor corticospinal tract involvement resulting in spasticity [upper motor neuron (UMN) weakness] or flaccidity [lower motor neuron (LMN) weakness]. Most of the authors prefer to keep gait instability resulting from motor weakness (flaccidity or spasticity) out of the terminology of ataxia. For example, children

TABLE 1: Comparison of clinical features of cerebellar, sensory, and vestibular ataxia.

	Cerebellar ataxia	Sensory ataxia	Vestibular ataxia
Ataxia	Limb or truncal ataxia	Limb ataxia	Truncal ataxia
Dysarthria	Present	Absent	Absent
Nystagmus	Present	Absent	Present
Vertigo	Absent	Absent	Present
Hypotonia	Present	Absent	Absent
Deep tendon reflexes	Pendular	Absent	Normal
Romberg sign	Absent	Present	Absent
Vibration and position sense	Normal	Diminished	Normal

with spastic diplegic cerebral palsy can present with gait instability and repeated falls. Similarly, children with Duchenne muscular dystrophy can also present with repeated falls and waddling gait. These gait instabilities resulting from UMN or LMN weakness are not classified under ataxia.

Similarly, Guillain–Barré syndrome and Miller–Fisher syndrome can also present with acute ataxia. Ataxia, areflexia, and ophthalmoplegia with variable cranial nerve involvement are seen among children with Miller–Fisher syndrome. Movement disorders such as chorea, choreoathetosis, ballismus, and myoclonus can also result in gait disturbance and repeated falls. These disorders are discussed in **Chapter 17**. To re-emphasize, motor weakness and movement disorders are *not* labeled as ataxia and hence, not discussed further in this chapter.

LOCALIZATION OF LESION: NEUROANATOMY

Ataxia can result from a cerebellar, posterior column, or vestibular involvement **(Table 1)**. The involvement of the cerebellum and its afferent and efferent pathways, including spinocerebellar pathway and fronto-ponto-cerebellar pathway originating in frontal lobe, can result in ataxia.

- *Cerebellar hemispheric lesions* can result in tendency to fall in the direction of the affected hemisphere with decreased tone in the ipsilateral limb (*limb ataxia*). It may also lead to tremors, dysmetria, and speech abnormalities.
- Lesion involving *cerebellar vermis* results in *truncal ataxia* wherein the child is unable to sit still and moves the body to and fro with the bobbing of head (titubation).
- *Bilateral frontal lobe dysfunction* can also result in ataxia and is often indistinguishable clinically from those due to cerebellar hemispheric involvement.
- The presence of *unilateral ataxia* might suggest an underlying focal structural involvement of the cerebellum.

Posterior column disease can result in ataxia (*sensory ataxia*) wherein the child tends to walk carefully and keep looking at their feet for finding the location in space. It leads to high stepping gait (foot raises high with each step and falls heavily), and this gait worsens with the closing of eyes (*Romberg sign*). Ataxia, when associated with vertigo, dizziness, and lightheadedness, can be due to vestibular nerve or labyrinthine involvement (*labyrinthine ataxia*).

CLINICAL APPROACH TO CHILD WITH ACUTE ATAXIA

Common causes of acute ataxia in children include postinfectious acute cerebellar ataxia and drug-induced ataxia. **Box 1** provides a list of causes of acute ataxia in children. Evaluation of a child with acute ataxia requires baseline knowledge of the causes of acute ataxia. History and examination need to be focused to determine the etiology. Clinical pearls in acute ataxia have been summarized in **Table 2**.

History and Examination

Following points in the history and examination help in arriving at the clinical diagnosis of the cause of acute ataxia:
- Look for following *clinical features of cerebellar dysfunction:*
  - Ataxia (disturbance in the smooth performance of voluntary motor acts)
  - Intentional tremor (tremors of hands when the child attempts to make a directed movement)

BOX 1: Causes of acute/recurrent ataxia in children.

- *Drug ingestion:*
  - Anticonvulsant-like phenytoin
  - Antihistaminics
- *Postinfectious/immune causes:*
  - Acute postinfectious cerebellitis (acute cerebellar ataxia)
  - Miller–Fisher syndrome
  - Multiple sclerosis
  - Myoclonic encephalopathy/neuroblastoma syndrome
- *Trauma:*
  - Hematoma
  - Postconcussion
  - Vertebrobasilar occlusion
- *Migraine:*
  - Basilar migraine
  - Benign paroxysmal vertigo
- *Brainstem encephalitis genetic causes:*
  - Episodic ataxia type 1 and type 2
  - Hartnup disease
  - Maple syrup urine disease
  - Pyruvate dehydrogenase (PDH) deficiency
- *Other causes:* Brain tumor

TABLE 2: Clinical pearls to reach a diagnosis of acute ataxia.

Key features	Diagnosis
Acute cerebellar ataxia with preceding viral prodrome	Acute cerebellar ataxia (postinfectious)
Acute ataxia following drug overdosage	Phenytoin toxicity and AED toxicity
Acute ataxia, areflexia, hypotonia, and muscle weakness	Guillain–Barré syndrome
Ataxia, areflexia, and ophthalmoplegia	Miller–Fisher syndrome
Ataxia, ophthalmoplegia, cranial nerve palsy, and altered sensorium	Bickerstaff brainstem encephalitis
Ataxia, altered sensorium, and features of raised ICP	ICSOL (brain tumor) or posterior circulation stroke
Ataxia, irritability, and opsoclonus	Opsoclonus myoclonus ataxia syndrome
Ataxia, vomiting, nausea, and nystagmus	Labyrinthitis
Headache, ataxia, and vomiting with or without cranial nerve palsy	Basilar migraine

(AED: antiepileptic drugs; ICP: intracranial pressure; ICSOL: intracranial space-occupying lesion)

- Dysmetria (overshoot/undershoot of visual target: tested by finger-to-nose test, finger-to-finger test, and heel-to-shin maneuver)
- Dysdiadochokinesia (impaired performance of rapid alternating movement)
- Asynergia (decomposition of complex movement into isolated successive parts)
- Titubation (bobbing of head)
- Dysarthria (abnormality in articulation and prosody of speech)
- Slow, staccato, and scanning speech
- Hypotonia (decrease in muscle tone in response to stretch)
- Nystagmus
- Pendular knee jerk or hyporeflexia

- Look for following *clinical features of posterior column dysfunction:*
  - Impairment on foot tapping, heel and toe walking, and tandem walking
  - Positive Romberg sign
- Look for *clinical features of vestibular dysfunction:*
  - Vertigo maximal at the onset which can progress to ataxia when severe
  - Associated nystagmus
  - Episodic in nature

- *Progression of ataxia:*
  - Acute ataxia with rapid improvement (drug-induced and acute cerebellar ataxia)
  - Acute ataxia with a prolonged or intermittent course (myoclonic encephalopathy neuroblastoma syndrome, multiple sclerosis, and metabolic disorders)
- *Clinical points to establish the etiology of acute ataxia:*
  - Features of ipsilateral cerebellar signs, ipsilateral cranial nerve involvement, and contralateral weakness, with headache and altered sensorium, suggest *intracranial space-occupying lesion of cerebellum.*
  - History of drug intake (anticonvulsants such as carbamazepine and phenytoin, antihistaminic, and dextromethorphan) must be elicited. *Drug-induced ataxia* is often associated with downbeat nystagmus and vomiting.
  - History of head trauma/sport injury/injury to the neck (vertebrobasilar artery injury) should be obtained.
  - If a child with acute ataxia has severe throbbing headache associated with abrupt and transient loss of consciousness, visual loss, vertigo, tinnitus, hemiparesis, or paresthesia of fingers/toes/corners of the mouth, we need to think of *basilar migraine.*
  - Family history of migraine (*basilar migraine*)
  - History of preceding viral infection suggests postinfective/immune causes
  - Ataxia in a child with multiple cranial nerve palsy with or without altered sensorium and features of raised intracranial pressure would raise a possibility of *posterior circulation stroke.*
  - Nausea, vomiting, and nystagmus in a child with a history suggestive of otitis media are suggestive of *labyrinthitis.*
  - *Conversion reaction* can also present like acute ataxia. Neurological examination is usually unremarkable. A child with conversion reaction can usually sit without difficulty but when brought to stand, begins to sway from the waist.
  - Presence of ataxia along with ophthalmoplegia (involvement of upgaze followed by the lateral gaze and downgaze), areflexia, and associated motor weakness in limbs is a point to suggest *Miller–Fisher syndrome.*
  - Multiple cranial nerve palsy, antecedent febrile illness, and ophthalmoplegia in a child with acute ataxia when associated with altered sensorium suggest a possibility of *Bickerstaff brainstem encephalitis.*
  - In a child with recurrent episodes of ataxia lasting for <10 minutes with a complete recovery in between the episodes, one must consider a possibility of episodic ataxia type 1. This condition is often confused with seizure.
  - Past history of motor weakness or vision loss indicates prior demyelinating disease (*multiple sclerosis or neuromyelitis optica*).
  - Observe for clinical features of myokymia of face/hand/arm during the episodes of ataxia with hand posture resembling carpopedal spasm (*episodic ataxia type 1*).
  - History of developmental delay or regression points to underlying aminoaciduria [*Hartnup disease* or *maple syrup urine disease*, pyruvate dehydrogenase (PDH) deficiency, or biotinidase deficiency].

- Ask for a history of photosensitivity with pellagra-like rash after sunlight exposure (*Hartnup disease*).
- Abnormal urinary odor needs to be enquired (*maple syrup urine disease*)
- Look for features of chaotic eye movement (opsoclonus), ataxia, and irritability in a child younger than 3 years which strongly suggest the possibility of *opsoclonus myoclonus ataxia syndrome.*
- Failure to thrive, anemia, short stature, vomiting, diarrhea, and ataxia often point to *gluten-sensitive enteropathy.*

Investigations for Acute Ataxia

Investigation must be used judiciously for evaluating a child with acute ataxia. It will largely depend on the clinical possibilities raised by history and examination.

- *Drug screening* (measurement of drug levels in the blood) is a must in all suspected cases of drug-induced ataxia.
- *Neuroimaging* of the head is essential in all cases of acute ataxia to rule out intracranial space-occupying lesion, especially those involving cerebellum or posterior fossa lesions [magnetic resonance imaging (MRI) head] and cases with a history of head trauma [noncontrast computed tomography (NCCT) head]. Some of the common MRI findings in various causes of acute ataxia are summarized in **Table 3**.
- *Lumbar puncture* is indicated in suspected brainstem encephalitis [cerebrospinal fluid (CSF)] shows mononuclear pleocytosis and raised protein and Miller–Fisher syndrome (in early stages, CSF shows lymphocytic pleocytosis and later protein elevation).
- *Electroencephalogram* (EEG) has a limited role in evaluation, except in children with suspected pseudoataxia (where epilepsy presents like ataxia), which shows prolonged, generalized 2–3 Hz spike-wave complex with frontal dominance. EEG can show occipital intermittent delta activity in basilar migraine.
- *Brainstem-evoked auditory response audiometry* (BERA) can show prolonged interpeak latencies in cases of brainstem encephalitis.
- *Urinary excretion of homovanillic acid* (HVA) and *vanillylmandelic acid* (VMA) is elevated in myoclonus encephalopathy and neuroblastoma syndrome. Children with opsoclonus myoclonus ataxia syndrome (OMAS) are screened for occult neuroblastoma using urinary VMA and

TABLE 3: Magnetic resonance imaging (MRI) findings in children with acute ataxia.

MRI findings	Possible diagnosis
Bilateral asymmetric white matter lesion, variable cerebellar, basal ganglia, and thalamus involvement	Acute disseminated encephalomyelitis and clinically isolated syndrome
Contrast enhancement of cochlea	Labyrinthitis
Cerebellar hyperintensity with diffusion restriction	Acute cerebellitis
T2 hyperintense lesions in brainstem	Brainstem encephalitis (enteroviral, varicella, and listeria)
T2 hyperintensity in pons, midbrain, thalamus, and cerebellum	Posterior circulation stroke
Normal MRI study	Basilar migraine, pseudoataxia, opsoclonus-myoclonus-ataxia syndrome, conversion reaction, and acute cerebellar ataxia

HVA levels. These levels can be normal among children with OMAS.
- *Electromyography* (EMG) can show continuous motor unit activities in hands in children suspected of episodic ataxia type 2.
- *Lactic acid levels* are elevated in children with PDH deficiency and other mitochondrial disorders.
- *Metabolic screen:* Urine amino acid, plasma amino acid, lactate, pyruvate, cholesterol, and lipoprotein estimation may be required to rule in/out genetic/metabolic disease.

Diagnosis

Majority of the final diagnosis is based on a cluster of symptoms, signs, and findings on neuroimaging. **Flowchart 1** provides a general outline on the approach to a child with acute ataxia. Following clinical points may help to arrive at the diagnosis of children with acute ataxia:

When to think of postinfectious cerebellar ataxia and cerebellitis?
- Sudden onset of cerebellar ataxia in children following an infectious illness such as varicella, Epstein–Barr virus (EBV), and *Mycoplasma* infection in toddlers (mean age 2–4 years)
- Latency from infection to ataxia ranges from mean of 9–11 days.
- Majority of these children recover within few months from onset.
- If imaging evidence reveals cerebellar edema and clinical features of raised intracranial pressure are present, then "cerebellitis" needs to be kept as a differential diagnosis. MRI may reveal cerebellar hyperintensities in acute cerebellitis **(Figs. 1A and B)**. Cerebellitis may result in obstructive hydrocephalus that needs to be recognized. Moreover, a majority of patients with cerebellitis will have an ongoing fever and may demonstrate CSF pleocytosis.

When to think of clinical isolated syndrome or acute disseminated encephalomyelitis as cause of ataxia?
- The first demyelinating central nervous system (CNS) event with [acute disseminated encephalomyelitis (ADEM)] or without [clinically isolated syndrome (CIS)] encephalopathy can present with

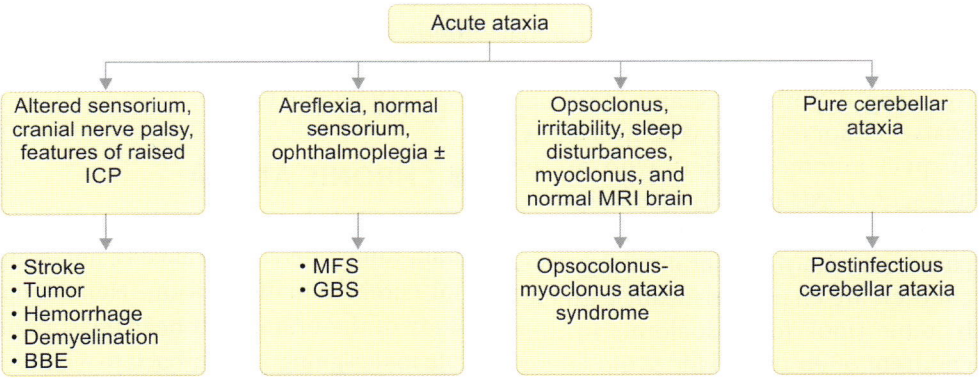

Flowchart 1: Clinical approach to a child with acute ataxia.

(BBE: Bickerstaff brainstem encephalitis; GBS: Guillain–Barré syndrome; ICP: intracranial pressure; MFS: Miller–Fisher syndrome)

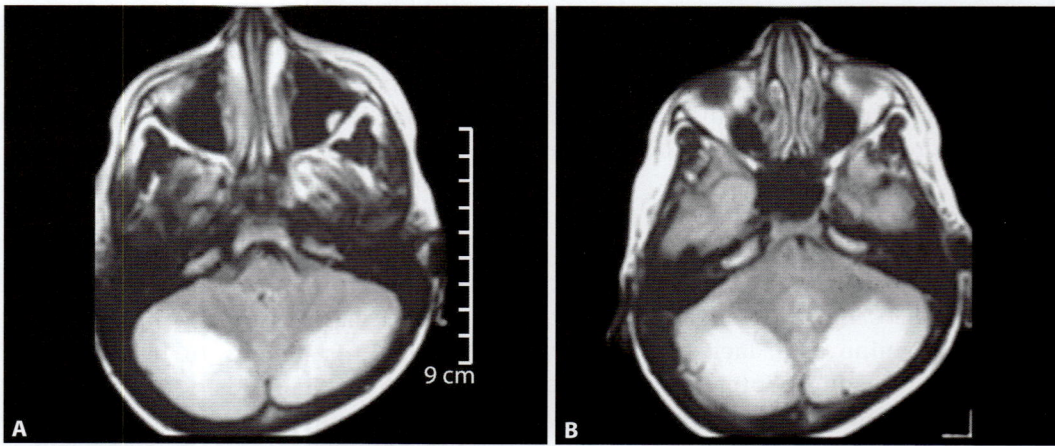

Figs. 1A and B: Magnetic resonance imaging (MRI) brain T2 axial showing bilateral symmetrical hyperintensities in cerebellar hemispheres suggestive of acute cerebellitis.

acute ataxia. If there is a past history of the demyelinating event, the possibility of multiple sclerosis needs consideration.
- Encephalopathy can present with irritability, sleepiness, obtundation, or coma. The presence of encephalopathy differentiates it from postinfectious cerebellar ataxia and warrants neuroimaging as well.
- MRI brain showing asymmetric, discrete white matter lesions in cerebrum and cerebellum

When to think of opsoclonus-myoclonus ataxia syndrome?
- Presence of ataxia, opsoclonus (rapid chaotic multidirectional including diagonal movement of eyeball), extreme irritability, sleep disturbances, and prominent coarse tremor recognized as myoclonus
- Suspect among toddlers who present like acute ataxia but either not improving or ataxia having waxing and waning course with normal neuroimaging. These children are characteristically extremely irritable (look for opsoclonus in these children; often these kids avoid looking straight and prefer keeping their eyes shut).

Ataxia not explainable by any of the above etiology should always be evaluated for autoimmune/paraneoplastic cause, including anti-Ho/anti-Yo antibody and anti-TPO antibody (Hashimoto disease). One should also look for systemic causes such as celiac disease and HIV infection.

When to think of episodic ataxia?
Presence of multiple brief episodes of wobbliness often associated with dizziness and vomiting should raise the possibility of episodic ataxia. These episodes are commonly misinterpreted as focal seizures. **Table 4** outlines the key differences between the two most common types of episodic ataxia (EA-1 and EA-2).

■ CHRONIC ATAXIA

Causes of chronic/progressive ataxia include brain tumor, hereditary ataxias, and congenital cerebral malformation. Neuroimaging study of the brain (MRI head) has a crucial role in designing an approach to a child with chronic ataxia. Causes of chronic ataxia are enumerated in **Box 2**. Broadly, we can divide

TABLE 4: Key differences between episodic ataxia type 1 and type 2.	
Episodic ataxia type 1	**Episodic ataxia type 2**
KCNA1 gene mutation	*CACNA1A* gene mutation
Late childhood	Late childhood/adolescents
Brief attacks of ataxia, dysarthria, weakness, tremors, with loss of coordination that lasts for seconds to minute often confused with focal seizures	Longer attacks of ataxia, headache, vertigo, nystagmus, dysarthria, and diplopia lasting for hours to days
It is often precipitated by sudden change in posture	50% have migraine
Interictal myokymia over face, arm, and hands	Interictal nystagmus, pursuit, and saccadic eye movement
Dramatic response to acetazolamide/phenytoin	Poor response to acetazolamide; phenytoin to be avoided
MRI brain normal; CPK normal	MRI brain may show progressive cerebellar atrophy

(CPK: creatine phosphokinase; MRI: magnetic resonance imaging)

BOX 2: Differential diagnosis of a child with chronic or progressive ataxia.

- Brain tumor:
  - Cerebellar astrocytoma
  - Cerebellar hemangioblastoma (von Hippel–Lindau disease)
  - Ependymoma
  - Medulloblastoma
  - Supratentorial tumors
- Hereditary ataxia:
  - *Autosomal recessive inheritance*:
    - Abetalipoproteinemia
    - Ataxia telangiectasia
    - Friedreich ataxia
    - Hartnup disease
    - Juvenile GM2 gangliosidosis
    - Refsum disease
    - Wilson disease
    - MSUD (maple syrup urine disease)
    - Pyruvate dehydrogenase deficiency
    - Ramsay–Hunt syndrome
  - *Autosomal dominant inheritance*:
    - Olivopontocerebellar degeneration
    - Machado–Joseph disease
  - *X-linked inheritance*:
    - Adrenoleukodystrophy
    - Leber's optic neuropathy
- Congenital malformations:
  - Basilar impression
  - Cerebellar aplasia
  - Dandy–Walker malformation
  - Vermal aplasia
  - Chiari malformation

chronic ataxia as *progressive ataxia* versus *nonprogressive ataxia*. We consider congenital malformations of cerebellum including cerebellar aplasia, Chiari malformation, Dandy–Walker malformation, vermal aplasia, and Joubert syndrome to present with nonprogressive ataxia. Progressive ataxia includes brain tumors (astrocytoma, hemangioblastoma, ependymoma, and medulloblastoma) and hereditary disorders such as ataxia telangiectasia (AT), Friedreich ataxia (FA), and ataxia with oculomotor apraxia. Based on the predominant clinical feature, chronic ataxia can be divided into pure cerebellar ataxia or those with other clinical features (complicated ataxia) **(Flowchart 2)**.

Metabolic disorders that can present with progressive ataxia include mitochondrial disorders, peroxisomal disorders (Refsum disease and adrenoleukodystrophy), leukodystrophy (Canavan, Alexander, Pelizaeus–Merzbacher disease, and vanishing white matter disorder), lysosomal storage disease (Krabbe disease, metachromatic leukodystrophy, and Niemann–Pick disease type C), congenital disorders of glycosylation,

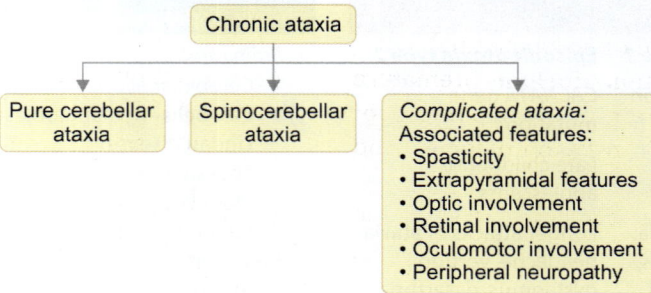

Flowchart 2: Clinical features of chronic ataxia.

TABLE 5: Treatable causes of chronic ataxia.	
Etiology of ataxia	**Possible treatment**
Abetalipoproteinemia	Vitamin E
Ataxia with vitamin E deficiency	Vitamin E
Biotinidase deficiency	Biotin
Cerebrotendinous xanthomatosis	Chenodeoxycholic acid
Coenzyme Q (CoQ) deficiency	CoQ
Episodic ataxia type 1/2	Acetazolamide
Friedreich ataxia (Not treatable)	Possible role of CoQ, vitamin E, and idebenone
Hartnup disease	Nicotinamide
PDH deficiency	Ketogenic diet

(PDH: pyruvate dehydrogenase)

and abetalipoproteinemia. One of the main objectives of the evaluation of a child with chronic ataxia is *not* to miss treatable causes **(Table 5)**. The most common causes of chronic ataxia include AT, ataxia with oculomotor apraxia, Friedreich ataxia, and spinocerebellar ataxia (SCA). Among these, Friedreich ataxia is the most common hereditary form of chronic and progressive ataxia. Some of the key clinical, radiological, and laboratory features of these common conditions are summarized here.

BOX 3: Causes of early onset cerebellar ataxia.
- Ataxia telangiectasia
- Ataxia with oculomotor apraxia
- Adrenomyeloneuropathy
- Hartnup disease
- Niemann–Pick disease type C
- Metachromatic leukodystrophy
- Sialidosis

Diagnosis

When to think of ataxia telangiectasia?
- Progressive early-onset cerebellar ataxia with onset in the 1st year of life once the child learns to walk **(Box 3)**.
- The clinical features of progressive cerebellar ataxia with oculomotor apraxia (disruption of smooth pursuit movement) and oculocutaneous telangiectasia (site—auricle, nasal bridge, and antecubital fossa) point to ataxia–telangiectasia.
- Presence of choreoathetosis/dystonia in the early phase when the child learns to walk is common; by 10 years of age, they have truncal ataxia, tremors, dysarthria, dysphagia, peripheral neuropathy, and most are bedridden by 12 years of age.
- An important feature of AT is preserved cognition till end.
- Features that strongly suggest AT include recurrent sinopulmonary infections (leading to chronic bronchitis) (decrease

in IgA and IgE) and propensity for lymphoreticular malignancy (Hodgkin disease, leukemia, and lymphoma).
- Rare presentations include premature graying of hair, hypertrichosis of forearm, insulin-resistant diabetes, and hypogonadism.
- MRI brain shows cerebellar and vermian atrophy
- Serum AFP (α-fetoprotein) levels and CEA (carcinoembryonic antigen) levels are elevated (AFP may be normal in first 2 years).
- Sequencing of the *ATM* gene or immunoblotting for ATM protein are required for diagnosis.
- Treatment is mainly supportive. The immunological status can be improved by the plasma transfusion of thymosin. These patients are highly sensitive to chemotherapy and radiotherapy, which might impose a significant hurdle in their management in case the child develops lymphoreticular malignancy.

When to think of ataxia with oculomotor apraxia?
- Onset at 4–5 years (AOA1) or later 12–20 years (AOA2) with the presence of progressive cerebellar ataxia, nystagmus, slow saccades (oculomotor apraxia), and dysarthria with areflexia (peripheral neuropathy) that progress to the nonambulatory stage by 7–10 years of age.
- Extrapyramidal features such as choreoathetosis and dystonia can develop in the late stage. Pyramidal features can also be seen in 20% of AOA1.
- Variable cognitive impairment
- Laboratory investigations that support AOA1 are cerebellar atrophy on MRI brain, sensorimotor axonal neuropathy, raised serum AFP level, raised CPK level, hypoalbuminemia, and raised serum cholesterol.
- Genetic diagnosis by confirmation of *APTX* gene mutation (AOA1) and *syntaxin* gene mutation (SETX) (AOA2)
- A possible role of coenzyme Q supplementation in AOA1

Clinical features that are common to AT and AOA are genetically autosomal-recessive inheritance, progressive ataxia with oculomotor apraxia, cerebellar atrophy on imaging, sensorimotor axonal neuropathy, and raised AFP level. Preserved cognition and presence of immunodeficiency with a propensity to recurrent sinopulmonary infection favor AT over AOA.

When to think of Friedreich ataxia?
- Late onset (<10 years) of progressive ataxia (autosomal-recessive inheritance) characterized by slowly progressive gait ataxia associated with nystagmus, slow saccades, absent deep tendon reflexes, and extensor plantar reflex with impaired posterior column dysfunction (Romberg sign). **Box 4** summarizes the key clinical features of conditions that have FA like presentation.
- Other features include cranial nerve involvement [cranial nerve 7 (facial weakness), 9, 10 (dysarthria and dysphagia), scoliosis (60–80%), pes cavus (50–75%), and weakness of lower limb (65–90%)].
- Other features that can be seen in children with FA include retinitis pigmentosa,

---

BOX 4: Differential diagnosis of Friedreich ataxia-like presentation.
- Ataxia with vitamin E deficiency (AVED)
- Refsum disease
- Late onset Tay–Sachs disease
- Cerebrotendinous xanthomatosis
- Infantile-onset spinocerebellar ataxia

cataract, optic atrophy, auditory dysfunction, cardiomyopathy, and diabetes mellitus.
- MRI brain can be normal in the early stages. Atrophy of the cerebellum and spinal cord can be seen late.
- Laboratory investigations that support the diagnosis of FA include sensorimotor axonal neuropathy on nerve conduction study, raised CSF protein.

Features that are common to FA and ataxia with vitamin E deficiency (AVED) are ataxia, dysarthria, areflexia, age at onset, but AVED has no cardiomyopathy, no peripheral neuropathy, and no diabetes. AVED is slowly progressive, and patients have decreased visual acuity. Serum vitamin E levels are low. Mutation in the tocopherol transfer protein gene (*TTPA* gene) is diagnostic. *Refsum disease* is characterized by retinal degeneration, cerebellar degeneration, chronic sensorimotor polyneuropathy, sensorineural hearing loss, ichthyosis, and cardiac abnormalities associated with raised serum phytanic acid.

When to think of spinocerebellar ataxia?
As the name suggests, it refers to a group of genetic disorders with autosomal-dominant inheritance characterized by progressive ataxia and cerebellar atrophy on imaging. It has variable age at onset, can be seen in late childhood, adolescents, and adults. It can result from CAG triplet expansion (SCA 1, 2, 3, 6, 7, and 17) with larger the number of repeats, severe is the phenotype. SCA can also result from a point mutation (SCA types 4, 5, 14, and 37). **Table 6** summarizes the clinical phenotype specific to each type of SCA. Childhood-onset SCA includes SCA 2, 7, 13, 27, and dentatorubral-pallidoluysian atrophy (DRPLA).

TABLE 6: Common clinical features of spinocerebellar ataxia (SCA).

Clinical features	Types of SCA
Slow saccades	SCA2 and –7
Ophthalmoplegia	SCA3, –2, and –1
Downbeat nystagmus	SCA6
Parkinsonian features/spasticity	SCA3 (Machado–Joseph)
Extrapyramidal features	SCA 1, 2, *SCA 3*, 12, 21, 27, DRPLA (chorea)
Areflexia	SCA2, –3, and –4
Seizures	SCA10, DRPLA (myoclonus), SCA7, and –17
Cognitive decline/psychosis	SCA13, SCA17, 21, 27, and DRPLA
Tremors	SCA2, –8, and –12
Pigmentary retinal changes and maculopathy	SCA7
Dopa-responsive dystonia	SCA3
Dysphonia and palatal tremor	SCA20

(DRPLA: dentato-rubro-pallido-luysial atrophy)

When to think of abetalipoproteinemia?
- Abetalipoproteinemia has an autosomal-recessive inheritance, which manifests with fat malabsorption and progressive deficiency of vitamins A, E, and K.
- Infants present with failure to thrive from the beginning with recurrent loose stools and vomiting.
- Psychomotor developmental delay from the beginning
- Ataxia and dysmetria develop in the first decade.
- Loss of proprioceptive sensation in hands and feet

- Retinitis pigmentosa and nystagmus are common in children with abetalipoproteinemia
- Laboratory parameters show anemia, acanthocytosis, low plasma cholesterol, low plasma triglyceride, and absence of apolipoprotein B in plasma.
- Vitamin E supplementation and dietary fat restriction are the available treatment options.

Do not miss vitamin B_{12}-related ataxia (subacute combined degeneration of spinal cord): They commonly present with ataxia with loss of vibration and proprioception. It is sensory ataxia with the presence of Romberg sign. A variable degree of spasticity may be seen. Serum vitamin B_{12} levels may be normal or low. It is one of the most common reversible causes of progressive ataxia.

Brain Tumor Causing Ataxia

Posterior fossa tumors constitute most brain tumors causing ataxia, which includes cerebellar astrocytoma, brainstem glioma, ependymoma, and primitive neuroectodermal tumors (medulloblastoma). Cerebellar astrocytoma most commonly presents in the age group of 5–9 years with headache, unsteadiness of gait, vomiting, papilledema, and signs of cerebellar dysfunction.

Tables 7 and 8 summarize the key clinical features for various etiology of chronic ataxia.

Steps in Clinical Approach to Chronic Ataxia

1. *Static or progressive:* If ataxia was there ever since child started walking and now the same is improving, and imaging reveals congenital malformation of the cerebellum, this is likely to be static etiology for chronic ataxia. No further evaluation will be required for other

TABLE 7: Key clinical features of etiology for chronic ataxia.

Clinical features	Disease
Ichthyosis	Refsum disease
Pellagra-like rash	Hartnup disease
Telangiectasia	Ataxia telangiectasia
Sensorineural hearing loss	Friedreich ataxia and mitochondrial disorders
Abnormal fat distribution	CDG (congenital disorders of glycosylation)
Short stature	Kearns–Sayre syndrome
Diabetes mellitus	Friedreich ataxia
Cataract	Cerebrotendinous xanthomatosis and Marinesco–Sjögren syndrome
Retinitis pigmentosa	Abetalipoproteinemia and Refsum disease

TABLE 8: Clinical features in differential diagnosis of chronic ataxia.

Clinical features	Differentials of chronic ataxia
Extensor plantar	AOA2, FA, and AVED
Chorea and dystonia	AOA1, AOA2, and AT
Cognitive impairment	AOA1, AOA2, CDG, and DRPLA
Epilepsy	CDG, mitochondrial, and biotinidase deficiency
Myoclonus	MERRF and AOA2
Oculomotor apraxia	AT and AOA1/2
Slow saccades	KSS and SCA1/2
Tremors	AVED, AOA1/2, AT, and SCA12
Peripheral neuropathy	FA, AT, abetalipoproteinemia, and Refsum

(AOA: ataxia with oculomotor apraxia; AT: ataxia telangiectasia; AVED: ataxia with vitamin E deficiency; CDG: congenital disorders of glycosylation; FA: Friedreich ataxia; MERRF: myoclonic encephalopathy with ragged red fiber; KSS: Kearns–Sayre syndrome; SCA: spinocerebellar atrophy)

causes of ataxia in such cases, except for genetic workup for congenital malformation if deemed essential.

2. *Age at onset:* Early onset of progressive ataxia is limited to AT, ataxia with oculomotor apraxia, and metabolic causes of progressive ataxia. Late-onset ataxia includes Friedreich ataxia phenotype and spinocerebellar ataxia.
3. *Clinical phenotype:* Clinical phenotype needs differentiation into pure cerebellar type, spinocerebellar type, and complicated ataxia. Look for clinical features of spasticity, extrapyramidal features, oculomotor features, vision, hearing, cognitive decline, seizures, and myoclonus.
4. *Neurological examination:* The objective of neurological examination in a child with chronic ataxia is localization—cerebellar ataxia or sensory ataxia. Sensory ataxia would manifest with positive Romberg sign, loss of joint position sense and vibration, loss of deep tendon reflex (DTR). Common causes of sensory ataxia in children include vitamin B_{12}-related neurological manifestation, vitamin E deficiency, Friedreich ataxia, and Miller–Fisher syndrome.
5. *Summarizing the clinical findings:*
    - Acute/episodic/chronic ataxia
    - Nonprogressive or progressive ataxia
    - Cerebellar syndrome present or absent
    - Cognitive status
    - Clinical evidence of peripheral neuropathy
    - Posterior column sensation
    - Pyramidal, extrapyramidal features, and movement (choreoathetosis and dystonia)
    - Ocular signs (oculomotor apraxia and AT)
    - Age at onset

■ CASE VIGNETTES

A 7-year-old boy presented with wobbly gait and recurrent falls noticed for the last 3 years. He was born to nonconsanguineously married couple. His elder sister, who is 10 years of age, is perfectly fine and going to school. He attained age-appropriate motor milestones and was walking up to nearby school till 4 years of age. His intelligence and school performance are fine but have frequent school absenteeism owing to recurrent respiratory infections requiring hospitalization twice a year. He never had seizures. His examination revealed normal anthropometric variables. He had telangiectasia in both eyes. Higher mental functions were unremarkable. There were slow saccades with evidence of oculomotor apraxia. Motor examination revealed areflexia. Cerebellar signs were present. There were no meningeal signs. The rest of the systemic examination was normal.

Analysis of this Case

- *Age at onset:* 4 years (early onset); early motor development was normal that rules out congenital malformation or a static etiology. Moreover, ataxia is worsening with time. Hence, it is clearly progressive ataxia, which is early onset. Considering the age of onset, AT, AOA, mitochondrial, leukodystrophy, and late onset of gangliosidosis are possibilities. FA and AVED look less likely considering early-onset ataxia.
- *Family history:* Absence of family history, nonconsanguineous parents, and healthy siblings makes autosomal-recessive disorders less likely but does not rule out either.
- *Clinical phenotype of pure cerebellar signs:* Preserved cognition and intelligence with no decline, no seizure, and no pyramidal

or extrapyramidal features in the last 4 years makes other neurometabolic etiology such as mitochondrial disorders, leukodystrophy, gangliosidosis less likely but obviously imaging will clearly help in this regard. Presence of oculomotor apraxia strongly favors AT and AOA. This keeps genetic disorders such as AT and AOA more likely. Evidence of peripheral neuropathy could be possible considering areflexia but will require nerve conduction study. Presence of ocular telangiectasia is pathognomonic of AT in this case.

- *To summarize:* Chronic progressive ataxia with age at onset being 4 years with pure cerebellar ataxia and oculomotor apraxia with ocular telangiectasia, preserved cognition, no pyramidal or extrapyramidal features, possible evidence of peripheral neuropathy, no systemic features, preserved vision and hearing, and no significant family history. Clinical possibility, in this case, would be ataxia–telangiectasia. Other differentials will include ataxia with oculomotor apraxia.

Laboratory Investigations for Chronic Ataxia

- Neuroimaging head (MRI head) to rule out congenital malformation among those with static or nonprogressive ataxia. Most common MRI finding is cerebellar atrophy characterized by cerebellar cortex being thin, shrunken cerebellar folia, large cerebellar fissure, and vermis atrophy. It is seen among AT, AOA1, AOA2, cerebrotendinous xanthomatosis (CTX), SCA, and abetalipoproteinemia. It can also be seen in late-onset Tay–Sachs disease and CTX. Patients with Friedreich ataxia might have cervical spinal cord atrophy. DRPLA might have pontocerebellar atrophy. Cerebellar white matter signal changes can be seen in CTX. SACD (vitamin B_{12} deficiency) might also manifest with signal changes in the spinal cord (inverted U sign). Investigational approach to a child with chronic ataxia is depicted in **Flowchart 3**.
- Sensory and motor nerve conduction studies are required among patients with chronic ataxia. Sensory neuropathy is seen among cases of Friedreich ataxia, AVED, and abetalipoproteinemia. Axonal sensorimotor polyneuropathy can be seen in AT, AOA1, AOA2, and CTX. Refsum disease can have demyelinating neuropathy.
- Electrocardiogram (T-wave changes and features of ventricular hypertrophy) and echocardiography (cardiomyopathy) in cases with Friedreich ataxia.
- *Blood tests for individual clinical entities:*
  - Serum albumin (low) and serum cholesterol (high) (AOA1)
  - Serum α-fetoprotein (AT and AOA1)
  - Peripheral smear for acanthocytes (abetalipoproteinemia)
  - Vitamin E level (AVED and abetalipoproteinemia)
  - Very low-density lipoprotein (VLDL) and low-density lipoprotein (LDL) (abetalipoproteinemia)
  - Serum phytanic acid (Refsum disease)
  - Serum cholesterol and bile alcohol (CTX)
  - Lipoprotein and cholesterol levels (abetalipoproteinemia)
  - IgA, IgE, IgG2, and IgG4 levels (AT)
  - Very long-chain fatty acid levels (adrenoleukodystrophy)
  - Lactate and glucose–lactate tolerance (mitochondrial disorders)
- Urine amino acids (Hartnup disease and maple syrup urine disease)

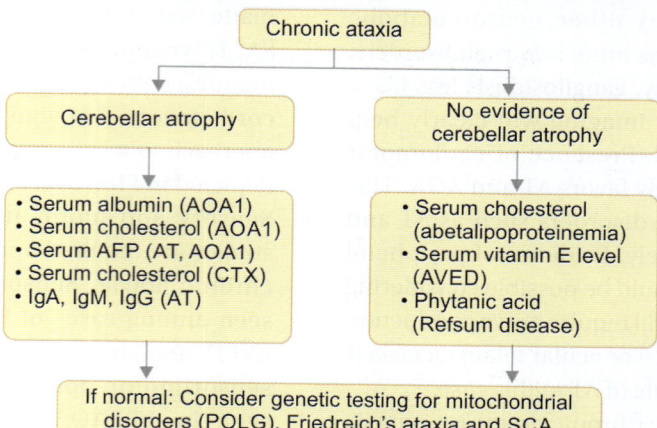

Flowchart 3: Laboratory approach to a child with chronic ataxia.

(AFP: α-fetoprotein; AOA: ataxia with oculomotor apraxia; AT: ataxia telangiectasia; AVED: ataxia with vitamin E deficiency; CTX: cerebrotendinous xanthomatosis; POLG: pathogenic polymerase gamma; SCA: spinocerebellar ataxia)

- Fibroblast activity of hexosaminidase (GM2 gangliosidosis) and phytanic acid (Refsum disease)
- Sea blue histiocytes are seen in bone marrow aspirates of neurovisceral storage diseases.
- Genetic studies (molecular genetic testing) for diagnosis of the type of spinocerebellar atrophy, Friedreich ataxia (*FRDA* gene), and ataxia–telangiectasia (*ATM* gene sequencing).

KEY MESSAGES

- Ataxia can be cerebellar, vestibular, or may be secondary to dysfunction of posterior column.
- Ataxia can present as acute ataxia, episodic ataxia, or chronic ataxia.
- Most common causes of acute ataxia include acute cerebellar ataxia and drug-induced ataxia.
- The most common cause of early-onset chronic ataxia includes ataxia-telangiectasia (AT), and late-onset chronic ataxia is Friedreich ataxia.
- Treatable disorders such as vitamin B_{12} deficiency, vitamin E deficiency, and biotinidase deficiency must not be missed.

CHAPTER 19: Approach to Diagnosis of Headache

■ INTRODUCTION

Headache is defined as pain located in the head, above the orbit-meatal line and nuchal ridge [International Classification of Headache Disorders (ICHD-3)]. It is one of the most common somatic complaints requiring referral to pediatric neurology services. There has been an increase in its incidence considering a significant change in the lifestyle of children. A headache often affects the quality of life, results in school absenteeism, poor academic achievements, decreased school activities, poor sleep, poor memory, and personality change. Prevalence of headache increases throughout childhood with peak at 11–13 years of age. Headache although at outset looks benign can turn to be an ominous symptom. Hence, a systematic evaluation of headache would be essential in all children.

Clinical evaluation of headache is often restricted to history and examination. Investigations have a limited role in the management of a child with headache. Tension-type headache (TTH) is the most common type of primary headache. Sinusitis is the most common cause of secondary headache.

■ TYPES OF HEADACHE

Headache can be broadly divided into a *primary headache* and *secondary headache*.

Primary Headache

Headache that is not attributable to any other causes is labeled as primary headache. **Table 1** outlines the ICHD-3 classification of primary headache. **Table 2** describes the other primary headaches apart from migraine. Among childhood migrainers, prepubertal boys and girls are equally affected. Postpubertal girls are more affected. Migraine without aura is more common than migraine with aura.

Chronic Daily Headache

Chronic daily headaches are those that persist daily or nearly daily. Chronic headache is often associated with fatigue and dizziness. It occurs at least 15 days a month, at least 4 hours a day for a duration of more than 3 months. There are three main types of chronic headache—(1) chronic migraine, (2) chronic TTH, and (3) new-onset persistent headache. If out of 15 days, on at least 8 days a month the headache that occurs has features of migraine headache, it would be considered chronic migraine. If the child has tension headache on at least 15 days a month, it would be considered a chronic tension headache. New-onset persistent headache is a persistent headache daily from the beginning. Pain is moderate, pressing with no associated nausea and vomiting with preceding viral illness. They have no symptoms or signs of

TABLE 1: International Classification of Headache Disorders (ICHD-3).

Types of headache	Classification
Primary headache	
Migraine	• Migraine without aura • *Migraine with aura:* Typical aura, brainstem aura, hemiplegic migraine, and retinal migraine • Chronic migraine • *Complications of migraine:* Status migrainosus, persistent aura without infarction, migrainosus infarction, and migraine aura-triggered seizure • *Probable migraine:* With or without aura • *Episodic syndromes associated with migraine:* Cyclic vomiting syndrome, abdominal migraine, benign paroxysmal vertigo, and benign paroxysmal torticollis
Tension-type headache (TTH)	• Infrequent episodic TTH • Frequent episodic TTH • Chronic TTH • Probable TTH
Trigeminal autonomic cephalgia	• Cluster headache • Paroxysmal hemicranias • Short-lasting unilateral neuralgiform headache attacks (SUNCT) • Hemicrania continua • Probable trigeminal autonomic cephalgia
Other primary headaches	Cough headache, exercise headache, thunderclap headache, cold stimulus headache, external pressure headache, primary stabbing headache, nummular headache, hypnic headache, and new daily persistent headache
Secondary headache	
	Headache attributed to: • Trauma to head/neck • Cranial or cervical vascular disorder • Nonvascular intracranial disorder • Substance abuse or withdrawal • Infection • Disorder of homeostasis • Disorder of cranium, neck, and eyes • Psychiatric disorder

raised intracranial pressure (ICP) or any progressive neurological disease. They are often associated with stress in the family (such as separated parents). By convention, episodic migraines are more common in early childhood, whereas a chronic migraine and chronic TTH are more common in adolescents.

Secondary Headache

Secondary headaches (as per ICHD-3) include those due to trauma to head/neck, cranial or cervical vascular disorder, nonvascular intracranial disorder, substance abuse, infection, a disorder of homeostasis, and a disorder of cranium, neck, eyes, ears, and nose. Headaches secondary to a brain tumor,

TABLE 2: Clinical features of primary headaches.

Primary headache	Description
Cluster headache (uncommon among children and adolescents)	Frequent attacks of severe, unilateral (periorbital and temporal) lasting for 15–180 minutes often associated with ipsilateral conjunctival congestion, lacrimation, nasal congestion, rhinorrhea, forehead/facial sweating/flushing, miosis, and ptosis
Paroxysmal hemicranias (uncommon among adolescents and children)	Frequent attacks of unilateral headache of similar character as cluster headache that lasts for 2–30 minutes, occurring multiple times a day with dramatic response to indomethacin
Short-lasting unilateral neuralgiform headache attacks (SUNCT)	Attacks of moderate-to-severe strictly unilateral headache that lasts for seconds to minutes, occurring at least once a day with prominent lacrimation and redness of ipsilateral eye
Primary cough headache	Headache precipitated by coughing or other Valsalva maneuver but not by prolonged physical exercise in absence of intracranial disorder
Primary exercise headache	Headache precipitated by any form of exercise in absence of intracranial disorder
New daily persistent headache	Persistent headache with acute onset, distinct and clearly remembered onset with pain becoming continuous and unremitting within 24 hours, persisting for more than 3 months

meningitis, and raised ICP are uncommon among children. Secondary headaches are often progressive when compared to primary headaches that are nonprogressive or acute recurrent.

■ CLINICAL EVALUATION

History

The aim of the history should be to differentiate primary from a secondary headache.

The first episode of an acute headache needs to be distinguished from acute recurrent headache. There are four patterns of headache in children—(1) acute single, (2) acute recurrent, (3) chronic progressive, and (4) chronic nonprogressive. Majority of primary headaches have acute recurrent or chronic nonprogressive headaches.

In contrast, secondary headache usually has a single event of acute headache or chronic progressive. Points in the history of headache are highlighted in **Box 1**. History often determines the need for an investigation. For example, in a child with acute headache presenting to casualty, history of possible toxic exposure to carbon monoxide (sleeping in a closed room with room heater in winter months) would warrant estimation of the carboxyhemoglobin level. The most common cause of acute recurrent headache in children is migraine.

Headache Diary

In a child with the previous history of a headache, a headache diary is immensely useful in determining the trend and response to medication. A headache diary must contain headache duration, frequency and degree of disability, and the need for medication. A headache diary must be able to document the severity of a headache, the pattern of headache, associated symptoms, any aggravating or relieving factor, and need for abortive medication. The severity

BOX 1: Points in history for childhood headache.

- Onset of headache (sudden or insidious onset)
- Duration of headache and frequency (daily, weekly, and monthly)
- Location of headache (frontal, temporal, and occipital)
- Severity of headache (mild, moderate, and severe)
- Type of headache (one type or more than one type)
- Static or progressive based on the frequency/severity of headache
- Associated nausea and vomiting
- Associated photophobia and phonophobia
- Relation to specific circumstances, food, and medication
- Is the child able to perform his/her activities despite headache?
- Past medical history—minor head trauma, viral infection, surgery, and stress
- History of drug intake (anticonvulsants, anticoagulants, and asthma medication)
- History of school experiences, dietary habits, and family relationships
- History of dental pain, nasal discharge, and facial pain
- History of seizure, altered sensorium, vertigo, gait abnormality, weakness, vision, and hearing difficulties
- Family history of headache

of headache can be documented regarding the pain rating scale or visual analog scale. A child with a daily persistent headache can be differentiated from migrainers. A broad approach to clinical diagnosis of acute headache is presented in **Flowchart 1**. Diagnosis of medication abuse can also be diagnosed with a headache diary. A sample headache diary is presented in **Figure 1**.

When to Think of Migraine in a Recurrent Headache?

Children with migraine will not have a constant headache; they have episodes of attacks. There are two main types of migraine—(1) migraine without aura and (2) migraine with aura. The transient focal neurological symptom that precedes or accompanies a headache is an aura. The most common aura is a visual aura (zigzag figure). Aura may consist of a premonitory symptom such as hyperactivity, fatigue, difficulty in concentration, sensitivity to light or sound, depression, and craving for certain food followed by a headache that ends with a headache-resolution phase. The presence of family history (seen in 60–75%) is supportive for diagnosis of migraine.

Think of migrainous headache when headache is moderate to severe in intensity, unilateral (mostly bilateral in younger children), pulsating, frontotemporal located, often associated with photophobia, phonophobia, nausea, and vomiting. The duration of migraine may last from 2 to 72 hours. If the child sleeps with trouble and wakes up fresh, the duration of sleep is counted in the duration of headache. Children during a headache often get cranky, prefer to go to sleep, and routine activities are stopped; they want silence (*phonophobia*—get irritated when someone makes noise) and prefer dark and cold room (*photophobia*—get irritated when the light is switched on). They are often accompanied by cutaneous allodynia. Criteria for a migraine with and without aura are shown in **Boxes 2 and 3**, respectively If a child has had less than five episodes of such headache, it is labeled as a probable migraine without aura. A diagnosis of "probable migraine" is used when all but one criteria for migraine are fulfilled, and headache is not better accounted by other headache disorders.

Severe and persistent headache with intractable nausea and vomiting lasting for more than 72 hours is called status migrainosus. In-between, the child may sleep

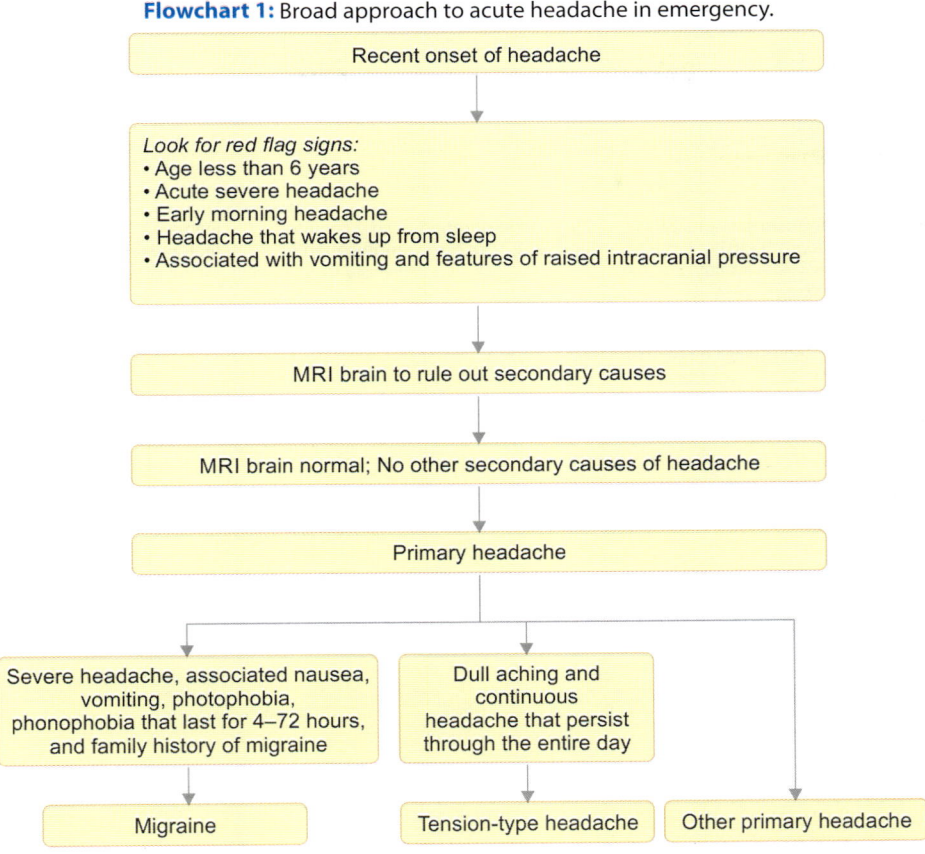

Flowchart 1: Broad approach to acute headache in emergency.

or can have a transient response to analgesic medication. The history of previous similar attacks of lesser duration is common in these children. Analgesic medication usage more than 15 tablets a month for more than 3 consecutive months would be considered medication abuse. This is one of the most common precipitating factors for status migrainosus in children.

The most common cause of an acute headache in children is upper respiratory tract infection accounting for 57% of cases presenting with acute headache in the emergency department (ED). This is followed by a migraine without aura, viral meningoencephalitis, shunt malfunction, postconcussion headache, and postictal headache. We need to consider these common causes of acute headache among children presenting to emergency room.

When to Think of Tension-type Headache?

Tension-type headache is typically bilateral, pressing or tightening quality, mild to moderate in intensity, and not aggravated by physical activity with absence of nausea, vomiting, photophobia, or phonophobia. The duration can vary between a minimum of 1 hour and a maximum of up to 7 days.

Headache diary (सरदर्द की डायरी)

Name (नाम):

Age/Gender (आयु/लिंग):

Address (घर का पता):

Phone Number (फोन नम्बर):

Month/Year				
Date तारीक	Headache intensity (score 0–10) सरदर्द कितना तेज था? 1. Mild/हल्का (0–3) 2. Moderate/तेज (3–7) 3. Severe/बहुत तेज (8–10)	Headache duration सरदर्द कितनी देर रहा?	Did it require medication? क्या दवाई की जरुरत पड़ी?	Remarks (Any precipitating factors?) क्या कोई सर दर्द का कारन था?

Fig. 1: Sample headache diary.

BOX 2: Diagnostic criteria for migraine with aura.

A. At least two attacks fulfilling criteria B and C
B. One or more of the following fully reversible aura symptoms: Visual, sensory, speech and/or language, motor, brainstem, and retinal
C. At least two of the following four characteristics:
   1. At least one aura symptom spreads gradually over 5 minutes and/or two or more symptoms occur in succession
   2. Each individual aura symptom lasts 5–60 minutes
   3. At least one aura symptom is unilateral
   4. The aura is accompanied, or followed within 60 minutes, by headache
D. Not better accounted for by another International Classification of Headache Disorders (ICHD-3) diagnosis, and transient ischemic attack has been excluded

> **BOX 3:** Diagnostic criteria for migraine without aura.
>
> A. At least five attacks fulfilling criteria B and D
> B. Headache attacks lasting 2–72 hours (untreated or unsuccessfully treated)
> C. Headache has at least two of the following four characteristics:
>   1. Unilateral location
>   2. Pulsating quality
>   3. Moderate to severe pain intensity
>   4. Aggravation by or causing avoidance of routine physical activity (e.g., walking or climbing stairs)
> D. During headache, at least one of the following:
>   1. Nausea and/or vomiting or
>   2. Photophobia and phonophobia
> E. Not better accounted for by another International Classification of Headache Disorders (ICHD-3) diagnosis

TTH can be *episodic* or *chronic* TTH. The frequency of episodes can be less than once a month (*infrequent episodic TTH*) or could be 1–14 days a month for a duration of more than 3 months (*frequent episodic TTH*) or more than 15 days a month for more than 3 months (*chronic TTH*). Coexisting TTH should be identified among migrainers. TTH can be associated with a pericranial tenderness that is evident on manual palpation.

New Daily Persistent Headache

New daily persistent headache (NDPH) is a continuous daily headache (mild to moderate), which is bilateral, pressing, and not aggravated by a routine physical activity where the patient can remember the exact date when the pain started. This can be associated with the migrainous symptom as well. The frequency of symptoms is daily right from the onset. It is considered one of the most difficult primary headaches with limited treatment options. It has a female predominance.

Benign Raised Intracranial Pressure or Idiopathic Intracranial Hypertension

Presence of severe throbbing headache with nausea, vomiting, and visual blurring or transient visual obscuration (TVO) is highly suggestive of headache of idiopathic intracranial hypertension (IIH), especially when associated with papilledema on fundus evaluation. Examination may reveal a decrease in visual acuity, visual field defects, or bilateral sixth cranial nerve palsy (feature of raised ICP). There is a wide list of causes—infectious [Epstein–Barr virus (EBV), *Coxsackie* B, Lyme disease, and malaria], drug induced (nitrofurantoin, tetracycline, vitamin A, and phenytoin), and medical conditions (Guillain–Barré syndrome, vitamin D deficiency, and chronic anemia) that predispose to IIH. Similarly, epidemiological data suggest postpubertal females and those with obesity are at a high risk for IIH.

History to Other Primary Headaches

Presence of autonomic symptoms such as conjunctival congestion, excessive lacrimation, and sweating often points to short-lasting unilateral neuralgiform headache attacks (SUNCT) or trigeminal neuralgia, especially when symptoms confine to the distribution of trigeminal nerve. Similarly, when the headache is associated with transient weakness of one side of the body (hemiplegic migraine), vertigo or tinnitus (basilar migraine), difficulty in movement of eyes with diplopia (ophthalmoplegic migraine), or transient blindness or scotomas (retinal migraine), it can often point to other types of primary headache **(Table 3)**.

History to Suggest Secondary Headache

We need to suspect secondary headache when the headache is occipital in origin (associated cervical muscle spasm), associated with

TABLE 3: Clinical pearls in headache evaluation.

Points in clinical history/examination	What does it suggest?
Unilateral headache with ipsilateral autonomic features such as eyelid droop, lacrimation, or rhinorrhea	Trigeminal autonomic cephalgia
Symptoms of behavioral change, irritability, and fatigue for a few days prior to the onset of symptoms	Prodromal phase of migraine with aura*
Headache that gradually increases in intensity (never maximal at onset) with or without nausea, photophobia, phonophobia, unilateral (older children), or bilateral (younger children)	Migraine attacks
Children prefer to sleep during headache and not able to perform routine activities	Migraine attacks
Headache associated (before or during the headache) with unilateral motor weakness with or without sensory symptoms and affected speech	Hemiplegic migraine
Occipital headache with vertigo, tinnitus, ataxia, and dysarthria	Basilar migraine
Presence of headache with ipsilateral oculomotor palsy	Ophthalmoplegic migraine
Episodes of unresponsiveness, confusion, agitation, speech difficulty, and disorientation with or without headache	Acute confusional migraine†
Predictable timing of intense nausea and vomiting associated with pallor and lethargy	Cyclical vomiting syndrome‡
Repeated attacks of monocular visual disturbances including scintillations, scotoma, and blindness associated with migraine	Retinal migraine
Recurrent attacks of moderate-to-severe midline abdominal pain associated with vasomotor symptoms, nausea, and vomiting that last for 2–72 hours; usually not associated with headache	Abdominal migraine‡
Recurrent brief attacks of vertigo without any warning signs lasting for minutes to hours with either of nystagmus, ataxia, vomiting, pallor, or fearfulness	Benign paroxysmal vertigo‡
Recurrent episodes of head tilt lasting for few minutes associated with one of following: Pallor, irritability, malaise, vomiting, or ataxia	Benign paroxysmal torticollis‡

*If these symptoms persist for more than 1 week, it would be called "persistent aura without infarction" provided the neuroimaging is normal.
†Not included in ICHD-3, but recognized as a separate type of headache in children.
‡Episodic syndromes associated with migraine.

profuse projectile vomiting (a feature of raised ICP), new onset of severe headache (possible intracranial space occupying lesion such as neurocysticercosis), and associated blurring of vision or decreased vision (possible ocular cause). Similarly, presence of risk factors such as repeated upper respiratory tract infection (sinusitis) can give a clue to an underlying cause. Children with cyanotic congenital heart disease can occasionally present with headache secondary to venous sinus thrombosis or brain abscess. Similarly, history of chronic drug intake (steroids and antibiotics that lead to benign raised ICP), history of chronic ear discharge (brain abscess), or history of head trauma (chronic subdural hematoma) must raise suspicion of secondary headache **(Table 4)**.

TABLE 4: When to think of secondary causes of headache?

Clinical clue	What should I think?
Presence of nasal discharge or morning cough for more than 2 weeks with an initial improvement followed by return of above symptoms or severe onset of above symptoms in association with fever	Sinusitis
History of ear discharge, pain in ears, and fever (otitis media)	Brain abscess or cerebral venous sinus thrombosis
History of trauma, vasculopathy, or on anticoagulants	Subdural hematoma
Recent use of steroid or tetracycline	Benign intracranial hypertension
Dehydration, heart disease, nephrotic syndrome, systemic lupus erythematosus (SLE), and malignancy	Cerebral venous sinus thrombosis

Examination

Majority of children presenting with isolated headache often have a normal neurological examination. Critical points on examination are enumerated in **Box 4**. It is evident that the presence of altered sensorium, nuchal rigidity, papilledema, abnormal eye movement, and ataxia in the presence of a headache must be considered ominous signs for further evaluation.

BOX 4: Focused examination for children with headache.

- General physical examination
- Cervical spine examination
- Palpation of bones and muscles
- Ears including external auditory meatus
- Temporomandibular (TM) joint, throat, and dental examination
- Examination of 9th to 12th cranial nerve
- Blood pressure measurement
- Height (short stature often points to endocrinal causes)

Analysis

At the end of history and examination, it is prudent to differentiate a primary and secondary headache. Similarly, presence of red flag signs such as early morning headache, occipital headache, headache that wakes up a child during sleep, or those with other features of raised ICP must be identified and evaluated accordingly **(Flowchart 1)**. Once secondary headaches have been ruled out based on history and examination (such as normal blood pressure, absence of sinus tenderness, and absence of neck muscle spasm), an attempt should be made to elicit and fit it into one of the types of primary headache. It is a good idea to use ICHD-3 classification to classify the type of headache. We need not memorize the entire classification; keep that print in your office and use it repeatedly to classify the type of headache. This may not be possible in the first consultation, so encourage the parents to maintain a headache diary **(Fig. 1)**. Hence, at the end of history and examination, analysis can be done under the following headings:

- Is it an acute headache, acute recurrent headache, or chronic headache?
- Are the symptoms causing significant impairment in activities of daily living?
- Are there any red flag signs of headache?
- Does this fit into any known secondary headache?
- If not, can you classify into any known primary headache?
- If not, it remains an unclassified headache, which often requires follow-up.

■ INVESTIGATIONS

There is no role of investigations in an established primary headache such as migraine. However, investigations are often performed to rule out other secondary causes when pointed by history and examination. Two most common investigations include neuroimaging and lumbar puncture.

Neuroimaging

Presence of nontraumatic headache in a setting of normal neurological examination does not warrant investigation. New and sudden onset of a severe headache (a thunderclap headache) always warrants a neuroimaging to look for features of subarachnoid hemorrhage. Red flag signs for evaluating a child with an acute headache are highlighted as a mnemonic in **Box 5**. One of the most common causes for subarachnoid hemorrhage in children includes ruptured aneurysm, arteriovenous malformation, or coagulation disorders. It would be preferable to get a noncontrast computed tomography (NCCT) scan over magnetic resonance imaging (MRI) brain in such a situation.

The yield of neuroimaging is around 3–4% among those with uncomplicated migraine, whereas the yield may be 15% among those with a chronic daily headache.

Most of the findings are incidental such as an arachnoid cyst **(Figs. 2A to D)**, Chiari I malformation, sinusitis, occult vascular malformation, and dilated Virchow–Robin space. Majority of them do not require any surgical intervention. It has been observed

> **BOX 5:** Red flag signs in children presenting to emergency with acute headache (mnemonic: SNOOPY).
>
> **S**ystemic:
> - Fever
> - Altered sensorium
> - HIV infection
> - Anticoagulation
>
> **N**eurological signs:
> - Cranial nerve palsy
> - Motor deficit
> - Cerebellar signs
> - New-onset seizure
>
> **O**nset:
> - Recent onset
> - Thunderclap headache
>
> **O**ccipital:
> - Occipital headache
>
> **P**attern:
> - Precipitated by Valsalva
> - Positional
> - Progressive
> - Lack of family history
>
> **Y**ears:
> - Age <6 years

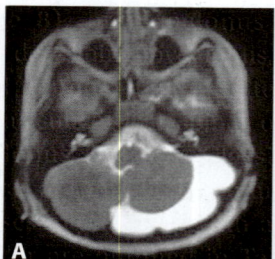 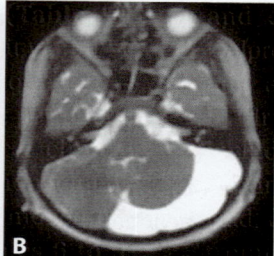 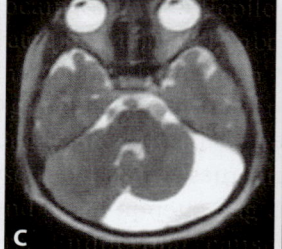 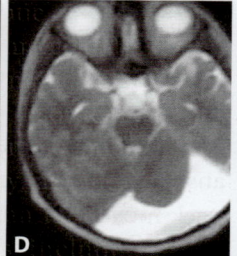

Figs. 2A to D: MRI brain (T2 axial) showing a left-sided arachnoid cyst appearing as a bright cyst behind the cerebellum.

that all patients with surgically remediable lesions had objective neurological findings. Presence of neurocutaneous markers and microcephaly in a child who presented with headache warrants neuroimaging. Patients with suspected IIH may show flattening of posterior globe, empty sella, distention of perioptic subarachnoid space, and transverse venous sinus stenosis on MRI brain. Optical coherence tomography and B-scan ultrasonography are useful in investigating children with IIH. MR venography is essential to exclude venous sinus thrombosis before establishing diagnosis of IIH. Routine use of neuroimaging among children aged more than 6 years with a migraine or chronic daily headache with normal neurological examination is not justified.

Indications for Neuroimaging

- First severe new-onset headache
- Headache in an immunocompromised patient
- Headache that wakes up the child from sleep associated with vomiting
- Early morning headache with severe vomiting or headache associated with straining
- Subacute headache that progresses rapidly (change in type of headache)
- Associated fever, neck rigidity, vomiting, irritability, seizure, alteration of behavior, or altered sensorium or development of any focal neurological deficits including gait abnormality.

Lumbar Puncture

Lumbar puncture is indicated only among those with fever, neck rigidity, and meningeal signs and those with the immunocompromised state. It is useful for diagnosis of pseudotumor cerebri and subarachnoid hemorrhage. Subarachnoid hemorrhage is diagnosed on neuroimaging, and ideally lumbar puncture is contraindicated in the same. However, presence of fresh blood on lumbar puncture raises a possibility of subarachnoid hemorrhage. Diagnosis of IIH is made on documentation of raised CSF opening pressure (>280 mm H_2O) based on the age. The American Academy of Neurology has published evidence-based recommendations for evaluating a child with recurrent headache **(Boxes 6 and 7)**.

BOX 6: American Academy of Neurology (AAN) recommendations for evaluation of a child with recurrent headache.

- Obtaining a neuroimaging study on a routine basis is not indicated in children with recurrent headaches and a normal neurologic examination (Level B; class II and class III evidence)
- Neuroimaging should be considered in children with an abnormal neurologic examination (e.g., focal findings, signs of increased intracranial pressure, and significant alteration of consciousness), the coexistence of seizures, or both (Level B; class II and class III evidence)
- Neuroimaging should be considered in children in whom there are historical features to suggest the recent onset of severe headache, change in the type of headache, or if there are associated features that suggest neurologic dysfunction (Level B; class II and class III evidence)

BOX 7: Tips for the management of acute migraine headache in children.

- Abortive medications are started as soon as the headache is reported by the child
- The most used abortive medications for acute migraine include ibuprofen (10 mg/kg/dose) or paracetamol (15 mg/kg/dose). Restrict the use to less than 3 times a week
- Triptans can be tried among those who fail to respond to nonsteroidal anti-inflammatory drugs (NSAIDs). Rizatriptan 5–10 mg can be tried orally among children older than 6 years. Alternatively, intranasal sumatriptan or zolmitriptan is useful among children older than 12 years
- Few children with prominent nausea and vomiting can respond to antiemetic medications including prochlorperazine and metoclopramide
- Maintaining good hydration helps children with acute migraine
- Children who do not respond to oral medications might require intravenous metoclopramide or prochlorperazine along with NSAID like ketorolac. Other medications that may be used in emergency setting include intravenous valproate, subcutaneous sumatriptans, and dihydroergotamine
- Prophylactic medications are recommended among those with frequent headache (more than once a week) or severe disabling headaches
- Common drugs used for prophylaxis of migraine include flunarizine (5–10 mg), propranolol (10–20 mg), topiramate (25–50 mg), and amitriptyline (1 mg/kg/day)
- Biobehavioral therapy including biofeedback and relaxation therapy are useful in chronic cases and among children with TTH

KEY MESSAGES

- It is essential to differentiate a primary from secondary headache.
- Migraine without aura and chronic TTH are the two most common causes of primary headache in children.
- Investigations have limited role in evaluation of headache in children except in presence of red flag signs of headache.
- Use ICHD-3 classification of headache to categorize the type of primary headache in every patient.
- Headache diary is a useful tool to arrive at the diagnosis and helps in reaching classification of primary headache.

CHAPTER 20

Approach to a Child with Macrocephaly and Microcephaly

■ MACROCEPHALY

Macrocephaly is defined as abnormally large head with occipitofrontal circumference (OFC) >2 SD [97th percentile] for the age and gender. Since many typically developing children will also have OFC between +2 and +3 SD, many clinicians consider a cut-off of > 3 SD to be "clinically relevant" macrocephaly. We know that normal head circumference increases by 2 cm/month (0–3 months), 1 cm/month (3-6 months), 0.5 cm/month (6–12 months), 1 cm every 6 months (1–3 years), and 1 cm per year (3–5 years).

Broadly, macrocephaly can be primary or congenital (at birth or in utero) or secondary (postnatal). Macrocephaly must be differentiated from megalencephaly which refers to large, oversized, and overweight brain (>2 SD). Megalencephaly can be secondary to increase size/number of neurons (anatomical/developmental megalencephaly) or accumulation of abnormal metabolic substance (metabolic megalencephaly). Macrocephaly results from several causes like megalencephaly, skeletal dysplasia, hydrocephalus, and subdural collection. Large head is macrocephaly and large brain is megalencephaly.

Focused History in a Child with Macrocephaly

- *Birth history:*
  - History of prematurity could suggest post-intraventricular hemorrhage (IVH) hydrocephalus.
  - History of neonatal seizures and encephalopathy suggestive of neonatal meningitis could suggest postmeningitic hydrocephalus as the possible cause of large head.
  - History of a term baby with excessive crying, bulging fontanelle and seizure is suggestive of intracranial bleed and this could have resulted in secondary hydrocephalus with resultant large head.
- *Onset of macrocephaly:* If head was large at the time of birth it is likely to be primary macrocephaly and if it develops subsequently after birth, it is secondary macrocephaly. Most of the acquired etiologies such as meningitis, intracranial bleed would result in secondary macrocephaly. Conditions such as congenital aqueductal stenosis would present as primary macrocephaly.

- *Development history:* Developmental history in a child with macrocephaly gives a lot of clinical clues **(Flowchart 1)**. Presence of isolated macrocephaly in a typically developing child could suggest benign enlargement of subarachnoid space (BESS). MRI brain showing evidence of enlarged subarachnoid spaces with normal or dilated ventricles is suggestive of BESS. As the name suggests, BESS is a benign condition and does not require any surgical or medical intervention. It usually stabilizes by 12–18 months. Majority of children with macrocephaly may have associated developmental delay, intellectual disability, or features of autism spectrum disorder (ASD). We need to remember that almost 15–20% of children with ASD will have macrocephaly. If the developmental history is suggestive of developmental regression in a child with macrocephaly, one must think of neurometabolic disorders such as glutaric acidemia type 1.

- *Features of raised intracranial pressure (ICP):* Presence of excessive irritability, bulging fontanelle with progressive increase in head circumference are common features of raised ICP in infants. In older children, raised ICP may manifest with history of repeated vomiting, difficulty in walking, or altered sensorium and seizures. Presence of raised ICP in a child with macrocephaly often indicates hydrocephalus that would require intervention. Hydrocephalus must be differentiated from *Hydranencephaly. Hydranencephaly* refers to complete absence of cerebral tissue with the entire intracranial cavity occupied with cerebrospinal fluid (CSF). Hydranencephaly often results from bilateral fetal internal carotid obstruction. This needs to be differentiated from hydrocephalus, as there is no role of surgical intervention in hydranencephaly.

- *Family history:* Family history of macrocephaly may suggest benign familial

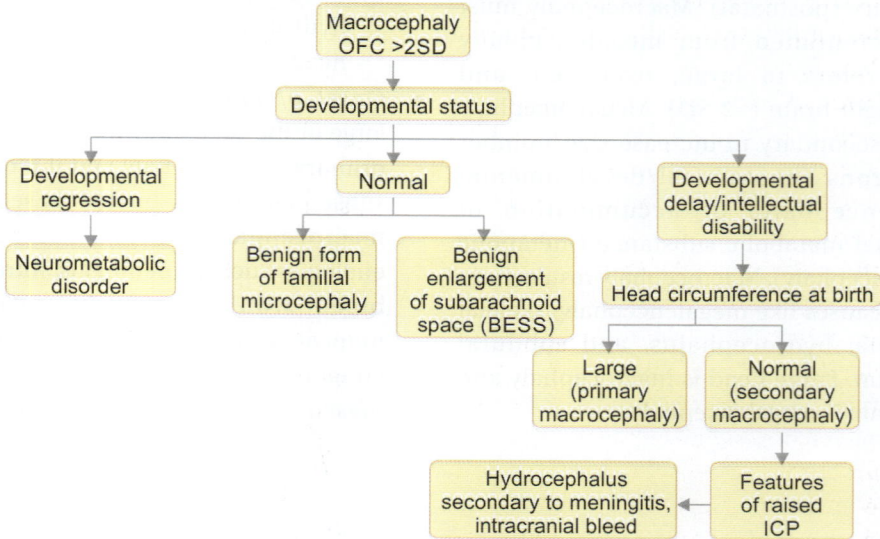

Flowchart 1: Algorithmic approach to macrocephaly.

(ICP: intracranial pressure; OFC: occipitofrontal circumference; SD: standard deviation)

macrocephaly. History of consanguinity, recurrent sibling loss may suggest neurometabolic disorder with autosomal recessive inheritance. History of recurrent abortions and stillbirth may point to chromosomal disorders. Family history of neurofibromatosis may also be noted.

Focused Examination in a Child with Macrocephaly

- Head circumference measurement must be accurate and must measure maximum circumference from occiput to nasion using a nonstretchable tape. Compare the measurement using the World Health Organization (WHO) growth charts. Head circumference >2 SD would point to macrocephaly.
- *Facies:* Abnormal coarse facies in a child with macrocephaly could point to lysosomal storage disorder such as mucopolysaccharidosis. Presence of elongated ears in a child with intellectual disability and macrocephaly may suggest fragile X syndrome, especially when associated with macroorchidism (large testes) and heart lesion (mitral valve prolapse).
- *Skeletal abnormality:* Large head with presence of frontal bossing, rachitic rosary, and wide wrist would point to rickets. Large head in a child with anemia requiring repeated blood transfusion would suggest thalassemia. Presence of ribcage abnormality and vertebral abnormality would point to underlying skeletal dysplasia. Presence of short stature with macrocephaly must raise suspicion of skeletal dysplasia.
- *Neurocutaneous markers:* Presence of café-au-lait macules, axillary frecklings, and neurofibroma may suggest neurofibromatosis type 1. Remember to examine the parents (autosomal dominant inheritance). Look for ash-leaf macule, shagreen patch which could suggest tuberous sclerosis. Facial milia with palmar pits may suggest Gorlin syndrome.
- Presence of tall stature (>+2 SD) along with macrocephaly (>2 SD) with or without facial features would suggest overgrowth syndrome. There may be segmental overgrowth or hypertrophy of limbs with or without other cutaneous manifestations and vascular features.
- *Organomegaly:* Presence or organomegaly in a child with macrocephaly and developmental regression could suggest lysosomal storage disorder. The key clinical features are summarized in **Flowchart 2**.

BROAD APPROACH TO A CHILD WITH LARGE HEAD

1. *Is it macrocephaly? If yes, is it hydrocephalus or megalencephaly?*
2. *If megalencephaly, is it metabolic or syndromic megalencephaly?*
   Megalencephaly could be secondary to metabolic conditions such as Canavan disease, Alexander disease, or it could be syndromic cause such as neurofibromatosis **(Flowchart 3)**.
3. *If hydrocephalus, is it congenital or acquired?*
   Onset at birth or within the first 6 months is often considered congenital hydrocephalus. Onset beyond 6 months of age often points to acquired hydrocephalus.
4. *What could be cause of hydrocephalus?*
   - *Preterm infants:* Intraventricular bleed
   - *Term infants:* Dandy–Walker malformation, Arnold–Chiari malformation type II, arachnoid cyst, vein of Galen malformation, intrauterine infection, and Aqueductal stenosis

Flowchart 2: Clinical clues in a child with macrocephaly.

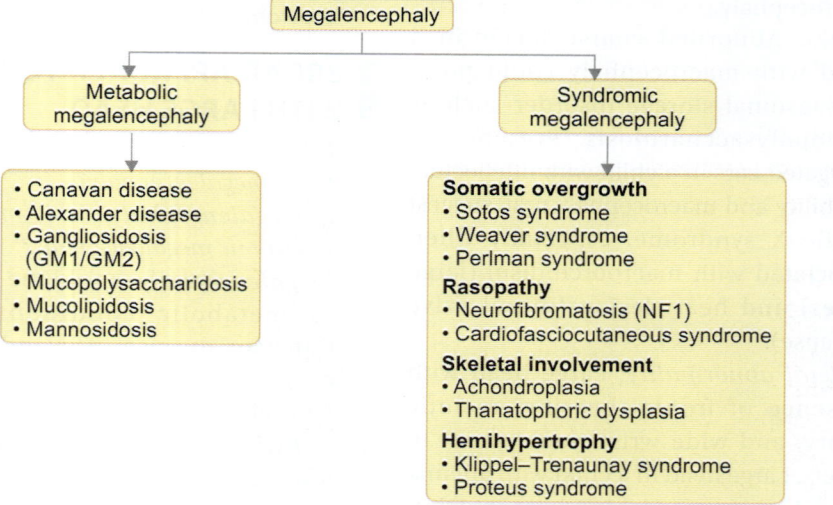

(DD/ID: developmental delay/intellectual disability)

Flowchart 3: Broad classification of megalencephaly.

- Older children: Tumor (obstructive hydrocephalus), trauma, and infection (e.g., tubercular)
5. Are there any clinical features of hydrocephalus?
   - Infants: Failure to thrive, developmental delay, irritability, poor feeding, vomiting, apneic spells, bulging tense anterior fontanelle, distended scalp veins, cranial sutures splayed, transillumination sign (if cortex is very thin), sixth cranial nerve palsy, upgaze palsy (Sun-setting sign) **(Fig. 1)**, nystagmus, optic atrophy (chronic), spasticity.
   - Older children: Intellectual disability, early morning headache, projectile vomiting, diplopia, behavioral

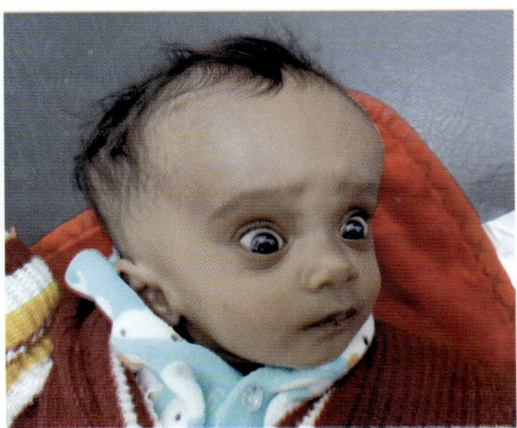

Fig. 1: Infant with congenital hydrocephalus with large head and Sun-setting sign.

disturbances, squint, papilledema (more common in acquired hydrocephalus rather than congenital hydrocephalus), Parinaud syndrome (light near dissociation, convergence retraction nystagmus, and eyelid retraction), hypothalamic/pituitary dysfunction (gigantism, obesity, delayed puberty, and primary amenorrhea)

Investigating a Child with Macrocephaly

- Investigations will be determined by the broad group of etiology that we are considering based on clinical evaluation. It is good to prioritize investigating for treatable cause such as rickets (X-ray wrist, serum vitamin D level), beta-thalassemia (Hb electrophoresis), and hydrocephalus (MRI brain).
- Neuroimaging is useful in diagnosis of hydrocephalus. Three important radiological signs include enlargement of the anterior and posterior recess of the third ventricle, dilatation of temporal horns of lateral ventricles, effacement of cortical sulci **(Fig. 2)**. Periventricular ooze can be appreciated around the ventricles in obstructive hydrocephalus **(Fig. 3)**. Dilation of fourth and third ventricles along with the above signs indicates communicating hydrocephalus. However, the presence of normal or small fourth ventricle suggests obstructive hydrocephalus. Brain atrophy must always be differentiated from hydrocephalus with former having prominent sulci/gyri, irregular ventricular margin, lack of periventricular ooze, and periventricular white matter volume loss.
- Magnetic resonance imaging (MRI) brain is also useful in identifying BESS, megalencephaly (overgrowth syndrome), and unidentified bright objects (UBO) (neurofibromatosis) **(Fig. 4)**.
- Macrocephaly with features of autism spectrum disorder may warrant testing for *PTEN* mutation and other *PIK 3CA*, *MTOR*-related disorders
- Children with segmental overgrowth with vascular/cutaneous manifestation may warrant testing for *PIK 3CA* gene/*AKT 1* gene mutation.
- In absence of vascular malformation in overgrowth syndrome, methylation study

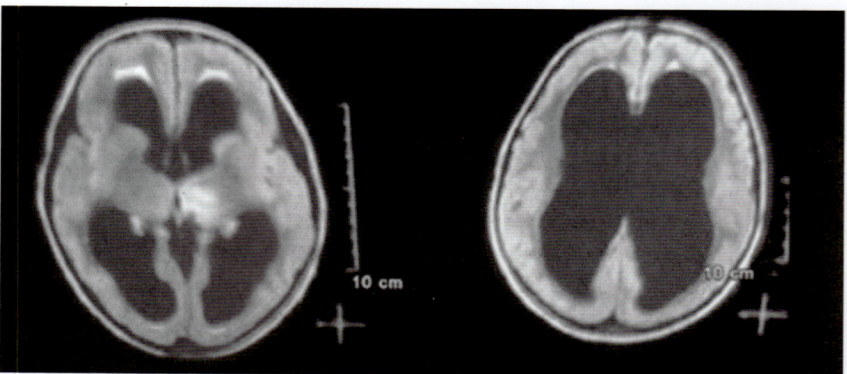

Fig. 2: MRI brain (T2/FLAIR) reveals dilated lateral ventricles with presence of periventricular ooze. (FLAIR: fluid attenuated inversion recovery; MRI: magnetic resonance imaging)

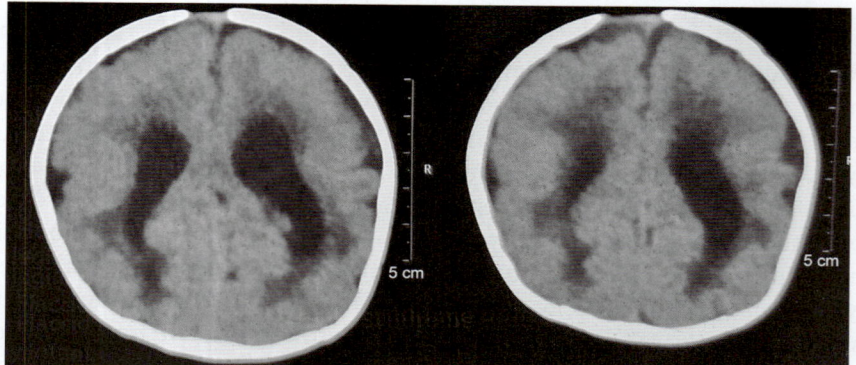

Fig. 3: CT scan showing hydrocephalus (dilated lateral ventricles with periventricular ooze). (CT: computed tomography)

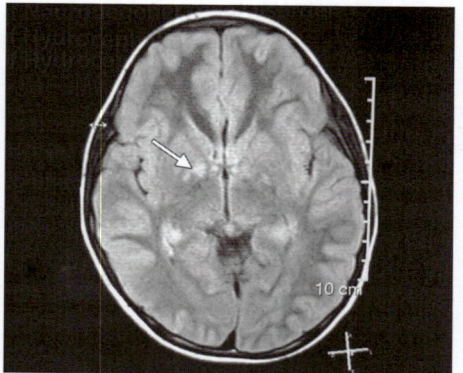

Fig. 4: MRI brain (T2/FLAIR) reveals unidentified bright object (UBO) in the basal ganglia in a child with neurofibromatosis type 1. (FLAIR: fluid-attenuated inversion recovery; MRI: magnetic resonance imaging)

will be required to diagnosis Beckwith–Wiedemann syndrome.
- The presence of features of achondroplasia would require targeted genetic testing.
- Chromosomal microarray/exome sequencing/macrocephaly gene panel testing would be useful among those with isolated macrocephaly and intellectual disability.

Management

- Identifying and treating rickets with vitamin D supplementation, beta-thalassemia with bone marrow transplantation/

repeated blood transfusion with appropriate chelation is essential.
- Management is largely supportive (occupational therapy/physiotherapy/speech therapy), and multidisciplinary approach is required for appropriate management.
- *Management of comorbidities:* Epilepsy (antiseizure medication), and spasticity (baclofen and tizanidine)
- Few overgrowth syndromes with neurocutaneous syndrome will require surveillance for malignancy.
- Congenital hydrocephalus, especially obstructive hydrocephalus (with periventricular ooze, papilledema, and signs of raised ICP), requires surgical intervention for CSF diversion. Two options include shunt (ventriculoperitoneal or ventriculoatrial) surgery or endoscopic third ventriculostomy (ETV) with or without choroid plexus cauterization. By convention, ETV is a preferred choice beyond infancy considering high failure rates in infancy. Children who have mild arrested hydrocephalus, those with cortical mantle size <1 cm, associated malformations often do not require surgical intervention. Three main complications with shunt surgery include shunt failure, shunt infection, and slit ventricle syndrome **(Table 1)**.

TABLE 1: Key features of shunt malfunction, shunt infection, and slit ventricle syndrome.

Clinical parameters	Shunt failure	Shunt infection	Slit ventricle syndrome
When to suspect	Development of new-onset headache, vomiting, seizures, neck retraction, tense bulging anterior fontanelle, papilledema in a shunted child must raise suspicion of shunt malfunction	Development of fever, seizure, headache, and vomiting within a few months of shunt surgery should raise suspicion of shunt infection	Development of intermittent symptoms of headache, vomiting, and seizures in a shunted child with chinked ventricles on imaging must raise suspicion of slit ventricle syndrome
Clinical signs	Shunt chamber may not be compressible but fill immediately (distal block); if the shunt chamber is easy to compress but refill slowly then it indicates proximal block at the ventricular level	Signs of inflammation may or may not be seen in subcutaneous shunt chamber	No local signs
Neuroimaging findings	Imaging may reveal an increase in ventricular size compared to previous scans	Imaging may reveal an increase in ventricular size compared to the previous scan	Imaging reveals small chinked ventricles owing to lack of compliance of ventricle wall
Management	Shunt revision is the only option. Often the shunt is broken or blocked	Intravenous (IV) antibiotics, shunt exteriorization, and shunt revision	Difficult to manage often requires surgical expertise

MICROCEPHALY

The term microcephaly is used when OFC is <2 SD below the mean for age and gender. When OFC <3 SD, the term "severe microcephaly" is used. Similar to the term megalencephaly, the term "microencephaly" refers to small-sized brain. Microcephaly can be in concordance with reduction in weight and height (proportionate or symmetrical) or there can be disproportionate or asymmetrical microcephaly. Microcephaly can be genetic or primary microcephaly when microcephaly is present at birth and presumed to be secondary to genetic factors. In contrast, secondary or acquired microcephaly could be secondary to environment influence **(Flowchart 4)**.

Clinical History and Examination

- *Antenatal history:* Maternal fever, rash, lymph node swelling [TORCH (toxoplasmosis, rubella, cytomegalovirus, herpes, and other agents) infection]; radiation exposure; drug intake (antiseizure medication), alcohol or tobacco intake, maternal history diabetes
- *Birth history:* History of prematurity, perinatal asphyxia, intracranial bleed, hypoglycemia, and neonatal meningitis would be useful.
- *Developmental history:* Majority of children with microcephaly will have developmental delay/intellectual disability. History of motor regression with presence of hand stereotypies might suggest possibility of MECP-2-related Rett syndrome.
- *Comorbidities:* Many children with microcephaly will have one or more of following: squint, vision abnormality, hearing abnormality (kernicterus, TORCH infection); spasticity/dyskinesia (cerebral palsy).
- *Family history:* History of recurrent abortions/stillbirth would suggest

Flowchart 4: Approach to a child with microcephaly.

```
                    Microcephaly
                    OFC <2SD
           ┌───────────┴───────────┐
    Genetic or primary         Secondary
       microcephaly           microcephaly
    ┌──────┴──────┐         ┌──────┴──────┐
Syndromic   Nonsyndromic  Antenatal factors   Perinatal insult
e.g., Angelmann syndrome,                e.g., TORCH infection,    Asphyxia,
Cornelia-de-Lange syndrome,              Maternal PKU,             Meningitis,
Rubinstein-Taybi syndrome                Maternal alcohol, tobacco, Hypoglycemia,
                                         Maternal radiation,       Birth trauma
                                         Maternal Zika virus infection,
                                         Maternal uncontrolled diabetes
```

- Chromosomal abnormality, e.g., Trisomy 13, Trisomy 18, Ring chromosomes
- Malformation of cortical development, e.g., Lissencephaly, polymicrogyria, PV nodular heterotopia
- Primary microcephaly (monogenetic)
- Craniosynostosis

Autosomal recessive
- MCPH1
- ASPM

Autosomal dominant

X-linked

(OFC: occipitofrontal circumference; PV: periventricular; SD: standard deviation; PKU: phenylketonuria)

chromosomal disorders. History of consanguinity, with recurrent abortions would point to autosomal recessive microcephaly.
- *Dysmorphism:* Presence of dysmorphic features in a child with microcephaly points to syndromic causes of microcephaly. An attempt to fit into one of known syndromes such as Williams syndrome, Angelman syndrome, Rubinstein–Taybi syndrome would be useful.
- *Skull shape:* Overriding of sutures with closure of fontanelle is seen in children with microcephaly and craniosynostosis.
- *Systemic features:* Presence of aortic stenosis (Williams syndrome); syndactyly of 2nd and 3rd toe (Cornelia-de-Lange/Smith–Lemli–Opitz syndrome); cataract (congenital rubella syndrome); and chorioretinitis (CMV infections) could provide clue to underlying cause of microcephaly.

Investigations

- Neuroimaging provides significant information to underlying etiology. Computed tomography (CT) brain is useful in detecting calcifications **(Fig. 5)**. MRI brain is better modality for identifying underlying cortical malformation **(Flowchart 5)**.
- Among children with syndromic microcephaly, karyotype or chromosomal microarray would be useful.
- Exome sequencing is useful among those with nonsyndromic primary microcephaly, especially those with suspected *MCPH* mutation.
- Metabolic testing using urinary gas chromatography/mass spectrometry (GC/MS) is not routinely recommended unless there is strong possibility in view of consanguinity, recurrent sibling loss, and unexplained encephalopathy.

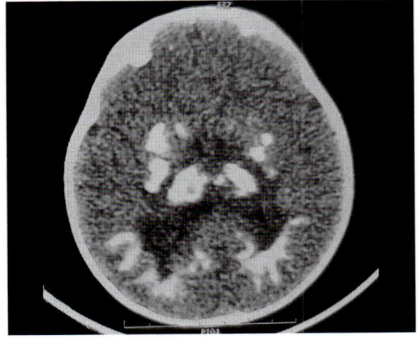

Fig. 5: Periventricular chunky calcification in a child with congenital CMV infection. (CMV: cytomegalovirus)

Flowchart 5: Neuroimaging in a child with microcephaly.

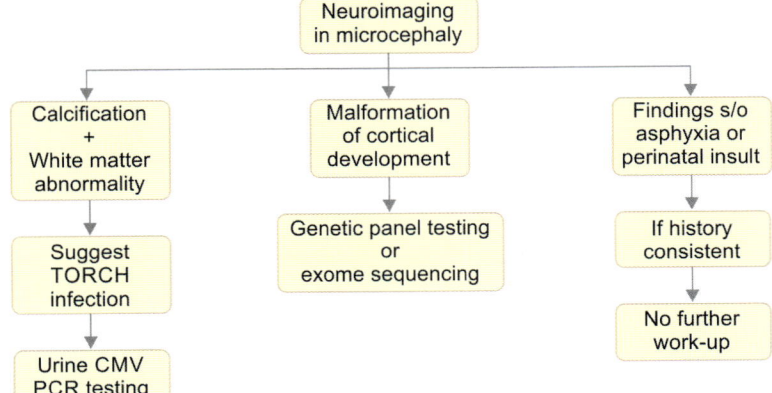

(CMV: cytomegalovirus; PCR: polymerase chain reaction; TORCH: toxoplasmosis, rubella, cytomegalovirus, herpes, and other agents)

KEY MESSAGES

- Macrocephaly refers to abnormally large head with head circumference >2 SD for age. This must be differentiated from megalencephaly that refers to large size of the brain.
- Common causes of macrocephaly include megalencephaly, skeletal dysplasia, hydrocephalus, and subdural collection.
- Macrocephaly could be primary or secondary to meningitis, or intracranial bleed.
- Microcephaly is used when head circumference is <2 SD, and when <3 SD, the term severe microcephaly is used.
- Karyotype or chromosomal microarray is useful among those with syndromic microcephaly. Exome sequencing is useful among those with nonsyndromic microcephaly to detect single-gene disorders.

CHAPTER 21: Approach to Neural Tube Defects

INTRODUCTION

Neural tube defects result from abnormal embryonic development of central nervous system. A flat neural plate folds with cranial and spinal neural fold to form a neural tube, a process called neurulation **(Fig. 1)**. To understand the embryonic basic of neural tube defect, an analogy of jacket is used. Imagine a Jacket that has four buttons and zips in between these buttons. Button 3 is at junction of hindbrain/cervical boundary, button 2 at forebrain/midbrain boundary, button 1 is rostral end of neural tube, and button 4 is caudal end of neural tube **(Fig. 2)**. On day 17 postfertilization, button 3 is closed first followed by closure of button 2 and button 1 and finally button 4. Between day 17 and day 28, the pores between button 3-2, button 2-1 and button 3-4 are zipped. This entire process is called primary neurulation. If button 3, does not close, it results in *craniorachischisis*. If button 2 does not close, it results in *anencephaly* and if button 1 does not close, it results in split face. If button 4 does not close, it results in *open spina bifida*. Hence, these disorders are called primary neurulation defects.

Once the jacket is closed, the cells in tail end undergo canalization to form lumen in lower sacral/coccygeal area. This process is secondary neurulation. Disturbance of secondary neurulation-like tethering

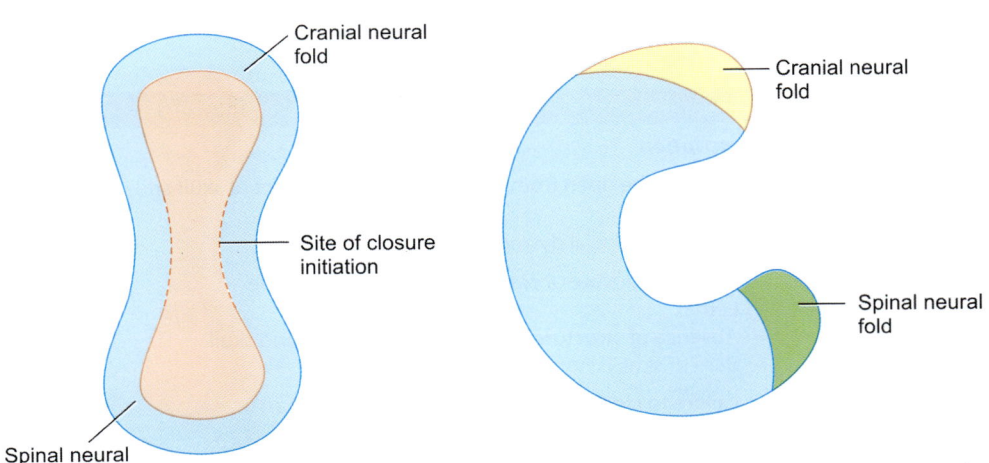

Fig. 1: Formation of neural tube.

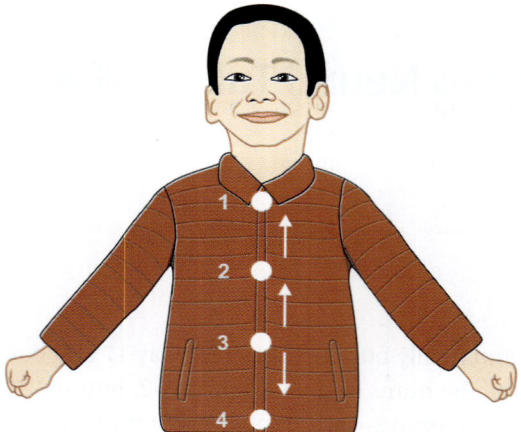

Fig. 2: Analogy to understand neural tube closure.

of spinal cord with associated lipoma are usually covered with skin as the jacket is closed now. Once neurulation is complete, sealing of last gaps are done at around 4 months after fertilization. Any defect at this time is called postneurulation defect, e.g., encephalocele, where hindbrain and meninges herniate through the gap that was not sealed. The classification of neural tube defect is depicted in **Flowchart 1**. The neural tube defects can be open **(Table 1)** or closed neural tube defects **(Table 2)**. The common neural tube defects include spina bifida occulta (A), meningocele (B) and myelomeningocele

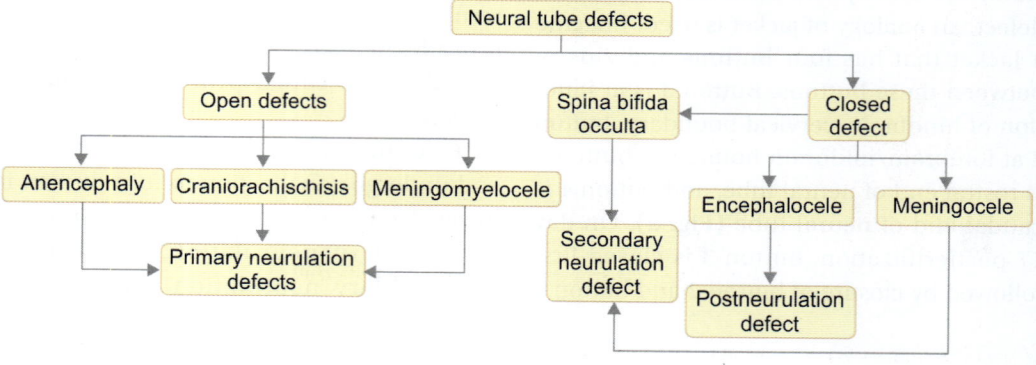

Flowchart 1: Classification of neural tube defects.

Neural tube defect	Description
Craniorachischisis	• Neural tube open from midbrain to spine (defect of skull and vertebra) • Lethal, rare • Neck short, facial dysmorphism
Anencephaly	• Failure of closure of cranial portion of neural tube • Lethal • Absence of structure derived from forebrain and skull • Base of skull is normal
Meningocele	• Failure to close posterior spinal portion (lumbar) • Defect in vertebral arch
Myelocele	• No meningeal sac • Open defect involves spinal cord

TABLE 1: Types of open neural tube defects.

TABLE 2: Types of closed neural tube defects.	
Neural tube defect	Key feature

Encephalocele	• Sac like protrusion of brain and meninges through opening in skull
	• What herniates
	  – Only meninges (meningocele)
	  – Meninges and brain (encephalomeningocele)
	  – Meninges, brain, ventricles (encephalomeningocystocele)

Meningocele	Herniation of meningeal sac through vertebral column
Spinal bifida occulta	• Abnormal development of embryonic tail bud (lower lumbar/sacral) • Closed defect with incomplete vertebral arches • Associated with sacral agenesis

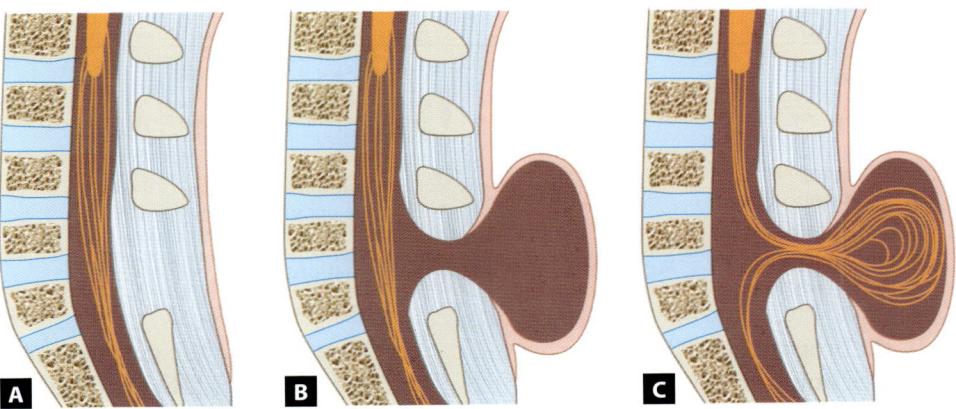

Figs. 3A to C: Common types of neural tube defects.

(C) **(Figs. 3A to C)**. Open myelomeningocele and myelocele are often associated with Arnold-Chiari malformation type II, hydrocephalus, and clubfeet. Other spinal cord malformations include tethered cord syndrome, split cord malformation, and syringomyelia **(Fig. 4)**.

BROAD APPROACH TO NEURAL TUBE DEFECTS

- What is level of defect? Is it at the level of cranium or is it at the level of spinal cord. If it is at the level of spinal cord, is it at cervical, thoracic, lumbar, or sacral level?
- Is the neural tube defect an open defect or closed defect? Open defects needs urgent surgical intervention to prevent central nervous system (CNS) infections.
- Is it associated with large head and hydrocephalus? If yes, it is likely to be associated with Arnold-Chiari malformation type II.
- What are the associated neurological deficits in the child with neural tube defect?
  • Is there involvement of bladder and bowel (incontinence and dribbling)?
  • Is there weakness and spasticity in legs?
  • Is there any zone of sensory loss in the legs?
- What are the associated deformities/complications in a child with neural tube defects?

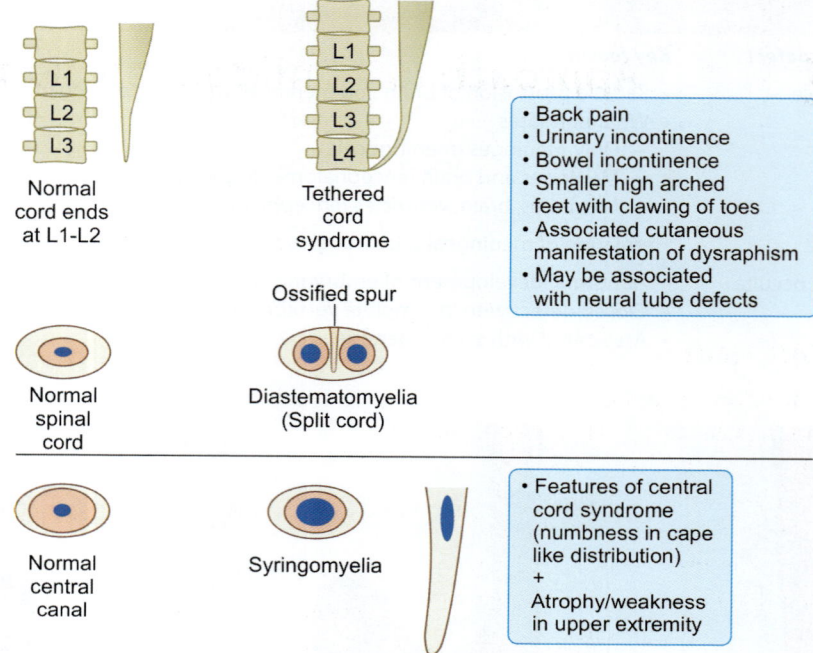

Fig. 4: Other spinal cord malformations.

- Is there associated hip deformity, talipes equinovarus, calcaneus foot deformity, rocker bottom foot, or scoliosis?
- Are there any bed sores/ulcers?
■ Is there a family history of neural tube defect (recurrence)? If one sibling gets affected, the chances of neural tube defect is 3–5% and if there are two affected pregnancies, then the chances increases to 10%. Intake of folic acid during the pregnancy can be useful.
■ Are there any evident risk factors (maternal folate intake, maternal hyperthermia, maternal malnutrition, maternal diabetes, and maternal obesity) to predict recurrence of neural tube defect in subsequent pregnancies?

KEY MESSAGES

- Open neural tube defects include craniorachischisis, anencephaly, meningocele, and myelocele.
- Closed neural tube defects include encephalocele, meningocele, and spina bifida occulta.
- Primary neurulation defects include anencephaly, craniorachischisis, and meningomyelocele. Spina bifida occulta and meningocele are secondary neurulation defects. Encephalocele is a postneurulation defect.
- Neural tube defects are commonly associated with hydrocephalus, spasticity in lower limbs, and urinary dribbling.
- Congenital talipes equinovarus, hip deformity, calcaneus foot deformity, rocker bottom feet, and scoliosis are common deformities associated with neural tube defects.

CHAPTER 22: Approach to a Child with Vision Loss

INTRODUCTION

Vision loss in children is one of the most problematic symptoms that require prompt evaluation and management. A systematic approach to a child with vision loss will help the clinician prioritize the investigation and provide appropriate intervention. The vision loss can be acute (presenting in an emergency setting) or long-standing chronic.

APPROACH TO A CHILD WITH ACUTE VISION LOSS

- *Is it monocular or binocular?*
  In general, monocular vision loss is considered ocular in origin, and binocular vision loss is considered cortical (embolic or ischemic).
- *Onset of vision loss:* Vision loss could occur within minutes, hours, or a few days. Sudden onset of vision loss that develops within seconds to minutes suggests retinal vascular disorder [central retinal artery occlusion (CRAO) or retinal vein occlusion (RVO)]. Migraine may present with vision loss that develops over hours. Most optic nerve disorders such as optic neuritis have an insidious onset of vision loss.
- *Is it a painful or painless vision loss?*
  CRAO presents as sudden onset, painless vision loss, whereas conditions such as optic neuritis present with painful eye movement. Similarly, traumatic ocular conditions will also be painful.
- *Is there a history of trauma?*
  A history of trauma to the head or eye followed by acute vision loss is one of the typical presentations in an emergency setting **(Flowchart 1)**. Ocular trauma can

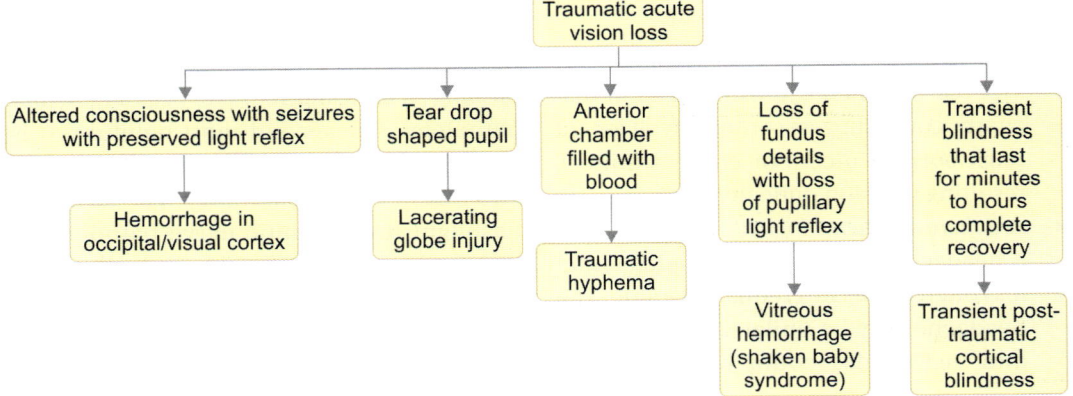

Flowchart 1: Traumatic acute vision loss.

result in globe rupture, retinal detachment, vitreous hemorrhage, or lens dislocation. Injury to the brain could result in hemorrhage in the region of the visual cortex that may result in cortical blindness. The simplest way to differentiate cortical blindness from ocular blindness is the pupillary (light) reflex, which is preserved in the former. History of floaters, smoky haze, and flashing lights/photos are common symptoms children with ocular trauma report.

- *Is there a fluctuation in vision loss?*
  When the child complains of vision loss but is inconsistent in time and place, the possibility of hysterical blindness cannot be ruled out. For example, a child with hysterical blindness might not bump into any objects in the room and can manipulate and move carefully without getting hurt.
- *Is it a transient or permanent vision loss?*
  Acute vision loss in children could be transient with complete recovery. Transient vision loss occurs following trivial head trauma (transient post-traumatic cerebral blindness), hypoglycemia, retinal migraine, and occipital lobe epilepsy. In adults, transient monocular vision loss is often an indicator for ischemic insult (amaurosis fugax), especially in the presence of cardiovascular risk factors.
- *Are there any other ocular symptoms?*
  The red inflamed eye with purulent discharge could suggest corneal involvement (e.g., corneal ulcers or corneal injury), resulting in vision difficulty.
- *Are there any neurological symptoms?*
  A headache preceding or following vision loss often points to a retinal migraine. The headache may be unilateral or bilateral, and vision loss could be monocular (on the same side of the headache) or binocular. The presence of weakness, numbness, and loss of consciousness must suggest a neurological cause of vision loss, especially ischemic. Magnetic resonance imaging (MRI) brain is often warranted in the evaluation of these children. Transient vision loss with seizure could point to benign occipital epilepsy. Features of raised intracranial pressure (ICP) would suggest pseudotumor cerebri.
- *Is there a family history?*
  A family history of migraine in a child with vision loss might help us to consider the possibility of retinal migraine.
- *Is there a history of drug or modification use?*
  Drugs, including ethambutol, hydroxychloroquine, chloramphenicol, and streptomycin can result in sudden, acute binocular vision loss. With drug intake, children may complain of patchy areas of blackness in the visual field (central or paracentral scotoma).

EXAMINATION

Assessment of visual acuity is challenging. Children are often uncooperative for formal ocular examination. The majority of information on visual acuity is obtained by observation of the child as to whether he avoids the bright lights and whether he fixates or follows human faces. A *pin-hole test* is beneficial; if vision improves through a *pin-hole*, it indicates refractory error or ocular pathology. The second most helpful test is *light reflex*, preserved in cortical vision loss and lost in ocular pathology. The swinging flashlight test for optic nerve pathology is the third most beneficial one. In this test, when the light is swung from the healthy eye to the affected eye, in a child with optic nerve pathology, there is pupillary dilation instead of constricting to the flashlight. The fourth fundamental examination is a fundoscopic examination for papilledema (Pseudotumor cerebri), papillitis (optic neuritis), or any signs of ocular injury. Broad approach to a child with vision loss is shown in **Flowchart 2**. The plan of investigations in a child with acute vision loss is outlined briefly in **Flowchart 3**.

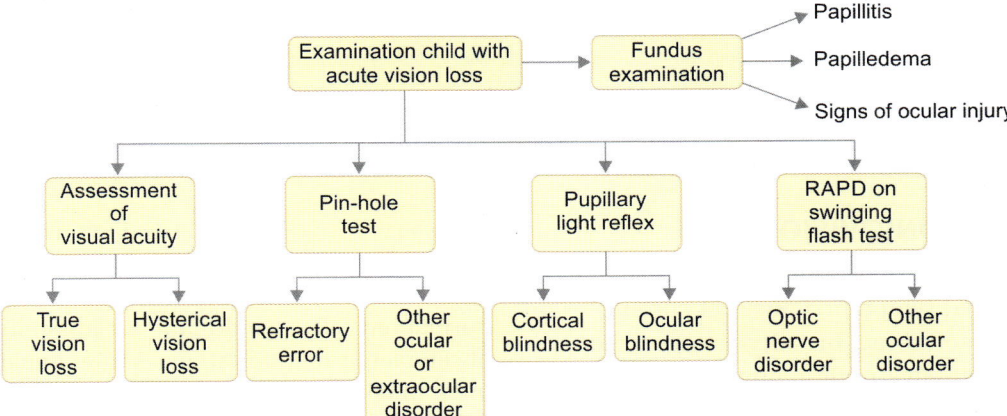

Flowchart 2: Broad approach to vision loss.

(RAPD: Relative apparent pupillary defect)

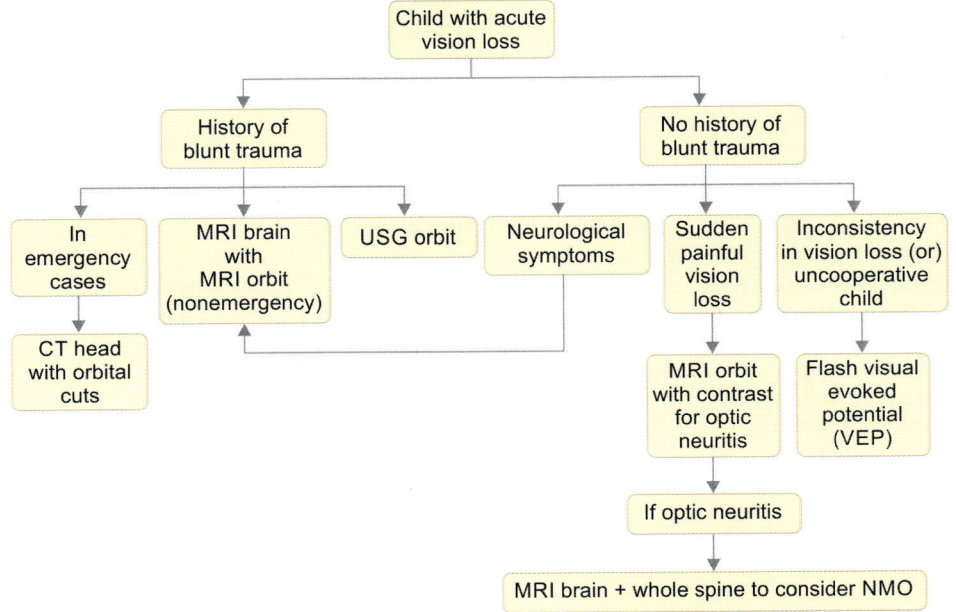

Flowchart 3: Investigating a child with acute vision loss.

(CT: computed tomography; MRI: magnetic resonance imaging; NMO: neuromyelitis optica)

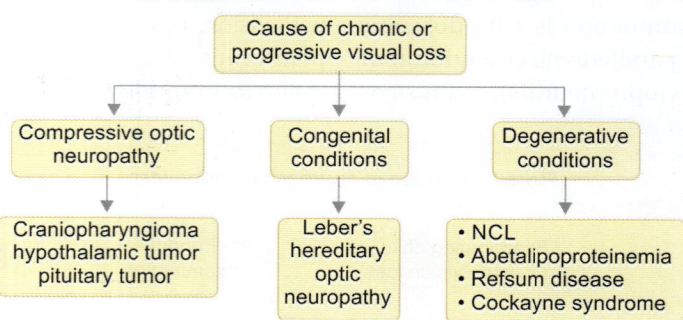

Flowchart 4: Causes of chronic vision loss.

(NCL: neuronal ceroid lipofuscinoses)

CHRONIC VISION LOSS

Chronic vision loss in children is seldom an isolated symptom. Causes of chronic vision loss could be broadly categorized into compressive optic neuropathy, congenital conditions, and degenerative conditions (**Flowchart 4**). Majority of times, it is associated with features of raised ICP, short stature, endocrine abnormality (craniopharyngioma/pituitary adenoma). In others, vision loss is a part of gray matter degeneration with cognitive loss with seizure as in *neuronal ceroid lipofuscinosis*. Uncommonly, vision loss starts in infancy with nystagmus, mid facial hypoplasia, and enophthalmos as in *Leber's hereditary optic neuropathy*. Loss of normal red reflex would indicate possibility of cataract or retinoblastoma. Visual impairment in children with global developmental delay would indicate chorioretinitis [TORCH (*Toxoplasma gondii*, other agents, rubella, cytomegalovirus, and herpes simplex virus) infection], optic atrophy or cortical blindness (structural damage to occipital cortex). Presence of papilledema in a child with vision loss often raises possibility of benign raised ICP (pseudotumor cerebri).

KEY MESSAGES

- Retinal vascular disorders present with sudden onset of painless vision loss whereas optic neuritis present with painful vision loss.
- Transient vision loss may occur in migraine, hypoglycemia, or following trivial head trauma.
- The presence of weakness, numbness, and loss of consciousness must suggest a neurological cause of vision loss.
- Vision loss in a child with papilledema may suggest a possibility of benign raised ICP.
- Rapid alternating swinging flash test can differentiate optic nerve disorder from other ocular disorders in a child with vision loss.

23. Approach to a Child with Hearing Loss

INTRODUCTION

Hearing loss refers to loss of hearing with decibel loss exceeding 25 dB as obtained by an average at 500 Hz, 1000 Hz, 2000 Hz and 4000 Hz (WHO definition of hearing impairment). The hearing loss could be divided into conductive hearing loss, sensorineural hearing loss, or mixed hearing loss. Majority of congenital hearing loss is secondary to sensorineural hearing loss, which could be syndromic (30%) or nonsyndromic monogenic disorder (70%) **(Flowchart 1)**. The nonsyndromic congenital deafness could have autosomal dominant (20%) inheritance or autosomal recessive inheritance (80%). Depending on the affected gene, severity of hearing loss and age at clinical presentation would vary. The most common implicated genes are *connexin 26 (GJB2), GJB6,* and *SLC26A4.*

APPROACH TO A CHILD WITH HEARING LOSS

- *Is it a hearing loss?* Any impairment in the ability to hear 10 Hz sounds at threshold considered normal is a hearing loss. By definition, pure tone threshold >25 dB at 500; 1,000; 2,000; and 4,000 Hz is considered hearing loss.
- *What is developmental status of child?* Children with isolated hearing loss have impairment in speech and language development. Hearing impairment could be a comorbidity in a child with global developmental delay or cerebral palsy. Majority of genetic syndromes, chromosomal disorder (trisomy 13/18), or acquired insult [TORCH (*Toxoplasma gondii*, other agents, rubella, cytomegalovirus, and herpes simplex virus) infection]

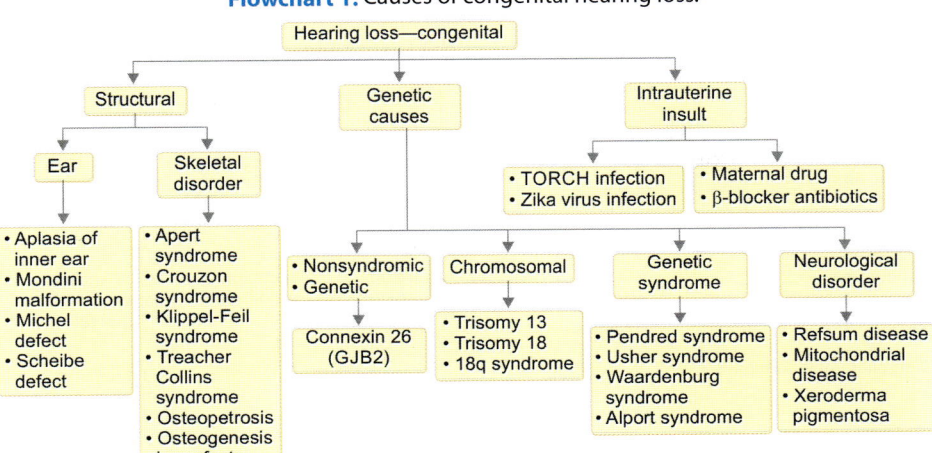

Flowchart 1: Causes of congenital hearing loss.

would result in global developmental delay and hearing loss. However, structural malformation (aplasia of inner ear, Mondini defect) or nonsyndromic hereditary hearing loss (*GJB2, GJB6,* and *SLC26A4*) would result in isolated hearing loss.

- *What is the age at onset?* Hearing loss could be identified in the neonatal period (congenital hearing loss) or delayed onset (identified at a later age but attributable to causes present at birth). Acquired causes of hearing loss such as meningitis, encephalitis, kernicterus, drug induced (e.g., aminoglycoside) would often present at a later age. Hence, delayed-onset hearing loss could be congenital or acquired. Congenital hearing loss is now identified at birth owing to robust neonatal hearing screening program. Neonatal hearing screening involves oto-acoustic-emission (OAE). If the test reveals "refer" on OAE, then auditory brainstem-evoked response (ABR) is conducted to defect hearing loss.

It is also important to remember than many nonsyndromic hearing loss may pass the neonatal screening and their hearing loss worsens over the time. For example, congenital CMV may pass neonatal hearing screening.

- *Are there any associated features for syndromic hearing loss?* One must look for associated ocular, renal, cutaneous and endocrine markers of underlying syndromic hearing loss **(Flowchart 2)**.
- *Are there any risk factors for acquired hearing loss?*
  - History of trauma to temporal bone can injure cochlea. Cochlear nerve injury can result in hearing loss (sensorineural).
  - History of excessive noise exposure can also damage outer hair cells (sensorineural hearing loss).
  - History of infection like *measles* and *mumps*
  - History to suggest pyogenic *meningitis,* especially *Haemophilus influenzae*
  - History of *drug exposure* [(aminoglycoside, macrolide (azithromycin), cisplatin/anticancer drug) and furosemide (loop diuretic)] in antenatal period or infancy
  - Antenatal history of fever, rash, and lymph node swelling (TORCH infection/zika virus infection)
- *What are characteristics of hearing loss?*
  - *Severity of hearing loss:* Hearing threshold 26–40 dB (mid), 41–55 dB (moderate), 56–70 dB (moderate-severe), 71–90 dB (severe), >90 dB

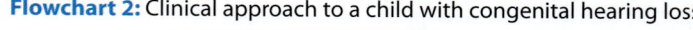

Flowchart 2: Clinical approach to a child with congenital hearing loss.

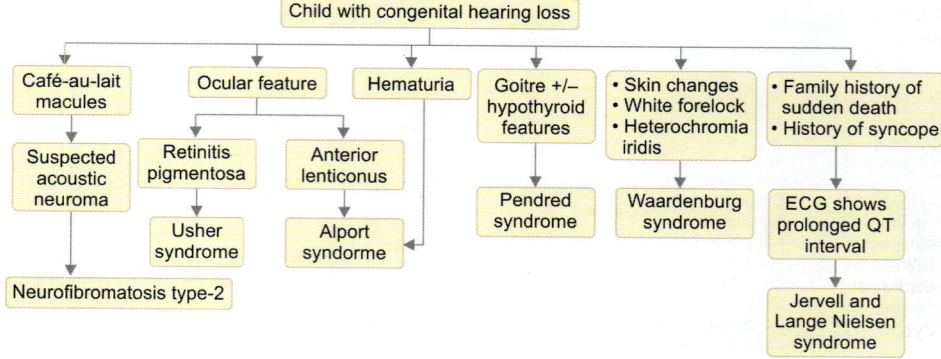

(profound) mild-moderate hearing loss requires bilateral hearing aid. Those with moderate-severe and severe may require bimodal treatment (cochlear implant in one ear and hearing aid in the other ear). Those with profound hearing loss will require bilateral cochlear implant.

- *Is it unilateral or bilateral?* Majority of unilateral hearing loss is acquired otological causes or structural malformation of ear.
- *Is it progressive hearing loss?* Most of nonsyndromic hereditary hearing loss is progressive in nature and hearing loss worsens with time. One may consider autoimmune hearing loss in progressive delayed-onset hearing loss.

BROAD APPROACH TO INVESTIGATING A CHILD WITH HEARING LOSS

Three main investigations for evaluation of a child with hearing loss include imaging (MRI temporal bone/CT temporal bone, CMV diagnostic and targeted genetic testing). A broad approach in investigating a child with hearing loss is depicted in **Flowchart 3**.

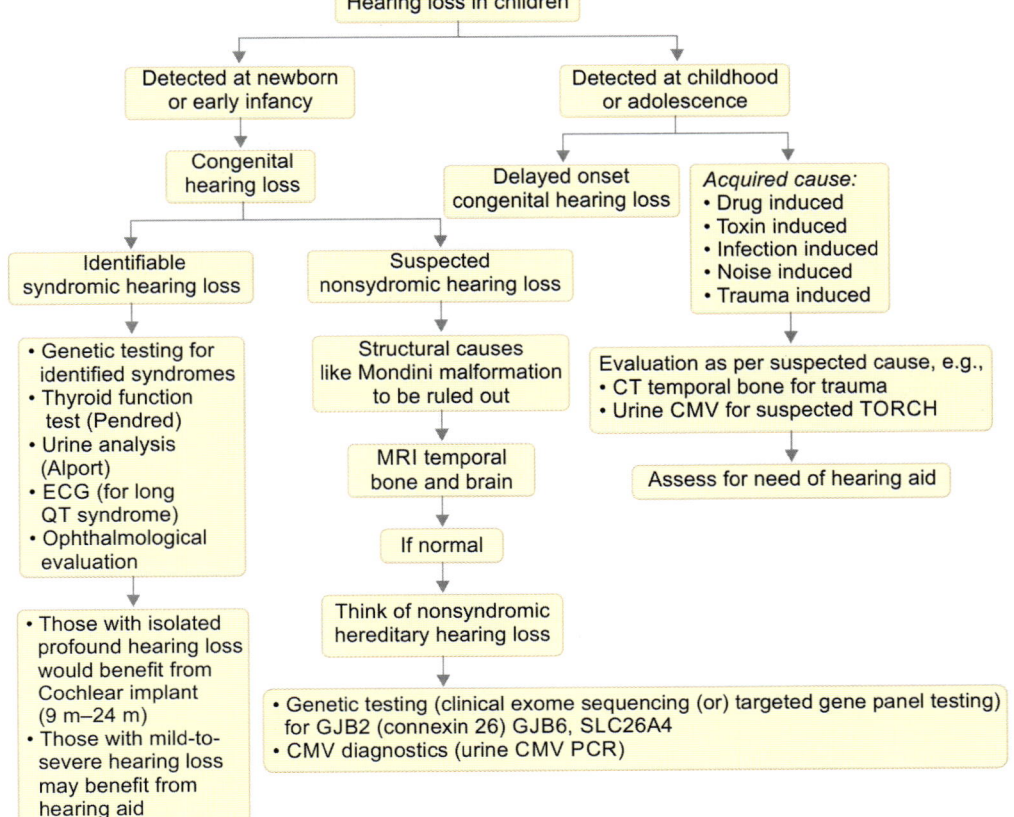

Flowchart 3: Investigating a child with congenital hearing loss.

(CMV: cytomegalovirus; PCR: polymerase chain reaction: TORCH: *Toxoplasma gondii*, other agents, rubella, cytomegalovirus, and herpes simplex virus)

SECTION 2: Neurological Approach to Diagnosis

KEY MESSAGES

- Hearing loss in children is defined when the hearing threshold exceeds 25 dB.
- Hearing loss could be congenital (detected at newborn or delayed-onset) or acquired.
- It is essential to identify syndromic causes of congenital hearing loss.
- Structural or anatomical causes of congenital hearing loss is detected on MRI temporal bone.
- Genetic causes (monogenic) are one of leading causes of nonsyndromic congenital hearing loss. The three most common genes are *GJB2 (connexin 26), GJB6,* and *SLC26A4*.
- All children with unilateral or bilateral sensorineural hearing loss should be screened for congenital CMV infection.
- Children with mild-severe hearing loss respond to hearing aids and those with profound hearing loss respond only to cochlear implants.

SECTION 3

Residents' Corner: Exam-oriented Cases

24. A Case of Cerebral Palsy
25. A Case of Tubercular Meningitis
26. A Case of Acute Hemiplegia
27. A Case of Paraplegia
28. A Case of Acute Flaccid Paralysis/Guillain–Barré Syndrome
29. A Case of Floppy Infant
30. A Case of Muscular Dystrophy
31. A Case of Neurodegenerative Disorder
32. A Case of Hydrocephalus

24. A Case of Cerebral Palsy

HISTORY TAKING

This chapter helps in bedside case presentation of a child with cerebral palsy. Cerebral palsy is static encephalopathy, and the most frequent presenting complaint is developmental delay. Symptoms usually start from the birth, although parents often notice the delay late. If the child has faltered in development after initial normal development, this suggests neuroregression and should be dealt with in a different manner.

The presenting complaints of "developmental delay from birth" are followed by the history of presenting illness. The history of presenting illness will thus start from the antenatal period followed by birth history, developmental history, and history of comorbidities. This is followed by immunization history, nutritional history, family history, and socioeconomic history.

Presenting Complaints

It will be good to keep the following points in your mind while framing presenting complaints:
- Number of presenting complaints can be 2–3 (avoid more than 4 presenting complaints).
- They must be in a chronological order of appearance.
- Avoid the use of medical terminology as far as possible.

Children with cerebral palsy usually have 3–4 presenting complaints.

First complaint is often *developmental delay,* which can be expressed as:
- Delayed attainment of developmental milestones
- Nonattainment of developmental milestones since beginning
- Inability to sit and speak till now
- Inability to sit and speak as per his/her age

Second complaint could be related to *motor weakness or tone abnormalities,* which can be expressed as:
- Tightness of both lower limb and upper limb noticed since 8 months of age
- Abnormal twisting postures of upper limb and lower limb noticed since 9 months of age
- Paucity of movement of right upper and lower limbs noticed since 1 year of age

Third complaint could be one of *comorbidities* such as seizure, vision loss, hearing impairment, recurrent chest infections, and inability to gain weight. The following complaints could be framed to depict positive comorbidities present:
- Multiple episodes of convulsions/fits since 3 months of age
- Three episodes of convulsion in the last 2 months with the last episode 2 days back
- Inability to focus with eyes noticed since 3 months of age

- Poor visual regard noticed since 3 months of age
- Poor response to sound or hearing impairment noticed since 3 months of age
- Multiple episodes of fever, cough, and fast breathing lasting for 5–6 days over the last 2 years
- Poor weight gain since the beginning

Fourth complaint could be an *acute presentation* for which the child has been brought to medical attention such as fever, cough, loose stools, vomiting, or convulsion. It is not essential to form only these presenting complaints; it will obviously depend upon case to case. **Table 1** outlines a few common clinical scenarios and model presenting complaints.

History of Presenting Illness

Start the history with antenatal history, as the presenting complaints are often from the beginning of life in a child with cerebral palsy.

TABLE 1: Complaints in different type 1 cerebral palsy (CP).

Clinical situation	Presenting complaints
Spastic diplegic cerebral palsy	• Inability to walk properly till now • Tightness of both legs with crossing of legs while walking
Spastic quadriplegic cerebral palsy	• Inability to sit or speak till now (or delay in attainment of developmental milestones) • Tightness noticed across the lower limb and upper limbs since the age of 4 months • Three episodes of convulsions over last 2 months
Dyskinetic cerebral palsy	• Inability to sit or speak till now • Abnormal twisting postures of both hands and legs with arching of back noticed since 8 months of age • Cough and fever for 3 days

Antenatal History

Brief and relevant antenatal history about the case of cerebral palsy must include maternal age, whether the conception was spontaneous/in vitro fertilization, previous abortions/stillbirths, ultrasonography scan for fetal malformation and monitoring of fetal growth, regular antenatal visits, and vaccination (tetanus). Besides, detailed individual trimester-wise history (rationale in bracket) should be elicited:

- *T1 (first trimester):* Bleeding per vaginum (threatened abortion), leaking per vaginum (chorioamnionitis), drug history (especially antiepileptic or antipsychotic drugs like fetal valproate syndrome), smoking, radiation, alcohol exposure (fetal alcohol syndrome), fever with rash and swelling in neck/axilla [TORCH (toxoplasmosis, others—syphilis and hepatitis B, rubella, cytomegalovirus, herpes simplex) infection], excessive vomiting, burning micturition [maternal urinary tract infection (UTI) is an independent risk factor for cerebral palsy].
- *T2 (second trimester):* Time at which fetal movements were perceived (excessive fetal movements may indicate intrauterine seizure as seen in nonketotic hyperglycinemia; paucity of fetal movement may indicate fetal onset of hypotonia as in spinal muscular atrophy or congenital myopathy and congenital muscular dystrophy), paleness of body or excessive lethargy, history of headache or raised blood pressure records or deranged blood sugar records during antenatal visit [maternal anemia, pregnancy-induced hypertension (PIH), and gestational diabetes are risk factors for asphyxia].
- *T3 (third trimester):* Bleeding per vaginum, premature rupture of membranes, maternal fever (chorioamnionitis),

burning micturition (UTI), time taken to delivery (prolonged labor predisposes to asphyxia), need for medication for labor induction/instrumentation (indicator of intrauterine asphyxia), and any precipitous labor (prone to intraventricular bleeds)

Birth History

History of mode of delivery, birth weight, whether the baby cried immediately at birth, need for resuscitation, history of neonatal encephalopathy, neonatal seizures, and neonatal jaundice must be elicited. History of neonatal intensive care admission—need for mechanical ventilation, need for inotropic support, history of phototherapy or exchange transfusion for neonatal jaundice, duration of neonatal intensive care unit (NICU) stay, and need for nasogastric feeds must also be recorded.

Neonatal encephalopathy, neonatal seizures, hypoglycemic insult, intraventricular bleed, preterm brain injury, neonatal jaundice requiring exchange transfusion, and prolonged ventilation (hypoxic injury) are some of the most common causes of neonatal brain injury. It is essential to screen for these adverse neonatal events. Remember that delayed cry at birth is not equivalent to birth asphyxia. It is important to elicit history of neonatal encephalopathy following delayed cry at birth, which may be considered a significant clinical brain injury.

Clinical Status at the Time of Neonatal Discharge

At the time of discharge, ask whether the baby was accepting direct breastfeeds well, was having adequate weight gain, was alert and active, or remained dull/lethargic. This gives us an idea about the degree of encephalopathy or neurological deficit at the time of discharge. For instance, if the baby was dull, lethargic with a paucity of limb movement, and had difficulty in feeding, it is more likely that the baby had signs of encephalopathy.

Developmental History

Developmental history becomes the history of presenting illness, as the presenting complaint is delayed attainment of milestones. Developmental history may be presented in a chronological manner (age-wise) as per the developmental milestone attained across each domain. This is in contrast to a separate heading of developmental history wherein we present the developmental history in the domain-wise manner. Presenting the history should be in a chronological manner.

Example: The baby attained social smile by 3 months. By the age of 6 months, he could hold his neck and could open the hands. By 9 months, he could recognize parents and start cooing. At the present age of 12 months, the child can turn from prone to a supine position, tries to reach for objects, smiles at the mirror image, and has started babbling. These developmental milestones are suggestive of global developmental delay with an approximate developmental age of 5–6 months in the gross motor sphere, 4–5 months in the fine motor sphere, 6–7 months in the cognitive sphere, and 4–5 months in the language sphere against a chronological age of 12 months.

In the cognitive and social domains, it is essential to elicit a history of self-care, learning, communication, acceptance in society, and participation in domestic life. This evolves from the concept of impairment, activity limitation, and participation restrictions as per the international classification of functioning, disability, and health of the World Health Organization (WHO).

History of Early Signs of Cerebral Palsy

There is no separate heading called "early signs of cerebral palsy" while presenting the history, but early markers of cerebral palsy must be identified in history. This can be presented along with the chronological age of its appearance while presenting the above developmental history, as these complaints again form a part of presenting illness **(Practical Box 1)**. The following early signs may be elicited:

- Lack of alertness and interest in surrounding (a sign of encephalopathy)
- Excessive irritability and poor quality of sleep (a sign of encephalopathy)
- Reduced spontaneous limb movement or asymmetry of limb movement (a sign of encephalopathy)
- Constant fisting of hands (a sign of encephalopathy)
- Early handedness (an early sign of hemiplegic cerebral palsy)
- Small growth of head or small head (indicates poor growth of the brain)

Microcephaly or small head at birth should always be enquired. This often indicates intrauterine or antenatal insult such as TORCH infection and congenital malformation. This must be differentiated from acquired microcephaly, which often results from perinatal brain insult. Head circumference at birth will be useful in this regard, if parents were informed about the same. Hence, every small head size at birth is not a result of perinatal asphyxia. Static intrauterine insults, such as TORCH infection or congenital malformation, are also an important cause of cerebral palsy.

History of Comorbidities

Salient comorbidities that need to be screened include vision, hearing, feeding difficulty, excessive drooling of saliva, recurrent vomiting, recurrent chest infection, constipation, perception of sensation, seizures, or abnormal body movement **(Table 2)**.

History of Motor Deficits

Motor deficits constitute the most important aspect of cerebral palsy history. History of motor deficits enables us to classify the type of cerebral palsy as hemiplegic, diplegic, spastic, quadriplegic, and dyskinetic **(Table 3)**.

Description of Gait (History)

In ambulatory children with a cerebral palsy, description of gait becomes an important part of history as well as examination. From the gait description, it needs to be clear what type of cerebral palsy we are dealing with. Few examples of description of gait in the history are given in **Practical Boxes 2 and 3**.

Description of Speech (History)

Speech can be described briefly in one line while describing the language milestones in the history of presenting illness among those who are able to communicate with a good vocabulary. It is essential to differentiate between spastic and extrapyramidal dysarthria. Children with isolated spastic dysarthria might have strained quality of

---

PRACTICAL BOX 1: An example of history of presenting illness.

During the initial 6 months, the baby had lack of alertness and was not responsive to sound. He remained lethargic and had paucity of spontaneous limb movements. By the age of 6 months, he had developed neck holding. His hands were constantly fisted till almost 12 months of age; now he opens his hands intermittently but does not hold the object held in his hand

TABLE 2: Eliciting history of comorbidities.

Comorbidity	Salient points in history
Vision	Ability to fix on object, ability to follow or track objects and persons appropriately, and any evident jerky movements of eyes or any obvious deviation of eyes
Hearing	Ability to respond to name, turning to sound, and excessive startles to sound
Feeding	Difficulty in swallowing both solids and liquids (*pseudobulbar effect*), keeps them in mouth for long periods then spitting it (*oropharyngeal incoordination*), persistent drooling of saliva, abnormal tongue thrusting movement (*choreoathetoid movement of tongue*), abnormal chewing/grimacing/pouting or lip smacking movement (*oromotor dyskinesia*)
Bowel habits	Any history of constipation or passage of hard stools or straining at stool
Seizures	History of episodes of vacant stare (*dialeptic seizures*), jerky movement of limbs (*clonic seizures*), abnormal tight posturing followed by jerky movement of limbs (*generalized tonic-clonic seizure*), forced turning of face/head (*focal seizure*), sudden shock-like jerk of body (*myoclonus*)
Sleep	Difficulty in sleep onset, sleep duration in hours, and frequent daytime naps
Behavior	Aggressive, stubborn, temper tantrum, disruptive behavior

TABLE 3: Salient points in history of motor deficits.

Salient points in history	This indicates
Early handedness and paucity of movement of one side of the body	Hemiplegia
Tightness noticed across hips while changing the nappies (*hip adductor spasticity*), scissoring of legs on attempt to make him stand (*hip adductor spasticity*), on attempt to sit he/she sits with his legs crossed under his/her thighs resembling an English letter "W", on attempt to crawl he/she drags his/her body, as if crawling by soldier commando (*commando crawl*)	Diplegia
Tightness noticed across both upper limb and lower limb joints	Quadriplegia
Fixed contractures/deformities across joints	Contractures/deformity
Abnormal twisting movements of hands while reaching for an object, abnormal arching of the back or abnormal twisting postures of lower limbs on an attempt to bear weight/walk	Dystonia
Abnormal slow writhing movement (*athetosis*), abnormal flowing, bizarre movement (*chorea*), or violent flinging movement (*ballismus*)	Choreoathetoid movement

PRACTICAL BOX 2: An example of description of hemiplegic gait.

While walking, he holds his right arm tightly glued to his body with decreased swing of the right upper limb. At the same time, he drags the right foot and scrapes the toes swinging the right lower limb in semicircular fashion (this description favors right hemiplegic gait)

PRACTICAL BOX 3: An example of description of diplegic gait.

While walking, he keeps the lower limb in such a manner that knees cross in front of each other with each step with hips being held close together. He takes short and narrow steps dragging both the legs and scraping the toes against the floor. It often appears as if feet are stuck to the floor (this description favors scissoring or diplegic gait)

voice and appear as if they are speaking from their stomach with poor clarity of speech. This speech is often associated with excessive drooling of saliva with a child keeping his tongue protruded. Extrapyramidal dysarthria will have poor clarity of speech and slurred, irregular, and jerky speech with a poor articulation of words. The rest of the detailed speech description can be provided in the examination at the time of the higher mental function (HMF).

Etiological History

The majority of etiological history is already covered in antenatal and birth history. Further, metabolic disorders that can present in this manner should be ruled out. History of abnormal urinary odor, episodes of excessive lethargy (*inborn errors of metabolism*), fluctuations, or worsening with febrile illness (*mitochondrial/organic acidemia*) must be elicited. Any history of postnatal brain injury in the form of head trauma and meningitis (fever, seizure, and altered sensorium) may be useful.

Treatment History

History of investigations including neuroimaging and electroencephalography, if performed, must be described. The nature of supportive treatment including physiotherapy, use of night splints/braces, and occupational and speech therapy, if any, may be mentioned. Any medications for tightness (spasticity/dystonia) and seizures can be mentioned in this history. The name of medications can be mentioned, if parents are able to recollect their name or else it may be mentioned that *"child is receiving drugs for control of seizure, nature of which is not known"*. Since history starts from the beginning, the conventional title of "past history" may not be applicable in this case. Hence, include all relevant medical and surgical illnesses in the history of presenting illness.

Other Conventional Pediatric History

Other history includes immunization history, nutritional history, family history, and socioeconomic history. Three-generation pedigree must be made. History of consanguinity, sibling loss, and family history of similar illness or any other neurological or systemic illness must be elicited. Depending on the gender of affected sibling and presence or absence of consanguinity, the mode of inheritance such as autosomal-recessive or X-linked recessive must be suggested.

Summary of History

Example

A 3-year-old boy, a product of nonconsanguineous marriage, presented with complaints suggestive of global developmental delay with a developmental age of 5–7 months in all the domains. The mother complained of tightness involving all the four limbs along with associated feeding difficulties and excessive drooling of saliva. The child has intact vision, intact hearing, no seizures, no history suggestive of extrapyramidal movement disorders, and no fixed deformities or contractures. There is no significant family history, and nutritional history reveals a calorie deficit of 400 kcal/day. The child belongs to a nuclear family with lower middle socioeconomic status.

The probable etiology of this illness could be perinatal asphyxia, neonatal seizures, and prolonged neonatal mechanical ventilation.

Other differentials/etiological possibilities include:
- Perinatal insult secondary to intrauterine TORCH infection
- Neurometabolic disorders including organic acidemia, mitochondrial disorders, urea cycle defects, and peroxisomal disorders
- Structural malformation of central nervous system (CNS) such as schizencephaly, lissencephaly, and polymicrogyria

Thinking about Differential Diagnoses at the End of History Taking

It is a good idea to keep broad differentials and set up points for and against each differential diagnosis kept. In the case discussed above, the etiologies that could be considered are given in **Table 4**.

■ FOCUSED EXAMINATION

The sequence of presenting examination findings includes opening remark, vital signs, anthropometry, general physical examination (GPE), developmental examination, and CNS examination. Kindly refer to "*Clinical Methods in Pediatrics by Piyush Gupta*" for detailed methods of examination.

However, salient points in each part of these examinations are summarized here:
- *Opening remark:* This reflects the findings that are obvious even before you touch the child. It is considered as "first look findings". It is desirable to comment on the posture, alertness, overall built, and nutrition and if any medical gadgets (IV cannula and nasogastric tube) attached **(Practical Box 4)**.
- *Vital signs:* These signs will include temperature, heart rate, respiratory rate,

TABLE 4: Differentials and points for and against each differential diagnosis.

Differential diagnosis	Points for (+)	Points against (−)
Perinatal asphyxia	• History of asphyxia • History of neonatal seizure • History of neonatal encephalopathy • Global developmental delay (GDD) from beginning • *Static insult:* Slowly gaining developmental milestones • Spastic quadriparesis	
TORCH infection	• GDD from beginning • Static insult slowly gaining • Spastic quadriparesis (±)	No history of antenatal fever/rash
Neurometabolic disorder	• GDD from beginning • Static insult slowly gaining • Spastic quadriparesis (±)	• No consanguinity (A-R) • No sibling loss (A-R) • No history suggestive of metabolic error such as the abnormal smell of urine • No fluctuations in illness
Structural malformation	• GDD from beginning • Static insult slowly gaining • Spastic quadriparesis (±)	No seizures (±)

Note: ± means that this point may favor or disfavor this differential.
(A-R: autosomal recessive)

> **PRACTICAL BOX 4:** An example of description of opening remark.
>
> Child is sitting comfortably in mother's lap; he is alert, smiling, and showing reasonable interest in surroundings with evident tight posturing of both upper and lower limbs with intermittent twisting postures of hands. He is of average built and nutrition. He has IV cannula secured in his right hand

> **PRACTICAL BOX 5:** Vital sign description.
>
> - *Temperature:* 99°F right axilla as measured for 3 minutes
> - *Heart rate:* 80 beats/min and pulse is regular, rhythmic, synchronous, all peripheral pulses palpable
> - *Respiratory rate:* 26 breaths/min, regular, and abdominothoracic
> - *Blood pressure:* 90/62 mm Hg as measured in right arm supine position
> - Capillary refill time is <3 seconds

blood pressure, capillary refill time, and SpO_2, if applicable. Most of these children are often admitted for respiratory tract infection **(Practical Box 5)**.

- *Anthropometry:* Children with cerebral palsy are prone to malnutrition secondary to feeding difficulties, gastroesophageal reflux disease, and recurrent chest infections. Detailed anthropometric measurements and interpretations including weight, length, head circumference, and mid-arm circumference are required.

  In children with spastic quadriplegia, exact length measurement might be difficult owing to fixed contractures or deformities; the same may be acknowledged during the case presentation.

- *GPE:* Conventional head-to-toe GPE with emphasis on the following parameters is expected:
  - Signs of malnutrition, anemia, and vitamin deficiency
  - *Head shape:* Presence of overriding sutures, craniosynostosis, and abnormal skull shape must be commented.
  - Any evidence of *neurocutaneous markers* such as café-au-lait macules, port-wine stain, ash-leaf macules, and axillary fold freckling
  - Any obvious *bony deformities* such as scoliosis and kyphosis must be commented.
  - Any evidence of *hip subluxation* can be commented (spastic diplegic children are prone to hip subluxation). Although it is mentioned under musculoskeletal examination, it can be mentioned in GPE as well.
- *Developmental examination:* The focus of developmental examination in a child with cerebral palsy is to confirm the findings of developmental history. At the end of the developmental examination, we can conclude that *"developmental examination findings corroborate with a developmental age of 5–6 months as elicited by history in all domains"*. Detailed developmental examination as per the age can be read from *"Clinical Methods by Piyush Gupta, 4th edition"*. It is obvious that only relevant examination as per developmental and chronological age will be performed and this will be decided on a case-to-case basis. *Primitive reflexes* including the presence of asymmetric tonic neck reflex, palmar grasp, and Moro reflex can be described as a part of the developmental examination.

  The developmental examination is described under the headings of gross motor domain, fine motor skills, cognition, and adaptive skills **(Practical Boxes 6 and 7)**.

> **PRACTICAL BOX 6:** Description of developmental examination.
>
> A 3-year-old boy with global developmental delay with spastic quadriplegia and history revealing overall developmental age of 5–6 months
> *Gross motor:*
> - *Pull to sit:* Head control was complete
> - *Prone positioning:* He could lift his head and chest off the couch and elbow extended
> - *Vertical suspension:* Intermittent scissoring of legs was noticed
> - *Supine position:* He could turn from prone to side position
> - Overall gross motor age is 16–20 weeks
>
> *Fine motor skills:* He could reach for the cubes but could not transfer from one hand to the other. Grasp of the cubes was immature and was masked by dystonic posturing of hands (fine motor age 4–5 months)
> *Cognitive:* He turned to mother's voice and looked at mother when asked to point at her, he gets excited when mother reaches for him, and he looks eagerly at the toys offered to him but is afraid to hold them
> *Language:* He was observed to babble but did not speak any meaningful monosyllables (4–5 months)
> Overall development of the child is 4–5 months as against a chronological age of 36 months

> **PRACTICAL BOX 7:** Presenting developmental examination of a 6-year-old child with spastic diplegia.
>
> - *Gross motor:* He can walk, run, and climb stairs with one foot per step while going up, but uses two per step while coming down (4–5 years)
> - *Fine motor skills:* He can draw hexagon, build bridge using cubes, and draw three parts in draw-a-man test
> - *Cognition:* He could do simple verbal additions, but cannot do subtraction, can count 1–25; he could identify all colors; he can differentiate small and big size; in the picture book, he can point to more than five objects and name up to four objects
> - *Language:* He can narrate a rhyme with normal fluency and articulation with no evidence of dysarthria during his spontaneous conversation
>
> *Impression:* Gross motor age 4–5 years against expected 7 years; the rest of milestones are age appropriate and correspond to developmental age assessed as per history

- *Gross motor skills* will include maneuvers like pull to sit, ventral suspension, vertical suspension, prone positioning, ability to sit independently, ability to stand from sitting position, ability to stand and walk independently, and so on. Among those who are ambulatory, gait needs to be described in the motor examination.
- *Fine motor skills* will be tested using rattle, red ring, cubes, pencils/crayons, picture cards, colors, thread beads, simple form boards, and draw-a-man test.
- *Cognition:* Few of cognitive assessment that can be done bedside includes mature pointing, looking for hidden toy, pointing to body parts, pointing to named object/person, identifying shapes, colors, size, concept of numbers, answering questions from the story, counting 1–10, telling days of week, doing simple arithmetic calculation, and so on.
- *Speech:* Correlate the history of speech milestones with the observation of spontaneous speech.
- At this stage, one can mention the persistence of *primitive reflexes* including asymmetric tonic neck reflex, palmar grasp, crossed extensor, and Moro reflex. Many examiners prefer primitive reflexes as a part of reflexes in motor system examination.

- *CNS examination:*
  - *HMFs:* Most of the HMFs cannot be assessed objectively in children with cerebral palsy. It is a good idea to comment on appearance, behavior, consciousness, and speech **(Practical Box 8)**. Other components of HMF including orientation, attention span, abstract thinking, memory, insight, perception, calculation, and fund of information are difficult to assess in these children. Components of language assessment include fluency, articulation, comprehension, reading, writing, repetition, and naming. Also, we may comment on content, volume, and the pitch of speech. Refer to **Chapter 1** on clinical neuroanatomy to understand the components of speech and types of dysarthria.
  - *Cranial nerves:* Focus of cranial nerve examination is to comment on visual acuity (presence of visual fixation and following), fundus (to look for evidence of chorioretinitis and optic atrophy), deviation of eyes (paralytic squint/concomitant squint), nystagmoid eye movement, hearing response, and integrity of oropharyngeal coordination (drooling of saliva, poor gag reflex, oromandibular dystonia, oromotor dyskinesia, tongue-thrusting movement, difficulty in sucking/swallowing, and tonic bite reflex) **(Practical Box 9)**.

PRACTICAL BOX 8: Description of speech of a 7-year-old child with dyskinetic cerebral palsy.

On assessment of spontaneous conversation, there is reduced clarity of speech with poor articulation of words with constant drooling of saliva. There is a marked restriction of speech output. The child prefers gestural communication to indicate for his needs. The content of speech is appropriate, as his mother can understand what he wishes to convey. Comprehension of verbal commands, naming, and repetition is preserved. However, reading and writing could not be assessed in this child. This speech could indicate extrapyramidal dysarthria

PRACTICAL BOX 9: Cranial nerve (CN) description of a 7-year-old child with dyskinetic cerebral palsy.

- *First CN:* Could not be tested
- *Second CN:* Visual fixation and following are preserved. However, formal visual acuity could not be performed. Color vision and field of vision could not be tested. Fundus reveals primary optic atrophy
- *Third/fourth/sixth CN:* There is right eye esotropia evident on primary gaze; conjugate eye movements are preserved in all cardinal plane; and saccadic eye movements are preserved with no evidence of oculomotor apraxia. Pupils are normal size and reactive to direct light reflex. Accommodation reflex could not be tested. There are no evident nystagmoid movements
- *Fifth CN:* Jaw movements are preserved, but there is evidence of difficulty in opening the jaw owing to oromandibular dystonia. The sensory component of 5th CN could not be commented
- *Seventh CN:* Facial symmetry is preserved. Other parts of 7th CN examination including taste sensation in anterior two-thirds and testing for tear production were not tested
- *Eighth CN:* He could localize to whisper and respond appropriately
- *Ninth/tenth CN:* There was difficulty in opening the mouth. There was constant drooling of saliva and difficulty in deglutition. However, I could not observe the movements of soft palate and uvula, nor was he cooperative for gag reflex testing
- *Eleventh CN:* Could not be tested
- *Twelfth CN:* He intermittently protrudes the tongue with drooling of saliva. Individual tongue movements could not be tested. There are no obvious tongue fasciculations

> **PRACTICAL BOX 10:** Description of posture and gait.
>
> *A 3-year-old child with spastic quadriplegic cerebral palsy (CP): Posture:* Child is lying supine with both upper limbs flexed at elbow, and wrist joint with pronation of forearm. The lower limbs are extended at hip, knee, and ankle joint with intermittent arching of the back
>
> *A 6-year-old child with spastic diplegia:*
> *Gait:* He walks with short steps, keeping his both thighs tight close to each other, dragging each foot with narrow base and scraping the floor with his toes with normal arm swing. While he is walking, it seems as if both his feet are sticking to the floor. There is no difficulty in initiation of gait; he could stop abruptly when asked to do so and can negotiate turn on either side (to rule out parkinsonian features)

- *Motor system examination:* Components of motor system examination include gait/posture, bulk of muscle, tone of muscle, power of muscle, deep tendon reflexes (DTRs), superficial reflexes, and abnormal movement and coordination. Posture is described among those children who are nonambulatory and gait is described among the ambulatory children **(Practical Box 10)**.

Details of patterns of *gait* described in cerebral palsy including scissoring gait, jump gait, equines gait, crouch gait, and stiff knee gait can be read from standard textbooks.

Tone assessment is the most crucial step in the examination of children with cerebral palsy. It is essential to look for evidence of spasticity and rigidity and differentiate them from dystonia. This helps in classifying the type of cerebral palsy. One should also comment on evidence of contractures or spasticity in a specific group of muscles.

- *Upper limb:* Flexors, adductor, and internal rotators are the most commonly affected.
- *Lower limb:* Hip flexor (crouched), knee flexor (flexed knee), hip adductors (scissoring), and knee are internally rotated and gastrocnemius (on the toe).

The most common mistake that happens during the case presentation is to differentiate spasticity from rigidity and dystonia. Dystonia is a movement disorder and not a tone abnormality **(Table 5)**.

Contractures, if any, should be commented on dynamic or fixed contractures. Any obvious deformities must not be missed. These include kyphoscoliosis; hip subluxation and dislocation; equinus, varus, and valgus deformity; and femur internal and external torsion. It will be good to grade tone across the individual joints as per modified Ashworth grading of tone **(Table 6)**. Other methods including Tardieu scales are also acceptable.

In children less than 2 years, angles (adductor angle, ankle dorsiflexion angle, and popliteal angle) may be measured using a goniometer and mentioned under tone assessment while describing the motor system examination and compared with age norms **(Table 7)**.

- *Power examination:* Most of the formal power testing will be difficult in children with cerebral palsy owing to limited cooperation and muscle contractures. But a rough functional assessment of upper limb muscles including the maturity of grasp and release will be useful. Power must be tested across individual joints, and a rough estimate of assessment must be made. If the child is able to move across the joint against gravity, the power is *"at least 3/5"* across that joint for that particular movement. It is often not possible to test all movements across the joints, and this must be acknowledged while presenting the case. Functional assessment is more

TABLE 5: Differences between spasticity, dystonia, and rigidity.

Features	Spasticity	Dystonia	Rigidity
Important feature	Velocity-dependent resistance	Sustained abnormal twisting posture	Independent of speed or posture
Increase speed of passive movement	Resistance increases	No effect	No effect
Presence of fixed postures	No	Yes	No
Effect of emotions	No	Yes	No
Direction	Unidirectional	Bidirectional	Bidirectional
Upper motor neuron signs (brisk reflexes and extensor plantar)	Present	Absent	Absent

TABLE 6: Modified Ashworth grading of tone.

Grade	Feature
Grade 0	No increase in tone
Grade 1	Slight increase in tone with a catch or minimal resistance at the end of range
Grade 2	Minimal resistance through the range but with catch
Grade 3	More marked increase tone through ROM (range of motion)
Grade 4	Considerable increase in tone, passive movement difficult
Grade 5	Affected part is rigid

TABLE 7: Angles for assessment of tone.

Age (months)	Adductor angle (°)	Popliteal angle (°)	Ankle dorsiflexion (°)	Scarf sign
0–3	40–80	80–100	60–70	Elbow does not cross midline
4–6	70–110	90–120	60–70	Elbow crosses midline
7–9	110–140	110–160	60–70	Elbow goes beyond axillary line
10–12	140–160	150–170	60–70	–

important in children with cerebral palsy than individual movements.

Gross motor function classification system (GMFCS):
- Walks without restrictions
- Walks without assistive devices but limitations in community
- Walks with assistive devices
- Transported or uses powered mobility
- Severely limited dependent on wheelchair

Manual ability classification system (MACS) (4–18 years) for upper limb function:
- Handles objects easily and successfully
- Handles most of objects but decreased quality and speed
- Handles objects with difficulty, needs help to prepare or modify activity
- Handles limited selection of easily managed objects in adapted situation
- Does not handle object at all and inability to perform simple action

TABLE 8: Description of movement disorder in children.

Movement disorder	Description (keywords are marked in italics)
Athetosis	Slow, *distal, writhing*, continuous, and involuntary movements. They are commonly associated with chorea (choreoathetosis)
Ballismus	Involuntary, *high-amplitude*, and *flinging* movements that typically occur proximally
Chorea	Involuntary, *semipurposive, bizarre*, and *chaotic* movement
Dystonia	Dystonia is a syndrome of sustained muscle contractions, frequently causing abnormal twisting and repetitive movements, or abnormal postures
Myoclonus	Quick, very brief, involuntary, and nonsuppressible shock-like movements of one or more muscles
Parkinsonism	*Presence of two or more of the cardinal features of Parkinson's disease:* Tremor at rest, bradykinesia, rigidity, and postural instability
Stereotypies	Involuntary, patterned, coordinated, repetitive, nonreflexive movements that occur in the same fashion with each repetition
Tics	Sudden, rapid, abrupt, repetitive, and nonrhythmic movement
Tremors	Oscillating and rhythmic movements about a fixed point, axis, or plane that occur when antagonist muscles contract alternately

Power assessment is followed by an examination of DTRs, superficial reflex, and assessment of abnormal movement including choreoathetosis, dystonia, and ballismus **(Table 8)**. Coordination testing is often limited owing to limited cooperation, and the same can be acknowledged. Brisk DTR is an indicator of pyramidal tract involvement. DTR is difficult to elicit among those with generalized dystonia.

Other Neurological Examination

- *Sensory system examination:* The majority of sensory system examinations cannot be performed among children with cerebral palsy unless cognition is relatively preserved.
- *Cerebellar signs:* It is again difficult to elicit individual cerebellar signs among these children. In the presence of choreoathetosis and dystonia, cerebellar signs should not be overinterpreted.
- Meningeal signs may be difficult to elicit.
- *Skull and spine examination* with a focus on skull shape, craniosynostosis, and evidence of raised intracranial pressure (McEwan sign).

Musculoskeletal Examination

The focus of musculoskeletal examination includes joint range of motion (ROM) (slow and smooth), deformity including dynamic deformity (only on posture such as standing), contractures, balance, posture, sitting, and gait **(Table 9)**.

SUMMARY OF CASE (TEMPLATE)

A 3-year-old boy, product of nonconsanguineous marriage with no significant family history, presented with:
- Global developmental delay (developmental age of 5–6 months against 3 years of age)

TABLE 9: Musculoskeletal examination.

Examination	Focus of examination
Back	Scoliosis and kyphosis
Hip	Femoral anteversion, hip flexion, hip adductor contracture, and hip subluxation
Knee	High-riding patella, posterior capsular tightness, and popliteal angle
Ankle	Varus/valgus deformity, leg length discrepancy, and gastrocnemius/soleus contracture
Sitting balance	Free sitting/hand-dependent sitting/propped sitter

- Mixed signs of spasticity (Ashworth grade 4) and dystonia
- Fixed contractures involving bilateral ankle joint and dynamic hip adductor contracture
- GMFCS (level 2), MACS (level 3)
- Preserved vision, hearing, and right esotropia
- Feeding difficulties secondary to oromandibular dystonia and oromotor dyskinesia
- Excessive drooling of saliva
- No epilepsy/seizures
- Wasting and no stunting by the WHO classification
- Presence of anemia

Possible etiological differentials:
- Perinatal asphyxia
- Structural malformation of CNS
- Perinatal TORCH sequelae
- Neurometabolic disorders such as phenylketonuria and organic acidemia

KEY MESSAGES

- Bedside case presentation of a child with cerebral palsy may start from the antenatal period, natal period, and postnatal period followed by the history of early signs of cerebral palsy.
- Developmental history is a part of history of presenting illness and may be presented as per the chronological age rather than presenting domain-wise.
- History of comorbidities including vision, hearing, seizures, contractures, feeding difficulties, constipation, and recurrent chest infections must always be elicited.
- Domain-wise developmental examination, measurement of angles (in infants), the examination of primitive reflexes, and advanced postural reactions are additional examinations that must not be missed during case presentation of cerebral palsy.
- The summary of the case must always mention the functional status in terms of GMFC and MACS.

CHAPTER 25: A Case of Tubercular Meningitis

■ INTRODUCTION

Chronic meningitis is a leptomeningeal inflammation that persists beyond 4 weeks. Tubercular meningitis is the most common cause of chronic meningoencephalitis in Indian children. Other causes include partially treated pyogenic meningitis, cryptococcal meningitis, and neoplastic causes. **Table 1** enumerates the causes of chronic meningitis. The present chapter deals with a bedside case presentation of a child with tubercular meningitis.

■ HISTORY PRESENTATION

TABLE 1: Causes of chronic meningitis.

Infectious causes	
Bacterial	Tuberculosis, brucellosis, borreliosis, listeriosis, leptospirosis, and syphilis
Viral	HIV, cytomegalovirus, and mumps
Fungal	Cryptococcal, histoplasmosis, blastomycosis, and nocardiosis
Parasitic	Cysticercosis and toxoplasmosis
Noninfectious causes	
Neoplastic	Leukemia, non-Hodgkin lymphoma, and primary brain malignancy
Vasculitis	SLE, Sjögren syndrome, Behçet disease, and sarcoidosis

(HIV: human immunodeficiency virus; SLE: systemic lupus erythematosus)

Presenting Complaints

A 2-year-old boy was brought with fever for 15 days. He developed multiple episodes of convulsions 4 days back and has altered consciousness since then. He had lost 3 kg weight in the last 1 month and has not been eating well. Mother has a history of active tuberculosis and is on antitubercular drugs for last 2 months.

His presenting complaints include:
- Loss of weight and appetite for last 1 month
- Fever off and on for last 15 days
- Multiple episodes of convulsions 4 days back followed by altered consciousness for last 4 days

We have included a complaint of loss of appetite and weight loss for 1 month to emphasize on the fact that the duration of illness was 1 month and not 15 days. Moreover, weight loss of 3 kg in 1 month is a significant loss and cannot be ignored. The inclusion of this complaint in the presenting complaints makes us think of chronic illness rather than acute neurological illness.

If the child described in the situation above was admitted 15 days back (15th day of illness) and he had developed right hemiparesis after 3 days of hospital admission (18th day of illness); fever has subsided, and sensorium has improved and he has started

accepting oral feeds. Presenting complaints as on today (30th day of illness) will include:
- Fever off and on for last 30 days
- Multiple episodes of convulsions and altered consciousness (or sensorium) for last 18 days
- Paucity of movement of the right upper limb and lower limb for the last 12 days

There are two ways to present this case. One way is to present as on the day of presentation to the hospital and the second way is to present as on today. Both are acceptable. If new clinical symptoms have emerged during the hospital stay that could probably change the hypothesis (as in this case, right-sided hemiparesis), then it would be better to present as today.

Note that we have dropped that complaint of "loss of weight and appetite" to restrict the number of complaints to three. Moreover, the duration of the above complaints already points to long-standing subacute or chronic illness. We have added "paucity of movement of right upper and lower limb", as this points to a focal neurological deficit that could indicate vascular insult. The presenting complaints should include all complaints that could help us to narrow the differentials. If right-sided hemiparesis was noticed on examination, you can go back to history to include the same.

History of Presenting Illness

History of presenting illness (HOPI) must always be presented in chronological order as if narrating a story of what exactly happened. This is similar to a suspense story where the sequence of events is very important with a detailed description of the relevant development. One of the common errors is to elaborate on the presenting complaints and describe negative history at the end. This method often called "history of presenting complaints" might often miss the sequence of events.

While presenting the HOPI, day of illness can be used as a tag to describe the sequence of events **(Practical Box 1)**. It is important to elaborate the events such as fever, seizure, and altered sensorium, but at the same time, not to miss the sequence of events.

Negative History

The concept of negative history needs to be very clear. Negative history does not mean all complaints in the body that are not present in the child. It is a common misperception that the longer the list of negative history better is the case presentation. Even if one or two negative histories are asked, one should be able to defend the rationale behind it. Negative history helps us to analyze the hypothesis and rule out possibilities. For example, in the case discussed above, history

---

PRACTICAL BOX 1: An example of the history of presenting illness.

Child was apparently well a month back when he developed fever that was high grade, documented to 104°F, not associated with rigors, and was often relieved with medication for few hours only to reappear. Fever persisted for the next 18 days despite medications. By the 11th day of illness, he developed flurry of multiple episodes of convulsions that consisted of jerking of all the four limbs with uprolling of eyeballs, frothing from the mouth and clenching of teeth, with no associated bladder bowel incontinence. Each episode lasted for 20–30 minutes with a brief period of recovery followed by the next episode of convulsion. He was in altered sensorium in the form of no eye opening, not responding to verbal commands, not recognizing the parents and not indicating for bladder/bowel needs. Child was admitted in another medical center for 4 days before he was brought on the 15th day of illness. Within 3 days of hospital admission (18th day of illness), parents also noticed paucity of movement of the right upper and lower limb

of ear discharge (a risk factor for brain abscess), rash (meningococcal and measles), and diarrhea (enteroviral encephalitis and *Shigella* encephalopathy) will be useful.

History to Determine the Extent of Involvement

- *History related to higher mental function:* In a child with subacute-to-chronic encephalopathy, we need to determine the degree of altered sensorium by this history whether the child is comatose or in a minimally conscious state (*see* **Chapter 11**). History of altered sensorium is elaborated in the form of the preserved sleep–wake cycle, presence of eye opening, verbal response, ability to follow simple commands, ability to recognize parents, showing reasonable interest in surrounding, indicating for hunger, bladder, and bowel needs. An example of a child in a minimally conscious state is described in **Practical Box 2**.
- *History related to cranial nerves:*
  - History of visual fixation and visual tracking of objects (cranial nerve II) (preserved visual fixation in a child with encephalopathy depicts a better sensorium) (visual loss is uncommon in children with tubercular meningitis unless there is opticochiasmatic arachnoiditis or drug-induced visual toxicity)
  - History of recent abnormal deviation of eyes or jerky movements of eyes or drooping of eyelids (cranial nerves III, IV, and VI) (we use the word "recent" to differentiate it from pre-existing squint) [presence of bilateral sixth nerve palsy is an indicator of raised intracranial pressure (ICP); in such situation, other histories of raised ICP such as repeated vomiting and headbanging would be useful].
  - History of difficulty in opening the mouth or loss of sensation in the face (cranial nerve V) (if the child is in coma, this history may be omitted).
  - History of inability to close the eyes, deviation of face in the form of deviation of angle of mouth or drooling of saliva from one side (cranial nerve VII) [presence of unilateral seventh cranial nerve palsy prompts us to explore the history of associated hemiparesis, as it would indicate a vascular insult in a child with tuberculous meningitis (TBM) such as basal ganglia infarct].
  - History of inability to respond to verbal commands despite normal sensorium (cranial nerve VIII) (if the child is in coma, obviously he will not respond, so may omit this history).
  - History of nasal regurgitation of feeds, drooling of saliva, difficulty in swallowing and alteration in voice (cranial nerves IX and X) (lower cranial nerve palsies are uncommon in children with TBM, presence of the lower cranial nerve palsy must provide a hint to alternate diagnosis such as brainstem tumor).

> **PRACTICAL BOX 2:** An example of how to present the history of consciousness.
>
> Child is in altered sensorium in the form of intermittent eye opening, but no vocalization, does not recognize parents, shows no meaningful interest in surroundings, does not indicate for bladder, and passes urine in bed itself. But mother has noticed that he opens eyes intermittently and then sleeps again suggestive of preserved sleep–wake cycle. In addition, while the child has eye opening, when mother attempts to talk to him, she feels he makes occasional meaningful gestural communication such as nodding "yes" when asked "do you want water?"

- History related to motor system involvement:
  - *History of posture:* History of posture comes along with description of altered sensorium. The posture of the child can be described in history if the child is lying in a constant posture. Postures that are pertinent in history will include decorticate posturing, decerebrate posturing, or hemiplegic posture **(Practical Box 3)** (Decorticate or decerebrate posturing in a child with TBM is an indicator of raised ICP/impending herniation; hemiplegic posture would indicate cortical involvement on the contralateral side).
  - *History of tone:* History of flaccidity of limbs or flabbiness of muscle or tightness of limb muscles noticed by parents while caring for child must be noted. (Tightness is noticed more often than flaccidity in children with TBM; tightness could be because of pyramidal or extrapyramidal tract involvement)
  - *History of muscle power:* History of the paucity of movement of one side of limbs and its ability to lift the limbs off the bed (indicates hemiparesis: translates into muscle power of more than 3/5) (Hemiparesis is an indicator of contralateral cortical involvement).
  - *History of abnormal movement (indicates extrapyramidal involvement):*
    - History of distal slow writhing movements of hands (athetosis)
    - History of flowing dance such as abnormal involuntary movement (chorea)
    - History of abnormal twisting postures of limbs (dystonia)
    - History of shock-like jerks in trunk or limbs (myoclonus)
    - History of violent flinging movements of limbs (ballismus)
- *History related to the sensory system:* This history will be limited among those with coma or minimally conscious state.
- *History related to cerebellar system:* History of clumsiness or overshooting while trying to reach for an object (among those with normal consciousness), history of jerky eye movements.
- *History related to autonomic nervous system:* History of excessive or decreased sweating, dizziness with a sudden change of posture (among those with preserved consciousness) (autonomic features predominate among those with autoimmune encephalitis that may present as subacute encephalopathy).
- *History of bladder involvement* to differentiate upper motor neuron (UMN) bladder (uninhibited bladder with urge incontinence) from lower motor neuron bladder (history of bladder retention). Bladder retention is uncommon among patients with TBM; its presence indicates a possible spinal cord pathology such as arachnoiditis.
- *History of raised ICP:* History of repeated vomiting, headbanging, irritability, or

> **PRACTICAL BOX 3:** An example of how to present history related to posture.
> - Child lies in bed with extended posture of both upper limb and lower limb with arching of back and neck, lifting the body off the level of bed (*decerebrate posturing*)
> - Child lies in bed with both upper limbs flexed, and lower limbs extended with occasional arching of back (*decorticate posturing*)
> - Child lies in bed with paucity of movement of right upper and lower limb that remains flaccid and could not be lifted away from the bed (*hemiplegic posturing*)

headache (among those with preserved consciousness).
- *History related to meningeal signs:* History of neck stiffness noticed by parents.

Etiological History

In a child who presents with subacute-to-chronic onset of febrile encephalopathy with or without focal neurological deficits and raised ICP such as TBM, following additional history can point toward a specific etiological diagnosis:

- History of rash in the body (meningococcal or measles) (*Measles often triggers the onset of TBM; illness could have started with measles-like rash. Measles being an immunocompromised state could possibly trigger latent tuberculosis*)
- History of associated or preceding diarrhea (enteroviral encephalitis and enteric fever) (*Untreated or partially treated enteric fever could progress to subacute febrile encephalopathy*)
- History of bleeding from any other site (bleeding diathesis presenting with intracranial bleeds), history of ear discharge (*chronic suppurative otitis media*), or history suggestive of sinus infections (*brain abscess*)
- History of head trauma in the recent past (*chronic subdural hemorrhage may present with subacute encephalopathy that mimics TBM*)
- History of upper respiratory infection or diarrhea few weeks prior to onset of this illness or history of recent vaccination (*indicates a trigger for demyelinating or autoimmune process*)
- History of yellowish discoloration of eyes and urine (*hepatic encephalopathy*)
- History of blood transfusion or history suggestive of multisite infection (*HIV infection-associated encephalopathy*)
- History of joint pain, swelling, and rash in past (*points toward underlying vasculitis*)
- History of bony pains, mass in the abdomen, unremitting fever, and swellings in the neck (cervical lymphadenopathy) indicate underlying malignancy
- Past history of abnormal urinary odor, unexplained lethargy, profuse vomiting, and fluctuating illness in the form of worsening with febrile illness points to metabolic inborn errors of metabolism including mitochondrial disorders.
- History of recent travel to a hilly region or any possible tick bite (*rickettsial infection*)
- History of prolonged drug intake or possible toxin exposure such as exposure to lead (occupation of parents: working in lead factory) (*lead encephalopathy*)

At the end of history, we should have a fair idea on the duration of illness, the chronology of events, the extent of neurological involvement, and possible etiology.

■ FOCUSED EXAMINATION

Opening Statement

We start describing the examination by an opening remark on findings that are obviously evident. Here, we may describe the sensorium, posture, overall built and nutrition, and any medical gadgets if attached.

Sensorium: Formal assessment of sensorium is a part of higher mental function in central nervous system (CNS) examination. However, a brief mention of sensorium at outset becomes relevant before we proceed for formal examination. At this stage, we do not have to commit on Glasgow coma scale scoring but could use its terms of eye opening, motor response, and verbal response to describe the sensorium **(Practical Box 4)**.

Posture: Description of posture must be made in the form of position of limbs,

> **PRACTICAL BOX 4:** An example of how to present sensorium in the opening statement.
>
> "He is sleeping comfortably right now, but while I examined him 15 minutes ago, he was irritable, restless, agitated with occasional spontaneous eye opening, nonpurposive motor movements, and mumbling meaningless vocalization"

> **PRACTICAL BOX 5:** An example of description of posture.
>
> *Posture can be described as follows:* Child is lying supine in the bed with both arms being adducted at shoulder joint, flexed at elbow, and wrist joint. Lower limbs are extended at hip, knee, and ankle joint with intermittent arching of back, suggestive of decorticate posturing

trunk, and head. Gross impressions that are expected include hemiparesis, quadriparesis, decorticate, or decerebrate posturing. These findings obviously will be confirmed while doing motor system examination, but posture gives us a fair idea of motor deficit **(Practical Box 5)**.

Vital Signs

Vital signs will include temperature, heart rate, respiratory rate, blood pressure, and oxygen saturation. Analysis of vital signs in a neurological patient is of utmost importance. The presence of bradycardia with or without hypertension would point toward features of raised ICP. The presence of tachycardia with poor pulse volume and hypotension indicates signs of shock. Use the right size of blood pressure cuff while measuring blood pressure. Ideal blood pressure cuff must cover two-thirds of arms' length and at least 80% of arm circumference. The respiratory pattern is extremely helpful in assessing the site of lesion (Read **Chapter 11**). It might be useful to mention SpO_2 in sick children. (Handheld battery-driven saturation probes can be purchased and should be used in daily practice)

Anthropometry

Weight in a child with encephalopathy has to be measured by bringing weighing scale bedside and calculated by subtracting the weight of parent + child and weight of parents alone. While measuring the length of the child (height measurement is practically not possible among children with tubercular meningitis), it is essential to understand that the presence of decerebrate posturing and fixed flexion contractures can underestimate the length. Hence, it is important to acknowledge that the length was approximate and not accurate.

General Physical Examination

In addition to routine head-to-toe general physical examination, few important clinical signs that may point to underlying diagnosis must be looked into **(Table 2)**. Presence of neurocutaneous markers could indicate neurocutaneous syndromes. One should always comment on the presence or absence of a Bacille Calmette–Guerin (BCG) scar. Look for evidence of bedsores, contractures, poor hygiene, extravasation in cannula site, and evidence of thrombophlebitis.

Neurological Examination

- *Higher mental function:* Level of consciousness needs to be described in higher mental function **(Practical Box 6)**. Kindly read **Chapter 11** on "Approach To A Child With Altered Sensorium and Coma." The rest of the higher mental examination including orientation, memory, attention span, abstract thinking, spatial perception, fund of information, and calculation is often not possible in an unconscious child. Speech can be described only among those with a comprehensible verbal response. Consciousness is described in terms of eye opening, motor movements, verbal response, and sleep–wake cycle. In chronic neurological patients, Glasgow coma scores have limited utility. Hence, it is better to describe the sensorium verbatim and conclude in terms of conscious child, minimally conscious child, a child in coma or vegetative state **(Table 3)**. Other methods of describing consciousness have been discussed in **Chapter 11**.

- *Cranial nerve:* Cranial nerve examination in a child with altered sensorium is challenging, as it is difficult to test most of the cranial nerves in a comatose child. An example of the description of the cranial nerve has been illustrated in **Practical Box 7**.
- *Motor system examination:*
  - *Posture:* Description of posture comes again hereafter mentioning in the opening statement. If the opening statement has described it thoroughly, one can commit that description of posture was already made and is suggestive of decorticate posturing, decerebrate posturing, hemiplegic posturing, etc. **(Practical Box 5)**
  - *Bulk:* Bulk of muscle appears symmetrical on both sides with no evidence of focal atrophy or hypertrophy. We do not expect any asymmetry to develop in the short span of 1 month. Children with TBM are cachectic and have poor muscle bulk.
  - *Tone:* The tone of the muscle is tested by resistance to passive flexion. It must be assessed across the proximal and distal joints of the upper limb as well as the lower limb. In children

TABLE 2: Clinical signs on general physical examination (GPE) and neurological illness.

Sign on GPE	Neurological illness
Pallor	Intracranial bleed and cerebral malaria
Icterus	Hepatic encephalopathy, leptospirosis, and complicated malaria
Rash	Meningococcemia, measles, and rickettsial infection
Petechiae	Dengue, viral hemorrhagic fever, and meningococcemia
Head and scalp hematoma	Head trauma

PRACTICAL BOX 6: An example of description of higher mental function.

Child has intermittent eye opening, no verbal response, and withdraws to pain with preserved sleep–wake cycle. He makes reproducible and consistent meaningful response, e.g., when his mother asks him "do you want water?", he replies by nodding his head to indicate yes. Hence, sensorium is suggestive of minimally conscious state

TABLE 3: Various states of consciousness.

	Minimally conscious state	*Vegetative state*	*Coma*	*Brain dead*
Wakefulness (sleep–wake cycle)	Preserved	Preserved	Absent	Absent
Awareness	Partial	Absent	Absent	Absent
Brainstem reflex	Preserved	Preserved	Preserved	Absent

> **PRACTICAL BOX 7:** An example of description of cranial nerves (CNs).
>
> - *1st CN:* Could not be tested
> - *2nd CN:* Visual fixation or tracking is absent; field of vision and color vision could not be tested; fundus examination reveals that optic disk is bright with clear margin, optic cup is visualized, there are no hemorrhages, exudates, or evidence of choroid tubercles
> - *3/4/6 CN:* On oculovestibular reflex (Doll's eye response), there is conjugate movement of eyes in opposite direction to head movement with no evidence of 6th CN palsy. Pupils are normal in size and position and reactive to light. Accommodation reflex could not be tested. There is no evidence of nystagmus
> - *5th CN:* Corneal reflex is preserved bilaterally. Rest of motor and sensory parts of 5th CN could not be tested
> - *7th CN:* There is deviation of angle of mouth to left side with flattening of right nasolabial fold. There is drooling of saliva from the left side. He is able to close both eyes, with no evidence of Bell's phenomena. These findings are suggestive of right-sided upper motor neuron type of facial palsy
> - *8th CN:* 8th CN could not be tested
> - *9th/10th CN:* Uvula is central in position, elevates symmetrically on testing palatopharyngeal reflex (gag reflex) with symmetrical constriction of posterior pharyngeal wall suggestive of intact 9th and 10th CNs
> - *11th CN:* Could not be tested
> - *12th CN:* Could not be tested although tongue shows no evidence of atrophy or fasciculation

with TBM, increased tone with evidence of spasticity (feel of "catch" on passive movement) indicates a feature of raised ICP with pyramidal tract involvement. In the presence of abnormal dystonic posturing, the tone may be variable (it may appear to be increased when he is awake/crying and decreased when he is asleep).

- *Power:* Detailed power examination is often not possible in a child with encephalopathy. However, one can comment on the presence or absence of antigravity movement (power of at least 3/5). If a child is unable to move limbs against gravity, one can reposition to eliminate the gravity and reassess for the presence of the power of 2/5 or power of <2/5 depending on the ability to move with gravity being eliminated. Hence, in a child with coma, one can grade the power as "at least 3/5" or "power of 2/5" or "power of <2/5". Individual joints cannot be tested in a child with altered sensorium but a gross functional assessment of proximal and distal joints of upper limb and lower limbs is acceptable.
- *Deep tendon reflex (DTR):* All DTRs should be tested including biceps jerk, triceps jerk, supinator jerk, knee jerk, and ankle jerk. In the presence of contractures, DTRs may be difficult to elicit. Brisk DTRs indicate pyramidal tract involvement. Similarly, in the presence of dystonia, DTRs may become difficult to elicit.
- *Superficial reflexes:* It is expected that all superficial reflexes, including abdominal, cremasteric reflex will be absent in UMN lesion as in TBM. Plantar response (using Babinski method) is essential to record in terms of fanning of all other toes and direction of movement of the great toe as extensor, flexor, or mute response. An extensor plantar response will consist of an extension of the great toe along with fanning of all other toes. We need to be careful not to misinterpret a withdrawal response as extensor plantar response. In the withdrawal Babinski response, there will be dorsiflexion of the feet

along with an extension of the great toe, whereas, in extensor plantar response, there will be no dorsiflexion of the feet. It is good to reconfirm the plantar response using other methods such as Oppenheim, Gordon, and Chaddock reflex. In the presence of extrapyramidal features, extensor plantar response needs to interpret cautiously as children often have hyperextension of great toe even in the absence of any stimuli (called striatal toe).
- *Abnormal movements:* The presence or absence of extrapyramidal movements such as chorea, athetosis, dystonia, myoclonus, and ballismus must be commented.
- *Other neurological examination:*
  - *Sensory system* examination is often limited among children with altered sensorium.
  - *Cerebellar system* examination is restricted to the presence or absence of nystagmus. The rest of the coordination testing of the upper limb and lower limb is not possible among children with altered sensorium.
  - *Meningeal signs:* It would be good to comment on all the three meningeal signs, including neck rigidity, Kernig's sign, and Brudzinski sign.
  - *Skull and spine examination* must focus on the presence or absence of McEwan sign or crackpot sign.

SUMMARY

Read **Chapter 4** on "Making a Clinical Neurological Diagnosis" to understand the analysis of the history and examination findings to arrive at a clinical diagnosis. An example of how to summarize a case has been illustrated here.

A 2-year-old boy born to nonconsanguineously married couple who presented with a long-standing febrile illness involving the central nervous system. He presented with a history of fever, weight loss, seizures, and altered sensorium for 30 days. The child belongs to lower socioeconomic status and is unimmunized with a calorie gap of 770 kcal as per the nutritional history. He has severe wasting and stunting as per the World Health Organization (WHO) classification with mild anemia and no signs of vitamin deficiency. The child is in a minimally conscious state with right-sided UMN facial palsy, right-sided hemiparesis with UMN signs of spasticity, hyperreflexia, and extensor plantar response with features suggestive of raised ICP. There are no clinical signs of extrapyramidal, cerebellar, or meningeal involvement. There is no other systemic involvement.

Anatomical site of localization: Presence of altered sensorium, seizures, features of raised ICP along with right-sided hemiparesis and ipsilateral facial palsy suggests an involvement of cerebral cortex with a possible insult (vascular) in the left cerebral hemisphere.

Possible etiology: Infective etiology (bacterial, fungal, viral, or protozoal)

Differential diagnosis:
- Tubercular meningoencephalitis
- Partially treated pyogenic meningitis
- Chronic meningoencephalitis (Amebic, cryptococcal, HIV, enteroviral, and arboviral)
- CNS vasculitis
- Demyelinating illness

Further management of the patient could be discussed as into immediate management, urgent investigations, and investigations for etiological work-up, treatment, rehabilitation, and follow-up plan for the ease of presentation **(Table 4)**.

TABLE 4: Management strategy of a child with suspected tubercular meningitis (TBM).	
Steps	**Details**
Immediate management and urgent investigation	- *Ensure patent airway, breathing, and circulation* (This is the most vital step in the management of children with altered sensorium)
- *Secure intravenous cannula* (Procure urgent samples for blood sugar to rule out hypoglycemia, serum sodium/potassium to look for dyselectrolytemia, blood urea and creatinine for renal functions, hemoglobin level to look for the degree of anemia, total leukocyte count for leukocytosis, and platelet count to rule out thrombocytopenia)
- *Treat seizures:* Load with phenytoin @20 mg/kg followed by maintenance @5 mg/kg
- *Treat raised ICP:* Start mannitol @5 mL/kg loading followed by 2 mL/kg 6 hourly
Investigation for etiological work-up	- *CECT brain:* CT scan to look for evidence of basal exudates, tuberculoma, and hydrocephalus for tubercular meningitis; rule out brain abscess. If the patient is sick and intubated, then CECT brain would be a quicker option when compared to MRI brain but for the risk of radiation exposure
- *Fundus (if not done earlier):* To look for evidence of papilledema
- *Lumbar puncture (once features of raised intracranial pressure settle):* Cytology, protein, sugars, culture, TB-PCR, cryptococcal antigen, wet mount for *Acanthamoeba*, viral (arboviral, enteroviral) panel if required
- *MRI brain with contrast:* MRI brain must be considered over CECT in nonemergent clinical conditions. Posterior fossa structures, brainstem structures, and white matter pathology including demyelination can be delineated better on MRI brain
- *Tubercular work-up:* Mantoux, chest X-ray, gastric aspirate for acid-fast bacilli (AFB), and parental screening for tuberculosis
Management	- *If there are clear imaging and CSF evidence of TBM:* Antitubercular drugs along with IV dexamethasone should be started
- Neurosurgical consultation for the need of urgent shunt surgery
- *If the imaging findings and/or CSF findings are not supportive of tubercular meningitis:* Empirical treatment with broad-spectrum antibiotic and acyclovir should be initiated
Supportive care	- *Nutrition:* Nasogastric feeding
- *Care of bladder to prevent urinary tract infection:*
- *Care of bowel:* To prevent constipation
- *Care of eyes:* To prevent corneal scarring
- *Care of back:* To prevent bedsores
Discharge and follow-up	Once the child is able to tolerate feeds well, fever has settled, sensorium has started improving, the mother is trained for supportive care, we can plan discharge on ATT, steroids, and acetazolamide among those who were not shunted. Follow-up would be done after 2 weeks to reassess the sensorium, residual neurological deficit, initiation of occupational therapy, and physiotherapy and address any feeding issues if present.

(ATT: antitubercular treatment; CECT: contrast-enhanced computed tomography; CSF: cerebrospinal fluid; ICP: intracranial pressure; PCR: polymerase chain reaction)

KEY MESSAGES

- The presenting complaint must be framed keeping in mind the entire course of illness and must avoid medical jargons.
- History of presenting illness must focus on the chronology of symptoms, and the symptoms must be described based on the day of illness.
- History of the extent of neurological involvement must be presented before arriving at etiological history.
- Examination of a child with TBM must be focused to determine the level of consciousness, any cranial nerve deficits, any motor deficits, presence of meningeal signs, and other signs of raised ICP.
- Summarize the history in terms of duration of symptoms (chronic), extent of neurological involvement (encephalopathy, cranial nerve, or motor deficit), possible neuroanatomical site of lesion (cortical and pyramidal tract involvement), and possible etiology (infective).

26. A Case of Acute Hemiplegia

■ INTRODUCTION

Hemiplegia refers to weakness of one side of the body. Common causes of acute hemiplegia are enumerated in **Box 1**. Refer to **Chapter 37** for an approach to a child with vascular stroke. This chapter focuses on how to present a bedside case of a child with acute hemiplegia.

■ PRESENTING COMPLAINTS

The presenting complaints could be one or more of the following:
- Sudden onset of weakness of right side of body
- Sudden onset of weakness of right upper limb and lower limb
- Paucity of movement of right upper and lower limb

BOX 1: Common causes of hemiplegia in a child.
- Vascular stroke (arterial, venous, or hemorrhagic)
- Mineralizing angiopathy following trivial head trauma
- Space-occupying lesion such as tuberculoma, neurocysticercosis, brain tumor, and abscess
- Todd's paralysis
- Migraine
- Demyelination (acute disseminated encephalomyelitis or clinically isolated syndrome)
- Reversible posterior leukoencephalopathy syndrome
- Rasmussen encephalitis

- Deviation of face toward left side
- Deviation of eyes or double vision
- Altered consciousness and single/multiple episodes of convulsion

Most children with stroke often present with sudden onset of symptoms. Hence, it is often acceptable to use this phrase "sudden onset" while framing the presenting complaints. Weakness in layman term might mean fatigue or asthenia. Alternatively, one can use the term "paucity of movement" to depict motor weakness. Weakness of one side will result in difficulty in walking. However, we do not use such broad presenting complaints like "walking difficulty", which often could lead to confusion, as it might result from any of the following—spasticity, flaccidity, movement disorder, motor weakness, ataxia, and so on.

History of Presenting Complaints

Clinical Presentation

- Clinical presentation of *arterial ischemic stroke* could include focal weakness, speech disturbance, gait instability (ataxia), sensory symptoms, and visual field defects. Encephalopathy is uncommon in arterial ischemic stroke unless there is a dense infarct with cytotoxic edema. Majority of children rather present with weakness of limbs, speech disturbance, or gait instability (ataxia).

- *Venous strokes* often present with seizure, altered sensorium, and focal weakness. Encephalopathy, seizures, and features of raised intracranial pressure (ICP) are prominent in children with venous stroke. Although arterial strokes can also present with features of raised ICP, they are more frequent in venous strokes.
- Children with insidious onset of motor weakness, cognitive regression, and neuropsychiatric manifestations might point toward small vessel central nervous system (CNS) vasculitis.

Onset of Weakness

Onset of weakness: It can be hyperacute (within minutes), acute (within few hours), or insidious (within hours to days). *Hyperacute onset* often indicates hemorrhagic stroke. *Acute onset* is characteristic of embolic stroke. Thrombotic stroke is usually *insidious* in onset.

Description of onset must depict the preceding events prior to the onset of weakness. A child who develops seizures and focal weakness immediately following cardiac surgery is more likely to have a hyperacute onset secondary to cardiogenic embolic stroke.

"He slept well in the night and when he woke up in the morning, parents noticed that he was stumbling and was not able to bear weight on his right leg. At the same time, they noticed that there was paucity of movement of right upper limb as well." This clearly depicts an acute onset of weakness, which could be arterial ischemic stroke.

Progression of Weakness

It is essential to maintain the chronology while describing the progression of weakness. Time to reach nadir of weakness needs to be described. Nadir of weakness indicates the maximum motor deficit at any point of time. In the example given in **Practical Box 1**, it is clear that nadir of the weakness was achieved on day 3 of illness and the weakness did not progress further. It remained static till day 8 followed by gradual recovery.

> **PRACTICAL BOX 1:** Description of progression of weakness.
>
> Parents noticed clumsiness in walking when he woke up in the morning. Gradually by day 2 of illness, he was unable to bear weight on his right leg, although he could drag and walk few steps. But by the next day (day 3), he stopped standing and could only sit with his own support. His weakness remained static till day 8 of illness, when he started gradually improving and he could resume standing by day 10 and started walking with support by 14th day of illness

Extent of Weakness

Most of children with vascular stroke develop hemiparesis rather than hemiplegia. The extent of weakness needs to be determined in the following domains:

- Whether it is *distal predominant* weakness or *proximal predominant* weakness [most upper motor neuron (UMN) lesions result in predominant distal weakness]
- Whether *both upper limb and lower limb are affected* equally or is *upper limb affected more than lower limb*. (Most UMN lesions have upper limb involvement more than lower limb considering the cortical representation)
- Is there a *tightness* or *flabbiness* in the affected limb?
- Are there any *abnormal bizarre flowing movements* or *fixed twisting postures* of the affected limbs? (To indicate extrapyramidal involvement; presence of hemidystonia or hemichorea could indicate a contralateral basal ganglia lesion)

- Is there a *truncal weakness*? (Difficulty in getting up from lying position, difficulty in turning from one side to other side while lying down)
- Is there any history of *cranial nerve (CN) involvement* [difficulty in vision (2nd), deviation of eyes, diplopia, malalignment of eyes (3rd, 4th, and 6th CN), deviation of face, drooling of saliva (7th CN), nasal regurgitation of feeds, altered voice, and difficulty in swallowing (9th and 10th CN)]?
- Is there a history to suggest *difficulty in field of vision* (difficulty in seeing on one side)? (older children can often convey such symptoms)
- *Cortical involvement*: Is there history of convulsion, altered sensorium (altered awareness and wakefulness), and altered behavior (excessive irritability, aggressive behavior)?
- *Speech disturbance:* Older children with arterial ischemic stroke involving left (dominant) hemisphere could present with inability to speak (aphasia), effortful speech as if speaking deep from the stomach (spastic dysarthria)
- Is there a history of *gait instability* or wobbliness while walking? (indicates cerebellar involvement)
- History of vertigo, tinnitus, or occipital headache (posterior circulation stroke)
- Is there a history to suggest raised ICP? (headache, vomiting, altered sensorium, and excessive head banging)

Functional Status

It is essential to incorporate functional status while describing the extent of weakness **(Practical Box 2)**. Functional status is expressed in terms of ability to walk, stand, or sit independently, activities of daily living such as eating, dressing, and hand preference.

> **PRACTICAL BOX 2:** Description of current functional status.
>
> Child presented on day 5 of illness at the nadir of weakness. At admission, he was nonambulatory, not able to stand or bear weight on his legs, and was dependent on parents for toilet care. He was unable to lift his right arm or use his right hand for eating and is being fed by his parents

Etiological History

- *History of trauma to head (severe or trivial) in recent past:* Trivial head trauma such as fall from bed is also associated with mineralizing angiopathy resulting in focal neurological deficit such as hemiparesis and hemidystonia in infants and toddlers.
- History of injury inside the mouth by hard objects like pencil, history of injury to neck to suggest carotid artery dissection
- History of sensation of aura or history of any frank seizure at the onset of hemiplegia (predicts focal seizure followed by Todd's palsy)
- History of severe headache at the onset of weakness (hemiplegic migraine)
- History of ongoing fever or recent history of fever, vaccination (demyelination: clinically isolated syndrome). Children with focal cerebral arteriopathy might also have history of recent infection in past
- History of fever and rash in recent past (to rule out varicella vasculopathy)
- History suggestive of cardiac symptoms (bluish discoloration of lips, suck-rest-suck cycle, and feeding diaphoresis) or history of recent cardiac procedure (at risk for embolic stroke)
- History of easy fatigability, paleness of body, and poor appetite (iron deficiency anemia as a risk factor for arterial ischemic stroke)
- History of progressive paleness of body requiring multiple blood transfusion (sickle cell anemia)

- History of fever, rash, photosensitivity, and joint pain [to rule out systemic lupus erythematosus (SLE) as a cause of small vessel vasculitis]
- History of developmental delay, fluctuating clinical course with worsening with febrile illness (waxing and waning course), failure to thrive [indicates mitochondrial disorders such as MELAS (mitochondrial encephalopathy with lactic acidosis and stroke)]
  - History of bleeding from any other site indicates underlying bleeding diathesis that predisposes to hemorrhagic stroke.
  - Past history of similar episodes of transient hemiparesis is a very strong pointer toward a bilateral pathology such as moyamoya arteriopathy. Same-sided recurrent episodes of hemiplegia with associated headache also points toward hemiplegic migraine. Most of children with alternating hemiplegia of childhood often present with extrapyramidal movement disorders such as choreoathetosis and dystonia.

EXAMINATION

Opening Statement

Opening statement may mention paucity of movement of one side of the body. Any evident dystonia may also be commented on the opening statement of examination.

Vital Signs

Look for evidence of bradycardia and hypertension as features of raised ICP. Clinical signs of raised ICP are observed in venous hemorrhagic stroke or a massive arterial stroke. Presence of tachypnea and tachycardia could indicate an underlying cardiac illness. Children with hemorrhagic stroke can present in shock with hypotension and tachycardia.

Anthropometric Parameters

Anthropometric evidence of malnutrition often indicates an underlying chronic pathology such as mitochondrial disorder or underlying cardiac lesion.

General Physical Examination

- Presence of pallor (may indicate iron deficiency anemia or sickle cell anemia). Sudden onset of severe anemia in an infant or a child with focal neurological deficit favors hemorrhagic stroke.
- Look for evidence of varicella scar marks (postvaricella vasculopathy).
- Look for signs of malnutrition and failure to thrive (underlying mitochondrial disorders).
- Presence of clubbing and cyanosis indicates cyanotic congenital heart disease.
- In older children, look for signs of infective endocarditis (risk for embolic stroke).
- Presence of lens dislocation in a child with intellectual disability and Marfanoid habitus who presented with stroke could often point to homocystinuria.
- Presence of hemolytic facies could point to chronic hemolytic anemia such as sickle cell anemia.
- Presence of neurocutaneous markers such as hemifacial port-wine stain indicates underlying Sturge–Weber syndrome. Children with Sturge–Weber syndrome often present with chronic hemiplegia rather than acute hemiplegia. Presence of café-aulait macules indicates neurofibromatosis, which predisposes a child to developing moyamoya vasculopathy.
- Presence of malar rash and photosensitivity suggests SLE.

Higher Mental Function

Consciousness

Presence of wakefulness with awareness of self and surroundings indicates a conscious state. Features of encephalopathy in a child with focal neurological deficit indicate a diffuse cortical involvement or features of raised ICP. To reemphasize, venous strokes are more likely to present with altered sensorium and seizures.

Speech

Involvement of speech is dependent on the dominant hemisphere. In majority of children, the left side of the brain is the dominant hemisphere. Hence, left-sided strokes (present with right-sided hemiparesis) have prominent aphasia. One common mistake that residents often commit is to comment on aphasia in an encephalopathic child. Aphasia is a disorder of language, which is described only among conscious patients. Speech is a very important component of higher mental function in hemiplegic children as presence of aphasia often points to involvement of dominant hemisphere, whereas presence of spastic dysarthria would indicate corticospinal tract involvement.

Other Higher Mental Functions

Other parts of *higher mental function* include orientation, memory (temporal lobe), attention span, spatial perception, insight (frontal lobe), abstract thought, fund of information, and calculation (parietal lobe). These higher mental functions give an idea of the affected lobes of the brain. Children with long-standing moyamoya vasculopathy and small vessel vasculitis can develop cognitive decline that can be detected on higher mental function examination.

Cranial Nerve Examination

Cranial nerve examination is of utmost importance in hemiplegic patients. It is required for localization of the lesion. In general, ipsilateral cranial nerve palsy and contralateral hemiparesis (crossed hemiparesis) indicate a brainstem lesion whereas ipsilateral hemiparesis and same-sided cranial nerve palsy indicate a lesion in corticospinal and corticobulbar fibers in the contralateral side above the level of nucleus of cranial nerves in brainstem. Read **Chapter 1** on basics of neurology to understand the principles of localization. Few points are re-emphasized:

- *Optic nerve:* Involvement of optic nerve resulting in loss of visual acuity indicates a possibility of optic neuritis. Presence of optic neuritis in a patient with hemiplegia gives a hint toward a demyelinating cause (clinically isolated syndrome) for hemiplegia. Field of vision testing can be performed in older children with hemiplegia by confrontation test. If one side of visual field is affected, it is called hemianopia. If the same half of visual field (say right side) is affected in both eyes, then it is called homonymous hemianopia (this indicates pathology or lesion at the level of optic nerve). If only one quadrant (one-fourth of visual field) is affected, it is called quadrantanopia. If the upper quadrant is affected, it is called superior quadrantanopia (this happens in a temporal lobe lesion), whereas inferior quadrantanopia results from a parietal lobe lesion. Fundus must be evaluated to look for evidence of papilledema (raised ICP) or papillitis (optic neuritis).
- *3rd, 4th, and 6th CNs:* Test the extraocular movement in all cardinal gaze. Presence of bilateral 6th nerve palsy in a child with

hemiplegia would indicate features of raised ICP. Ipsilateral 6th cranial nerve palsy with contralateral hemiplegia would indicate an ipsilateral pontine lesion (Raymond syndrome). Similarly, ipsilateral 7th cranial nerve palsy with contralateral hemiplegia would also point to a pontine lesion (Foville syndrome). Millard–Gubler syndrome would mean both 6th and 7th CN palsy. Presence of miosis and anhidrosis (Horner syndrome) would point toward carotid arterial dissection.

Note: When you ask the child to look at right, right eye's 6th CN (lateral rectus) and left eye's 3rd CN (medial rectus) act together to enable the child to look at right. This is called conjugate gaze. This conjugate gaze is taken care at pons level [paramedian pontine reticular formation (PPRF)] and frontal lobe [frontal eye field (FEF)]. As we know from the chapter on localization **(Chapter 1)**, left FEF governs right PPRF that in turn stimulates right 6th CN and through medial longitudinal fasciculus (MLF) stimulates left 3rd CN. Hence, when left FEF is stimulated, it will result in conjugate movement of eye to the right side. Hence, if there is right-sided tonic conjugate gaze palsy (eyes are tonically deviated to right), it could be an irritative left frontal lesion such as seizure activity or could be secondary to lesion in the right pons affecting PPRF. It could also be due to unopposed left FEF activation in right-sided destructive lesion like brain abscess. We also know that 3rd and 4th CN nucleus are at midbrain level and 6th CN nucleus is at pons level. Hence, any nuclear or infranuclear lesion would result in isolated cranial nerve palsy. Such palsies do not affect conjugate eye movement; rather, it affects monocular eye movement (dysconjugate palsies).

You need to remember that corticobulbar fibers govern the nucleus of 3rd, 4th, and 6th CN on both the sides. Hence, monocular palsies could either result from a nuclear/infranuclear lesion or involvement of corticobulbar fibers. This also means that it has to be a bilateral lesion of corticobulbar fibers to cause isolated cranial nerve palsy, which often happens in raised ICP. Remember that nuclear or infranuclear lesions will have absent brainstem reflexes, whereas supranuclear lesion (lesion in corticobulbar fibers) will have preserved brainstem reflexes.

- *5th CN:* In children with hemiplegia, we are interested in corneal reflex (brainstem reflex; 5th afferent and 7th efferent), jaw jerk (exaggerated in pseudobulbar palsy with bilateral corticobulbar fibers)
- *7th CN:* Children with hemiplegia often have a UMN type of facial palsy. Crossed hemiparesis with facial palsy often indicates a pontine lesion. All corticobulbar fibers have bilateral innervations from both sides except for lower half of 7th CN and 12th CN, which have only contralateral hemispheric innervations.
- *9th and 10th CN:* Bilateral corticobulbar lesion (supranuclear) would result in detectable weakness involving absent gag reflex. Unilateral weakness often indicates infranuclear lesions. Remember that uvula deviates toward the normal side. It is easy to remember 10 + 7 = 17—both 7th and 10th will deviate toward the normal side. 5 + 12 = 17—both 5th and 12th CN will deviate toward the affected side.

Motor System Examination

- *Gait:* A hemiplegic child will have his arms adducted, elbow flexed, forearm pronated, and wrist and fingers flexed. His lower limb will be extended at the hip, knee, and ankle compelling the child to

circumduct his legs while walking. This is called circumduction or hemiplegic gait. In a UMN lesion, upper limbs are often more involved than lower limbs.
- *Bulk* is often preserved in acute hemiplegia. However, past history of similar episodes as in children with moyamoya vasculopathy might result in hemiatrophy.
- *Tone* is often increased in the affected limb with signs of spasticity, hyperreflexia, and extensor plantars. Presence of these findings indicates a UMN sign (pyramidal tract involvement). Tone may be normal or decreased in the acute phase of hemiplegia before UMN signs of specialty, hyperreflexia, and extensor plantar are evident.
- *Power*: Formal individual muscle power testing is often difficult, but power can be tested across the joints in older children. If there is selective weakness of deltoid, triceps, wrist extensor, finger extensor and abductor along with weakness of hip flexor, knee flexor and ankle dorsiflexor, it is highly suggestive of a UMN lesion (involvement of antigravity muscles). UMN weakness will have distal predominant weakness. In infants and young children, observation of shoulder and hand movement along with posture of hand can give a clue to the extent of weakness.
- *Abnormal movements* including choreoathetosis and dystonia need to be ruled out as hemidystonia or hemiballismus often mimics or accompanies hemiparesis.

Sensory System

Impairment of cortical sensation such as graphesthesia, stereognosis, and tactile extinction indicates a contralateral cortical parietal lesion. Involvement of parietal lobe can also result in impairment of both cortical and primary sensation such as pain/temperature and joint position/vibration.

Meningeal Sign

Presence of meningeal signs in a hemiplegic child strongly supports the diagnosis of acute meningoencephalitis.

Establishing the etiology: Common clinical clues are depicted in **Table 1**. A broad approach to clinical diagnosis is shown in **Flowchart 1** and localization in **Flowchart 2**.

Clinical approach, plan of investigation, and management of acute vascular stroke are discussed in **Chapter 37**.

■ SUMMARY AND ANALYSIS

Summary must include the following:
- Acute/hyperacute/insidious onset
- Hemiparesis or hemiplegia (which side)
- Associated impairment of consciousness (encephalopathy) and seizures
- Associated cranial nerve palsy
- Features of raised ICP
- Most likely etiology (vascular, infective, demyelinating, and structural)
- *If vascular:* Arterial or venous stroke?
- *If arterial:* Does it look like anterior circulation stroke (anterior and middle cerebral artery) or posterior circulation stroke (posterior cerebral artery)?
- *If vascular:* Does it look like a vasculopathy, coagulopathy, secondary to cardiac, metabolic, or hemoglobinopathies?
- *If coagulopathy:* Does it look like thrombotic or thromboembolic?

Answer to the last four questions are often not very clear on the basis of clinical evaluation alone; it needs radiological correlation.

TABLE 1: Clinical clues to cause of acute hemiplegia in children.

Clinical feature	What to think?
Acute hemiparesis with abrupt onset of headache and vomiting with altered sensorium	Intracranial hemorrhage
Abrupt onset hemiparesis with history of preceding vaccination, chickenpox, febrile illness	Arterial ischemic stroke (local cerebral arteriopathy)
Acute onset hemiparesis, altered sensorium in setting of fever, headache, vomiting with or without neck stiffness	Acute meningoencephalitis or acute disseminated encephalomyelitis
Acute hemiparesis with seizures, vision difficulty with altered sensorium in a child with chronic drug intake (cyclosporine) or nephrotic syndrome	Posterior reversible leukoencephalopathy syndrome (PRES)
Acute hemiparesis with severe headache and positive family history	Hemiplegic migraine
Acute hemiparesis following a seizure (focal)	Postictal Todd's paralysis
Acute hemiparesis in a child with known sickle cell disease or cardiac condition	Arterial ischemic stroke
Recurrent episodes of transient hemiparesis in one or both sides	Moyamoya disease
Recurrent episodes of hemiparesis with dyskinetic movement involving one or both sides of body	Alternating hemiplegia of childhood (AHC)

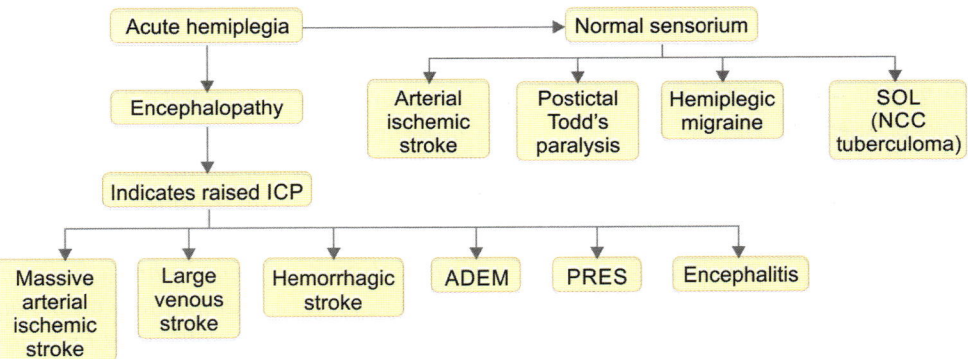

Flowchart 1: Broad clinical approach to a child with acute hemiplexia.

(ADEM: acute disseminated encephalomyelitis; ICP: intracranial pressure; NCC: neurocysticercosis; PRES: posterior reversible leukoencephalopathy syndrome; SOL: space-occupying lesion)

■ CASE VIGNETTES

Case 1

Summary

A 1½-year-old boy presented with a history of sudden onset of hemiparesis and encephalopathy for 2 days. There was history of preceding diarrheal illness for 3 days prior to the onset of these symptoms. There was no history of fever. Examination revealed signs of raised ICP, bilateral 6th cranial nerve palsy, hypertonia, hyper-reflexia, and extensor

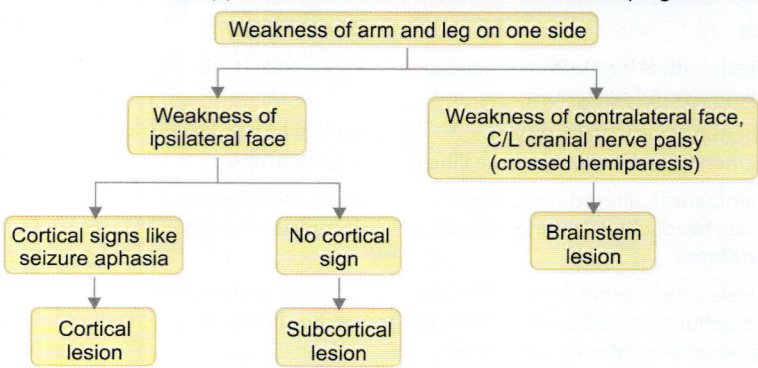

Flowchart 2: Approach to localization in childhood hemiplegia.

plantar response with fundus showing papilledema.

Analysis

Analysis	Result
Type of onset	Acute onset
Clinical presentation	Right hemiparesis and encephalopathy
Encephalopathy and/or seizures	Encephalopathy
Cranial nerve deficit	Bilateral 6th nerve palsy
Motor deficit	Right hemiparesis
Features of raised ICP	Present
Etiology	Vascular
Arterial or venous	Probably venous
Anterior or posterior circulation	Does not look like arterial stroke, so this question is not relevant in this case
Thrombotic or embolic	Thrombotic (acute onset)
Underlying risk factor	Dehydration secondary to diarrhea and vomiting

Learning Points

Children with venous stroke secondary to venous sinus thrombosis often present with seizures, encephalopathy, focal neurological deficit (hemiparesis and cranial nerve palsy), and signs of raised ICP. Risk factors for venous sinus thrombosis include preceding diarrhea, vomiting (dehydration), underlying cyanotic congenital heart disease, and other prothrombotic states with similar history in past.

Case 2

Summary

A 7-year-old boy presented with sudden onset of right-sided weakness, inability to speak, and two episodes of vomiting for 1 day. There was no history of trauma, fever, seizure, or alteration in consciousness. There was gradual improvement in hand function by 5th day of illness. Examination on the day of admission revealed right-sided hemiparesis and subtle right-sided UMN facial palsy and aphasia. His fundus examination was normal. There was no underlying cardiac problem or history to suggest repeated blood transfusion. At 6 months follow-up, he is doing well and hemiparesis has improved dramatically.

Analysis

Analysis	Result
Type of onset	Acute onset
Clinical presentation	Right hemiparesis, right 7th CN palsy, and aphasia
Encephalopathy and/or seizures	Absent
Cranial nerve deficit	7th nerve palsy
Motor deficit	Right hemiparesis
Features of raised ICP	Not sure (only two episodes of vomiting)
Etiology	Vascular
Arterial or venous	Arterial
Anterior or posterior circulation	Anterior circulation stroke
Thrombotic or embolic	Looks more like arteriopathy (focal cerebral arteriopathy) rather than coagulopathy
Underlying risk factor	Almost none

Learning Points

We consider arterial stroke when there is involvement of one or more of the following: Hemiparesis (and not hemiplegia), aphasia (involvement of dominant speech language), sensory deficit (cortical and/or peripheral sensation), and visual field deficit (quadrantanopia). Presence of these findings on history and examination suggests a cortical involvement supplied by middle or anterior cerebral artery. Children with isolated posterior circulation stroke often present with ataxia and cerebellar signs with or without visual deficit (cortical blindness). Arteriopathy is one of the most common causes of arterial stroke in children. It is often suspected among those with no risk factors for prothrombotic states. Among those with recurrent such episodes, possibility of moyamoya arteriopathy must always be kept. Recurrent stroke must also prompt us to think of mitochondrial disorders such as mitochondrial encephalopathy with lactic acidosis and stroke (MELAS), procoagulant states such as protein C, protein S, and antithrombin III deficiency.

KEY MESSAGES

- In a child with acute hemiplegia, type of onset of weakness, presence of features of raised ICP and other cranial nerve deficits would be useful in analysis.
- History must focus on differentiating between arterial ischemic stroke, venous stroke, and hemorrhagic stroke.
- Any child with recurrent hemiplegia must always be evaluated for the possibility of moyamoya vasculopathy.
- Acute hemiplegia in a child with preexisting cardiac disease prompts us to the possibility of a venous stroke or thromboembolic stroke.
- Presence of severe anemia in a child with acute hemiplegia must be evaluated for sickle cell anemia or iron deficiency anemia; both are important risk factors for arterial ischemic stroke.

CHAPTER 27: A Case of Paraplegia

■ INTRODUCTION

Paraplegia refers to the weakness of both lower limbs. It usually results from spinal cord lesions, which could be a compressive or noncompressive lesion **(Table 1)**. Readers are advised to understand localization in spinal cord lesions from **Chapter 1** on the basics of neurology. This chapter focuses on how to present a bedside case of a child with paraplegia.

■ HISTORY-TAKING

Presenting Complaints

Children with paraplegia will often present with weakness of lower limbs with or without bladder involvement. Common presenting complaints among these children include the following:
- *Motor complaints:* Weakness of both lower limbs, difficulty in walking and

TABLE 1: Clinical clues (history points) for various etiologies.

History points	Possible etiology
History of rash, joint pain, and photosensitivity	Small-vessel vasculitis [systemic lupus erythematosus (SLE), antiphospholipid antibody (APLA) syndrome]
History of visual loss or blurring of vision	Neuromyelitis optica
History of swelling in the neck and recurrent chest infection	Sarcoidosis
History of rash along with a dermatomal distribution	Varicella zoster infection
Family history of tuberculosis	Tuberculosis
History of animal or tick bite and recent travel	Borreliosis and tick paralysis
Pure vegan diet	Vitamin B_{12} and vitamin E deficiency
History of bony pain, swelling over the neck, and abdominal mass	Malignancy (leukemia and non-Hodgkin lymphoma)
History of trauma to back or injections	Traumatic myelopathy or traumatic neuritis
History of radiation exposure	Radiation myelopathy
Toxin or industrial exposure	Lead-induced neuropathy
Family history of paraparesis	Hereditary spastic paraparesis (HSP)

standing, progressive increasing difficulty in walking, or clumsiness in walking
- *Sensory complaints:* Presence of anesthesia (lack of sensation), paresthesia (abnormal sensation), girdle-like sensation, pain in the legs radiating from the back (radiating pain), or deep-seated pain (vertebral pain)
- *Dorsal column sensation:* Dizziness or instability when eyes are closed
- *Bladder involvement:* Dribbling or retention of urine

History of Presenting Complaints

Description of Weakness

- *Extent of weakness:* Weakness of lower limb muscles can be proximal or distal. Proximal weakness can be elicited by asking for the difficulty in climbing upstairs, going downstairs, getting up from squatting position (indicates hip abductor and hip extensor weakness) or buckling of the knee while walking (indicates quadriceps weakness). Distal weakness is often elicited by asking for a history of repeated falls with twisting of ankle, slipping of chappals or tripping on small objects on the floor. Additional truncal weakness should be enquired as difficulty in getting up from lying down position with the help of hand support or difficulty in turning around in the bed. The majority of children with acute paraplegia are bedridden, and it is difficult to differentiate proximal from distal weakness.
- Is the weakness *symmetrical or asymmetrical* (asymmetric flaccid weakness points to poliomyelitis or traumatic neuritis)?
- Ask for history of *flabbiness or tightness* of lower limb [flaccid weakness could represent lower motor neuron (LMN) lesion or stage of spinal shock; tightness could represent spasticity of limbs indicating upper motor neuron (UMN) lesion]
- *Current functional ability:* Is the patient ambulatory or nonambulatory? If ambulatory, describe his/her gait in terms of balance. If nonambulatory, describe the best functional ability (e.g., *"he is bedridden, can take turns but cannot get up from bed without assistance"* or *"he can get up and sit in the bed independently but cannot stand without assistance"*).
- Gross *wasting of muscles* of lower limb will give clue to chronicity of problem (global atrophy often indicates neuronopathy and distal atrophy indicates neuropathy.)
- *Abnormal twitching movements* noticed in the muscle (fasciculations indicate neuronopathic process, i.e., anterior horn cell pathology)

Note: The above points correspond to motor examination—bulk, tone, and power; so, it is easy to remember to ask them in the history as well.

Onset and Progression of Weakness

It is essential to determine whether the paraplegia has an acute, subacute, or insidious onset. Spastic diplegic cerebral palsy, hereditary spastic paraplegia, and craniovertebral junction anomaly are common causes of long-standing weakness in lower limbs. We are not dealing with longstanding paraparesis in this chapter. Case presentation of acute flaccid paralysis is discussed in **Chapter 28**. Causes of acute/subacute onset or insidious onset are listed in **Table 2**.

History of Neuraxis Involvement

History of sensory involvement: History of girdle-like sensation or zone of hyperalgesia

TABLE 2: Causes of acute/subacute onset or insidious onset.

Acute/subacute onset	Insidious onset
• Transverse myelitis • Traumatic paraplegia • Anterior spinal artery syndrome	• Tubercular spine • Spinal epidural abscess • Spinal cord tumors

with loss of touch and pain sensations below any level indicates a lesion in the spinal cord. History of radicular pain that starts from the back radiating to lower limbs that often increases with coughing or sneezing also needs to be elicited (indicates radiculopathy). Vertebral pain that is dull aching confined to the spine points to inflammatory or traumatic pathology to the spine. Funicular pain has been described as ill-defined dull aching deep-seated pain along the spine seen among patients with intramedullary lesions. History of swaying while standing with eyes closed (e.g., while washing his face in the bathroom or walking in the dark) often indicates impairment of posterior column function.

History of bladder complaints: History of urinary dribbling, urgency, frequency, and hesitancy must be elicited among older children who have normal intelligence and had achieved bladder control. Bladder involvement can be of two types—*spastic bladder* (if the lesion is above S2-S4) and *flaccid bladder* (if the lesion is at S2-S4 level). The child with spastic bladder will have urgency, frequency, and hesitancy with variable residual urine in the bladder. In contrast, flaccid bladder will have large residual urine but lack of urinary urgency and frequency, although hesitancy may be present. Constant urinary dribbling is a feature of sensory bladder (interruption of sensory supply to bladder). Readers are advised to understand the bladder physiology from **Chapter 9**.

Constipation or bowel incontinence: History of constipation or bowel incontinence must be elicited to determine the extent of neurological involvement. Loss of perianal sensation is specific for cauda equina/conus medullaris lesion.

History of higher mental function and cranial nerves:
- History of altered sensorium or convulsion (brain lesions are uncommon causes of paraplegia. Anterior cerebral artery infarct or sagittal sinus thrombosis rarely presents with weakness of lower limb.)
- History of difficulty in vision (optic neuritis is associated with transverse myelitis)
- History of deviation of eyes (squint) and drooping of eyelids (ptosis) (presence of ptosis in a paraplegic child suggests the possibility of myasthenia)
- History of facial deviation or drooling of saliva or difficulty in deglutition (7th/9th/10th cranial nerve) (uncommon in paraplegic children)

Etiological history:
- Any prior vaccination (polio vaccine and antirabies vaccine) or recent febrile illness (transverse myelitis)
- History of rash and fever (herpes infection and chickenpox infection-induced myelopathy)
- History of fever, back pain, and radicular pain (epidural abscess)
- History of rash, joint pain, photosensitivity to sunlight (SLE or other connective tissue disease)
- History of unexplained fever, bony tenderness, abdominal distension, mass in the abdomen, swellings in the neck (malignancy—leukemia causing compressive myelopathy)
- History of trauma to the spine (traumatic myelopathy or fracture vertebra with resultant compression)

- History of swelling or deformity with or without contact history of pulmonary tuberculosis (Pott's paraplegia)
- Any previous such episodes of short-lasting weakness (hypokalemic periodic paralysis)
- History of chronic diarrhea or passage of greasy stools (malabsorption) leading to vitamin E deficiency
- History of a tick bite (borreliosis)
- Dietary history to screen for possible vitamin B_{12} deficiency (pure vegans)
- History of pica and residence in industrial factories (lead neuropathy)
- Family history of paraparesis (hereditary spastic paraparesis).

TABLE 3: Causes of compressive vs. noncompressive myelopathy.

Compressive myelopathy	Noncompressive myelopathy
• Pott's spine • Epidural abscess • Epidural malignancy • Leukemia/lymphoma • Post-traumatic compression	• Transverse myelitis • Neuromyelitis optica • Multiple sclerosis • Infective myelopathy (varicella zoster, herpes simplex, enterovirus, *Listeria, Borrelia, Mycoplasma*, and neurocysticercosis) • Anterior spinal syndrome • Vitamin B_{12} deficiency

Finding the Etiology

Etiology can be broadly classified into infective (bacterial, viral, protozoal, and fungal), parainfectious/demyelinating [transverse myelitis, Guillain–Barré syndrome (GBS), neuromyelitis optica (NMO), and multiple sclerosis], vascular (anterior spinal artery occlusion), nutritional (vitamin B_{12} deficiency and vitamin E deficiency), malignancy (leukemia and lymphoma), genetic (hereditary spastic paraparesis and spinal muscular atrophy). It could also be classified as compressive (tubercular spine, lymphoma, and leukemia) or noncompressive (transverse myelitis, NMO, and anterior spinal artery syndrome). Clues in history for various disorders leading to paraparesis are shown in **Table 3**.

Summarizing the History

Summarize the history under the following heads:
- Acute/subacute/insidious onset
- Extent of weakness with current functional ability
- Sensory system involvement
- Bladder and bowel involvement
- Involvement of higher mental functions along with cranial nerve
- Possible neuroanatomical site of lesion (level of lesion, compressive vs. noncompressive, and extramedullary versus intramedullary lesion)
- Possible underlying etiology

PHYSICAL EXAMINATION
Posture and Gait

The posture (nonambulatory) or gait (ambulatory) of the child may be described in the opening statement as follows: *On examination, he is lying supine on the bed and is comfortable. There is paucity of movements of lower limbs, lying flaccid with lateral side of the foot touching the bed.*

Vital Signs

The presence of fever often indicates ongoing infection. Respiratory distress may indicate diaphragmatic or intercostals muscle weakness. A child with GBS can have autonomic involvement in the form of hypertension, tachycardia, and bradycardia.

General Physical Examination

Presence of lymphadenopathy, organomegaly, and bony tenderness may indicate underlying malignancy or disseminated tuberculosis. Spine tenderness and spinal deformity must always be examined. The presence of bedsores or any obvious deformities may indicate chronicity of the condition.

Focused Neurological Examination

The majority of children with paraplegia will have preserved higher mental functions and intact cranial nerve examination. The focus of cranial nerve examination would include visual acuity, the field of vision, and color vision. The presence of visual symptoms in a child with acute onset of paraplegia often points to a demyelinating cause such as neuromyelitis optica (NMO).

- *Bulk of muscle:* Presence of atrophy indicates a long-standing illness. If the distal foot muscles are atrophied with exaggerated arch of the foot, it indicates a neuropathy. If the atrophy is more evident in proximal muscles than distal muscles, it indicates a neuronopathy.
- *Tone of muscle:* Presence of hypertonia in lower limb muscles indicates UMN lesion, whereas flaccidity might indicate stage of spinal shock.
- *Power of muscle:* Power charting across individual joints indicates extent of weakness of lower limbs. In addition, presence of weakness of truncal muscles must be recorded. Upper limb muscles are relatively spared in paraplegic patients. Formal muscle power charting is often not possible among young children where we perform the functional assessment.
- *Deep tendon reflexes (DTRs):* All individual DTRs (biceps, triceps, supinator, knee, and ankle jerk) must be elicited. By principle, DTR is absent at the level of the lesion and exaggerated below the level of the lesion. We know the root value of all DTRs: biceps, supinator jerk C5-C6, triceps reflex C7, knee reflex L2-L3, ankle reflex L5-S1. Hence, if there is a loss of biceps and supinator jerk (C5-C6) with exaggerated knee and ankle reflex, we presume site of lesion to be at the C5-C6 level. Similarly, an inverted supinator jerk indicates lesion at the C5-C6 level.
- *Superficial reflexes:* Superficial reflexes are absent below the level of lesion with preserved reflexes above the level. The plantar response is usually extensor unless the patient is in spinal shock where it may be mute. The root value of superficial reflexes includes—abdominal reflex (T7-L1) and cremasteric reflex is L1-L2. T10 corresponds to the umbilicus. Hence, if the upper abdominal reflex is preserved, lower abdominal reflex and cremasteric reflex are absent, plantars are extensor, then root value is probably T10. Lesion at this level results in Beevor sign (umbilicus moving down while getting up).
- *Sensory examination:* Localization of site of lesion is best done by sensory system examination. There is zone of sensory hyperalgesia in a dermatome corresponding to the site of lesion with sensory loss below the same. Sensation should be tested separately for pain/temperature and position/vibration sense. We know that lateral spinothalamic sensation (pain and temperature) crosses at same level whereas posterior column sensation (vibration and position sense) ascends at same side and crosses at higher level. Hence, right-sided spinal

cord lesion would result in left-sided loss of pain and temperature sensation and loss of right-sided vibration and joint position sense below that level. In posterior column, cervical fibers are lateral and sacral fibers are medial. It is the reverse in lateral spinothalamic tract (sacral fibers are lateral). Hence, an extrinsic compressive lesion will affect sacral fibers of spinothalamic tract before it affects cervical fibers.
- *Lhermitte sign:* Forward flexion of neck would result in pain in back indicates cervical cord involvement.

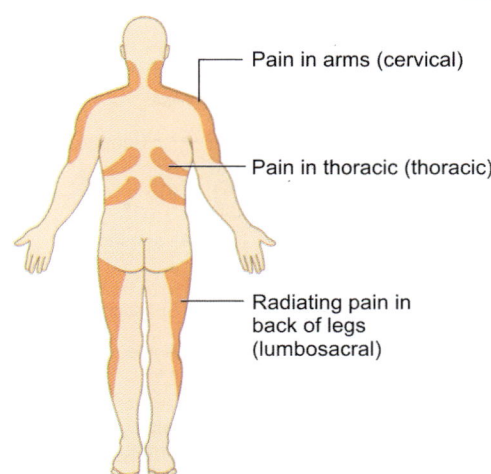

Fig. 1: Band-like sensation

Localization (Points to Remember)

- Presence of pyramidal signs (hyperreflexia, extensor plantars) with or without sensory loss points to a spinal cord pathology
- Establishing pattern of sensory loss is challenging in children as compared to adults.
- In acute phase of spinal cord injury, there may be areflexia and absent plantar response (spinal shock) which may persist for 1–2 weeks or may be longer
- Band-like radicular pain in the history can help in localization **(Fig. 1)**
- Girdle-like sensation have poor localizing value, e.g., lesion at thoracic cord may result in girdle sensation at hip.
- If weakness of lower limb is associated with edema, it indicates impaired vasomotor tone.
- We can identify the pattern of weakness **(Fig. 2)**.
- If it is a myelopathy, we can identify if it is compressive or non-compressive **(Figs. 3A and B)**.
- If compressive, is it extramedullary or intramedullary compression **(Figs. 4A and B)**.
- General rule is LMN involvement (areflexia) at the level of lesion and UMN involvement (hyperreflexia, spasticity) below the level of lesion **(Fig. 5)**
- Identify broad group of etiology—infective, demyelinating, vascular, systemic/autoimmune
- Broad clinical approach to a child with paraplegia is summarized in **Flowchart 1**
- Broad approach to investigating a child with paraplegia is summarized in **Flowchart 2**.

■ SUMMARY AND ANALYSIS

- Acute/subacute/chronic paraparesis or paraplegia
- Extent of weakness (proximal or distal weakness)
- Is it a single lesion or does it look multifocal? (multifocal or patchy involvement often favor demyelinating lesion such as transverse myelitis)
- UMN weakness or LMN weakness:
  - Spastic weakness or flaccid weakness
  - DTR brisk or not elicitable
  - Plantar response extensor or flexor

408 | **SECTION 3:** Residents' Corner: Exam-oriented Cases

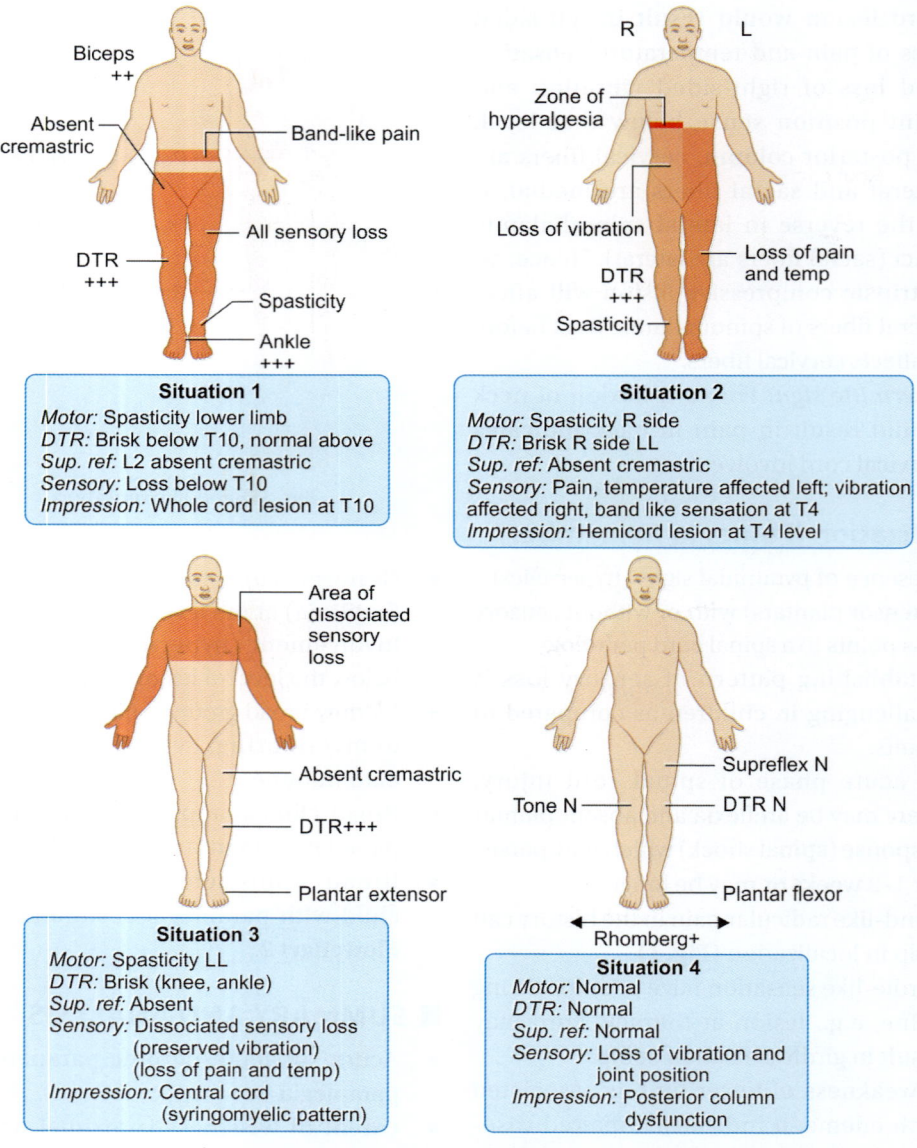

Fig. 2: Pattern of weakness. (DTR: deep tendon reflex)

- Current functional status (ambulatory or nonambulatory)
- Associated truncal weakness, upper limb weakness, cranial neuropathy, and any impairment of higher mental function
- Sensory loss (lateral spinothalamic tract or dorsal column)
- UMN or LMN type of bladder involvement, if any
- Localization of site of lesion (site of lesion)
- *Type of lesion:* Compressive or noncompressive lesion; if noncompressive, is it an intramedullary or extramedullary lesion?

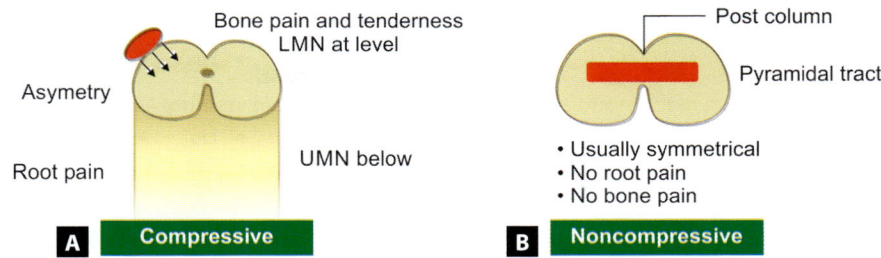

Figs. 3A and B: (A) Compressive versus (B) noncompressive myelopathy. (LMN: lower motor neuron; UMN: upper motor neuron)

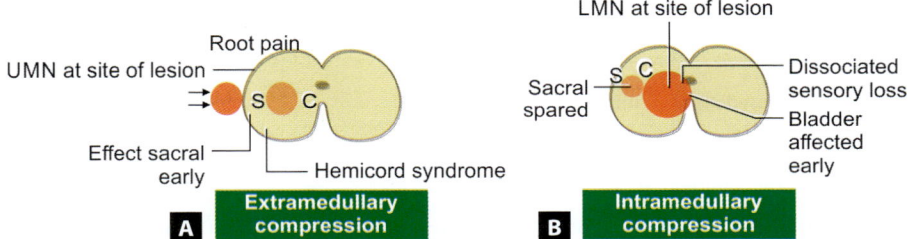

Figs. 4A and B: (A) Extramedullary versus (B) intramedullary lesion. (LMN: lower motor neuron; UMN: upper motor neuron)

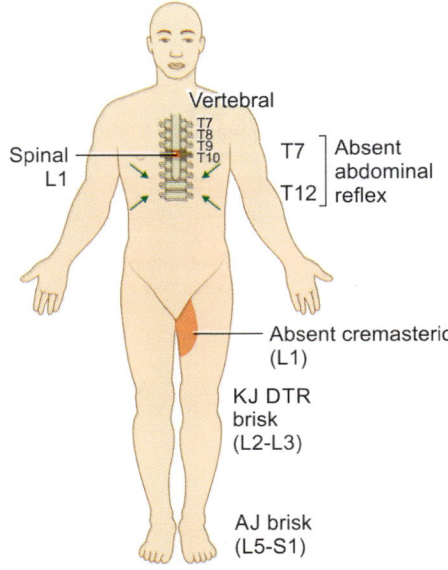

Fig. 5: LMN at the level of lesion and UMN below the level of lesion. (DTR: deep tendon reflex; LMN: lower motor neuron; UMN: upper motor neuron)

SECTION 3: Residents' Corner: Exam-oriented Cases

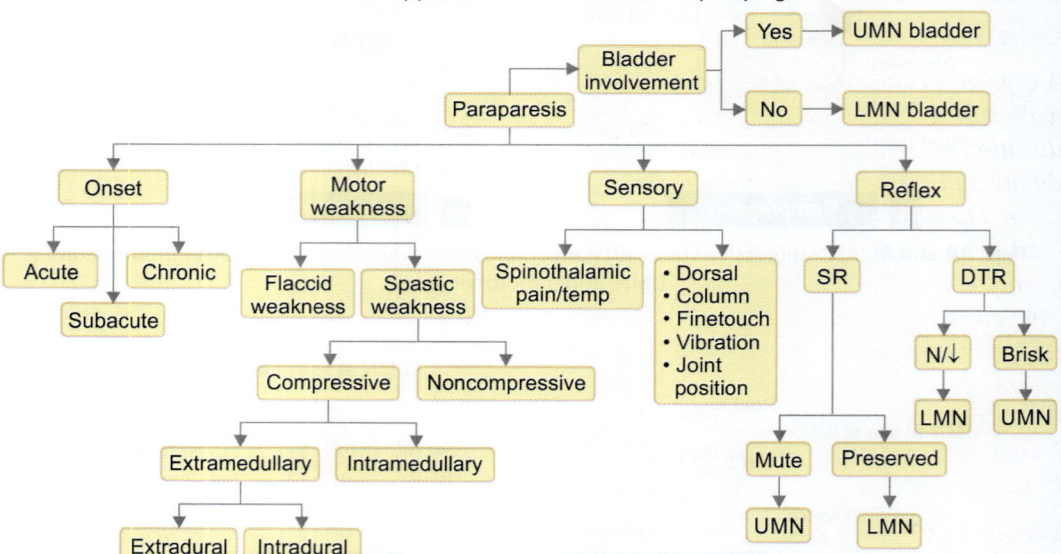

Flowchart 1: Approach to a child with acute paraplegia.

(DTR: deep tendon reflex; LMN: lower motor neuron; SR: superficial reflex; UMN: upper motor neuron)

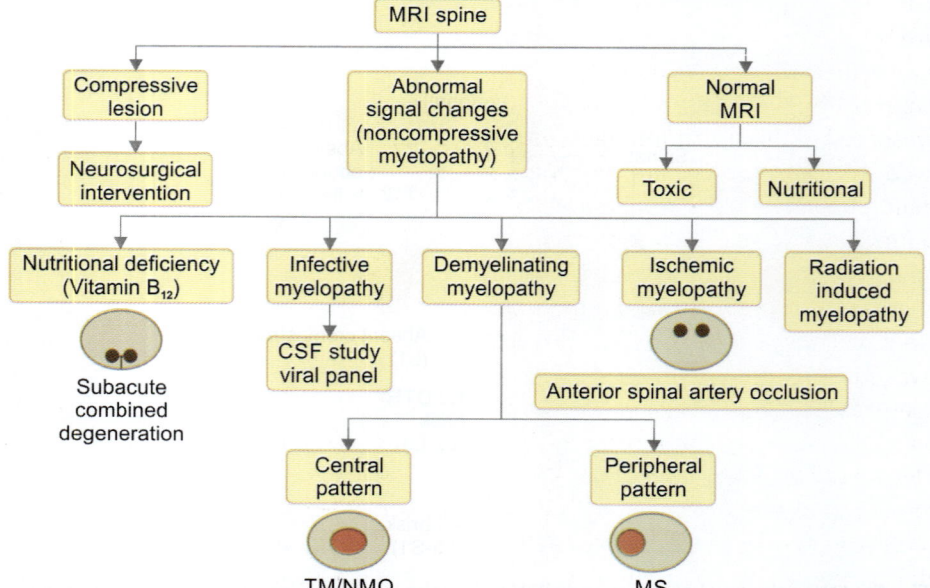

Flowchart 2: Approach to investigating a child with paraplegia.

(MS: multiple sclerosis; NMO: neuromyelitis optica; TM: transverse myelitis)

CASE VIGNETTES

Case 1

A 6-year-old boy presented with inability to walk and stand or bear weight on his legs for duration of 5 days. This was associated with diffuse dull aching pain in the back along with fever. There were no sensory symptoms, or bladder or bowel involvement. There was no history of trauma or intramuscular injection. The child was developmentally normal. Physical examination revealed bilateral symmetrical weakness of both lower limbs involving both proximal and distal muscles. Knee DTRs were absent and ankle DTRs were brisk. Plantars were extensor.

How do I summarize?

This 6-year-old typically developing boy presented with insidious onset of paraparesis for 5 days associated with fever. There is symmetric weakness involving both proximal and distal groups of muscles of the lower limb with signs of spasticity, brisk DTR, and extensor plantars. There is no definitive sensory or bladder involvement. Current functional ability is that he is bedridden with preserved ability to sit independently, preserved upper limb function, no cranial nerve palsy, preserved cognition, and higher mental functions. There is a lack of radicular or funicular pain. There is dull aching pain in the back, which is ill localized and could indicate a vertebral pain. His abdominal reflex was preserved and cremasteric reflex was absent. Knee DTR was absent and ankle DTR was brisk. Hence, the most probable site of lesion is L1-L3. Based on the clinical symptoms and signs, the lesion looks like a noncompressive intramedullary lesion. Considering the presence of ongoing fever, vertebral pain, a strong possibility of infective myelitis, or transverse myelitis involving lumbosacral region has to be considered.

Explanation

Sensory localization in a 6-year-old child might be difficult. Absent knee DTR and brisk ankle DTR points to the root value of L2-L3, as DTRs are absent at the affected level and brisk below that level. Superficial reflex is absent at that level (cremasteric absent at L1-L2) with normal abdominal reflex (hence the lesion is below T12) with extensor plantar (UMN lesion). The most likely site of lesion is L1-L3. It is essential to remember that the acute stage of the spinal cord could have decreased tone and absent DTR. This stage of flaccidity is followed by a stage of spasticity and hyperreflexia. Absence of radicular pain and no spinal tenderness makes extrinsic compression less likely. Presence of fever and noncompressive lesion with root localization often points to focal inflammatory pathology such as transverse myelitis. Vascular pathology cannot explain the ongoing fever, although malignancy can present with fever. The presence of a very short history for 5 days goes against malignancy. Other causes of infective compressive pathology such as epidural abscess and tubercular spine could be kept as one of differential diagnoses but there is a lack of compressive signs and symptoms on examination.

Case 2

A 10-year-old boy presented with complaints of progressive difficulty in walking for 6 months, associated with a history of on-and-off fever. He has difficulty getting up from the floor and can hardly take 1–2 steps with support. She requires assistance to get up from the bed. There is no weakness in hands. There is no history to suggest any cranial nerve palsy or impairment of cognition. Examination revealed a malnourished child. Lower limb power is <2/5 across both proximal and distal joints. The tone is decreased. Knee DTRs are brisk and ankle DTR is brisk. Plantars are extensor. Cremasteric reflex is absent. The abdominal reflex is absent. There is severe tenderness in the spine at the thoracolumbar space. Straight leg test elicits severe pain. There is a symmetrical loss of pain and temperature sensation below the abdomen. Joint position sense is absent bilateral in the great toe. Vibration sense is absent when tested in bilateral medial malleolus.

Interpretation

The presence of spinal tenderness points to the extrinsic compressive lesion. Brisk knee and ankle DTR with extensor plantars point that lesion is above L1-L2 (knee DTR L1-L2). Since cremasteric reflex (L1) and abdominal reflex (T7-T12) is absent, most probable site of lesion will be from T7 to L1. Since there is spinal tenderness at this point, the probable site of the lesion remains T7-L1. Loss of all sensation below L1 dermatome points to lesion above the same. Since all sensations, both lateral tract, and posterior tract are affected, it needs to be a dense lesion involving the spinal cord. Now we know that the L1-L2 spinal level corresponds to the D10 vertebra. Hence, it looks like a compressive pathology involving lower thoracic (T10) vertebra. Since there is an ongoing fever for 6 months, it could be a chronic infection such as tuberculosis or malignancy such as non-Hodgkin lymphoma.

Case 3

An 8-year-old boy presented with complaints of urinary incontinence for a duration of 7 days. There is subtle difficulty in walking with twisting of the ankle while walking. In addition, there is dull aching backache. There are no sensory symptoms. Examination reveals bilateral symmetrical distal predominant weakness with brisk ankle DTR. He is currently ambulatory with assistance.

Extensor plantar response was observed. There was no definitive sensory involvement, except for the loss of sensation in the perianal area.

Explanation

The presence of only subtle distal predominant weakness with loss of perianal sensation and early bladder involvement often favors conus medullaris lesion. In contrast, cauda equina lesions have predominant radicular pain with asymmetric spastic weakness involving both limbs with late bladder involvement.

Case 4

A 12-year-old girl presented with difficulty in walking and sways while walking for the last 3 months. There is motor weakness (power 4/5) across proximal and distal muscles. DTRs preserved. Plantars response is flexor. Pain and temperature sensations are preserved. There is loss of vibration and joint position sensation with positive Rhomberg sign.

Interpretation

It is a chronic motor weakness with dissociated sensory loss (loss of vibration with preserved pain sensation) suggestive of dorsal column dysfunction. In an adolescent girl, vitamin B_{12} deficiency must be strongly considered.

■ PLANNING INVESTIGATIONS

- Magnetic resonance imaging (MRI) spine with contrast would help to differentiate compressive or noncompressive myelopathy. Presence of contrast enhancement

indicates infective or inflammatory pathology.
- Children with longitudinally extensive transverse myelitis (LETM) (involvement of more than three consecutive spinal segments is called LETM) should be additionally screened for MRI brain and orbit to look for evidence of NMO.
- A lumbar puncture will support or refute the spinal cord inflammation. Cerebrospinal fluid (CSF) oligoclonal band and serum NMO antibody levels can be estimated to look for acquired demyelination.
- Acquired demyelination can be screened by additional evoked potentials.
- Infective screening would include serology for Epstein–Barr virus (EBV), *Mycoplasma*, and herpes simplex virus (HSV).
- Thyroid-stimulating hormone (TSH) and anti-thyroid peroxidase (anti-TPO) needs to be screened.
- Other supportive investigations include Mantoux test, chest X-ray for latent tuberculosis, and NMO antibody for transverse myelitis.
- Other vasculitic workup including antinuclear antibody, anti-dsDNA antibody, anticardiolipin antibody, and anticytoplasmic antibody is required among children with transverse myelitis.
- One might have to screen for serum homocysteine level, hemoglobin, mean corpuscular volume, and serum vitamin B_{12} levels.

■ MANAGEMENT

Supportive management includes nursing in a neutral position. Bladder care is essential to prevent urinary tract infection. Methods including clean intermittent catheterization are useful. Bedsores can be prevented with regular change of posture. Definitive management will depend on etiology—antitubercular drugs for the tubercular spine, methylprednisolone for transverse myelitis, and antineoplastic drugs for leukemia/lymphoma. Transverse myelitis is often treated with pulse methylprednisolone (30 mg/kg/day for 3–5 days) followed by tapering steroids (prednisolone 1 mg/kg/day for 14–21 days). Alternate therapy includes intravenous immunoglobulin and rituximab. Poor prognostic factors include complete paraplegia at the onset, duration of <24 hours to the maximum deficit, sphincter disturbance, and younger age at onset.

KEY MESSAGES

- Acute onset of weakness of lower limbs in the presence of bladder retention is a strong pointer to possible cord pathology.
- The nature of pain can vary depending on the underlying problem in patients with paraplegia such as funicular pain in an intramedullary lesion, radicular pain in GBS, deep-seated pain, or vertebral pain can be seen in compressive myelopathy.
- Localization of lesion in a patient with paraplegia could be arrived based on a sensory level, extent of motor weakness, deep tendon reflexes, and superficial reflexes.
- Presence of vision loss (optic neuritis) in a patient with paraplegia always raises a possibility of NMO.
- The most common cause of acute-onset paraplegia in children includes transverse myelitis (idiopathic) and GBS.

28. A Case of Acute Flaccid Paralysis/Guillain–Barré Syndrome

■ INTRODUCTION

Acute flaccid paralysis (AFP) refers to acute onset (<14 days), weakness of limbs or any part of body in a child <15 years of age, or any paralytic illness in a person in whom polio is suspected [World Health Organization (WHO) case definition for AFP]. AFP can result from involvement of central nervous system, spinal cord lesion, anterior horn cell pathology, peripheral nerve pathology, neuromuscular junction disorder, or muscle pathology **(Table 1)**. Four most common differentials of AFP include acute poliomyelitis, Guillain–Barré syndrome (GBS), acute transverse myelitis (ATM), and traumatic neuritis. The variants of GBS include acute motor axonal neuropathy (AMAN), acute motor sensory axonal neuropathy (AMSAN), acute inflammatory demyelinating polyneuropathy (AIDP), and Miller–Fischer syndrome (MFS) variants. Other uncommon variants of GBS include pharyngo-cervico-brachial (PCB) variant, pure sensory ataxic variant, and polyneuritis cranialis (PC) variant. In addition, AFP may result from viral myositis, acute flaccid myelitis (AFM), tick paralysis, botulism, drug-induced peripheral neuropathy, hypokalemia, drug-induced myopathy, and myasthenic crises. The key clinical features of common causes of AFP are summarized in **Table 2**.

■ HISTORY-TAKING

Presenting Complaints

Presenting complaints will depend on the extent of muscle weakness. Few common

TABLE 1: Causes of acute flaccid paralysis.

CNS causes	Anterior horn cell	Peripheral nerve	Neuromuscular junction	Muscle
• ADEM • NMO • CVST • Brainstem encephalitis • Tumor • Abscess • Hematoma	• Poliomyelitis • Nonpolio enterovirus • Rabies • Varicella zoster • JE virus	• GBS • CMV infection • Tick paralysis • Porphyria • Drug-induced (chemo therapeutic drugs) • Critical illness polyneuropathy	• Myasthenia • Botulism • Snakebite • Organophosphorous poisoning • Borreliosis	• Viral myositis • Hypokalemic periodic paralysis • McArdle disease • Polymyositis • Critical illness myopathy

(ADEM: acute disseminated encephalomyelitis; CMV: cytomegalovirus; CVST: cerebral venous sinus thrombosis; GBS: Guillain–Barré syndrome; JE: Japanese encephalitis; NMO: neuromyelitis optica)

TABLE 2: Key clinical features of common causes of acute flaccid paralysis.

Conditions	Key features
Acute poliomyelitis	Asymmetric pure motor ascending paralysis with no sensory involvement, history of intramuscular injection or fever at onset of weakness, and unimmunized child
Guillain–Barré syndrome (GBS)	Symmetrical ascending motor and/or sensory weakness with or without bulbar, respiratory, or facial weakness. Deep tendon reflexes (DTRs) are usually absent, but may be preserved in 10–15%; history of preceding febrile illness or vaccination in the preceding few weeks
Acute transverse myelitis (ATM)	Symmetric weakness with a sensory level; early bladder involvement; history of preceding febrile illness; DTRs are absent in spinal shock stage and then become exaggerated
Acute flaccid myelitis (AFM)	Sudden onset of flaccid weakness with areflexia and multiple cranial neuropathies are often associated with enterovirus infection
Postdiphtheritic polyneuropathy	Onset of bulbar weakness with descending appendicular weakness and history of preceding sore throat or bull neck
Botulism	Sudden onset of flaccid weakness with ptosis and extraocular muscle weakness in infants following ingestion of contaminated food products
Tick paralysis	Insidious onset, slowly progressive pure motor weakness with ocular involvement, pupil abnormality (dilated pupil), dysarthria; presence of eschar mark, occurrence during the rainy season and history of recent travel are supportive
Acute intermittent porphyria	Predominant neuropsychiatric manifestation with features of autonomic instability
Critical illness polyneuropathy	Development of flaccid weakness in an intensive care unit (ICU) patient with prolonged mechanical ventilation with or without need for neuromuscular relaxants or corticosteroids
Myasthenic crises	Sudden onset flaccid paralysis with ptosis, history of diurnal variation, and sudden worsening with febrile illness
Traumatic neuritis	Onset of weakness in one limb with areflexia following intramuscular injection
Hypokalemic pseudoparalysis	Sudden onset of flaccid weakness of neck muscles and limbs following heavy carbohydrate meal that recovers completely in a few days. Patient may have such recurrent episodes
Rabies	Onset of ascending weakness with autonomic instability; development of ptosis following a bite by a rabid dog on the face, especially when the child has received only antirabies vaccine and not rabies-specific immunoglobulin
Viral myositis	Pain and weakness in limb muscles with muscle tenderness

presenting complaints in children with AFP (usual duration of these complaints is 2–4 days) include one or more of the following:
- Inability to walk and stand
- Weakness of lower limbs and upper limbs
- Severe pain in the limbs with inability to stand and walk
- Weakness of lower limbs progressing to weakness of upper limbs
- Breathing difficulty

- Inability to swallow food and water
- Altered voice
- Deviation of face toward one side

History of Presenting Illness

History of presenting illness (HOPI) needs to focus on the onset, progression, and extent of the weakness before arriving at etiological history. The sequence of events must be presented in a chronological manner to understand the pattern of muscle weakness in a child with suspected GBS **(Practical Box 1)**.

Onset and Progression of Weakness

Onset of weakness (hyperacute, sudden, or insidious) could provide clinical clue to underlying etiology. Hyperacute onset (weakness that develops within few minutes to hours) with pain often points to vascular pathology such as anterior spinal artery thrombosis. Sudden-onset weakness such as weakness that is evident on waking up in the morning can be seen in GBS, acute poliomyelitis, and ATM. Children with ATM can also have insidious onset of weakness that develops over few days. In the example provided in **Practical Box 1**, the child had sudden onset of weakness.

History of progression of weakness from the onset to its nadir (maximum weakness) needs to be recorded. The weakness in children with GBS can progress rapidly within few hours to as slow as 2–3 weeks to reach a nadir beyond which weakness remains static with subsequent slow recovery. The sequence of muscle weakness can also provide a vital clue. Ascending paralysis from lower limb to upper limb involvement can be seen in GBS. In contrast, botulism and postdiphtheritic paralysis will have descending paralysis starting from bulbar muscles down to upper limb and then to lower limb muscle. Children with hypokalemic periodic paralysis can have episodic weakness where the child recovers completely in between the episodes. Similarly, children with CACNA1A-related channelopathies including familial hemiplegic migraine can have recurrent episodes of muscle weakness. GBS is unlikely to present with recurrent flaccid paralysis.

Extent and Symmetry of Weakness

Extent of involvement (lower limb, upper limb, truncal, neck flexor, bulbar, ocular, and respiratory weakness) will guide the diagnosis and treatment strategy. See **Chapter 15** on approach to neuromuscular weakness to understand the pattern of muscle weakness. If the child has isolated lower limb weakness with complete sparing of truncal and upper limb muscles, it would raise suspicion of ATM. If the weakness started from lower limb and then progressed

> **PRACTICAL BOX 1:** Example of history of presenting illness.
>
> The child was apparently well till 4 days back when he started complaining of severe pain in the legs and was unable to walk. Gradually within the next 6 hours, his pain worsened, and he could not stand or bear weight on his legs. By the next morning, he was bedridden and required assistance to get up from the lying-down posture (*indicative of truncal weakness on day 2 of illness*). On the same day, his parents noticed that he was unable to use his hands to hold the spoon to eat (*indicative of distal upper limb weakness on day 2*) nor was he able to lift his arm to wear his shirt (*indicative of proximal upper limb weakness*). There was no breathing difficulty (*respiratory weakness*), no difficulty in swallowing or alteration of voice (*bulbar weakness*), and no diplopia or deviation of eyes (*extraocular muscle weakness*). The weakness has been static and has not progressed further in the last 2 days (nadir of weakness was day 2)

to involve truncal muscles and upper limb muscles, this would be considered ascending paralysis. Ascending weakness is characteristic of GBS and the weakness may subsequently ascend to involve bulbar and respiratory muscles. Isolated bulbar weakness can be seen in postdiphtheritic polyneuropathy. Extensive weakness with predominant involvement of ocular and bulbar muscles with ptosis could be observed in children with myasthenia gravis presenting as myasthenic crises. While describing the extent of involvement, it is also essential to ascertain the involvement of sensory system (paresthesia and anesthesia), involvement of urinary bladder (bladder retention), and autonomic involvement (excessive sweating and postural hypotension).

Symmetry of weakness is a crucial information in HOPI. ATM and GBS would often result in symmetrical weakness. Asymmetrical patchy motor weakness is a classical feature of acute poliomyelitis and other nonpolio enterovirus infections. Till now, we know how the weakness started (onset), how fast did it progress (progression), and what all did it involve (extent of weakness). Now, let us recognize few patterns of muscle weakness.

Pattern of Weakness and Neurological Involvement

- If there is motor weakness, which is asymmetric and patchy with preserved sensations, such pure motor weakness with complete sensory sparing is classical of poliomyelitis. Children with GBS (AMAN variant) can also present with isolated asymmetrical pure motor weakness.
- Symmetric ascending motor weakness with or without sensory involvement is classical of GBS.
- Presence of ptosis, extraocular weakness, and diplopia often points to myasthenia gravis, especially when there is a history of diurnal variation (weakness minimal in the morning when the child gets up and it gets worse by evening). Children with myasthenia gravis can present as AFP (myasthenic crises).
- In a child with AFP, if the ptosis and extraocular muscle weakness are prominent, it must raise suspicion of snakebite intoxication and rabies (paralytic or dumb rabies). Dumb rabies may present with flaccid paralysis, especially if there is a history of dog bite in the recent past that was treated only with antirabies vaccination and not immunoglobulin.
- Bulbar onset of weakness should raise suspicion of postdiphtheritic polyneuropathy or botulism. History of preceding bull neck or sore throat would point to former and history of ingestion of canned food or contaminated honey can point to the latter.
- In a child with AFP, presence of multiple cranial neuropathies along with abnormalities of pupil can be seen following tick paralysis or in AFM. Sixth or seventh cranial nerve palsy can be also observed in children with GBS. There are few uncommon variants of GBS such as pharyngo-cervico-brachial (PCB) variant, which may present with isolated bulbar weakness, and PC variant, which may present with multiple cranial nerve palsy. Children with Lyme disease can have facial nerve paralysis. Hence, cranial nerve involvement in AFP can be seen in tick paralysis, polydiphtheritic polyneuropathy, GBS, AFM, and Lyme disease.
- Sudden onset of flaccid paralysis with evidence of cranial neuropathies should

also raise a clinical suspicion of AFM. This condition is clinically indistinguishable from GBS. However, neuroimaging reveals selective involvement of gray matter of spinal cord and brainstem in contrast to root enhancement in GBS.
- Urinary bladder can be involved in both ATM and GBS. Early involvement of bladder in the form of retention would suggest a possibility of ATM, although 10–15% of children with GBS might also develop bladder retention.
- Sensory involvement (positive sensory symptoms such as paresthesia) can be present in GBS, which is a polyradiculoneuropathy. Most of patients with polyradiculoneuropathy (GBS) will have severe radicular pains (pain that radiates along with the limbs) often masking these sensory symptoms.
- Majority of children with AFP will have normal sensorium. Presence of altered sensorium along with multiple cranial neuropathies should make us strongly think of brainstem encephalitis.
- In a child with episodic muscle weakness with behavioral symptoms, abdominal pain, and photosensitivity, a possibility of porphyria must be considered.
- Deep-seated pain in the back (funicular pain) can be seen in children with ATM. Pain in the muscles along with weakness is suggestive of inflammatory myositis such as viral myositis.

Etiological History (Specific)

- History of preceding febrile illness, diarrheal illness, or vaccination followed by onset of weakness is consistent with GBS.
- Fever at onset of illness is observed in acute poliomyelitis.
- History of preceding diarrheal illness prior to onset of AFP raises a possibility of enteroviral infection and AMAN variant of GBS.
- History of bull neck (swelling in neck), throat infection, and fever in preceding 2–3 weeks can be present in children with postdiphtheritic polyneuropathy. Immunization status must always be enquired for the same reason.
- Onset of weakness following intramuscular injection can be seen in acute poliomyelitis and traumatic neuritis.
- Trauma to spine or head must be elicited to look for possibility of traumatic myelopathy.
- History of dog bite in the preceding few years (rabies)
- History of recent travel to hilly or tropical thick forest areas, sleeping on the floor, or any evident history of insect bite (tick bite)
- History of ingestion of canned old food and ingestion of contaminated honey products (botulism)
- History of chemotherapeutic drugs such as vincristine and amiodarone can result in peripheral neuropathy. History of prolonged steroid intake could lead to steroid-induced myopathy. Most of drug-induced neuropathy or myopathy have subacute to chronic course instead of AFP.
- Predominant sensory symptoms (paresthesia, numbness, and tingling sensation) with abdominal pain should point us toward occupational hazards including arsenic or lead exposure.
- History of similar episodes in the past, presence of nonspecific abdominal pain, and history of photosensitivity should raise suspicion of porphyria.

- Onset of weakness immediately following a heavy exercise or running must raise a possibility of glycogen storage disorders.
- History of prolonged intensive care unit (ICU) stay, use of corticosteroids, and use of neuromuscular blockade such as vecuronium/rocuronium during ICU stay preceding the onset of AFP can suggest the possibility of critical illness polyneuropathy.
- Parental occupation and nearby industrial exposure (possible lead exposure)
- Sudden onset of weakness in the morning following heavy carbohydrate meal such as heavy dinner at a party (hypokalemic periodic paralysis).

EXAMINATION

Examination must be focused among children with AFP. The focus of each part of examination is outlined below:
- *Vitals:* Presence of fluctuating tachycardia, bradycardia, hypertension, or hypotension favors autonomic instability seen in children with GBS.
- *General physical examination:*
  - Look for eschars (tick bite)/snakebite/ dog bite marks in all children presenting with AFP. Always search for tick behind the ears, in scalp, and in nape of the neck.
  - Look for zoster vesicular lesions.
  - Presence of anemia along with nail changes, rash, and alopecia in children with chronic lead exposure.
  - Look for muscle tenderness in viral myositis.
- *Neurological examination:*
  - *Higher mental function:* Usually preserved in children with AFP
  - Cranial nerve involvement including pupil size and reaction and any evidence of papilledema on fundus examination.
- Focus of motor examination would be to determine the extent and degree of muscle weakness [muscle power must be graded by MRC (Medical Research Council)]. Extent of weakness may be described in terms of the following:
  - Proximal and distal lower limb weakness
  - Proximal and distal upper limb weakness
  - Truncal weakness
  - Neck flexor/neck extensor weakness
  - Bulbar weakness
  - Ptosis/extraocular muscle weakness
- Respiratory weakness (single breath count) (Once we splint the movement of the chest by placing our hands over the costal margins, it will restrict the movement of diaphragm, hence, if a child has intercostal muscle weakness, he was breathing because of intact diaphragm; once that diaphragm is also splinted, his respiratory distress worsens. This is a clinical method to identify intercostal and diaphragmatic weakness. If the respiratory distress worsens by splinting the intercostal muscles, then it is diaphragmatic weakness.)

In addition to muscle power grading, tone, deep tendon reflexes (DTRs), and superficial reflexes must be assessed. Hypotonia must not be equated to muscle weakness. A child can have hypotonia without muscle weakness. Similarly, one can have muscle weakness (spastic weakness) without hypotonia. Children with AFP often have both muscle weakness and hypotonia. DTRs are usually absent in children with GBS. However, 10–15% of children with GBS can have normal or rather exaggerated DTRs. Similarly, DTRs are usually expected to be

brisk in ATM, but paradoxically DTRs may be completely absent in stages of spinal shock.
- Sensory system examination
- Involvement of bladder
- Test cerebellar signs as acute cerebellar ataxia can mimic GBS-like presentation. Similarly, the Miller–Fischer variant of GBS can present as ataxia and ophthalmoplegia along with areflexia.
- Terminal neck rigidity can be seen in poliomyelitis and in few children with polyradiculoneuropathy (GBS).

Other relevant systemic examination includes hepatosplenomegaly, lymphadenopathy, and bony tenderness to look for possibility of malignancy with paraneoplastic or metastatic cord lesion presenting with AFP.

Analysis

It is important to synthesize the above history and examination to reach a clinical diagnosis or broad differentials so that appropriate investigations can be planned (**Practical Box 2**). Analysis can be done in terms of the following parameters:
- Onset and progression of weakness
- Extent of neuromuscular weakness
- Involvement of sensorium, cranial nerves, sensory, autonomic system, urinary bladder, cerebellar, and meningeal signs
- Any other systemic findings
- Possible neuroanatomical site of lesion
- Possible etiology
- Points in favor and against clinical diagnosis of GBS are summarized in **Box 1**.

■ PLANNING INVESTIGATION

Reporting

Once the airway, breathing, and circulation are established and a clinical possibility has been raised for AFP, immediate reporting to the AFP surveillance team must be sent.

PRACTICAL BOX 2: Analysis of case.
- *Summary:* A 4-year-old boy presented with sudden-onset, rapidly progressing, and ascending symmetrical motor weakness involving both proximal and distal muscles of upper limb and lower limb along with truncal weakness. There was no preceding febrile illness, vaccination, injections, or trauma. The weakness started 4 days back and reached its nadir on day 2 and has been static since then. There is flaccid motor weakness with MRC power of <2/5 in all the tested muscles. There is global areflexia, and the plantar response was mute. There is no neck flexor, bulbar, respiratory, or extraocular muscle weakness. There is no involvement of higher mental functions, cranial nerves, sensory system, and urinary bladder. The rest of systemic examination was unremarkable. Currently, the child is bedridden
- *Neuroanatomical site:* Considering flaccid motor weakness (symmetric) with areflexia and mute plantars, the possible neuroanatomical site could be anterior horn cell or nerve fibers
- *Etiology:* The possible differential diagnoses include Guillain–Barré syndrome (GBS), acute transverse myelitis, and poliomyelitis. Points that favor GBS include symmetric ascending paralysis, areflexia, static course after reaching a nadir, and no bladder involvement. However, there was no history of preceding febrile illness or vaccination. High cervical or longitudinally extensive acute transverse myelitis can also present with symmetric weakness of upper limb, lower limb, and trunk weakness. However, absence of bladder symptoms and sensory symptoms is a strong point against ATM. Since it is ascending paralysis, with bulbar sparing, other differentials like postdiphtheritic polyneuropathy and botulism are unlikely. Sparing of cranial nerves, in this case, disfavors postdiphtheritic polyneuropathy and acute flaccid myelitis. There was no history of muscle injection; traumatic neuritis seems unlikely

Nerve Conduction Study

Diagnosis of GBS is essentially clinical. Nerve conduction studies (NCS) are supportive investigations. Detailed description of

> **BOX 1:** Key clinical features of Guillain–Barré syndrome (GBS).
>
> *When to think of GBS?*
> - Symmetrical ascending weakness with or without sensory involvement
> - Progression up to 4 weeks
> - Deep tendon reflexes may be absent or preserved or rarely exaggerated
> - Severe cases can have bulbar or respiratory involvement
> - Presence of radicular pain in back and thighs
> - Absence of fever at the onset
> - May have autonomic instability
>
> *When not to think of GBS?*
> - Marked asymmetric weakness (*Poliomyelitis*)
> - Bulbar onset weakness (*Myasthenia*)
> - Sharp sensory level (*Acute transverse myelitis*)
> - Fever at onset of weakness (*Poliomyelitis*)
> - Predominant extraocular muscle weakness (*Myasthenia*)
> - Early respiratory weakness without limb involvement
> - Early urinary bladder involvement (*Acute transverse myelitis*)
> - Presence of pupillary abnormality (*Tick paralysis*)

NCS can be read from **Chapter 6** on "neurophysiological evaluation". There are two main patterns of abnormalities that are detected on NCS. One is axonal variant with predominant reduction of amplitude of compound muscle action potential (CMAP) and/or sensory nerve action potential (SNAP). In simple terms, if the amplitude of CMAP alone is reduced, then we think of AMAN. If the amplitude of both CMAP and SNAP are reduced, then we think of AMSAN. If there is an increase in distal latency with reduction of conduction velocity and evidence of temporal dispersion and conduction block, it indicates demyelinating pathology (AIDP).

Prognosis for recovery often is determined by degree of axonal loss. Children with AMAN/AMSAN might have a long time to recovery when compared to those with AIDP. In early stages of GBS, NCS can be normal or only F-wave abnormalities can be seen. Hence, a repeat NCS is suggested at 2nd to 3rd week of illness to establish the pattern of involvement. An interesting phenomenon of "sural nerve sparing" observed in many patients with GBS must be kept in mind while interpreting the NCS study. Apart from GBS, motor axonal polyneuropathy is observed in lead poisoning, porphyria, tick paralysis, critical illness polyneuropathy, and diphtheritic polyneuropathy. Children with HIV can have demyelinating polyneuropathy. Children with pharyngo-cervical-brachial variant of GBS usually have axonal neuropathy but may have normal NCS. Similarly, Miller–Fischer variant (ataxia, ophthalmoplegia, and areflexia) can also have normal NCS except for H-wave reflex abnormalities. **Table 3** and **Box 2** summarize clinical and electrophysiological differentiation of axonal and demyelinating polyneuropathy.

Cerebrospinal fluid (CSF) examination: Cerebrospinal fluid examination is often deferred till the 2nd week of illness and finding of albumin–cytological dissociation is supportive rather than confirmatory. In patients with GBS, by the 2nd or 3rd week of illness, CSF cytology shows <50 cells/mm^3 and CSF protein is more than normal range for the age. Albumin–cytological dissociation is also observed in patients with porphyria and postdiphtheritic polyneuropathy. Presence of CSF pleocytosis (>50 cells/mm^3) is strongly suggestive of alternative diagnosis including Lyme's disease, HIV infection, and sarcoidosis.

Neuroimaging

Magnetic resonance imaging (MRI) spine with contrast might reveal nerve root enhancement in GBS, evidence of ATM, evidence of isolated gray matter involvement

TABLE 3: Differentiating clinical features of axonal and demyelinating polyneuropathy.

Features	Axonal neuropathy	Demyelinating neuropathy
Onset of weakness to its nadir	Rapid progression to early peak of weakness	Progression can be gradual
Length-dependent involvement	Long axons of lower limbs are affected before upper limb nerves	Diffuse and patchy weakness although it can also start only in lower limb
Sensory symptoms	Clinical sensory symptoms common in AMSAN	Clinical sensory loss is minimal
Cranial neuropathy and dysautonomia	Uncommon	Frequent
Proximal versus distal	Distal predominant weakness	Proximal as well as distal weakness
Deep tendon reflexes (DTRs)	Proximal DTRs may be preserved in 10%	Global areflexia
Recovery	Slow recovery with residual deficits among those with axonal degeneration. Children with conduction block variant of AMAN recover faster with no deficits	Rapid recovery with no deficits

(AMAN: acute motor axonal neuropathy; AMSAN: acute motor sensory axonal neuropathy)

BOX 2: Electrophysiological criteria for motor axonal neuropathy and demyelinating polyneuropathy.

Criteria for acute inflammatory demyelinating polyneuropathy (AIDP):
- Presence of one or more of the following in at least two of the tested nerve provided the amplitude of compound muscle action potential (CMAP) >10%:
  – Reduced conduction velocity (<85–90%)
  – Increased distal latency (>110%)
  – Conduction block (proximal CMAP: Distal CMAP <0.5)
  – Temporal dispersion F-wave latency (>120%) or absent F wave

Criteria for acute motor axonal neuropathy (AMAN):
- Decrease in CMAP <80% of normal with none of the features of AIDP

of spinal cord and brainstem in AFM; and brainstem involvement in Bickerstaff brainstem encephalitis. It is important to emphasize that imaging is supportive and not diagnostic investigations.

Antiganglioside Antibody

Antiganglioside antibody testing is not routinely recommended in diagnosis of children with GBS nor do these antibodies have any prognostic importance. In exceptional cases with clinical ambiguity testing, these antibodies might support the clinical diagnosis. For example, GM1 and GD1a are elevated in AMAN, AIDP, and AMSAN; GT1a is raised alone in the pharyngo-cervical-brachial variant of GBS; GQ1b and GT1a are raised in Miller–Fisher syndrome and acute ataxic neuropathy; GQ1b and GT1a are elevated in Bickerstaff brainstem encephalitis; and GD1b is elevated in pure sensory ataxic variant of GBS.

Electromyography

There is no role of invasive investigations such as electromyography (EMG) in diagnosis of GBS. Positive sharp waves and fibrillations have been reported beyond 4 weeks of onset of GBS, which depict signs of acute denervation.

Other Supportive Investigations

Based on the etiology and clinical suspicion, specific laboratory investigations can be planned. It is usually not a good idea to order everything and get confused at the end. Investigations must be used judiciously. For example, blood lead levels can be planned only among those with suspected lead poisoning; urinary porphobilinogen (PBG) levels can be considered among those with acute intermittent porphyria and Lyme serology for children with suspected Lyme disease. The serum CPK level is elevated in viral myositis.

MANAGEMENT OF A CHILD WITH ACUTE FLACCID PARALYSIS

First Step in Management

Children with respiratory compromise need respiratory support in the form of oxygen, noninvasive, or invasive ventilation. Those with bulbar weakness require regular suctioning. Autonomic instability including hypertension needs appropriate management. Hypokalemia in periodic paralysis needs potassium supplementation. Children with cervical injury need cervical spine splinting.

TABLE 4: Specific treatment of conditions causing acute flaccid paralysis.

Condition	Treatment
Transverse myelitis	Methylprednisolone (30 mg/kg/day for 3–5 days)
Guillain–Barré syndrome and myasthenic crisis	Intravenous immunoglobulin (IVIG) 2 g/kg over 4–5 days. Alternatives include plasma exchange therapy. In case of no response, a second dose of IVIG may be considered
Lead poisoning	EDTA chelation therapy

(EDTA: ethylene diamine tetra-acetic acid)

Specific Treatment

Specific treatment for various conditions resulting in AFP has been summarized in **Table 4**.

Supportive Care

Children should be nursed in *neutral position* to prevent contractures. Regular change of posture and measures to prevent bedsores must be exercised. Children with urinary retention require clean intermittent catheterization. Pain needs to be addressed with analgesics and gabapentin. Physiotherapy needs to be initiated once the pain settles. Nutritional rehabilitation for children with prolonged hospital stay is a priority.

KEY MESSAGES

- Any child with AFP must always be reported to the AFP surveillance team.
- Rapidly progressive and symmetrical ascending paralysis with areflexia often suggests a possibility of GBS.
- AMAN variant has rapid progression, less cranial nerve involvement, less dysautonomia, and may have preserved deep tendon reflexes when compared to AIDP.
- Uncommon variants of GBS include Miller–Fischer variant, PC, pharyngo-cervical-brachial variant, and Bickerstaff brainstem encephalitis.
- Presence of pure motor weakness with pupillary abnormality must always raise a possibility of tick paralysis.

CHAPTER 29: A Case of Floppy Infant

■ HISTORY-TAKING

The common causes of floppy infant include spinal muscular atrophy (SMA), congenital myopathy, congenital muscular dystrophy, congenital myotonic dystrophy, and syndromic chromosomal disorders (**Table 1**). The clinical features of these conditions have been discussed in **Chapter 15**. The present chapter focuses on how to present a case of a floppy baby. Case presentation of a floppy infant will begin similar to case presentation of a child with cerebral palsy with presenting complaints starting right from birth.

■ PRESENTING COMPLAINTS

Common presenting complaints in a floppy child will include:
- Unable to hold the neck since beginning
- Paucity of movement of limbs when lying down (*indicates lack of antigravity movement and lack of muscle power*)
- Delay in the attainment of motor milestones
- Looseness or floppiness of arms and legs noticed since birth (*indicates hypotonia*)
- Recurrent episodes of fever, cough, and fast breathing requiring hospitalization in last few months (*floppy babies are prone to recurrent chest infections*)
- Difficulty in feeding with repeated episodes of vomiting and pooling of secretions and noisy breathing [*indicates predisposition to gastroesophageal reflux disease* (GERD)]
- Feeding difficulty, excessive perspiration, and swelling over the body and fast breathing noticed for the last 5 days (cardiac involvement)

As the floppiness started right from the birth, hence we use phrases such as "since birth" and "since the beginning", while framing presenting complaints. It is essential

TABLE 1: Common causes of floppy infant.

Site of lesion	Common causes
Central causes	Chromosomal disorders (such as Prader–Willi syndrome), cortical malformation, hypoxic-ischemic brain insult, and neurometabolic disorders
Anterior horn cell	Spinal muscular atrophy (SMA) and Pompe disease
Nerve	Congenital hypomyelinating neuropathy, early-onset hereditary motor sensory neuropathy (HMSN), and infantile neuroaxonal dystrophy (INAD)
Neuromuscular junction	Congenital myasthenic syndrome (CMS)
Muscle	Congenital myopathy, congenital muscular dystrophy, congenital myotonic dystrophy, and metabolic myopathy

not to miss the acute complaint, which brought the baby to pediatric emergency unit, e.g., fever, cough, and fast breathing for 4 days. It is also possible that the child has presented in the outpatient unit and has no active issue, except for floppiness and motor delay.

History of Presenting Complaints

Few neuromuscular causes such as spinal muscular atrophy type 0 and variants of congenital myasthenic syndromes may start manifesting from the antenatal period in the form of decreased fetal movements. They may require assisted delivery and have delayed cry at birth. The history of delayed cry at birth and the need for resuscitation at birth are, thus, important.

Antenatal History

- Consanguinity in parents, maternal age, gestation, live issues, and abortions (risk for autosomal recessive disorders and chromosomal disorders)
- Conception was spontaneous or by artificial reproductive techniques (there is no clear evidence to support that babies born out of artificial reproductive techniques are at the higher risk of genetic birth defects.).
- History of polyhydramnios and decreased fetal movement (indicates the antenatal onset of hypotonia)
- History of prolonged labor or precipitate labor

Example: Baby was born to nonconsanguineously married couple. The mother was 23 years old at the time of conception. It is her first baby with no previous abortion or stillbirth. The pregnancy was spontaneous conception. Regular antenatal checkup was done including antenatal ultrasonography. There was no history of polyhydramnios or decreased fetal movement. Baby was born by normal delivery with no history of prolonged labor or precipitate labor.

Birth History

- Mode of delivery (floppy babies with antenatal onset may have fetal distress warranting cesarean section)
- Gestation and birth weight
- Whether baby cried immediately at birth (respiratory muscle weakness can result in apnea at birth requiring resuscitation.)
- Feeding difficulty, prolonged mechanical ventilation, and difficulty in weaning from ventilator are specific markers of neonatal-onset respiratory muscle weakness.

Early Neonatal Period

During the early neonatal period, did parents perceive lack of movement of limbs? Parents often describe this as:

- "He used to lie supine and would remain in the same position unless we change his posture".
- "Paucity of limb movements with nearly no movement of limbs away from bed" [lack of antigravity movement is a strong indicator of lower motor neuron (LMN) weakness].

In addition to the paucity of limb movements and floppiness or looseness of limbs, parents also perceive feeding difficulties, recurrent vomiting, difficulty in breathing, and noisy breathing.

Development

Since motor delay is the presenting complaint, we can describe the gross and fine motor developmental milestones within the history of presenting illness. Age at the attainment of gross and fine motor milestones may be described with the last attained motor milestone. The focus is not on the sequence of attainment of milestones, rather on the weakness that has resulted in this motor delay. Weakness is to be described appropriately. For example, in a 9-month-old infant, we can describe that he/she has not yet attained neck holding with a paucity of limb movements and looseness of limbs. Then we go on to describe the extent of weakness.

The rest of the developmental history (cognition, speech, and social skills) including detailed fine motor skills can be described under the heading of developmental history. This is in contrast to presenting a case of cerebral palsy where all developmental domains become a part of history of presenting illness.

Extent of Weakness

Description of the extent of weakness is essential to ascertain the possible differentials. Find below clues in history that will describe the extent of weakness.

- *Proximal upper limb weakness:*
  - Inability to lift arms while changing his shirt
  - Inability to pick up a toy placed on the shelf
  - Difficulty in grooming or washing of hair
- *Distal upper limb weakness:*
  - Weakness of grip with difficulty in breaking chapatti
  - Clumsiness in holding his feeding bottle
  - Difficulty in opening door knob
  - Difficulty in using buttons/zippers
- *Neck flexor/extensor weakness:*
  - Difficulty in lifting the head off the bed
  - Head wobbles and flops to front or back when sudden breaks are applied while traveling
- *Truncal weakness:*
  - Difficulty in turning on the bed
  - Takes support of hands on an attempt to get up from lying down position
- *Proximal hip girdle weakness:*
  - Difficulty in running, climbing stairs, and getting up from sitting position on the floor
  - Difficulty in walking on slopes and even on flat surfaces
  - Buckling of the knee while walking (quadriceps weakness) or difficulty in getting up from kneeling down position (quadriceps weakness)
- *Distal lower limb weakness:*
  - Tripping on the ground with an ankle twist
  - Slipping of chappals
  - Dragging feet while walking

In infants, we cannot often delineate individual muscles, but we can mention that "there is a paucity of movement of both upper limbs and lower limbs with a limited movement away from the bed" (lack of antigravity movements indicates proximal upper and lower limb weakness). "He does not firmly hold toys offered to him in his hands" (distal upper limb weakness). "When lifted by his shoulders, he cannot hold his neck" (neck flexor weakness).

Extent of Neurological Involvement

In addition to muscle weakness, the child may have involved other parts of the neuraxis. Clues for specific neuraxis involvement are listed in **Table 2**.

History of the motor system and clues to underlying etiology: Apart from muscle weakness, it is essential to comment on other aspects of the motor system:

- History of muscle thinness over hands and legs (muscle atrophy, often a clue to *neuronopathy* or *neuropathy*)
- History of muscle looking bulky over shoulder and thigh (a clue to *congenital myotonia*)

TABLE 2: Clues for specific neuraxis involvement.

System involved	Symptoms on history
Sensory system involvement	Loss of sensation, tingling sensation, numbness, paresthesia (abnormal sensation), burning pain, and sensation of walking on cotton
Autonomic involvement	Dizziness on a sudden change of posture, lack of sweating with unexplained fever, history of urinary, and stool incontinence
Bulbar muscle weakness	Alteration in voice, difficulty in swallowing, and drooling of saliva
Respiratory muscle weakness	Difficulty in breathing, sudden night awakenings owing to breathlessness, excessive daytime sleepiness (owing to poor night sleep), difficulty in coughing, and noisy breathing
Cardiac involvement	Breathlessness on exertion, excessive perspiration, and swelling over body
Ocular involvement	Restriction in the movement of eyes, diplopia, apparent eye deviation, and drooping of eyelids
Facial muscle weakness	History of loss of facial expressions or deviation of face, ability to blow whistles, or drink using straw

- History of muscle stiffness (cramps are often a feature of *metabolic myopathy*)
- History of twitching movement noticed in the muscles [*myokymia* could represent denervation and fasciculations (could represent *neuronopathy*)]
- History of the passage of reddish-colored urine, especially after prolonged exercise (an indicator of *metabolic myopathy*)
- History of muscle pain (indicates *inflammatory myopathy*)
- History of fixed tightness at shoulder/elbow/ankle joints (*contractures*)
- History of easy fatigability (getting easily tired during activities, need to put extra efforts to perform the same activity compared to his age-matched peers) (a feature of *myopathy*)
- History of flabbiness/looseness of limbs noticed while changing his clothes or handling the baby (indicative of *hypotonia*)
- History of prolonged time to heal with formation of a scar on skin wounds (hypertrophic scar formation is a feature of *Ullrich muscular dystrophy*)
- History of fluctuations or diurnal variation in muscle weakness (indicates disorders of neuromuscular transmission). Children with congenital myasthenic syndrome may occasionally be better in the morning hours and are almost bedridden by the evening hours.
- History of worsening of weakness with febrile illness (seen among disorders of neuromuscular transmission or *mitochondrial myopathy*). The weakness worsens, and the child is completely bedridden during febrile illness and recovers to baseline weakness once the febrile illness subsides.
- History of prolonged time to open hands when a fist is made in the child or in his mother (indicates *myotonia*). Mothers of babies with congenital myotonic dystrophy may complaint of such clumsiness while using her hands.

History to Ascertain Other Systemic Features

- History of cognitive decline or global delay indicates the central cause of floppy baby rather than the neuromuscular

cause (except for neuromuscular causes such as syndromic congenital muscular dystrophy and mitochondrial myopathy where cognition can be affected).
- History of vision and hearing must be elicited (vision is affected in syndromic congenital muscular dystrophy and hearing may be affected in mitochondrial myopathy).
- Inability to gain weight or failure to gain adequate weight is often secondary to feeding problems, recurrent respiratory tract infection, and/or repeated vomiting.
- Excessive weight gain can be seen among non-ambulatory patients with voracious appetite.

Localization Based on History in Floppy Baby

Central cause: Global developmental delay, presence of cognitive delay, presence of seizures, facial dysmorphism, preserved anti-gravity movement, no facial or bulbar or ocular weakness, proximal–distal involvement, usually upper limb is more affected than lower limb but may be equally affected.

Anterior horn cell: Isolated motor delay, lack of antigravity movement, profound muscle weakness, presence of muscle wasting, presence of twitching movement in muscle, especially tongue (fasciculations).

Neuromuscular transmission: History of diurnal fluctuations, worsening of weakness with febrile illness, facial and ocular weakness, and history of drooping of eyelids

Nerve: Hereditary neuropathy is a rare cause of floppy baby (keep this etiology lower down). The presence of muscle wasting, distal predominant weakness, and presence of foot deformities favor neuropathic process.

Muscle: Proximal shoulder and hip girdle weakness, variable facial weakness, and preserved muscle bulk often point to muscle as a possible site of localization.

Summary of History

- Age and gender
- Product of consanguineous or nonconsanguineous marriage
- Static neuromuscular weakness or progressive weakness
- Extent of muscle weakness (proximal or distal upper limb, lower limb, neck muscles, truncal muscles, facial, ocular, bulbar and respiratory muscle weakness, and ptosis)
- *Any systemic involvement:* Cardiac and respiratory
- Nutritional status (degree of malnutrition)
- Contractures and deformities
- Any sensory or autonomic involvement
- Cognition, vision, hearing, and seizure
- Possible neuroanatomical localization

Read the chapter on neuromuscular weakness to understand the possible differential diagnosis. An example of how to summarize the history of a floppy child is provided in **Practical Box 1**.

■ EXAMINATION OF FLOPPY BABY

Posture

The opening remark will mention the posture of the baby while lying down **(Practical Box 2)**. The main purpose of observing the baby (before you commence formal examination) is to look for preserved or absent antigravity movement and whether obvious signs of hypotonia are present or not.

Vital Signs

Floppy infant often presents with respiratory tract infections. Vital signs are important to

> **PRACTICAL BOX 1:** Summary of history and its analysis.
>
> I am presenting a case of 2-year-old boy born to nonconsanguineously married couple. The child was brought with isolated motor delay with nonprogressive weakness of all the four limbs and floppiness. The child had both proximal and distal weakness with neck flexor and truncal weakness with contractures involving both ankle joints. Bulbar, ocular, facial, and respiratory muscles are spared. There is no cardiac involvement. Cognition, speech, vision, and hearing are preserved. There is no sensory or autonomic involvement
>
> *Neuroanatomical site of localization:* It could be anywhere in motor unit including anterior horn cell, nerve, or muscle involvement. Although, neuromuscular junction looks less likely considering absence of ptosis, diurnal fluctuations, but still cannot be ruled out on history alone
>
> Possible *differential diagnosis* will include:
> - Spinal muscular atrophy type 2
> - Congenital myopathy
> - Congenital muscular dystrophy
> - *Others:* Congenital myotonic dystrophy, congenital myasthenia syndrome, and mitochondrial myopathy

> **PRACTICAL BOX 2:** Opening remark in examination of a floppy infant.
>
> On examination, the baby is lying supine on the bed with paucity of movement of both upper and lower limbs. Upper limbs are lying abducted at shoulder with elbow being extended, wrist extended and supinated. Lower limbs are lying flaccid with both hips abducted, partly flexed on knee and ankle. There is lack of antigravity movement in an otherwise happy and cheerful baby. Baby is of average built and nutrition with an intravenous (IV) cannula in right hand

determine the severity of pneumonia. The presence of tachycardia out of proportion to tachypnea should alert to the possibility of underlying cardiac involvement (common in certain congenital myopathy). Type of breathing—thoracoabdominal or abdominothoracic respiration—also becomes essential to determine respiratory muscle involvement (diaphragmatic vs. intercostal muscle weakness).

Anthropometry

Anthropometric variables are essential to determine the extent of failure to thrive that may result from repeated respiratory tract infections, GERD, and recurrent vomiting.

General Physical Examination

Focus on contractures, deformities, bedsores, and signs of vitamin D deficiency. Children with Ullrich muscular dystrophy might have hypertrophic scar marks on the skin or formation of keloids, velvety feel of skin, and protuberant calcaneum. Facial weakness with lack of facial expressions, high-arched palate, and bitemporal hallowing can point to congenital myasthenic syndrome or congenital myopathy. Tented upper lip with wide-open mouth suggests congenital myotonic dystrophy.

Motor System Examination

- *Bulk:* Gross atrophy of both proximal and distal muscles of the upper and lower limb suggests the neuronopathic process. Atrophy can also be seen in late stages of congenital myopathy, congenital muscular dystrophy, and hereditary motor sensory polyneuropathy (early onset: CMT type 3/type 4).
- *Tone assessment:* There may be a gross reduction of both active tone and passive tone (active tone refers to tone generated by activation of the motor unit; passive tone refers to tone in the resting state owing to viscoelastic tension of muscle fiber). Tone as assessed by posture, feel of muscle, and resistance to passive movement across

both proximal and distal joints of the upper limb, and lower limb is often decreased. Evidence of hypotonia includes *frog-like posture* on supine position, *complete head lag* on the pull to sit, *ragdoll appearance* on ventral suspension, and *feel of slipping* over the shoulders when held in vertical suspension.

- *Power assessment:* Formal Medical Research Council (MRC) based power assessment is often replaced by functional power assessment in infants and young children. The absence of antigravity movement across the proximal shoulder and hip girdle joints indicates the power of <3/5. In such a case, movement is retested with gravity being eliminated. If the movement happens when gravity gets eliminated, this indicates the power of at least 2/5. The absence of antigravity movement often points to LMN lesion (especially neuronopathy). However, when antigravity movements are preserved, it indicates a power of "at least 3/5" across the proximal joints of the upper and lower limb. In such cases, it is not possible to differentiate whether it is 4/5 or 5/5. Comment on neck flexor or neck extensor weakness.
- *Deep tendon reflexes (DTRs):* Preserved or exaggerated DTR points to the central cause of hypotonia. The absence of DTR often indicates neuronopathy. DTR is sluggish in myopathy and may be absent in end-stage myopathy and neuropathy.

Sensory System Examination

Formal sensory system examination is often not possible among infants and young children. Localization or withdrawal to pain and temperature can be commented across the body dermatomes. Other sensations are often difficult to assess. Baby with sensory loss will often have signs of self-mutilation with self-biting of fingertips or lips (seen among babies with hereditary sensory autonomic neuropathy type III and in babies with Lesch–Nyhan syndrome). In addition, they can have loss of perspiration resulting in dry ichthyotic skin along with a history of unexplained fever.

■ SUMMARIZING THE CASE

At the end of history and examination, the case needs to be summarized based on the extent of neurological involvement, neuroanatomical site of lesion, and possible etiology or differentials **(Practical Box 3)**.

Based on the clinical points in favor and against each differential, the list of differential diagnosis can be revised and reorganized given in **Table 3**:

Table 3 is just giving an example and it is not a comprehensive guide; it will vary from one case to another case. However, the identification of points in favor and points against helps in rearranging the possibilities. In this case, differential diagnosis can be rearranged as:

- Congenital myopathy
- Nonsyndromic congenital muscular dystrophy
- *Others:* Congenital myotonic dystrophy, spinal muscular atrophy type II, and mitochondrial myopathy

It is possible that other differential diagnoses such as SMA type 2 can be ruled out owing to the absence of tongue fasciculations. At the end of the examination, we are often left with two or three most common diagnosis. Note that we are keeping a broad group such as congenital myopathy or nonsyndromic CMD at the end of clinical evaluation unless a very specific clinical sign clearly points to a possible underlying genetic mutation. For example, if the baby has protuberant calcaneum, soft velvety skin, joint hyperlaxity, and proximal joint

PRACTICAL BOX 3: Summary at the end of history and examination.
- A 2-year-old boy born to nonconsanguineously married couple with nonprogressive flaccid quadriparesis. There is neck flexor and truncal weakness with contractures involving both ankle joints. There is sparing of bulbar, ocular, facial, and respiratory muscle involvement with no evidence of ptosis. There is possibly no cardiac involvement. Cognition, speech, vision, and hearing are preserved. There is no sensory or autonomic involvement. There is no significant family history. Anthropometric variable reveal grade II PEM by the IAP classification with wasting and no stunting as per the WHO classification. The current functional status of GMFCS is level IV
- The flaccid quadriparesis has both proximal and distal weakness with hypotonia, areflexia, lack of tongue fasciculation, preserved muscle bulk, and flexor plantar response suggestive of LMN type of neuromuscular weakness with possible neuroanatomical site of lesion being muscle or neuromuscular junction or nerve. Considering lack of diurnal variation, lack of ocular involvement, or ptosis, the possibility of neuromuscular junction looks less likely. Similarly, lack of distal atrophy disfavors neuropathy although areflexia can very well go along. Hence, a possible neuroanatomical site is muscle. Possible differentials included at the end of history need to rearrange based on examination findings

(GMFCS: gross motor functional classification system; IAP: Indian Academy of Pediatrics; LMN: lower motor neuron; PEM: Protein-Energy-Malnutrition; WHO: World Health Organization)

TABLE 3: Revised and reorganized list of differential diagnosis.

Differential diagnosis	Points in favor	Points against
Congenital myopathy	Weakness, hypotonia, no tongue fasciculation, age at onset, benign or static course, early contractures, and preserved cognition	Areflexia and no facial involvement
Spinal muscular atrophy	Weakness > hypotonia, areflexia, age at onset, preserved cognition, and contractures may develop	No tongue fasciculation
Congenital myasthenic syndrome	Weakness and hypotonia	No facial weakness, no ptosis, no ophthalmoplegia, no fluctuations, and areflexia
Congenital myotonic dystrophy	Weakness and hypotonia	No myotonia in mother, late age at presentation, and no facial weakness
Nonsyndromic congenital muscular dystrophy (collagen VI-related CMD)	Weakness, hypotonia, contractures, nonprogressive, and nonambulatory till now	No skin involvement and areflexia
Mitochondrial myopathy	Weakness and hypotonia	No failure to thrive,* no systemic involvement, no fluctuations in course of illness, areflexia, and contractures
Pompe myopathy	Weakness and hypotonia	No hepatomegaly, no cardiac involvement, no previous hospitalization, age at presentation, nonconsanguineous couple, and no affected siblings

*The majority of children with mitochondrial disorders will have failure to thrive; hence, its absence is a point against mitochondrial disorder.

contracture then you can think of Ullrich type of collagen VI-related congenital muscular dystrophies. If such classical phenotypes are not discernible on examination, it is okay to keep broad differential like nonsyndromic CMD (syndromic CMD will have ocular and cognitive involvement as well which is clearly ruled out in this case).

INVESTIGATING A FLOPPY BABY

Creatine Phosphokinase Level

Total creatine phosphokinase (CPK) level can be borderline elevated in congenital muscular dystrophy; whereas, it will be normal in congenital myopathy and spinal muscular atrophy.

Molecular Diagnosis

If the phenotype is classical of a certain type of neuromuscular disorder, then we can directly confirm its molecular diagnosis. For example, if a baby had classical signs of weakness, profound hypotonia, lack of antigravity movement, areflexia, and tongue fasciculations, then we can straightaway order *SMN* gene deletion analysis. In the above case that was summarized, the phenotype is not classical of any disease; hence, we need to adopt a stepwise approach. Two options exist.

1. *Genetic panel versus clinical exome sequencing:* Clinical exome sequencing will screen stepwise for a possible genetic mutation in the case. However, the cost is prohibitive. Moreover, results such as variants of uncertain significance need to be interpreted cautiously by a trained geneticist in conjunction with a clinician. Another option is a genetic panel for congenital myopathy and congenital muscular dystrophy. This kind of genetic panel will test for all known genetic mutations responsible for congenital myopathy. The decision of genetic panel versus clinical exome sequencing needs to be prioritized based on clinical phenotype, cost, affordability, and availability of the test.
2. *Muscle biopsy-driven diagnosis:* In this era of genetic studies, invasive investigations such as muscle biopsy can be deferred. Muscle biopsy remains the investigation of choice among those who cannot afford genetic investigations. This may be followed by a specific single-gene mutation analysis.

Role of Electromyography

Electromyography (EMG) has a limited role in the diagnosis of floppy infant, except for establishing myotonia in mothers (congenital myotonic dystrophy). EMG can give a clue toward underlying etiology by establishing denervation potentials such as fasciculations in spinal muscular atrophy versus myopathic (low-amplitude motor unit action potentials (MUAPs) with early recruitment) potentials in congenital myopathy.

KEY MESSAGES

- Case presentation of a floppy baby must describe the extent of weakness (upper limb, lower limb, neck flexor, bulbar, ocular, and facial weakness).
- The floppiness could result from pathology of anterior horn cell (neuronopathy), nerve fiber, neuromuscular junction, or muscle. The central causes of floppiness are often associated with syndromic features.
- The presence of clinical signs of areflexia along with tongue fasciculation often points to neuronopathic problem such as spinal muscular atrophy.
- The summary of the case must describe extent of weakness, associated sensory system involvement, involvement of autonomic system, vision, hearing, cognitive abnormalities, and presence of contractures and deformities.
- Functional level in terms of gross motor functional classification system (GMFCS) must always be used in the summary.

CHAPTER 30: A Case of Muscular Dystrophy

■ INTRODUCTION

Common muscular dystrophies include Duchenne muscular dystrophy (DMD), Becker muscular dystrophy (BMD), limb-girdle muscular dystrophy (LGMD), and fascioscapular muscular dystrophy **(Table 1)**.

■ HISTORY-TAKING

Case presentation of muscular dystrophy differs from the case presentation of a floppy child, as parents perceive the onset of symptoms in early childhood rather than beginning from birth. The majority of

TABLE 1: Differentiating features of muscular dystrophy summarized.

Muscular dystrophy	Pattern of weakness	Characteristic features
DMD	Hip-girdle weakness (quadriceps and hip abductors), truncal weakness, neck flexor weakness	Onset 3–4 years, nonambulatory by 12 years, selective atrophy, hypertrophy, associated cardiomyopathy, restrictive lung disease, scoliosis
FSHD	Facial, biceps, triceps, and periscapular (scapular winging) but sparing of deltoids; late stages distal foot dorsiflexor weakness, and abdominal protuberance	Asymmetry is classical; triple hump sign (prominent deltoid)
EDMD	Weakness in the proximal upper limb, and distal lower limb (humeroperoneal weakness)	Early elbow contractures, ankle plantar flexor contracture, rigid spine, cardiac arrhythmia, and conduction block
Sarcoglycanopathy (LGMD type 2D-F)	Hip-girdle weakness (sparing of hip abductor) with maximal involvement of thigh adductors and knee flexors	Lumps and bumps in quadriceps, cardiac/cognition are normal
Dysferlinopathy (LGMD type 2B)	Distal onset (involvement of both tibialis and gastrocnemius), proximal weakness occurs late, and can have asymmetry or calf pain	Calf heads on trophy sign, biceps lumps, and diamond sign on quadriceps
Calpainopathy (LGMD type 2A)	Severe scapular winging, proximal weakness (hip extensor, knee flexor, and hip adductor)	Can have calf atrophy

(DMD: Duchenne muscular dystrophy; EDMD: Emery–Dreifuss muscular dystrophy; FSHD: facioscapulohumeral dystrophy; LGMD: limb-girdle muscular dystrophy)

muscular dystrophy have insidious onset (cannot clearly point to a date or month of onset of illness).

Presenting Complaints

Some of the common presenting complaints in children with muscular dystrophy include one or more of the following. The duration of the symptoms could have a different range, as per the type of dystrophy. In this example, we are presuming that the disease onset was occurring 3–4 years back.
- Difficulty in rising from the floor for the last 3–4 years
- Altered gait and repeated falls
- Problem in using the staircase
- Walking on the toes since early childhood
- Inability to run fast and tendency to repeated falls noticed for the last few months.

History of Presenting Complaints

Majority of these children present to outpatient except those who present with features of congestive heart failure owing to cardiomyopathy. In that case, the presenting complaint must include "cough, fever, and fast breathing" or "difficulty in breathing and excessive perspiration", depending on the clinical presentation.

The history often begins insidiously so the first line in the history of presenting illness would be "child was apparently well till around 3–4 years of age when parents noticed...". The 10 key points that need to be covered in the history of presenting illness in a child with suspected muscular dystrophy are listed below:
1. Is it *static* or *progressive*?
2. What is the *age at onset*?
3. The *extent of weakness* [lower limb (distal or proximal), upper limb (distal or proximal), trunk, neck flexor, neck extensor, facial, ocular, and bulbar muscle].
4. Are there any *other clinical markers* such as thinning or prominent group of muscles, muscle pain, history of the passage of red-colored urine following exercise, muscle cramps, any diurnal fluctuation, easy fatigability or exercise intolerance, fixed contractures in joints, and worsening or alleviating factors?
5. *Functional status:* Ambulatory with or without assistance, if ambulatory, how long is he able to ambulate unassisted, floor to standing time, dependency for activities of daily living such as dressing, feeding, and toilet care must be enquired.
6. Is there any *cognitive impairment* or *behavioral disturbances*?
7. Is any *other part of neuraxis* involved (sensory, bladder, bowel, autonomic, pyramidal or extrapyramidal, or cerebellar involvement)?
8. Are there any *systemic features* (cardiac, respiratory, and gastrointestinal)?
9. Is there a significant *family history*?
10. What are the broad differentials that you wish to consider?

Let us discuss these one by one.

Static or Progressive

If motor functions are worsening with time, then it is a progressive pathology. In neuromuscular illness, by convention, progressive disease is a dystrophic process and rest are usually static or very slowly progressive.

Age at Onset

The majority of children with dystrophinopathy (DMD) will have an onset of symptoms at 3–4 years of age and are usually nonambulatory by 12–13 years of age. Children with BMD and LGMD are ambulatory well beyond 16 years of age. Majority of muscular dystrophies such as facioscapulohumeral dystrophy (FSHD), Emery–Dreifuss muscular dystrophy (EDMD), and many variants of LGMD have an adult onset.

Extent of Weakness

- *Hip-girdle weakness:* Waddling gait, difficulty in rising from floor, climbing upstairs or going downstairs, climbing up with support on his thighs while rising from floor (dystrophinopathy), splaying of thighs while getting up from floor as if a sumo wrestler gets up (sarcoglycanopathy) (selective sparing of hip abductors with weakness of hip adductors), difficulty in getting up from kneeling-down position or buckling of knees while walking is indicative of quadriceps weakness (dystrophinopathies and sarcoglycanopathy), falls on uneven surfaces, and fall on ground with trivial push.

> **Example of History**
>
> A child was apparently well till 3–4 years of age when parents noticed he had difficulty in running and walking fast. He preferred slow walking taking broad steps keeping both feet apart with lurching of hip from one side to another side, keeping his abdomen protruded and buckling of knees while walking. Gradually over the next 6 months, parents noticed difficulty in other tasks including climbing upstairs, getting up from low-lying sofa, and toilet seats. When he sits on the floor, he takes the support of his hands on the knee to get up. Initially till 4 years, he used to get up within few seconds; now for the last 5–6 months, he takes a long time to get up and often refuses to get up without assistance.

- *Distal foot weakness:* Slippage and weak grip on slippers are common in dysferlinopathies (it is a type of LGMD) and EDMD. Majority of distal predominant weakness results from neuropathies except for these two muscular dystrophies, which can have distal predominant weakness apart from adult-onset myotonic dystrophy and late stages of FSHD.
- *Truncal weakness:* Difficulty in getting up from the bed, turning to the side, and taking the support of hand while getting up from bed are indicators of truncal weakness. Truncal involvement is common among children with dystrophinopathies. Rigid spine (weakness of trunk muscles and neck muscle leading to spine stiffness) noticed while getting up is a pointer toward EDMD.
- *Shoulder-girdle weakness* is manifested by difficulty in lifting the arm for dressing, lifting objects in the rack, or for combing his hair. Shoulder-girdle weakness is classical of FSHD and, when associated with tightness of elbow joints, is suggestive of EDMD.
- *Is it symmetrical weakness or asymmetrical weakness:* The majority of muscular dystrophies have symmetrical weakness except for dysferlinopathy and FSHD, which may have an asymmetric pattern.
- *Neck flexor/extensor weakness:* Turning to one side while lifting the head off the couch from lying-down position is suggestive of neck flexor weakness that is observed in dystrophinopathies and LGMD.
- *Facial weakness* can be noticed in the form of difficulty in using a straw to drink, difficulty in pursing the lips, difficulty in blowing candles, or loss of facial expressions. Facial weakness is characteristic of FSHD and childhood-onset congenital myotonic dystrophy.
- *Extraocular* or *bulbar muscle involvement* is uncommon in dystrophies except in oculopharyngeal muscular dystrophy (OPMD), which is an adult-onset

dystrophy. Presence of ptosis, prominent extraocular muscle involvement, always favors myasthenia or disorders of neuromuscular junction or congenital myopathy.

By this time, you should be able to determine the extent to which muscle weakness is involved in the given case. Is it proximal or distal predominant weakness? Does it involve lower limb muscles more than upper limb muscles? The majority of childhood-onset muscular dystrophy will have more involvement of lower limb muscles when compared to upper limb muscles.

Other Clinical Markers

- *Wasting or enlargement of a group of muscles:* This is better appreciated on an examination rather than on history unless the parents are concerned on the prominent calf muscle of their child. Ask for lumps and bumps in the quadriceps and biceps in patients with sarcoglycanopathy and dysferlinopathy, respectively.
- *Muscle pain:* The presence of prominent muscle pain is a feature of dysferlinopathy and inflammatory myopathy, especially dermatomyositis. The majority of children with DMD/BMD/other LGMD do not have muscle pain. Children with DMD can have discomfort in hypertrophied muscle.
- History of the passage of red-colored urine (myoglobinuria) following exercise and/or history of any muscle cramps is highly suggestive of metabolic myopathy such as McArdle disease. Children with DMD can occasionally present with such metabolic crises.
- *Diurnal fluctuation:* None of the dystrophies has diurnal variations, which are otherwise an indicator of myasthenia or metabolic (mitochondrial) myopathy.
- Easy *fatigability* or exercise intolerance often indicates low cardiac output that can be seen in children with dystrophinopathies or those with neuromuscular junction disorder.
- Fixed *contractures in* joints must always be enquired as children with DMD may develop toe walking with fixed ankle contractures early in the disease.

Functional Status

Determine functional status in terms of gross motor function classification (GMFC). History must be able to depict whether the child is ambulatory with or without assistance. If ambulatory, how long is he able to ambulate unassisted. It would be good to represent the progressive nature of illness while describing the functional status. Mention of floor to standing time gives a fair idea of progression. Similarly, increased dependency for activities of daily living such as dressing, feeding, and toilet care must be enquired.

Cognitive Impairment or Intellectual Disability

Children with dystrophinopathies and some congenital muscular dystrophy (POMT1 and Fukutin-related mutations in CMD) show variable severity of cognitive impairment. School performance and behavioral disturbances must be recorded.

Screening for Other Neuraxis Involvement

The involvement of pyramidal, extrapyramidal pathway, cerebellar, or autonomic system often points to alternative diagnosis rather than isolated muscular dystrophy.

Ask for Systemic Features

- *Cardiac involvement:* Ask for dizziness, orthopnea, syncope, and chest pain. They can vary from cardiomyopathy in dystrophinopathies to arrhythmia and conduction blocks in EDMD and autosomal-dominant LGMD.
- *Respiratory involvement:* Ask for breathing difficulty, morning headaches, and sleep disturbances. These can be observed in children with DMD with clinical features of restrictive lung disease or obstructive sleep apnea. Recurrent respiratory tract infection (cough, cold, and fast breathing) may be seen.
- *Others:* Children with DMD in a non-ambulatory stage can have associated gastroesophageal reflux disease (GERD).

Family History

We often start asking the family history by direct questions such as: "Is there anyone affected in the family?" The answer is always "no" unless they are very comfortable with the physician. None of the parents wish to disclose their entire family story at the first go. It is better to start making the pedigree by asking: "How many brothers do you have, how many children does the first brother have, are they fine?" By this process, parents often open up to disclose their family history and they understand that you are concerned. A direct question of "Are there similarly affected children in your family?" also invites a negative response. Hence, it is better to ask for family history of wheelchair dependence, skeletal deformities, polio-like illness, or any functional limitations. X-linked inheritance can be seen in DMD, EDMD, autosomal-dominant inheritance in FSHD, myotonic dystrophy, autosomal-dominant LGMD, and autosomal-recessive inheritance in sarcoglycanopathy.

Pattern Recognition

Analyze above history to reach a broad differential diagnosis in a child with suspected muscular dystrophy. Differentiating features of muscular dystrophy are given in **Table 1**.

■ FOCUSED EXAMINATION

Vitals

The presence of tachycardia, tachypnea, weak pulse volume, hypotension, and respiratory distress can be an early sign of cardiomyopathy in children with dystrophinopathies and EDMD. Look for pulse rate and rhythm to screen for cardiac rhythm abnormalities (EDMD). Children in a nonambulatory stage of DMD would have features of tachypnea and increased work of breathing owing to respiratory involvement (restrictive lung disease). Monitor blood pressure for hypertension among those on steroids.

Anthropometry

Obesity is prevalent among nonambulatory children with dystrophinopathies and those on long-term steroids. Body mass index (BMI) must be estimated among all children with muscular dystrophy. Estimation of height (ambulatory) and length (nonambulatory) in children with DMD is often erroneous among those with fixed joint contractures.

General Physical Examination

The presence of keratosis pilaris, keloids, and cigarette paper scars is common among children with congenital muscular dystrophy (Ullrich variant). The presence of heliotrope rash and Gottron papule are suggestive of juvenile dermatomyositis. The presence of scoliosis, pectus excavatum, and lumbar lordosis is common among children with dystrophinopathies, especially once they achieve nonambulation. Similarly, bedridden patients are prone to bedsores and pressure ulcers. Joint contractures at ankle, knee, and hip must be commented. Ankle contractures are common among patients with dystrophinopathies and calpainopathies (a type of LGMD). Early elbow contractures are often seen in patients with EDMD.

Central Nervous System Examination

- *Higher mental function, including mini-mental status examination:* Assessment of cognition and behavior is essential among children with DMD/BMD.
- *Cranial nerves:* The presence of extra-ocular muscle weakness and bulbar weakness is uncommon in muscular dystrophy except in adults with OPMD. Facial weakness is classical of FSHD and myotonic dystrophy. Hearing loss can be seen in FSHD. Tongue enlargement has been observed in children with DMD/BMD. The presence of tongue fasciculations suggests a neuronopathy such as a type II spinal muscular atrophy or late-onset Pompe disease. However, both these conditions are largely nonprogressive illness.
- *Motor system examination:*
  - Bulk of muscle: There is selective atrophy of biceps, triceps with hypertrophy of brachioradialis, deltoid, infraspinatus apart from classical calf muscles (gastrocnemius and tibialis anterior), and quadriceps hyper- trophy in children with DMD. Scapular winging is classical of calpainopathy **(Fig. 1)**. Children with FSHD will have significant atrophy of muscles of shoulder girdle, especially

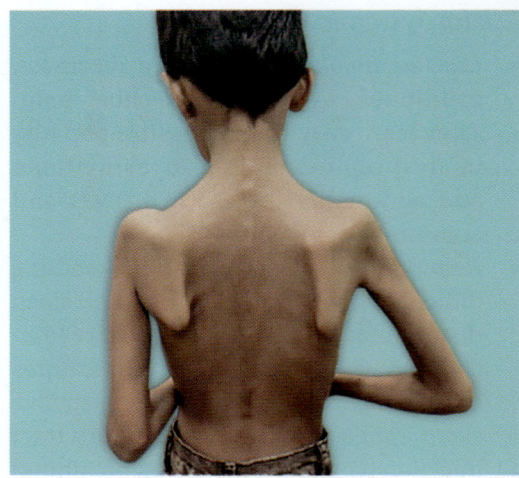

Fig. 1: Scapular winging.
Courtesy: Dr Rachana Dubey Gupta, Indore.

biceps and triceps, along with loss of facial expression **(Figs. 2A to C)**.
- *Classical signs in muscular dystrophy:*
  - Valley sign: To demonstrate this sign, the patient is asked to abduct the shoulder to 90°, with flexion of the elbow to 90° and hands directed upward. Back of the shoulder shows a depression or valley between two mounts (infraspinatus below and deltoid above) in children with dystrophinopathies (BMD/DMD) **(Fig. 3)**.
  - Calf on head trophy sign: It is seen in patients with Miyoshi myopathy. The patient is asked to abduct the shoulder, flex the elbow, and tighten the muscles. You can do this by asking the child to show his biceps muscles: "Let's see how strong you are!" We can observe the mounts of deltoid over scapular winging, atrophy of trapezius, sternocleidomastoid muscle, and supraspinatus, which resembles *calf on head trophy* **(Fig. 4)**.

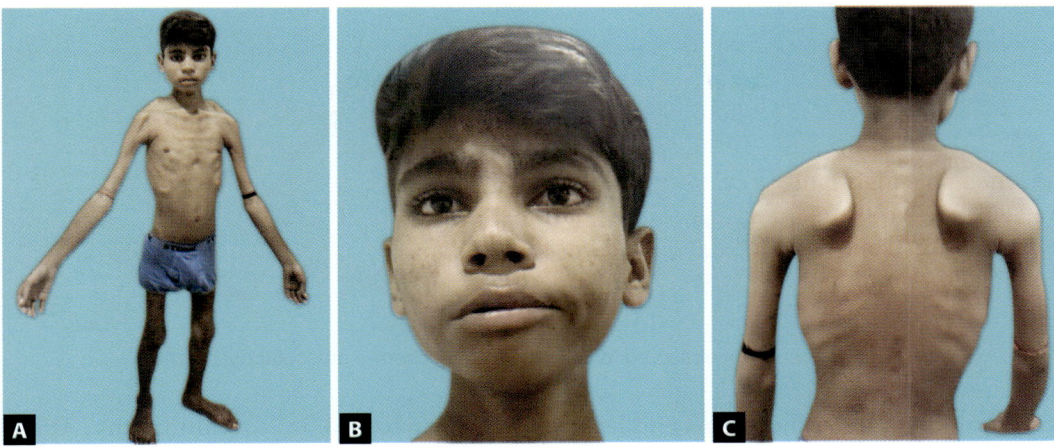

Figs. 2A to C: Child with facioscapulohumeral dystrophy (FSHD) showing atrophy of muscles of shoulder girdle, loss of facial expressions, and scapular winging.
Courtesy: Dr Rachana Dubey Gupta, Indore.

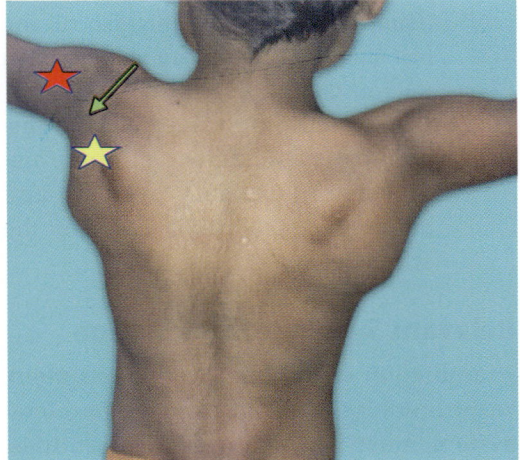

Fig. 3: *Valley sign:* A hollow or valley (arrow) is seen between infraspinatus (yellow star) and deltoid muscle (red star).
Courtesy: Dr Rachana Dubey Gupta, Indore.

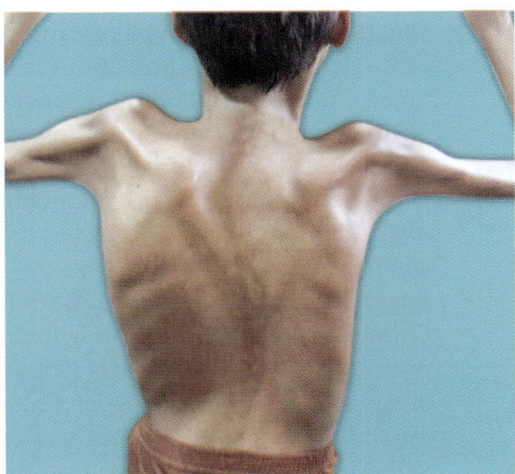

Fig. 4: Calf heads on trophy sign.
Courtesy: Dr Rachana Dubey Gupta, Indore.

- Biceps lumps can be observed in patients with dysferlinopathy. *Diamond sign* (bulge in quadriceps muscle when partly contracted) can be observed in patients with dysferlinopathies.
- *Gait:* Waddling gait is classical in children with dystrophinopathies (DMD/BMD) with hip abductor weakness. Selective loss of muscle power in quadriceps and hip abductors in children with DMD/BMD would result in using relatively spared muscles to get up from the sitting position called "*Gower sign*". Hence, on an attempt to get up from the floor, the child will roll

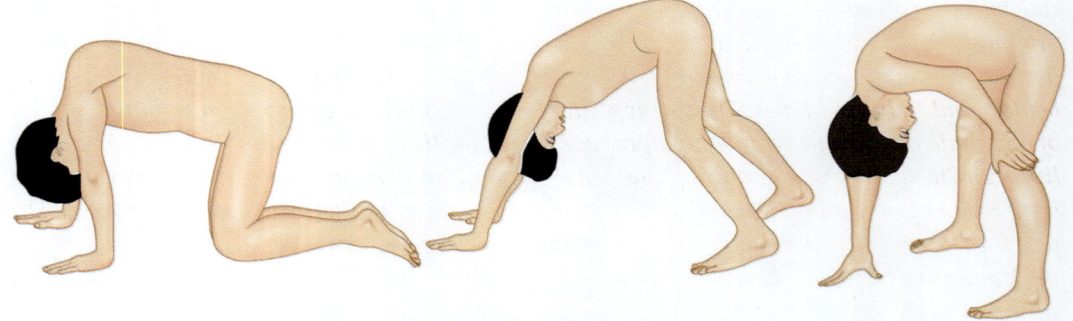

Fig. 5: Gower sign observed in children with Duchenne muscular dystrophy.

prone, extend their arms and legs far apart, and push the weight of trunk to extended legs, followed by keeping the arm over the thigh slowly extending the hip to rise to a standing position **(Fig. 5)**. In contrast, in patients with sarcoglycanopathy, hip abductors are spared with marked weakness of thigh adductors and knee flexors. This results in splaying of the thighs while getting up from the floor (*hip abduction sign*). This looks like as if a sumo wrestler is trying to get up.

- *Power assessment:* Medical Research Council (MRC) grading of individual muscle or group of muscles must always be elicited in all cases of muscular dystrophy. There is a selective weakness of a certain group of muscles that are specific to certain types of muscular dystrophy. Hip abductors, hip extensors, and quadriceps are classically involved in DMD/BMD. Hip adductors and knee flexors are classically weak with sparing of hip abductors in sarcoglycanopathy. Iliopsoas, hip adductors, quadriceps, and hamstring muscles are involved in the late stages of dysferlinopathy. Hip extensors, knee adductors, and knee flexors are involved in calpainopathy. Distal predominant weakness is a feature of dysferlinopathy, EDMD, and myotonic dystrophy.
- *Deep tendon reflexes (DTRs):* DTRs are usually preserved or sluggish till the last stages, and they are absent when the muscles undergo atrophy.
- Other neurological examinations, including assessment of abnormal movement, sensory system, and autonomic system, will be as per the scheme.

Relevant Systemic Examination

Examination of the cardiovascular system, respiratory system, and musculoskeletal system must be conducted. Deformities, including varus/valgus deformity, torsional deformity, and fixed/dynamic contractures, must be examined. This can be a part of the musculoskeletal system examination, or it can be mentioned at the end of the general physical examination.

■ FINAL ANALYSIS

A 14-year-old boy presented with difficulty in getting up from floor and difficulty in climbing stairs for the last 4 years. He has a history to suggest hip-girdle weakness, with relative sparing of the distal lower limb and upper limb muscles. There is possible truncal and neck flexor weakness but complete sparing of facial, ocular, and bulbar muscles. This is suggestive of a chronic progressive symmetrical proximal limb-girdle weakness involving the lower limb more than the upper limb. The current functional ability of the child is that he can walk independently for 100 meters and he often stumbles and falls. He has no other cardiac, respiratory, or gastrointestinal involvement. He is a school-going intelligent boy and has no behavioral issues. There are no other affected family members with similar illnesses.

His examination confirms proximal hip-girdle weakness with prominent weakness of hip abductors and hip extensor group of muscles with evidence of dynamic contracture of the ankle. There is selective hypertrophy of quadriceps, gastrocnemius, and brachioradialis muscle. DTRs are preserved. There is no evident fasciculation. The rest of the systemic examination is unremarkable. The clinical possibilities include the following:

The focus of examination would be differentiating selective weakness. Sarcoglycanopathy will have a typical weakness of hip adductors with sparing of hip abductors. In contrast, dystrophinopathies such as BMD will have a typical weakness of hip abductors. Other differentials, including Pompe disease and Bethlem myopathy, can also be entertained.

Differentials	Points in favor	Points against
Becker muscular dystrophy	Male gender, ambulatory beyond 12 years, proximal hip-girdle weakness, slowly progressive	No cardiac involvement at 14 years*; unaffected family members
Sarcoglycanopathy	Proximal hip-girdle weakness with sparing of others; no cardiac involvement, normal cognition	No consanguinity, unaffected family members; complete sparing of upper limb
Spinal muscular atrophy type III	Proximal hip-girdle weakness, slowly progressive	Selective atrophy and hypertrophy are never a feature of SMA, although they can have calf hypertrophy; absence of fasciculations or polyminimyoclonus; preserved DTR

*Cardiac involvement is subclinical in BMD, it may manifest in the third decade.
(DTR: deep tendon reflex; SMA: spinal muscular atrophy)

SUMMARIZE UNDER FOLLOWING HEADINGS

- Chronic/subacute/acute illness of neuromuscular disease
- Static or progressive (rapid or slow)
- Limb-girdle weakness or distal predominant weakness
- Any selective group of atrophy or hypertrophy
- Any selective weakness of any group of muscle
- Involvement of facial, ocular, bulbar, respiratory, and cardiac involvement
- Current functional status
- Most likely clinical differentials

SECTION 3: Residents' Corner: Exam-oriented Cases

KEY MESSAGES

- Case presentation of a child with suspected muscular dystrophy must start from the time parents noticed weakness in contrast to presenting a case of global developmental delay or cerebral palsy.
- History must focus on the pattern of the weakness (proximal or distal weakness; lower or upper limb predominant weakness; neck flexor weakness; facial, bulbar, and ocular weakness).
- Atrophy of certain groups of muscles (biceps and triceps) and hypertrophy of another group of muscles (gastrocnemius, quadriceps, deltoid, and brachioradialis) are very specific to clinical diagnosis of muscular dystrophy. In all other neuromuscular pathologies, we get uniform atrophy (spinal muscular atrophy or end stage of most neuromuscular or systemic illness) or hypertrophy of muscles (myotonia congenita).
- Formal Medical Research Council grading of group of muscles is an essential examination to determine and differentiate selective muscle involvement (hip abductors involved in DMD and spared in LGMD).
- Summary of the case must mention fixed contractures, deformities functional status in terms of GMFC system, nutritional status, and other extraneural symptoms/signs (if any).

CHAPTER 31

A Case of Neurodegenerative Disorder

■ INTRODUCTION

Neurodegenerative disorders (NDDs) have a myriad of clinical presentations. Overall, the clinical approach to the diagnosis of an NDD has been summarized in **Chapter 14**. This chapter focuses on points in the history and examination that need to be dissected while presenting a case of suspected neurodegenerative disease.

■ HISTORY-TAKING

The presenting complaint will depend on the part of neurological system that is affected. Most of the NDDs would often present with *loss of acquired milestones* along with symptoms pertaining to one or more parts of the neurological system. *For example*, in children with Wilson disease, a child could have lost the ability to walk and speak (regression of attained milestones) along with repeated twisting of the limbs (dystonia).

Presenting Complaints

Apart from "loss of attained milestones," presenting complaints in children with NDD will include one or more of the complaints listed below.

Motor System
- Paucity of movement of all the four limbs (quadriparetic weakness)
- Tightness of limbs noticed while handling the child (spasticity)
- Stiffness in the legs while walking (spastic legs)
- Wobbly gait or unstable gait or difficulty in walking (ataxia)
- Slowness of movement with the patient taking short steps to walk and move (parkinsonian features)

Abnormal Movement (Movement Disorder)
- Twisting or abnormal postures of the hands, neck, and legs (dystonia)
- Abnormal movements of the tongue and mouth (oromotor dyskinesia)
- Distal writhing movement involving both the hands (athetosis)
- Abnormal continuous flowing dance-like movement of limbs (chorea)
- Violent flinging movement (ballismus)
- Tremulous movement of hands and other parts of body (tremors)

Cognition
- Inability to recognize parents or fail to respond to simple parental commands
- Inability to understand simple gestures from parents
- Loss of ability to convey inner needs such as hunger, wet pants (bladder), or desire to pass stools

- Excessive inconsolable cry and irritability
- Lack of interest in the surroundings
- Deterioration in academic or school performance

Seizures
- Sudden violent jerks in the body resulting in falls and injury (myoclonus)
- Repetitive episodes of abnormal jerky movement of limbs and face that lasts for a few seconds to minutes (clonic seizure)
- Episodes of tight posturing that lasts for few seconds followed by jerky movement of limbs (tonic–clonic seizure)
- Episodes of abnormally prolonged staring (atypical absence seizure)

Behavior
- Hyperactive and restless behavior
- Aggressive behavior
- Disruptive behavior
- Stubborn with excessive temper tantrums
- Autistic features such as "being in his own world", reduced social interaction, lack of gestural communication, and motor stereotypies such as hand-flapping movement

Speech
- Loss of learned words (aphasia) or use of new meaningless words (paraphasia)
- Strained voice with reduced clarity of speech (spastic dysarthria)
- Speech with poor clarity of words (extrapyramidal dysarthria)
- Difficulty in speech with words sounding as if scanning the sentence (cerebellar dysarthria)

Sensory
Loss of ability to perceive the sensation of touch or pain in any part of the body.

Autonomic
- Loss of urinary continence (may be associated with cognitive decline)
- Decreased sweating and unexplained fever
- Sudden pallor, flushing, and temperature instability

Vision
- Difficulty in seeing objects
- Difficulty in seeing objects in the night or groping in the dark

Hearing
- Inability to respond to verbal commands
- Decreased hearing ability noticed by parents

History of Presenting Complaints

The following points need to be highlighted in the history of presenting illness—age at onset of symptoms, type of onset (sudden/insidious), rate of progression (rapidly progressive or slowly progressive), predominant clinical manifestation (cerebellar, extrapyramidal, cognitive decline, progressive myoclonic epilepsy, and pure pyramidal syndrome), current functional status, any significant family history, probable etiology (genetic or acquired), extent of involvement (extent of involvement of neuraxis), and possible neuroanatomical site of localization. An example has been provided in **Practical Box 1**. Important clinical features of common neurodegenerative diseases that present with the extrapyramidal syndrome are summarized in **Table 1**. Based on the cluster of symptomatology, clear differentiation into the gray matter and white matter degenerative brain disease is tricky, considering a marked overlap of symptoms. For example, children with

CHAPTER 31: A Case of Neurodegenerative Disorder

> **PRACTICAL BOX 1:** Focus of history of presenting complaint.
>
> A 3-year-old boy presents with insidious onset (*type of onset*) of rapidly progressive (*progression*) cognitive decline with myoclonus (*predominant clinical manifestation*) over a period of last 4 months (age at onset being 2 years 8 months) with no significant family history. There are no motor deficits and sensory deficits (*extent of involvement*). He is now bedridden and is dependent completely on parents for activities of daily living (*functional status*), the most probable neuroanatomical site being cerebral cortex (gray matter)

Krabbe disease (white matter degenerative disease) often present with mixed signs of spasticity (represents pyramidal tract involvement) and dystonia (represents basal ganglia involvement, which is a deep gray matter or extrapyramidal tracts) with or without cognitive decline (gray matter function).

Based on the predominant clinical manifestation in neurodegenerative disease, it could be broadly classified as extrapyramidal syndrome (dystonia and choreoathetosis), pyramidal syndrome (spasticity), cerebellar syndrome (ataxia), cognitive decline, or progressive myoclonic epilepsy phenotype (cognitive decline with myoclonus). A detailed analysis of each individual complaint is suggested in the following text.

History of Dystonia

- History of bizarre abnormal twisting postures (dystonia) that worsen on an attempt to perform an action and which subside in the sleep
- *Parts of the body involved:*
  - Spooning of all fingers in an effort to hold the object and associated with the trembling movement of the hands (upper limb)
  - Twisting of the legs on an attempt to stand or walk with feet unable to touch flat on the ground (lower limb)
  - Deviation of neck to one side (neck) with arching of the back (truncal)
  - Tongue thrusting movement keeping the mouth open or repeated closing and opening of the mouth with difficulty in chewing and swallowing. The patient often spits the food out after keeping it in the mouth (oromandibular dyskinesia).
  - Paucity of facial expression with a fixed smile (vacuous smile) on the face with preference to smile rather than to respond verbally to questions (facial)
  - Speech has a paucity of words with decreased clarity of spoken words. The child could comprehend the commands and respond in the right context. The patient prefers to communicate by gestures than to speak (speech).
- Was there a sequence of involvement of body parts? (Children with dopa-responsive dystonia often begin in one limb, then progress to all four limbs, and finally to trunk/neck muscles.)
- Any diurnal variation (dopa-responsive dystonia is better in morning hours and worsens by evening)
- Is it episodic (paroxysmal dyskinesia) or nearly continuous (present through the entire day and night)?
- Is there a fluctuation in the clinical course? (Clinical course in children with mitochondrial leukoencephalopathy worsens with a febrile illness, which recovers to baseline once the infection is treated.)
- Dystonia worsens with an emotional stressor and on an attempt to perform an action. It improves or subsides with sleep.

TABLE 1: Clinical diagnoses in children with predominant extrapyramidal features.

Disease	Key clinical features	Laboratory diagnosis
Wilson disease	Age at onset 7–10 years; predominant faciolingual–laryngeal rigidity (mask-like facies, open mouth, constant grimacing, dysarthria, and dysphagia); bizarre dyskinesia or unnatural posture; tremors of hands; generalized muscular rigidity; predominant neuropsychiatric manifestation and emotional lability; and presence of KF ring	• Serum ceruloplasmin <20 mg/100 mL • Serum copper >10 µg/dL • 24-hour urinary copper >100 g • Liver copper >250 µg/g dry weight • *ATP7B* gene mutation • MRI shows involvement of caudate, lenticular, thalamic, and dentate nucleus
Aceruloplas-minemia	Adult onset; slowly progressive dystonia, choreoathetosis, dysarthria, ataxia, dementia; diabetes mellitus; retinal pigmentary changes	• Low serum ceruloplasmin • Low serum iron • High serum ferritin • LFT is usually normal • MRI brain shows dentate nucleus and substantia nigra T2 hypointensity
Huntington disease (HD) (childhood onset)	Children <10 years present with cognitive decline, seizure, oromotor dysfunction, dystonia, bradykinesia, rigidity manifesting as gait disturbances, and positive family history; chorea is usually absent in childhood-onset HD	• MRI shows striatal atrophy • PET scan shows hypometabolism in caudate and putamen • *Genetic confirmation:* CAG repeat >60
Juvenile Parkinson disease	An uncommon condition, tremors at rest, rigidity, bradykinesia, mask-like facies, flexed postures of body, and normal intelligence	*PARK* gene mutation
Dopa-responsive dystonia (DYT5)	Starts with limb dystonia, classical diurnal variation (better in the morning); occasionally Parkinsonian features	• Normal MRI brain • Decreased CSF neopterin/HVA/tetrabiopterin • Dramatic response to trial of levodopa • Mutation in *GCH1* gene
Aromatic L-amino acid decarboxylase (LAAD) deficiency (neurotransmitter disorder)	Presence of orofacial dystonia, eye movement disturbances in infancy with autonomic dysregulation; no response to levodopa trial	• CSF HVA/HIAA reduced • Genetic confirmation
Pantothenate kinase-associated neurodegeneration (PKAN)	Onset < 10 years; progressive dystonia, rigidity, choreoathetoid movement, dysarthria, tremors, pigmentary retinal changes, and finally cognitive decline	• MRI shows hypointensity in globus pallidus with central hyperintensity (eye of tiger appearance) • *PANK-2* gene mutation
Neuroacanthocytosis	Orofacial–lingual and pharyngeal dyskinesia, uncontrollable tics, and seizures in one-third	• Acanthocytes in peripheral smear (>3%) • Raised CPK level
Spinocerebellar ataxia (type 3)	Dystonic-rigid-Parkinsonian features (type I); ophthalmoplegia, nuclear or supranuclear palsy	CAG repeat increased

(CPK: creatine phosphokinase; HIAA: 5-hydroxyindole acetic acid; HVA: homovanillic acid; KF: Kayser–Fleischer; LFT: liver function test)

- Many older children with dystonia will have sensory tricks. For example, if the child has cervical dystonia, he might attempt to hold his chin to one side that might probably relieve his dystonia in that posture. Children often find their own ways to relieve these symptoms temporarily. These are called sensory tricks or Geste antagoniste.
- Any associated sudden jerky movement (dystonia–myoclonus)
- *Etiological history:*
  - History of jaundice, polyuria, and polydipsia (Wilson disease)
  - History of diurnal variation and sequential involvement of limbs (dopa-responsive dystonia)
  - Any dramatic improvement with any drug like levodopa (dopa-responsive dystonia)
  - History of diminution of vision, groping in the dark, night blindness (neuronal ceroid lipofuscinosis)
  - Any associated history of severe sweating, excessive perspiration, and sleep disturbances [neurotransmitter disorders such as L-amino acid decarboxylase (LAAD) deficiency]
  - Any associated tics (neuroacanthocytosis)
  - Any abdominal swelling or mass (lysosomal storage disorders with hepatosplenomegaly)
  - History of any drug intake
  - Past history of measles-like infection (fever, cough, cold, and rash) in early childhood (subacute sclerosing panencephalitis)

History of Myoclonus

- Multiple episodes of violent sudden shock-like jerks of the trunk, head, and both upper and lower limbs
- *Parts of the body involved:*
  - Jerking or shrugging of shoulders with a resultant drop of objects held in hand, often resulting in the spilling of food or smearing the face with food while eating (upper limb)
  - Sudden jerk in lower limb resulting in sudden fall on to the ground with resultant injury (lower limb)
  - Sudden twitching movement in the face (face myoclonus in Unverricht–Lundborg syndrome)
  - Sudden jerk in the body resulting in fall while sitting (trunk)
- Does it increase with action (action myoclonus), touching a body part, or hearing a sound (reflex myoclonus)?
- Does such jerk result in sudden floppiness rather than tightness of limbs resulting in fall (negative myoclonus)? (Myoclonus is usually a sudden increase in the muscle tone, but there can be a brief loss of muscle tone in myoclonus, which is called as negative myoclonus.)
- Associated cognitive decline (progressive myoclonic epilepsy phenotype)
- *Etiological history:*
  - Does the child have visual hallucination and history of seizures with predominant visual symptoms suggestive of occipital seizures (Lafora disease)?
  - Associated muscle weakness and/or hearing loss [myoclonic epilepsy with ragged red fiber (MERRF)]
  - Associated upward gaze preference (Gaucher disease)
  - Associated abdominal swelling or mass (Gaucher disease)
  - Severe pain in the limbs (painful neuropathies in sialidosis)
  - Associated vision loss or night blindness (neuronal ceroid lipofuscinosis)

- History of measles in the past (sub-acute sclerosing panencephalitis)

History of Ataxia

- Difficulty in walking or abnormal gait. The child becomes wobbly when asked to stand in one place. The child has a tendency to fall owing to a lack of balance.
- The child has an unsteady gait; he walks like a drunken man.
- He might have tremulous movement of hands (action tremors of the cerebellum).
- He may have an alteration of the voice and drooling of saliva (dysarthria).
- Difficulty in seeing fast-moving objects, repeated eye blinking, or head thrusting movement (oculomotor apraxia in ataxia–telangiectasia)
- Decrease in vision and night blindness (Friedreich ataxia and ataxia with vitamin E deficiency)
- History of repeated sinopulmonary infections (ataxia telangiectasia)
- History of associated abnormal flowing movement of limbs or distal writhing movement of hands (ataxia telangiectasia or ataxia with oculomotor apraxia)
- History of breathing difficulty, cough, and respiratory distress (evidence of cardiomyopathy in Friedreich ataxia)

History of Cognitive Decline

- Decrease in scholastic performance, inability to read his books with any interest, cannot learn any new things, often forgets his very well-learned poems or facts which he used to recite
- Decreased ability to understand basic things at home to which he used to respond earlier. For example, inability to recollect or recite the happening in school when back home, lack of interest in songs or games which he used to like and not able to buy simple grocery items from a nearby shop.
- Decreased interest in surroundings or home, lack of interest in friends, television, or mobile phones which he used to enjoy, limited communication preferably by gestures.
- Many children with cognitive decline often have associated behavioral symptoms such as aggressive, disruptive (breaking things at home), temper tantrums, and hyperactive (inability to sit at one place) behavior.
- In terminal stages, he may fail to recognize the parents and will not indicate his/her bladder or bowel needs.

Impairment of functioning of activities of daily living is often seen in children with cognitive decline. Just a minor decline in school performances or poor memory must not be equated to cognitive decline.

History of Vision Difficulty

- Sudden loss of vision in both eyes (optic neuritis)
- Progressive loss of vision in both eyes noticed in the form of inability to read a letter written in the notebook (near vision) or blackboard in school (distant vision)
- History of double vision or deviation of eyes (weakness of extraocular muscle)
- History of halos around the bright light (glaucoma)
- History of floating spots or flashing lights (retinal detachment)
- History of distortion of words or lines (macular pathology)
- History of pain in moving the eyes with a sudden loss of vision (optic neuritis)

Difficulty in Walking

A child may have difficulty in walking owing to imbalance (ataxia), sudden jerks while walking (myoclonus), abnormal waddling and buckling of knee (myopathy), twisting of legs while walking (dystonia), abnormal twisting of the feet (distal weakness in neuropathy), and abnormal continuous flowing movements in legs (choreoathetosis). These histories need to be elicited to arrive at the right diagnosis when a patient presents with walking difficulty.

Difficulty in Feeding

A child with feeding difficulty may have difficulty in placing the food in the mouth owing to continuous movement of mouth (*oromotor dyskinesia*), or may have difficulty in opening the mouth (*oromandibular dystonia or trismus*), spitting the food immediately on placing the food in mouth owing to tongue thrusting movement, he may keep the food in the mouth for long before gulping it (*difficulty in deglutition*), and the child may vomit immediately after feeds (*gastroesophageal reflux disease*).

Difficulty in Speech

A child may not be able to speak because of loss of consciousness (altered sensorium), unable to speak or find the word to speak with intact consciousness (*aphasia*), able to speak with full efforts, slowly as if speaking from the depth of the stomach (*spastic dysarthria*), able to speak but lacks complete clarity owing to poor articulation of words (*extrapyramidal dysarthria*), and slow scanning speech (cerebellar dysarthria).

Family History

It is essential to draw a pedigree with three generations. The majority of children with NDDs have an autosomal recessive inheritance. Few have X-linked recessive inheritance (X-linked adrenoleukodystrophy) or maternal inheritance (mitochondrial disorders).

■ FOCUSED EXAMINATION

The examination needs to focus on the clinical thought or possibility suspected on the basis of history. The sequence of the examination remains the same—opening remark, vital signs, anthropometry, general physical examination, and neurological examination. Vitals must be carefully assessed, as many children with NDD present with a respiratory infection.

Anthropometry

In the presence of fixed contractures, measurement of height and length may be erroneous. Hence, anthropometry must be interpreted in the context of contractures. Short stature is often a feature of Kearns-Sayre syndrome. Presence of macrocephaly often narrows the clinical differentials (mucopolysaccharidosis, gangliosidosis, Tay-Sachs disease, Alexander disease, or Canavan disease).

General Physical Examination

It must focus on bedsores and contractures in bedridden patients. In addition, the clinical clue for the etiology of NDD must be ascertained. Extraneural manifestations have been enumerated in the chapter on approach to a child with neuroregression **(Chapter 14)**. Focused examination must be guided by the clinical syndromic possibility **(Table 2)**. For example, skin changes such as ichthyosis (Sjögren–Larson syndrome), subcutaneous lipoma (mitochondrial), and dark pigmentation (adrenoleukodystrophy) must be noted in a child presenting with pure pyramidal or spasticity.

TABLE 2: Focused examination in a case of neurodegenerative disease.

Clinical syndrome	Focused examination
Chronic progressive ataxia	Ocular telangiectasia and café-au-lait macules (ataxia–telangiectasia), ichthyosis (Sjögren–Larson syndrome and Refsum disease), pellagra-like rash (Hartnup disease), cataract (cerebrotendinous xanthomatosis), pigmentary retinopathy (MERRF and ataxia with vitamin E deficiency), signs of fat malabsorption (abetalipoproteinemia), abnormal fat pads (congenital disorders of glycosylation), pes cavus/scoliosis (Friedreich ataxia)
Progressive extrapyramidal (dystonia)	Pigmentary retinopathy (NCL and PKAN), Kayser–Fleisher ring (Wilson disease), and retinal degeneration (aceruloplasminemia)
Progressive myoclonic epilepsy	Pigmentary retinopathy (NCL), cherry red spot-on fundus (sialidosis), hepatosplenomegaly (Gaucher disease), and optic atrophy (mitochondrial)

(MERRF: myoclonic epilepsy with ragged red fiber; PKAN: pantothenate kinase-associated neurodegeneration)

Neurological Examination

The purpose of neurological examination is to determine the extent of neurological involvement and to confirm the findings of history.

- Higher mental function including assessment of cognition, behavior, and emotion gives a clue to degree of impairment of cognition and behavioral disturbances (presence of cognitive decline often indicates gray matter involvement)
- *Assessment of cranial nerve palsy:*
    - Vision assessment including fundus evaluation (vision loss is an indicator of white matter disease; retinal changes can give clue to an underlying disease)
    - *Extraocular muscle involvement:* Presence of gaze paralysis (upward gaze palsy in Gaucher disease) and impaired ocular saccades (oculomotor apraxia)
    - Facial weakness and lack of facial expression must be commented (Wilson disease).
    - Bulbar weakness and presence of oromandibular dyskinesia must be assessed.
- *Assessment of motor system:*
    - Presence of pyramidal signs (spasticity, hyperreflexia, and extensor plantars) indicates involvement of corticospinal tract.
    - Presence of dystonia and/or choreoathetosis (extrapyramidal syndrome) is suggestive of basal ganglia involvement.
    - Lack of coordination and ataxia is an indicator of cerebellar syndrome.
    - Presence of contractures and deformities must be confirmed.
- *Assessment of sensory system:*
    - Involvement of lateral spinothalamic tract (pain and temperature)
    - Involvement of dorsal column (loss of touch and vibration) as in children with vitamin B_{12} deficiency
- Assessment of cerebellar system (nystagmus, dysdiadochokinesia, and pendular jerk)

SUMMARY AND ANALYSIS

- Is it a neurodegenerative disease?
- What is the age of onset?
- Is it acute, intermittent, or chronic?
- Clinical presentation?
- Is it a gray matter or white matter disease?

- Is it central nervous system (CNS) involved alone or is peripheral nervous system also involved?
- Are there any extraneurological features?
- What clinical syndrome can it best fit (pure pyramidal syndrome, extrapyramidal syndrome, progressive cerebellar ataxia, and progressive myoclonic epilepsy)?
- What clinical differentials do you want to entertain?
- How will we plan the investigation to confirm?

KEY MESSAGES

- Case presentation of neurodegenerative disease must be able to depict the predominant clinical symptomatology (pyramidal syndrome, extrapyramidal syndrome, cognitive decline, cerebellar syndrome, and progressive myoclonic epilepsy).
- Age at onset of neurodegeneration and rate of progression, along with current functional status, must always be mentioned in the history of presenting illness.
- An attempt to localize the site of lesion (cortex, pyramidal tract, basal ganglia, cerebellum, and brainstem) will be useful in classifying and narrowing the differentials.
- Do not forget to draw a three-generation pedigree chart while presenting and analyzing a case of suspected neurodegenerative disease.
- There is a marked overlap in symptoms of white matter and gray matter degenerative brain disease. A clear differentiation based on clinical evaluation is often difficult.

32 A Case of Hydrocephalus

INTRODUCTION

Following questions need to be addressed while evaluating a child with hydrocephalus with or without neural tube defect:
- Is there a large head?
- Is the large head secondary to hydrocephalus?
- Is it congenital or acquired hydrocephalus?
- Is it syndromic or nonsyndromic?
- What is the most probable etiology for hydrocephalus?
- Are there clinical features to suggest features of raised intracranial pressure (ICF)?
- Is there an associated neural tube defect?
- What is the level of neural tube defect (if any); is it an open or closed defect?
- Are there any associated neurological, urological, or musculoskeletal problems?
- Is surgical treatment warranted for the child with hydrocephalus with or without a neural tube defect?

Let us understand broad clinical approach to a child with large head before we proceed to clinical history and examination.

BROAD APPROACH TO A CHILD WITH LARGE HEAD

- Is it macrocephaly? If yes, is it hydrocephalus or megalencephaly?

Macrocephaly refers to OFC (occipitofrontal circumference or head circumference) >+2 SD for age and gender. We know that normal head circumference increases by 2 cm/month (0–3 months), 1 cm/month (3–6 months), 0.5 cm/month (6–12 months), 1 cm every 6 months (1–3 years), and 1 cm/year (3–5 years). Macrocephaly can result from hydrocephalus (enlarged ventricles) or megalencephaly (large brain). Megalencephaly refers to the large size of brain parenchyma. Hence, all microcephalies do not result from hydrocephalus.
- *If megalencephaly, is it metabolic or syndromic megalencephaly?*

Megalencephaly could be secondary to metabolic conditions such as Canavan disease, Alexander disease, or it could be syndromic cause such as neurofibromatosis **(Flowchart 1)**.

Other important differentials of a large head:
- *Benign enlargement of subarachnoid space (BESS):* Large head in typically developing children, with MRI brain showing evidence of enlarged subarachnoid spaces with normal or dilated ventricles, is called BESS. As the name suggests, BESS is a benign condition and does not require any surgical or medical intervention. It usually stabilizes by 12–18 months.
- *Hydranencephaly:* It refers to complete absence of cerebral tissue with the entire intracranial cavity occupied with cerebrospinal fluid (CSF). Hydranencephaly often results from bilateral fetal internal carotid obstruction.

Flowchart 1: Broad classification of megalencephaly.

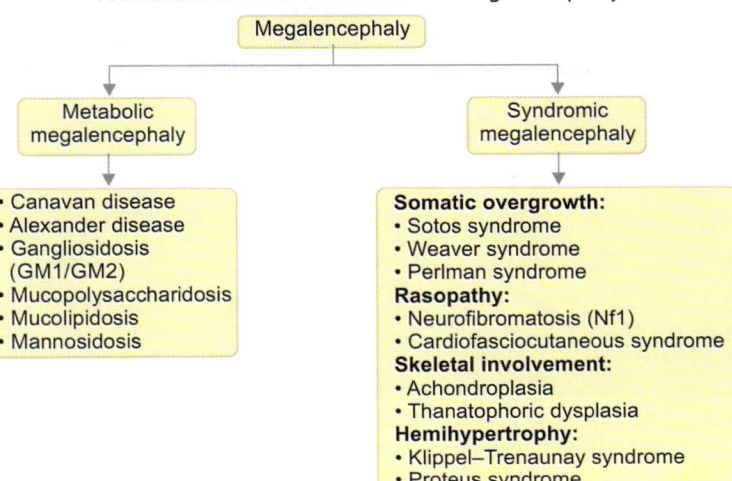

- Megalencephaly
  - Metabolic megalencephaly
    - Canavan disease
    - Alexander disease
    - Gangliosidosis (GM1/GM2)
    - Mucopolysaccharidosis
    - Mucolipidosis
    - Mannosidosis
  - Syndromic megalencephaly
    - **Somatic overgrowth:**
      - Sotos syndrome
      - Weaver syndrome
      - Perlman syndrome
    - **Rasopathy:**
      - Neurofibromatosis (Nf1)
      - Cardiofasciocutaneous syndrome
    - **Skeletal involvement:**
      - Achondroplasia
      - Thanatophoric dysplasia
    - **Hemihypertrophy:**
      - Klippel–Trenaunay syndrome
      - Proteus syndrome

This needs to be differentiated from hydrocephalus, as there is no role of surgical intervention in hydranencephaly.
- *Chronic subdural effusion:* It may result from meningitis or head trauma.
- *If hydrocephalus, is it congenital or acquired?*

Onset at birth or within the first 6 months is often considered congenital hydrocephalus. Onset beyond 6 months of age often points to acquired hydrocephalus.
- *What could be cause of hydrocephalus?*
  - *Preterm infants:* Intraventricular bleed
  - *Term infants:* Dandy–Walker malformation, Arnold–Chiari malformation type II, arachnoid cyst, vein of Galen malformation, intrauterine infection, and aqueductal stenosis
  - *Older children:* Tumor (obstructive hydrocephalus), trauma, and infection (e.g., tubercular)
- *Are there any clinical features of hydrocephalus?*
  - *Infants:* Failure to thrive, developmental delay, irritability, poor feeding,

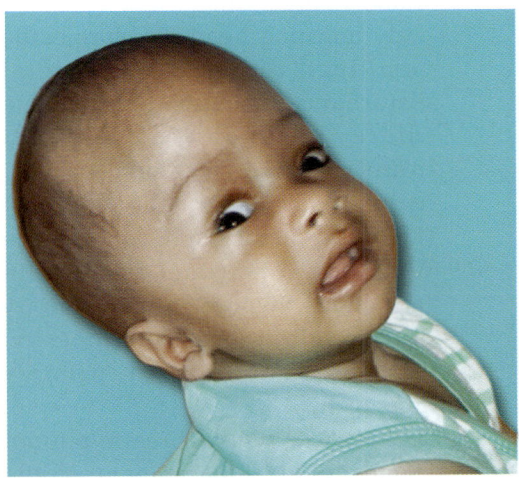

Fig. 1: Baby with congenital hydrocephalus with large head and sunsetting sign.

vomiting, apneic spells, bulging tense anterior fontanelle, distended scalp veins, cranial sutures splayed, transillumination sign (if cortex is very thin), sixth cranial nerve palsy, upgaze palsy (sunsetting sign) **(Fig. 1)**, nystagmus, optic atrophy (chronic), and spasticity

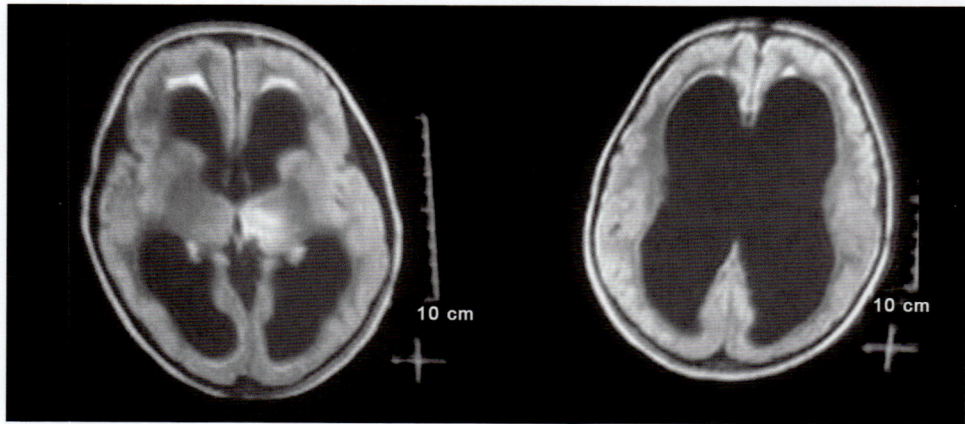

Fig. 2: MRI brain (T2/FLAIR) reveals dilated lateral ventricles with presence of periventricular ooze. (T2/FLAIR: T2-weighted-fluid-attenuated inversion recovery)

- *Older children:* Intellectual disability, early morning headache, projectile vomiting, diplopia, behavioral disturbances, squint, papilledema (more common in acquired hydrocephalus rather than congenital hydrocephalus), Parinaud syndrome (light near dissociation, convergence retraction nystagmus, and eyelid retraction), hypothalamic/pituitary dysfunction (gigantism, obesity, delayed puberty, and primary amenorrhea)
- *Radiological signs:* Three important signs include enlargement of the anterior and posterior recess of the third ventricle, dilatation of temporal horns of lateral ventricles, effacement of cortical sulci **(Fig. 2)**. Dilation of fourth and third ventricles along with the above signs indicates communicating hydrocephalus. However, the presence of normal or small fourth ventricle suggests obstructive hydrocephalus. Brain atrophy must always be differentiated from hydrocephalus with former having prominent sulci/gyri, irregular ventricular margin, lack of periventricular ooze, and periventricular white matter volume loss.
- *Does it require surgical intervention?*
- Congenital hydrocephalus, especially obstructive hydrocephalus (with periventricular ooze, papilledema, and signs of raised ICP), always requires surgical intervention for CSF diversion. Two options include shunt (ventriculoperitoneal or ventriculoatrial) surgery or endoscopic third ventriculostomy (ETV) with or without choroid plexus cauterization. By convention, ETV is a preferred choice beyond infancy considering high failure rates in infancy. Children who have mild arrested hydrocephalus, those with cortical mantle size <1 cm, associated malformations often do not require surgical intervention. Three main complications with shunt surgery include shunt failure, shunt infection, and slit ventricle syndrome **(Table 1)**.

TABLE 1: Key features of shunt malfunction, shunt infection, and slit ventricle syndrome.

Clinical parameters	Shunt failure	Shunt infection	Slit ventricle syndrome
When to suspect	Development of new-onset headache, vomiting, seizures, neck retraction, tense bulging anterior fontanelle, papilledema in a shunted child must raise suspicion of shunt malfunction	Development of fever, seizure, headache, and vomiting within a few months of shunt surgery should raise suspicion of shunt infection	Development of intermittent symptoms of headache, vomiting, and seizures in a shunted child with chinked ventricles on imaging must raise suspicion of slit ventricle syndrome
Clinical signs	Shunt chamber may not be compressible but fill immediately (distal block); if the shunt chamber is easy to compress but refill slowly then it indicates proximal block at the ventricular level	Signs of inflammation may or may not be seen in subcutaneous shunt chamber	No local signs
Neuroimaging findings	Imaging may reveal an increase in ventricular size compared to previous scans	Imaging may reveal an increase in ventricular size compared to the previous scan	Imaging reveals small chinked ventricles owing to lack of compliance of ventricle wall
Management	Shunt revision is the only option. Often the shunt is broken or blocked	IV antibiotics, shunt exteriorization, and shunt revision	Difficult to manage often requires surgical expertise

(IV: intravenous)

HISTORY-TAKING

Presenting Complaints

Children with hydrocephalus may present with one or more of the following:
- Increasing/large head size
- Excessive irritability, vomiting, and feeding difficulties
- Delayed attainment of developmental milestones
- Inability to gain weight according to the age
- Swelling noticed in the back since birth
- Multiple episodes of abnormal body movement in the past 3 months of age

History of Presenting Illness

The primary purpose of history would be determining whether it is congenital (right from the birth) or acquired hydrocephalus and to determine the presence or absence of features of raised intracranial pressure and to establish the most probable etiology. Start your history from the antenatal period, if the onset of the large head is right from birth or early infancy.
- *Antenatal history:* Maternal fever/rash [*Toxoplasma gondii*, other agents, rubella, cytomegalovirus (CMV), and herpes simplex virus (TORCH) or mumps infection]; maternal folate

intake (for prevention of neural tube defects); maternal drug intake (sodium valproate and phenytoin for neural tube defects); antenatal ultrasonography scans (for ventricular size/presence of associated neural tube defects); any prenatal screening [triple test or maternal α-fetoprotein (AFP) level estimation]
- *Birth history:* History of premature delivery (preterms are prone to intraventricular bleed with secondary hydrocephalus), history of perinatal asphyxia (white matter volume loss leads to large ventricle called hydrocephalus ex vacuo, which is often misinterpreted as hydrocephalus on neuroimaging; clinically they will not have macrocephaly), head circumference at birth (large head size at birth suggests congenital hydrocephalus), presence of swelling at the back (neural tube defect and a possibility of Chiari II malformation)
- *Postnatal history:* Head trauma (post-traumatic intraventricular hemorrhage resulting in secondary obstructive hydrocephalus), history suggestive of meningitis (postmeningitis-acquired hydrocephalus)
- *History of features of raised intracranial pressure:*
  - *Infants:* Excessive irritability, inconsolable cry, feeding difficulties, poor weight gain, vomiting and tightness of limbs
  - *Older children:* Headache, vomiting, neck pain, stiffness of limbs, and alteration in gait
- Sudden or insidious onset of headache, projectile vomiting and neck pain in a typically developing child could indicate a feature of raised intracranial pressure that could be seen in posterior fossa tumor causing obstructive symptoms.
- The presence of ongoing fever and neck stiffness often points to infective etiology. The majority of acquired causes, such as infective or malignant causes of hydrocephalus, do not result in macrocephaly.
- The presence of difficulty in breathing along with features of congestive heart failure in an infant with a large head and features of increased intracranial pressure often point to a possibility of the vein of Galen malformation.
- Family history of hydrocephalus or large head (X-linked hydrocephalus or AR hydrocephalus)
- *History of comorbidities:*
  - Vision impairment (long-standing hydrocephalus can be associated with optic atrophy)
  - Seizures (around 30% of children with hydrocephalus will have associated epilepsy)
  - Hearing impairment [can be seen in congenital *Cytomegalovirus* (CMV) infection]
  - Motor impairment in terms of:
    - Flailness or tightness of limbs (spasticity is indicative of corticospinal tract involvement as in raised intracranial pressure)
    - Paraparesis (weakness of both lower limbs with sparing of upper limbs often points to Chiari II malformation)
    - History of urinary bladder retention and/or urinary dribbling often points to the neurogenic bladder in children with neural tube defects

- History of recurrent unexplained febrile illness also points to recurrent urinary tract infections owing to vesicoureteral reflux and hydronephrosis
- History of constipation or fecal incontinence (neurogenic bowel) in children with neural tube defect
- History of foot and hip deformities can often point to associated neural tube defects

- Presence of hepatosplenomegaly and coarse facies (mucopolysaccharidosis and mucolipidosis)
- History of neuroregression, large head, and fundus showing cherry-red spot (GM2 gangliosidosis)
- Look for syndromic features of associated syndromes such as Noonan syndrome, Costello syndrome, cardiofaciocutaneous syndrome, VACTERL anomaly, Meckel–Gruber syndrome, and Walker–Warburg syndrome

■ FOCUSED EXAMINATION

Clinical Signs of Hydrocephalus

- *Infants:* Tense bulging anterior fontanelle with head circumference >2 SD; dilated scalp veins; splaying of cranial sutures with wide-open fontanelle; presence of transillumination sign; sunsetting sign with impaired upward gaze palsy owing to pressure on midbrain tectum; and sixth cranial nerve palsy (unilateral or bilateral)
- *Older children:* Percussion over skull reveals resonant note (crackpot sign) in children with bony closure of fontanelles; diplopia resulting from 6th cranial nerve palsy; symptoms of pseudobulbar palsy such as difficulty in deglutition and swallowing.

Clinical Signs for Other Causes of Megalencephaly

- Neurocutaneous markers (neurofibromatosis can result in megalencephaly, i.e., large size of the brain)
- Short stature (genetic conditions such as achondroplasia can have large head)
- Presence of features of overgrowth (Sotos syndrome as in somatic overgrowth syndromes associated with megalencephaly)

Clinical Signs in Children who have Undergone Shunt Surgery for Hydrocephalus

- Whether the shunt can be palpated in the subcutaneous plane of the neck (if the shunt is not palpable, the possibility of shunt migration needs consideration)
- Whether the chamber of the shunt is compressible (a clue to patency of shunt)
- Any surrounding signs of redness (erythema) along the path of shunt could point to shunt infection, especially in the presence of fever and within 3 months of shunt surgery.
- Presence of clinical signs of raised ICP in a shunted child often ignites the suspicion of shunt malfunction/block or shunt infection.

Clinical Signs of Neural Tube Defects

- Open or closed defect in the spinal cord; level of the lesion
- Presence or absence of paraparesis/spasticity in legs, hyperreflexia, and loss of sensation below the site of lesion
- Presence or absence of hip deformity, talipes equinovarus deformity, calcaneus

foot, rocker-bottom foot, and femoral or tibial torsion deformities (hip and foot deformities are commonly associated with neural tube defects)
- Any evidence of scoliosis (a symptom of hydromyelia)
- Pressure sores/ulcers and burn injury owing to loss of sensation below the level of the lesion
- Loss of anal sphincter tone can be observed in children with neural tube defects

■ CASE VIGNETTES

Case 1

A 6-month-old boy was brought with increasing head size since birth, failure to thrive, developmental delay, features of raised intracranial pressure (in the form of sunsetting sign), and evolving spasticity. He was born by cesarean section delivery and had a large head size at birth. He had an uneventful antenatal, natal, and postnatal period. There was no dysmorphism, neurocutaneous markers, or spina bifida. There was no significant history of similar illness in the family.

Analysis

Is there a large head?	Yes
Is the large head secondary to hydrocephalus?	Probably yes
Is it congenital or acquired hydrocephalus?	Congenital (onset at birth)
Is it syndromic or nonsyndromic?	Nonsyndromic (no features of dysmorphism or neurocutaneous syndromes)

Contd...

Contd...

What is the most probable etiology for hydrocephalus?	Considering that head size is gradually increasing, it is likely that hydrocephalus could be due to conditions such as aqueductal stenosis or Dandy–Walker malformation. Other conditions such as TORCH infection and postintraventricular bleed hydrocephalus are unlikely to progress until 6 months of age. The latter are static conditions, unless they result in obstructive hydrocephalus.
Are there clinical features to suggest features of raised intracranial pressure?	Yes (sunsetting sign, spasticity, and repeated vomiting)
Is there a neural tube defect?	No
What is the level of defect: is it open or closed?	Not applicable
Are there any associated neurological, urological, and musculoskeletal problems?	None

The index case has an onset right from the birth (it is congenital hydrocephalus) with no evidence of antenatal, natal, or postnatal insult (this probably rules out TORCH infection, maternal drug exposure, intraventricular bleed, or postnatal meningitis or trauma). Since the head size is rapidly increasing in size, it is more likely that we are dealing with hydrocephalus rather than any other cause of large head (megalencephalic head would increase as per the age and would not exceed the expected gain in head circumference). Progressive increasing of head size also points to conditions such as aqueductal stenosis, which are bound to increase if untreated. There are definitive features of raised intracranial pressure (thus warranting urgent surgical intervention; had there been a large head secondary to arrested hydrocephalus, surgeons often do not want to operate on such conditions despite large head). Arrested hydrocephalus means the hydrocephalus is not progressing further, there is no periventricular ooze, rather there is a paucity of periventricular white matter, so everything has become chronic, and there is no feature of raised ICP although there is a large head.

Impression

To summarize, we are probably dealing with a case of congenital nonsyndromic hydrocephalus with features of raised intracranial pressure that would require surgical intervention. Investigation of choice for this child will include MRI Brain. Child needs to be managed surgically (VP shunt or third ventriculostomy).

Analysis

Is there a large head?	Yes
Is the large head secondary to hydrocephalus?	Probably yes
Is it congenital or acquired hydrocephalus?	Congenital (onset at birth)
Is it syndromic or nonsyndromic?	Nonsyndromic
What is the most probable etiology for hydrocephalus?	Arnold–Chiari malformation type II
Are there clinical features to suggest features of raised intracranial pressure?	Probably yes (repeated vomiting)
Is there a neural tube defect?	Yes
What is the level of defect; is it open or closed?	Lumbosacral; open meningomyelocele
Are there any associated neurological, urological, and musculoskeletal problems?	Yes, spastic paraplegia, bilateral CTEV, and no urological issues till now

Case 2

A 2-day-old girl was born by cesarean section with open meningomyelocele in lumbosacral region with macrocephaly. She presented to the emergency room with repeated vomiting. There is no associated dysmorphism or any neurocutaneous markers. There is associated bilateral congenital talipes equinovarus (CTEV) and complete lack of mobility of both lower limbs. There is no previous affected sibling or any other significant family history.

Impression

The index case has open meningomyelocele, congenital nonsyndromic hydrocephalus with CTEV, and spastic paraplegia. These features are suggestive of Chiari II malformation. The possibility of active central nervous system (CNS) infection cannot be ruled out considering open meningomyelocele. This child will require urgent surgical intervention with priority to close the open defect and plan procedure for CSF diversion on a later date.

Case 3

A 12-month-old boy presented with global developmental delay, failure to thrive, macrocephaly, and epileptic spasms. He was born preterm (29 weeks) and had a stormy neonatal period with a need for mechanical ventilation, seizures, and recurrent apnea. Sonography during the neonatal period revealed intraventricular hemorrhage (IVH). Examination reveals hypotonia; there are no dysmorphism or neurocutaneous stigmata.

Analysis

Is there a large head?	Yes
Is the large head secondary to hydrocephalus?	Probably yes
Is it congenital or acquired hydrocephalus?	Acquired hydrocephalus secondary to preterm intraventricular bleeding
Is it syndromic or nonsyndromic?	Nonsyndromic
What is the most probable etiology for hydrocephalus?	Secondary to preterm intraventricular bleed
Are there clinical features to suggest raised intracranial pressure?	Probably no
Is there a neural tube defect?	No
What is the level of defect: is it open or closed?	Not applicable
Are there any associated neurological, urological, musculoskeletal, or nutritional problems?	Yes, failure to thrive (nutritional) and epileptic spasm (neurological)

Impression

It appears that the baby has a global developmental delay with epileptic spasms and failure to thrive secondary to hydrocephalus resulting from intraventricular hemorrhage of prematurity. Priority at this juncture would be to treat epileptic spasms and nutritional rehabilitation. There is a limited role of CSF diversion at this age for post-IVH hydrocephalus. The absence of features of raised intracranial pressure and the absence of pressure effects (such as periventricular ooze on neuroimaging) often discourage the neurosurgeon to intervene. Similarly, presence of fixed disabilities such as spastic paraplegia, neurogenic bladder, and high level (e.g., cervical) meningomyelocele are risk factor for poor outcome and surgical interventions are not very meaningful in these patients.

Management of Post-IVH Hydrocephalus

There are two options for management—direct ventricular drainage (Ommaya reservoir or subgaleal shunt) and ventriculoperitoneal (VP) shunt. VP shunting may be hazardous considering the risk of collapsed cortical mantle, risk of subdural hemorrhage, and marked cerebral conformational changes. Third option is repeated lumbar puncture which is considered in a few patients with a presumption that once CSF-containing blood is removed, it might allow normal resorption of CSF. Fourth option is intraventricular fibrinolytics which is practiced in few centers. Although, there is lack of clear consensus, Ommaya reservoir in infancy followed by VP shunting later is often practiced in many centers.

Case 4

A 10-year-old boy presented with multiple episodes of seizures. He has intellectual disability, macrocephaly, and multiple café-au-lait macules in the skin of his body. He has no dysmorphism or any motor deficit.

Analysis

Is there a large head?	Yes
Is the large head secondary to hydrocephalus?	Cannot say, it could be just megalencephaly; neuroimaging is essential to clarify
Is it congenital or acquired hydrocephalus?	Not relevant (this is probably not hydrocephalus, so no question of congenital or acquired). But yes, it started from birth, so can be considered a congenital process
Is it syndromic or nonsyndromic?	Probably syndromic
What is the most probable etiology for hydrocephalus?	Neurofibromatosis
Are there clinical features to suggest raised intracranial pressure?	Probably no
Is there a neural tube defect?	No
What is the level of defect; is it open or closed?	Not applicable
Are there any associated neurological, urological, musculoskeletal, or nutritional problems?	Yes, intellectual disability and epilepsy (neurological)

Impression

We are dealing with a syndromic cause of macrocephaly (neurofibromatosis) with no signs of raised intracranial pressure. The priority of management would be to control the seizures with antiepileptic drugs. Few neurocutaneous conditions such as tuberous sclerosis (subependymal nodule) can have obstructive hydrocephalus that requires either surgical intervention or medications such as everolimus. In other syndromic causes of hydrocephalus, there is a limited role of surgery.

POSTNATAL MANAGEMENT OF NEURAL TUBE DEFECT

- *Closure of meningomyelocele:* The first priority would be a closure of meningomyelocele within 24–48 hours of birth to prevent ascending infection and further nerve cell degeneration. This will result in the protection of neural tissue.
- *Shunt surgery:* CSF diversion surgery such as the placement of ventriculoperitoneal shunt is often required following the closure of the defect. The development of pseudobulbar palsy in children with Arnold–Chiari II malformation also warrants urgent surgical intervention.
- *Management of comorbidities:* Comorbidities including management of seizures (antiepileptic drugs), spasticity (physiotherapy and antispasticity medications such as baclofen or tizanidine) and contractures (orthopedic intervention) are essential.
- *Management of urological problems:* Children with neural tube defects are prone to the neurogenic bladder with resultant increased risk of vesicoureteric

reflux and hydronephrosis. They must be screened for regular urine cultures and vesicourethrocystogram. Renal ultrasonography must be performed to look for the development of hydronephrosis. Clean intermittent catheterization and urinary antibiotic prophylaxis are the mainstay of treatment for neurogenic bladder.
- *Management of constipation:* High-fiber diet supplementation, laxatives, and enema remain the cornerstone in the management of constipation among children with neural tube defects.
- *Management of orthopedic ailments* including hip dysplasia, CTEV, calcaneus deformity, rocker-bottom feet, femoral or tibial torsion, and varus deformity by appropriate surgical intervention is warranted.
- We should counsel the mother to take routine folic acid supplementation (4 mg/day) to prevent recurrence in the subsequent pregnancy. Recurrence risk after a single affected child is 4%, and with two previous affected siblings, it increases to 10%.

KEY MESSAGES

- Macrocephaly can result from hydrocephalus (enlarged ventricles) or megalencephaly (large brain).
- Hydrocephalus can be congenital or acquired. Most common cause of congenital hydrocephalus is aqueductal stenosis, and acquired hydrocephalus often results from intraventricular bleed or as a complication of meningitis.
- Clinical features of raised ICP in a child with hydrocephalus often warrant surgical intervention.
- The presence of neural tube defects with congenital hydrocephalus often point to Arnold–Chiari malformation type II.
- Three main complications with shunt surgery include shunt failure, shunt infection, and slit ventricle syndrome.

SECTION 4

Common Therapeutic Dilemmas

33. Antiseizure Medications
34. Management of Acute Seizure and Status Epilepticus
35. Treatment of Infections of Nervous System
36. Management of Raised Intracranial Pressure
37. Medical Management of Acute Vascular Stroke
38. Management of Developmental Disorders
39. Treatment of Neuropathies and Myopathies

CHAPTER 33: Antiseizure Medications

■ INTRODUCTION

It is well known that almost 20–40% of children with epilepsy continue to have seizures, despite optimal treatment with correct antiepileptic drugs (ASDs). ASDs are better called antiseizure medications. Conventional ASDs, despite having an advantage of lower cost and easy availability, are associated with significant side effects, often warranting withdrawal. Till nearly 10 years ago, there was a flood of second-generation ASDs, which partially challenged the traditional ASDs. Last decade has witnessed many third-generation ASDs. ASDs can be categorized as first-, second-, and third-generation ASDs **(Box 1)**.

The commonly prescribed *first-generation ASDs* include phenytoin (PHT), phenobarbitone (PB), carbamazepine (CBZ), and sodium valproate (VPA) **(Table 1)**. Second-generation ASDs include levetiracetam (LEV), zonisamide (ZSM), lamotrigine (LTG), and oxcarbazepine (OXC) **(Table 2)**. There are a large number of newer third-generation ASDs that have been introduced in the market. The approved indications for these newer ASDs have been summarized **(Table 3)**. Other investigational compounds under development for seizure and epilepsy include ganaxolone, bumetanide, darigabat, loraceserin, soticlestat, STK-001 and XEN 1101. Of them, ganaxolone has been approved by the Food and Drug Administration (FDA) for treatment of seizures associated with cyclin-dependent kinase like-5 deficiency.

Commonly prescribed benzodiazepines include clobazam, clonazepam, and nitrazepam. Benzodiazepines are never used as monotherapy. They are commonly used as add-on drugs for myoclonic seizure, atonic

BOX 1: Classification of commonly prescribed antiepileptic drugs.

First-generation ASD
- Phenytoin
- Phenobarbitone
- Valproate
- Carbamazepine

Second-generation ASD
- Vigabatrin
- Oxcarbazepine
- Lamotrigine
- Topiramate
- Gabapentin
- Levetiracetam
- Zonisamide
- Stiripentol
- Rufinamide

Third-generation ASD
- Eslicarbazepine
- Lacosamide
- Retigabine (Ezogabine)
- Brivaracetam
- Perampanel
- Cenobamate

(ASD: anti-seizure drug)

TABLE 1: First-line antiepileptic drugs: Indications and dose.

Drug	Maintenance dose	Clinical use (common)	Caution
Phenobarbitone (PB)	3–5 mg/kg/day (maximum 400 mg/day)	First line in neonatal seizure and used in status epilepticus. It is also useful in preventing recurrence of febrile seizures	Short-term concern of sedation; concerns of cognitive and behavioral problems (hyperactivity and aggressiveness); slow withdrawal with risk of recurrence; it can exacerbate porphyria
Phenytoin (PHT)	5–8 mg/kg/day (ceiling 300 mg/day)	• It is useful in generalized as well as focal seizures. It is used as second-line agent in status epilepticus. It is cheap, easily available, and effective medication. It is highly protein bound • Hence, serum PHT level can be very high in hypoalbuminic state. It follows first-order kinetics; once elimination pathway is saturated, drug levels increase exponentially with slight increase in dose	Long-term use is associated with concerns of gingival hypertrophy, coarse facies, hirsutism, and osteoporosis; it can rarely lead to Stevens–Johnson syndrome; toxicity results in ataxia, nystagmus, and incoordination
Valproic acid (VPA)	15–20 mg/kg/day; maximum can be 60 mg/kg/day (ceiling dose 3,000 mg/day)	Broad-spectrum antiepileptic drug often used as first-line drug in generalized seizures. It is one of first-line treatments for most of the epilepsy syndromes including epileptic encephalopathies, childhood absence epilepsy, and juvenile myoclonic epilepsy	Common side effects: tremors, sedation, and thrombocytopenia; major concerns are encephalopathy secondary to hyperammonemia, hepatitis, and pancreatitis; long-term use is associated with concerns of weight gain, hair loss, and polycystic ovarian cyst
Carbamazepine (CBZ)	10–35 mg/kg/day (maximum 1,600 mg/day)	Its primary indication is focal epilepsy. It is a cheap medication with good efficacy. It can precipitate absence and myoclonic seizures	HLA-B*1502 associated with severe cutaneous reaction such as Stevens–Johnson syndrome; it can cause dizziness, hyponatremia, diplopia, weight gain, and leukopenia
Ethosuximide (ETX)	15–40 mg/kg	It is the drug of choice for childhood absence epilepsy and juvenile absence epilepsy with generalized tonic-clonic seizure (GTCS)	Minor gastrointestinal disturbances such as nausea, vomiting, and diarrhea are reported

TABLE 2: Second-line antiepileptic drugs (ASDs): Indications, caution, and doses.

Drug	Maintenance dose	Clinical use (common)	Caution
Levetiracetam (LEV)	10–60 mg/kg	It is a broad-spectrum ASD effective in focal as well as generalized seizure and used in status epilepticus. Excellent oral bioavailability, no hepatic metabolism, and minimal drug interaction with other drugs	Major concern is behavioral symptoms. Common side effects include somnolescence, irritability, and dizziness
Lamotrigine (LTG)	0.15 mg/kg/day; increase gradually to 5–8 mg/kg/day. Dose must be limited to 2–3 mg/kg/day when used along with sodium valproate	Its primary indication is add-on to sodium valproate among children with drug-resistant epilepsy. It is also first line among adolescent girls with juvenile myoclonic epilepsy. It is a broad-spectrum ASD effective in focal and less effective in generalized seizures	Major concern is drug rash in 10–20% of children. Otherwise, a long-term side effect profile is favorable in terms of cognition and sedation
Topiramate (TPM)	Start at 1–3 mg/kg and can go up to 5–8 mg/kg/day (maximum 400 mg/day)	Broad-spectrum ASD useful in focal and generalized seizures including epileptic spasms. It is commonly used as add-on drug in drug-resistant epilepsy. Useful among epileptic children with associated migraine and obesity	Major concern with TPM is cognitive slowing, decreased attention, and memory. Weight loss, hypohidrosis, hyperthermia, metabolic acidosis, dehydration, and renal calculi are some of the other concerns. There is risk of hyperammonemia when combined with valproate
Oxcarbazepine (OXC)	Start with 10 mg/kg and can increase to 30 mg/kg/day	Approved drug for focal seizure	Major concerns include drug rash (1–4%) and hyponatremia [more common than carbamazepine (CBZ)]. It is better tolerated than CBZ
Zonisamide (ZSM)	Start at 2–4 mg/kg and increase to 10 mg/kg/day (maximum 400 mg/day)	It is a broad-spectrum ASD effective in generalized and focal seizures including epileptic spasms. It is commonly used as an add-on drug for drug-resistant epilepsy	My major concern is cognitive slowing, poor attention, and poor memory. Hyperthermia, metabolic acidosis, dehydration, and renal calculi are some of the other concerns
Vigabatrin (VGB)	Start with 50 mg/kg/day can increase to 150 mg/kg/day	Effective in short-term control of epileptic spasms, especially in children with tuberous sclerosis	Visual field defects are a major concern with the use of VGB. Other side effects reported with use of VGB include sedation, irritability, and hypotonia

TABLE 3: Key indications of newer antiepileptic drugs.

Drug	Indications
Stiripentol	Adjuvant in Dravet syndrome
Lacosamide	Adjuvant in refractory focal and generalized epilepsy
Rufinamide	Adjuvant treatment in refractory Lennox–Gastaut syndrome
Brivaracetam	Focal seizures (also available as injectable medication)
Eslicarbazepine	Focal seizure (beyond 4 years of age)
Perampanel	Focal seizures and adjunctive treatment of generalized seizure (beyond 4 years of age)
Retigabine	Focal epilepsy (approved for adults)
Cenobamate	Focal epilepsy (approved for adults)

seizure, atypical absence seizure, tonic seizures, and infantile spasms. Clobazam is particularly an effective add-on drug for Lennox–Gastaut syndrome, drug-resistant focal epilepsy, and epileptic spasms. Two major concerns with long-term use of benzodiazepines include tolerance (usually responds to increase in the dose) and possible adverse effect on cognition.

■ MECHANISM OF ACTION

Antiepileptic drugs act through various mechanisms. The two most common mechanisms include blocking an ion channel and activating the inhibitory γ-aminobutyric acid (GABA) pathway. Antiepileptics can work on one or more of the ion channels such as voltage-operated sodium channel (phenytoin and carbamazepine) or voltageoperated calcium channel (valproate and ethosuximide). The facilitation of GABA transmission could be achieved by GABA reuptake inhibition (tiagabine), GABA transaminase inhibitor (vigabatrin), or acting on the chloride channel (benzodiazepines and phenobarbitone) **(Table 4)**. Few ASDs have a combination of these mechanisms (e.g., levetiracetam), and few have a mechanism of action that is not very clear.

■ CHOICE OF DRUGS

Choice of Antiepileptic Drug in Acute Seizure

When a child is brought convulsing to emergency room, the first drug used for aborting the seizure is benzodiazepines (midazolam or lorazepam). There is no need of any ASD, if the seizure was secondary to hypoglycemia, hypocalcemia, hyponatremia, or hypernatremia. The underlying cause needs to be treated in such a situation. Management of acute seizure and status epilepticus is covered in **Chapter 34**. Once the seizures are controlled, a decision for ASD needs to be taken. Do we need to load with any ASD? If yes, which ASD will be suitable? Few common principles that we may adopt to decide the choice of ASD in emergency care are summarized in **Tables 1 and 2**.

- *Febrile seizure:* Children with simple febrile seizures should not be loaded with ASDs unless they have febrile focal seizures or febrile status epilepticus where sodium valproate would be the drug of choice.
- *First unprovoked seizure:* Phenytoin (15–20 mg/kg loading @ <1 mg/kg/h) or fosphenytoin is the drug of choice among those who present with first unprovoked seizure

TABLE 4: Mechanism of action of various antiepileptic drugs.

Main pathway/channel	Mechanism	Drugs
Sodium channel	Maintain Na channel in inactive state to prevent sodium influx into cells thus preventing repetitive firing	• Phenytoin (PHT) • Carbamazepine (CBZ) • Oxcarbazepine (OXC) • Lamotrigine (LTG) • Lacosamide (LCM) • Eslicarbazepine • Rufinamide
Calcium channel	T-type calcium channel blocker (acts on thalamus thus preventing rhythmic thalamocortical spike-wave pattern	• Ethosuximide (ETX) • Valproate (VPA)
	L-type calcium channel	• Lamotrigine (LTG) • Gabapentin (GBP) • Felbamate • Pregabalin
	N-type calcium channel	Levetiracetam (LEV)
GABA pathway	Inhibition of GABA-mediated chloride channel	• Benzodiazepine • Phenobarbitone (PB)
	GABA reuptake inhibition	Tiagabine
	GABA transaminase inhibitor	Vigabatrin (VGB)
Glutamate blockers	NMDA receptor blocker	Felbamate (FEL)
	AMPA receptor blocker	• Topiramate (TPM) • Perampanel (PER)
SV2A-binding site		Levetiracetam (LEV)
Carbonic anhydrase inhibitor		Acetazolamide and topiramate (TPM)
Potassium channel opener	Acts on KCNQ2/3	Ezogabine (Retigabine)

(GABA: γ-aminobutyric acid; NMDA: N-methyl-D-aspartate; AMPA: α-amino-3-hydroxyl-5-methyl-4-isoxazole propionate)

- *Seizures in a child with underlying developmental delay secondary to established cause:* Sodium valproate or levetiracetam may be preferred among those with pre-existing developmental delay secondary to an established cause such as perinatal asphyxia, especially when they have coexistent seizures such as epileptic spasms or myoclonic seizures. For example, a child with cerebral palsy, microcephaly secondary to prematurity presents to emergency with first seizure, and sodium valproate would be a good choice.
- *Seizures in a child with underlying developmental delay secondary to unknown etiology:* In a child with developmental delay who presents with seizures, if the etiology is not clear and neurometabolic etiology is a possibility, and it would be wise to avoid sodium valproate. In such a situation, levetiracetam is a good alternative.

- *Breakthrough seizure on suboptimal dose of ASD:* If the child was already on an ASD (submaximal dose) and had a breakthrough seizure despite good compliance, then same ASD can be loaded.
- *Breakthrough seizure on maximum dose of ASD:* If the child was already on maximal doses of ASD and presents with breakthrough seizure, the next best choice of ASD can be loaded
- *Poor compliance to ASD:* If the child was already on an ASD and parents had stopped the drug owing to poor compliance and the child was brought to emergency, the same ASD can be administered.

Choice of Antiepileptic Drug for Long-term Management of Epilepsy

Various factors determine the choice of ASDs. These include the type of seizure, epilepsy syndrome (if any), age of the patient, and comorbidities. Generalized seizures respond well to sodium valproate and levetiracetam; focal seizures respond well to carbamazepine, oxcarbazepine, phenytoin, levetiracetam, and topiramate (TPM). If a syndromic diagnosis has been established (based on seizure semiology, electroencephalography (EEG) findings, and age at onset), the choice of ASD can be based on the type of epilepsy syndrome:

- *Juvenile absence epilepsy* responds well to ethosuximide and sodium valproate. Other drugs include lamotrigine. Sodium valproate is the preferred choice when absence seizures are associated with GTCS.
- *Juvenile myoclonic epilepsy* responds favorably to valproate and lamotrigine.
- *West syndrome* responds well to ACTH (150 units/m^2)/oral steroids (prednisolone 4 mg/kg/day for 2 weeks followed by tapering) and vigabatrin. Other ASDs that are known to work in West syndrome include topiramate, zonisamide, and nitrazepam, or clonazepam
- *Lennox–Gastaut syndrome* responds well to sodium valproate, lamotrigine, topiramate, and rufinamide.
- *Dravet syndrome* responds to sodium valproate, clobazam, stiripentol, topiramate and zonisamide. Cannabidiol (5 mg/kg/day increased to 10 mg/kg/day) can be used in refractory cases.
- *Rolandic epilepsy* responds well to sodium valproate, carbamazepine, and oxcarbazepine. International League against Epilepsy (ILAE) 2013 guidelines for choice of ASDs are listed in **Table 5**.

In addition to the type of seizure and epilepsy syndrome, comorbidities and adverse effect profiles also determine the choice of ASDs **(Table 6)**. For example, in a 13-year-old girl diagnosed with juvenile absence epilepsy, despite sodium valproate being the drug of choice, one would prefer to avoid this drug in an adolescent girl for the fear of the risk of polycystic ovarian disease and weight gain. In such a case, ETX and LEV are reasonable alternatives.

Children with first unprovoked seizure, whose neuroimaging and EEG were normal, may not require long-term ASD. The recurrence risk can be explained to parents. Long-term ASDs are recommended in first unprovoked seizure among those with developmental delay, abnormal neuroimaging findings, and abnormality on EEG.

TABLE 5: International League Against Epilepsy (ILAE) choice of antiepileptic drugs (ILAE, 2013).

Clinical condition	Drug of choice with level of evidence (A–D)
Children with newly diagnosed or untreated partial-onset seizure for initial monotherapy	• OXC (level A) • CBZ, PB, PHT, TPM, VPA, and VGB (level C) • CLB, CLN, LTG, and ZNS (level D)
Children with newly diagnosed or untreated generalized-onset seizure for initial monotherapy	• CBZ, PB, PHT, TPM, and VPA (level C) • OXC (level D)
Children with absence seizure for initial monotherapy	• ESM and VPA (level A) • LTG (level C)
Children with benign childhood epilepsy with centrotemporal spikes	• CBZ and VPA (level C) • GBP, LEV, OXC, and STM (level D)
Children with juvenile myoclonic epilepsy	TPM and VPA (level D)

(CBZ: carbamazepine; LTG: lamotrigine; OXC: oxcarbazepine; PB: phenobarbitone; PHT: phenytoin; TPM: topiramate; VGB: vigabatrin; VPA: valproate acid; ZNS: zonisamide)

TABLE 6: Factors that determine the choice of antiepileptic drug.

Clinical/demographic factor	Antiepileptic drug to be avoided
Women and adolescent girls	Sodium valproate and phenytoin (cosmetic effects of gum hyperplasia)
Children with suspected neurometabolic disorder or those with unknown cause of global developmental delay	Sodium valproate (worsen metabolic crises)
Juvenile absence epilepsy and juvenile myoclonic epilepsy	PHT, CBZ, and OXC are known to worsen absence and myoclonic seizures
Lennox–Gastaut syndrome and West syndrome	PHT, CBZ, and OXC are known to worsen infantile spasms
Children with electrical status epilepticus in sleep (ESES)	CBZ and PHT are to be avoided, as they can worsen or exacerbate ESES
Children with excessive behavioral problems	Levetiracetam
Obese children	Sodium valproate

(CBZ: carbamazepine; OXC: oxcarbazepine; PHT: phenytoin)

GENERAL PRINCIPLES OF ANTIEPILEPTIC DRUG PRESCRIPTION

- Extended-release preparations of ASD can be used to improve the compliance with twice-daily dosing. There is no point in prescribing extended-release preparations in three or four times a day. Drugs with long $t½$ such as phenobarbitone (69 hours) and zonisamide (63 hours) may be prescribed in OD dose.
- *Extended or sustained-release preparations* or *Chrono preparations* have specific drug delivery system, and it will not be

appropriate to break these preparations. Ideally, even enteric-coated tablets also must not be broken. It is better to avoid prescribing ½ or ¾ tablets of chrono- or sustained-release preparation tablets.
- When switching from regular ASD to chrono- or extended-release preparation, the dose needs to be hiked by 10–20%.
- In case of seizure recurrence on ASD, the prescribed ASD should be hiked to a maximum tolerable dose before switching over to the next ASD.
- It is important to remember the ceiling doses of all ASDs, and do not to exceed the maximum allowable dose. So apart from mg/kg dosage, we also need to remember ceiling or maximum doses while prescribing drugs to adolescents. For example, the maximum dose of phenytoin is 300 mg, carbamazepine is 1,600 mg, and sodium valproate is 3,000 mg.
- Avoid polytherapy as much as possible; it is a good idea to withdraw the drug that did not work at the first go, especially once the second ASD has been introduced.
- Avoid drugs that have the same mechanism of action. For example, a combination of PHT and CBZ (both are sodium channel blockers) is not recommended.
- *Certain drugs work well together (synergistic effect):* VPA-LTG and VPA-TPM.
- Avoid combinations of PB and PHT, VPA and CBZ, VPA and PHT for the mutual drug interactions.
- Avoid repeatedly changing the brand of the ASD, especially in a child, where seizures are well controlled. Few brands of phenytoin such as syrup Dilantin has 25 mg/mL and syrup Eptoin has 30 mg/5 mL. One has to be careful always to prescribe mg/mL against the preparation of the drug.
- Avoid prescriptions in "(teaspoon full—tsf)". Always prescribe in milliliters (mL) and ask the parents to measure using a plastic disposable syringe.
- ASDs that are available as suspensions must always be shaken well before use.
- Selection of ASD could be based on the underlying genetic mutation. For example, high-dose phenytoin is useful in SCN8A, phenytoin in conventional dose is useful in SCN2A, carbamazepine useful in PRRT2, retigabine for KCNQ2, quinidine for KCNT1, memantine and dextromethorphan for GRIN2A. Few ASDs are contraindicated in certain genetic mutations such as phenytoin is avoided in SCN1A.

SIDE EFFECT PROFILE OF COMMON ANTIEPILEPTIC DRUGS

Parents must always be warned against the possible side effects of commonly prescribed ASDs. These are listed in **Table 7**. In case of adverse effect, parents should be asked to discontinue the drug immediately. There is a lot of interest in the cognitive side effects of ASDs. Memory impairment has been reported with phenobarbitone, attention deficit with PHT, CBZ, TPM, and mild psychomotor slowing with VPA. These may manifest with poor school performance. The drugs that have hepatic metabolism include VPA, PB, PHT, CBZ, and LTG. Caution needs to be exercised with their use in hepatic failure. Weight gain is a significant problem with VPA, CBZ, and gabapentin.

In contrast, weight loss is common with TPM, ZSM, and ETX. Irreversible visual field defect is a known side effect with VGB. Drugs such as CBZ, PHT, PB, ETX, and ZSM have been associated with serious side effects

TABLE 7: Common side effects of antiepileptic drugs.

Antiepileptic	Side effects
Sodium valproate	Menstrual disturbances, risk of polycystic ovarian disease, weight gain, and transient hair loss*
Carbamazepine	Drug rash (HLA-B* 1502 allele predispose), worsening school performance, weight gain, increased urinary frequency, osteoporosis, and hyponatremia
Oxcarbazepine	Somnolence, vomiting, and hyponatremia
Phenytoin	Cosmetic, bone, gum, hirsutism, acne, and hepatic failure
Phenobarbitone	Sedation, hyperactivity, cognitive impairment, and exacerbation of porphyria
Lamotrigine	Drug rash and Stevens–Johnson syndrome (very low dose is started and hiked gradually)
Levetiracetam	Behavior changes
Topiramate	Language deterioration, acidosis, hyperammonemia, renal stones, and oligohidrosis (unexplained fever)
Vigabatrin	Hypotonia, weight gain, excessive irritability, and visual field defects
Zonisamide	Renal stones and oligohidrosis (unexplained fever)
Rufinamide	Shorten the QT interval

*May respond to addition of biotin.

such as Stevens–Johnson syndrome. ZSM is associated with aplastic anemia. Drugs that cause sedation and somnolence include benzodiazepine, PB, CBZ, PHT, VGB, GBP, and TPM.

Tips on Use of Antiepileptic Drugs

- Few drugs such as levetiracetam have the least drug interactions.
- The majority of the ASDs have hepatic metabolism, except for levetiracetam and vigabatrin that have renal excretion and are safe in hepatic failure.
- The side effects of some drugs are used as an indication. For example, in an obese child with epilepsy, topiramate (weight loss) is preferred over valproate (weight gain).
- If the child has a comorbid migraine, then TPM or VPA will be useful, as it will work for both epilepsy and migraine.
- HLA phenotype (HLA-B 1502) can predict the cutaneous reaction such as Stevens–Johnson syndrome with carbamazepine and phenytoin.
- Lacosamide can prolong PR interval, and chronic therapy may result in tics and diplopia.
- Children on valproate and topiramate are very prone to the risk of hyperammonemia. In that case, carnitine supplementation may help.
- Routine blood testing such as complete blood count and liver function tests are not recommended except for felbamate where there is increased risk of hematological and liver damage. Most of the idiosyncratic reactions such as leukopenia with carbamazepine and transaminitis with sodium valproate occur within first 3–6 months of starting the treatment.

WHEN TO STOP ANTIEPILEPTIC DRUG?

Duration of Antiepileptic Drug Therapy

Duration of long-term ASD will depend on underlying cause. Conventionally, children with epilepsy are continued on ASD for a minimal duration of 2 years. The duration of ASD can be shorter among those with acute symptomatic seizures such as meningoencephalitis, posttraumatic seizure, and neurocysticercosis (NCC). For example, children with meningoencephalitis or head trauma with focal neurological deficits or those with abnormality on neuroimaging may be administered ASD for 3–6 months provided the EEG was normal. Similarly, among those with NCC, ASD can be withdrawn once the lesion has resolved. However, if the NCC becomes calcified, it is better to continue ASD for 2 years.

Discontinuing Antiepileptic Drugs

There is no definitive protocol on when and how to withdraw ASDs. By convention, among children with well-controlled epilepsy who have been seizure free for 2 years, ASDs can be safely withdrawn. EEG should be performed ideally before withdrawal of ASD. A normal EEG reduces the chances of recurrence after ASD withdrawal. ASD must be tapered slowly over 3–6 months duration. Fast tapering over 1 month must be discouraged. Parents must be explained that 30–35% of children may have recurrence, despite documentation of normal EEG findings and slow tapering.

Children with juvenile absence epilepsy, juvenile myoclonic epilepsy, and other epileptic syndromes may have higher risk of recurrence even after 2 years of seizure freedom. Similarly, those with structural malformation and abnormalities such as cortical dysplasia, gliosis, and mesial temporal sclerosis are at the higher risk of recurrence. Children with idiopathic epilepsy who had infrequent seizures, which were easily controlled with ASD, have fewer chances of recurrence.

If the child was on multiple ASDs, the first ASD to be introduced is to be withdrawn first and the last ASD must be the last to go. If the child was on add-on drug such as benzodiazepines, they must be withdrawn first before tapering the last conventional ASD. For example, if the child was well controlled for 2 years on LEV, VPA, and CLB, the sequence of withdrawal could be LEV, CLB, and then VPA. Each drug will be withdrawn slowly over 2–3 months. Hence, for those on multiple ASDs, tapering might take longer time.

Antiepileptic Drug Level Monitoring

Therapeutic drug monitoring (TDM) is expensive, and the facility is often not available in the majority of the institutions. It is theoretically useful when there is a breakthrough or refractory seizure to assess the compliance. It is useful for detecting antiepileptic drug toxicity, especially when the child is on phenytoin, which has dose-dependent pharmacokinetics. In clinical practice, the only indication of drug monitoring is to diagnose suspected clinical toxicity. In the majority of other indications, treatment decisions are often not based on TDM but on clinical response. Regular measurement of drug levels and liver function tests with sodium valproate is not required in case the child has well-controlled epilepsy and is asymptomatic for liver disease. In case the child in on multiple ASDs, which have drug interactions when given together, drug level measurement might guide for optimizing drugs and doses.

KEY MESSAGES

- Focal epilepsy responds well to carbamazepine, oxcarbazepine, levetiracetam, and phenytoin; whereas, generalized epilepsy responds well to sodium valproate and levetiracetam.
- Sodium valproate must be avoided in those with suspected metabolic or liver disorder; phenytoin and carbamazepine must be avoided in epileptic encephalopathy and those with genetic epilepsy with febrile seizure plus.
- Side effects must be explained to parents well ahead of prescription—drug rash and Stevens–Johnson with phenytoin, carbamazepine, and lamotrigine; weight gain and polycystic ovarian disease with valproate; behavioral side effects with levetiracetam.
- Avoid polypharmacy as much as possible, reach the maximum tolerable dose of the ASD before adding second ASD.
- There is a limited role of therapeutic drug monitoring (TDM) except for the diagnosis of suspected drug toxicity.

CHAPTER 34

Management of Acute Seizure and Status Epilepticus

◼ DEFINITION

Status epilepticus (SE) has been defined by the International League against Epilepsy (ILAE, 2015) as a condition resulting from the failure of mechanisms responsible for seizure termination, or from initiation of mechanisms which lead to abnormally prolonged seizures. There is a clear risk of neuronal death, neuronal injury, and alteration of neuronal network with SE depending on the type of seizure and duration of the seizure.

In the timeline, the ILAE has introduced two terms—T1 and T2. T1 refers to time beyond which seizure should be regarded as "continuous seizure activity" whereas T2 is a timeline beyond which there is a clear risk of long-term complications. The treatment must be initiated within the T1 time frame, considering that the majority of seizures last for less than T1 duration, and if prolonged beyond this time, it must be considered for treatment. T1 and T2 time frames are delineated as follows, depending on the type of seizures (tonic–clonic, focal, or absence):

	T1 (min)	T2 (min)
Tonic–clonic SE	5	30
Focal SE	10	60
Absence SE	10–15	Unknown

Operational definition of SE: Continuous seizure activity persisting beyond 5 minutes or two or more discrete seizures between which there is incomplete recovery of consciousness

Based on time from the onset, SE is classified as early SE (within 30 minutes), established SE (30–120 minutes), refractory SE (120 minutes to 24 hours), and super-refractory SE (beyond 24 hours).

Status epilepticus has also been classified on the basis of presence (*convulsive SE*) or absence of motor manifestation (*nonconvulsive SE*).

◼ CLASSIFICATION OF STATUS EPILEPTICUS

Four axes are used to describe the SE: Axis 1 (semiology), Axis 2 (etiology); Axis 3 (EEG descriptor), and Axis 4 (age) **(Table 1)**.

- Axis 1: The semiology axis is broadly divided into those with motor manifestation and those without motor manifestation and based on the degree of impaired consciousness.
- Axis 2: Etiology is classified into known etiology and unknown etiology.
- Axis 3: In facilities where ambulatory electroencephalography (EEG) could be performed, this axis would serve to see the EEG correlate for the clinical seizure. It is described based on its location (generalized, lateralized, bilateral independent, and multifocal), pattern

CHAPTER 34: Management of Acute Seizure and Status Epilepticus | 477

TABLE 1: Taxonomical classification of status epilepticus.

Axis	Classification	Subclassification
Axis 1 (semiology)	With prominent motor symptoms	Convulsive SE, myoclonic SE, focal motor SE, tonic status, and hyperkinetic SE
	Without prominent motor symptoms	NCSE with coma, NCSE without coma (generalized, focal, and unknown)
Axis 2 (etiology)	Known etiology	Acute etiology (e.g., stroke and encephalitis), remote etiology (postencephalitis and posthead trauma); progressive etiology (tumors and neurodegenerative diseases); SE in defined electroclinical syndromes
	Unknown etiology	Cryptogenic
Axis 3 (EEG correlate)	Location	Generalized, lateralized, bilateral independent, and multifocal
	Pattern	Periodic and rhythmic delta activity
	Morphology of waveform	Sharpness, phases, amplitude, and polarity
	Time-related factors, modulation, and effect of intervention	Prevalence and frequency, duration
Axis 4 (age)	Age	Neonate (till 28 days); infant (1 month to 2 years); childhood (>2–12 years); adolescence and adulthood (>12–59 years)

(EEG: electroencephalography; NCSE: nonconvulsive status epilepticus; SE: status epilepticus)

(periodic and rhythmic delta activity), morphology of the waveform, time-related factors (prevalence, frequency, and duration), modulation (stimulus-induced or spontaneous), and effect of an intervention.
- *Axis 4:* Age of the patient (neonate, infant, childhood, adolescence, and adulthood)

■ **CASE VIGNETTES**

Case 1

A 5-year-old child presented to casualty with focal seizure involving right upper limb and lower limb for the last 15 minutes. Neuroimaging subsequently revealed neurocysticercosis in the left parietal area with marked perilesional edema. The corresponding EEG at emergency room (ER) showed slowing in the left parietal leads.

Interpretation: Axis 1 (prominent motor symptoms, focal motor SE), Axis 2 (unknown etiology at presentation), Axis 3 (lateralized left parietal delta slowing), and Axis 4 (childhood). Here, we commit to unknown etiology as MRI was performed subsequently and not at the time of SE.

Case 2

A 2-month-old girl was brought to the pediatric casualty with multiple episodes of multifocal clonic jerks, each lasting for 2–3 minutes in the last 1 hour. Her blood glucose was 34 mg/dL at the time of the presentation. Corresponding EEG could not be performed.

Interpretation: Axis 1 (prominent motor symptoms and focal motor clonic), Axis 2 [known etiology, acute (hypoglycemia)], Axis 3 (cannot be commented), and Axis 4 (infant).

MANAGEMENT OF STATUS EPILEPTICUS

As per the American Epilepsy Society Guidelines (2016), the timeline for SE is divided into initial stabilization phase (0–5 minutes), initial therapy phase (5–20 minutes), second therapy phase (20–40 minutes), and third therapy phase (40–60 minutes).

Stabilization Phase (0–5 Minutes)

The initial stabilization phase is often considered a first-aid measure for acute seizure. It would include ensuring adequate airway, breathing, circulation, and oxygenation. The child needs to be monitored for vital signs, including oxygen saturation. Blood glucose needs to be assessed and hypoglycemia, if detected, needs to be corrected within this time frame. The majority of the seizures aborts within 5 minutes (T1) and may not require abortive medications such as benzodiazepines. In an out-of-hospital setting, the patient must be placed in the recovery position. It is a lateral decubitus position with arm closer to the floor being at the right angle to the body, the other arm placed under the cheeks, with the upper leg bent over the body creating stability to the convulsing child.

Initial Therapy Phase

The initial therapy phase would start from 5 minutes to a 20-minute endpoint. Benzodiazepines are the first line of treatment with an alternative of intravenous phenobarbitone (especially in neonates) **(Table 2)**. Intravenous diazepam, intravenous lorazepam, and intramuscular midazolam are the three drugs that have demonstrated level A evidence. IV lorazepam has a longer duration of action and fewer adverse effects when compared to the other two drugs. Other alternative benzodiazepines for prehospital management include intranasal midazolam (level B), buccal midazolam (level B), and rectal diazepam (level B). A maximum of two doses are allowed for diazepam and lorazepam. If the drug has been already administered in a prehospital setting, this dose must be considered for deciding on benzodiazepine. For example, if a child has

TABLE 2: Drugs for initial treatment of status epilepticus.

Drug and route of administration	Dose
Intravenous diazepam	0.15–0.2 mg/kg/dose (maximum 10 mg); may repeat once more in case of no clinical response
Intravenous lorazepam	0.1 mg/kg/dose (maximum 4 mg); may repeat once more in case of no clinical response
Intramuscular midazolam	0.2 mg/kg/dose AES guidelines: 5 mg (13–40 kg); 10 mg (>40 kg)
Rectal diazepam	0.2–0.5 mg/kg (maximum 20 mg)
Intranasal midazolam	0.2 mg/kg/dose (0.5 mg/single puff)
Buccal midazolam	0.3 mg/kg
Intranasal lorazepam	0.1 mg/kg
Intravenous phenobarbitone	15 mg/kg/dose

(AES: American Epilepsy Society)

TABLE 3: Drugs used during second phase therapy of status epilepticus.

Drug	Dose	Precaution
Phenytoin	15–20 mg/kg/dose (maximum 1,500 mg)	Rate @1 mg/kg/min
Fosphenytoin	20 mg PE/kg/dose (maximum 1,500 mg)	Rate @3 mg/kg/min
Sodium valproate	20–40 mg/kg/dose (AES guidelines mention 40 mg/kg) (maximum 3,000 mg)	Rate @20 mg/min infusion
Levetiracetam	30–60 mg/kg/dose (AES guidelines mention 60 mg/kg) (maximum 4,500 mg)	Rate @6 mg/kg/min
Phenobarbitone	15–20 mg/kg/dose	Rate @2 mg/kg/min

(AES: American Epilepsy Society; PE: phenytoin equivalent)

received intranasal midazolam once (in the prescribed dose) before reaching the hospital in SE, we can give only one more dose of benzodiazepine (midazolam, lorazepam, and diazepam).

Second Therapy Phase

This second phase starts at 20 minutes and ends at 40-minute cut-off. The three drug options include fosphenytoin/phenytoin, valproate, and levetiracetam. None have demonstrated any superiority over the other. Fosphenytoin has favorable pharmacokinetics with fewer adverse effects and the ability to be administered faster than conventional phenytoin. These drugs can be administered only once in the doses mentioned. There is no role of reloading the same drug at a lower dose. If none of the above three drugs are available, phenobarbitone can be administered, provided the same was not used in the initial treatment phase. Consider the risk of respiratory depression, when you administer phenobarbitone after administering benzodiazepine. The drug doses are summarized in **Table 3**.

Third Therapy Phase

The third phase begins at the end of 40 minutes and ends at 60 minutes. The phase beyond 60 minutes is labeled as refractory SE. There is level U evidence to attempt another second-line drug that has not been tried or move on to one of the anesthetic agents (midazolam, thiopental, propofol, or phenobarbital), provided the facility for continuous EEG monitoring is available **(Table 4)**.

TABLE 4: Drugs used in third phase for status epilepticus management.

Drug	Dose
Thiopentone	5 mg/kg bolus followed by 3–5 mg/kg/h
Midazolam	0.2 mg/kg bolus followed by 0.05–2 mg/kg/h
Propofol	1–2 mg/kg bolus followed by 1–2 mg/kg/h
Pentobarbital	5–15 mg/kg bolus, followed by 0.5–5 mg/kg/h

REFRACTORY STATUS EPILEPTICUS DEFINITION

Persistent seizure activity beyond 60–120 minutes or failure of conventional drugs is considered refractory status epilepticus (RSE). There is a lot of variability in the definition of RSE with variability in the duration of the seizure (60–120 minutes) and the number of antiepileptic drugs (AEDs) (two to three) that have failed. Continuous EEG monitoring is often required to monitor

> **BOX 1:** Indications of continuous electroencephalography (EEG) monitoring.
>
> *Indications for continuous EEG:*
> - Recent clinical seizure or status epilepticus with no return to baseline beyond 10 minutes
> - Coma including postcardiac arrest
> - Epileptiform activity or periodic discharges on initial 30 minutes EEG
> - Intracranial hemorrhage including subarachnoid hemorrhage, traumatic brain injury, and intracranial hemorrhage
> - Suspected nonconvulsive status epilepticus in patient with altered sensorium
>
> *Source:* Brophy GM, Bell R, Claassen J, Alldredge B, Bleck TP, Glauser T, et al. Guidelines for management of status epilepticus. Neurocrit Care. 2012;17(1):3-23.

the treatment response among those with RSE **(Box 1)**.

Treatment

Achievement of burst suppression pattern or cessation of electrographic seizures on EEG is often the goal of treatment in RSE. Intravenous pyridoxine in a dose of 100 mg should be attempted under EEG monitoring among all children aged <2 years of age with RSE.

Anesthetic drugs including propofol, pentobarbitone, and midazolam are treatment options. Midazolam is efficacious, short acting, easy to titrate, and has a lesser risk of hypotension compared to pentobarbitone. However, the latter has a lesser risk of breakthrough seizure following withdrawal as compared to midazolam. Propofol has a risk of propofol-related infusion syndrome (PRIS), which can be fatal. Vasopressors are often required to combat hypotension secondary to the administration of these drugs.

High-dose phenobarbitone (20 mg/kg loading followed by 5 mg/kg every 15–30 minutes till a maximum of 80 mg/kg or achievement of burst suppression on EEG) has been tried at many centers. Other drugs include inhalational anesthetic agents such as isoflurane and desflurane. Ketamine has been used in many centers among children with RSE. It is an N-methyl-D-aspartate (NMDA) receptor antagonist and has potential risk for neurotoxicity. It is also known to increase intracranial pressure and is contraindicated in those with raised intracranial pressure.

Newer Drugs

Newer AEDs used in RSE with variable success include oral topiramate (10 mg/kg/day for 2 consecutive days followed by maintenance therapy of 5 mg/kg/day), IV lacosamide (adult doses of 200–400 mg; limited pediatric experience using 10 mg/kg dose), oral perampanel [α-amino-3-hydroxy5-methyl-4-isoxazolepropionic acid (AMPA) receptor antagonist], and injectable brivaracetam. The literature pertaining to the utility of perampanel is restricted to adults and to retrospective studies and case series. Stiripentol (oral) is useful for Dravet syndrome and severe myoclonic epilepsy of infancy. There are no randomized controlled trials on these newer antiseizure medications (ASDs) in children. Neurosteroids including brexanolone are in clinical trials for RSE. Immunomodulatory therapy including pulse methylprednisolone and intravenous immunoglobulin or plasma exchange has been attempted in children with RSE with variable success. Medications other than antiseizure medications that are known to act on status epilepticus include dexmedetomidine, amantadine, mefloquine, and verapamil. Children with suspected autoimmune encephalitis such as NMDA receptor encephalitis, VGKC (voltage-gated potassium channel)-related encephalitis, and Hashimoto encephalitis are expected to improve and show clinical response to immunomodulatory therapy.

The *ketogenic diet* has been successful in many cases of children with febrile infection-related epilepsy syndrome (FIRES). Epilepsy surgery including hemispherectomies, multiple subpial transections, and corpus callosotomy has been attempted in few cases of RSE. Vagal nerve stimulation is an attractive alternative for generalized RSE (success rate of 75%) but for the prohibitive cost of the treatment. There are anecdotal reports of the possible role of therapeutic hypothermia, intravenous lidocaine, magnesium sulfate, neuroactive steroids (allopregnanolone), and electroconvulsive therapy in RSE in adults.

Super-refractory Status Epilepticus

Status epilepticus that continues or recurs 24 hours or more after the onset of anesthetic therapy are labeled as super-refractory status epilepticus (SRSE). It also includes cases that recur on the withdrawal of anesthetic drugs.

Mechanisms for Super-refractory Status Epilepticus

- In SRSE, there is rapid internalization of postsynaptic gamma-aminobutyric acid (GABA) receptors resulting in the reduction of a number of inhibitory neurotransmitter receptors (receptor trafficking). This possibly leads to nonresponse to benzodiazepines in SRSE. Tonic inhibition of extrasynaptic GABA (due to which, GABA is not able to exhibit its inhibition of seizure) leads to failure of seizure cessation.
- Excitatory GABA (GABA is usually inhibitory, it may become excitatory during SRSE may contribute to SRSE).
- Increase in the number of excitatory glutamate AMPA receptors, and prolonged and unregulated NMDA receptor activation.
- Mitochondrial insufficiency leads to failure of seizure termination.
- Inflammatory process is considered important in the persistence of SE. This inflammatory mechanism provides a window to a possible role of immunotherapy in SRSE.
- Breach of blood–brain barrier leads to free entry of albumin into the brain. Once the free albumin reaches the brain, it results in transformation of astrocytes making it hypersynchronous and excitotoxic.

New-onset refractory status epilepticus (NORSE) is defined as "state of persistent seizures with no identifiable etiology in patients without preexisting epilepsy that lasts longer than 24 hours, despite optimal therapy." There is a potential role of autoimmune basis for this clinical condition with a possible role of immunotherapy. FIRES is often considered a subset of NORSE. There is an emerging role of anakinra and tocilizumab in management of NORSE considering elevated cytokine levels following refractory seizures.

Non-convulsive status epilepticus must be considered among those with prolonged unresponsiveness following convulsive status epilepticus. This condition can be diagnosed using 24-hour video EEG monitoring. Untreated non-convulsive status epilepticus can lead to irreversible hypoxic brain injury.

Addressing the Underlying Etiology

Broadly, the etiology of RSE/SRSE can be clubbed under infectious, parainfectious, inflammatory, demyelinating, autoimmune, metabolic, traumatic, structural, and genetic causes. The common and uncommon causes of RSE are listed in **Table 5**. Traditionally, RSE was classified as symptomatic, if acute etiology such as stroke or encephalitis has been established as an etiology. RSE could also be seen in a child with a previous neurological insult such as perinatal asphyxia, intracranial bleed, or encephalitis

TABLE 5: Etiology of refractory status epilepticus.	
Broad group	**Etiology**
Common causes	Cerebrovascular diseases; CNS infection (bacterial meningitis, Japanese encephalitis, and herpes encephalitis); intracranial tumors; head trauma; withdrawal or low level of AED; hypoxic or anoxic related; metabolic disturbances (electrolyte imbalances, glucose imbalance, organ failures, and acidosis)
Uncommon causes for RSE	Anti-NMDA receptor encephalitis, paraneoplastic encephalitis, Hashimoto's encephalopathy, POLG mutation (mitochondrial disorder), HIV, genetic causes (ring chromosome 20 and Angelman syndrome), and drug/toxin induced (chemotherapeutic drugs)

(AED: antiepileptic drug; CNS: central nervous system; NMDA: N-methyl-D-aspartate; POLG: polymerase gamma; HIV: human immunodeficiency virus)

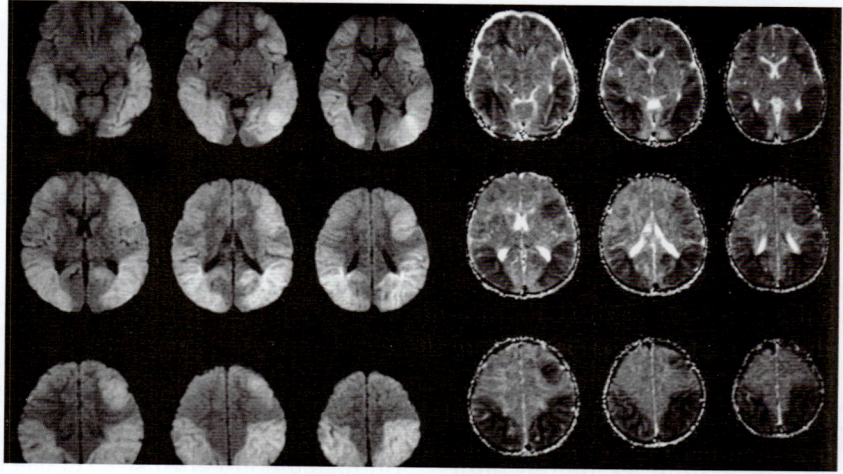

Fig. 1: MRI brain DWI images and ADC map showing hypoxic–ischemic brain injury following refractory status epilepticus (RSE). (ADC: apparent diffusion coefficient; DWI: diffusion-weighted imaging)

(remote symptomatic RSE). Similarly, RSE can occur as a manifestation of ongoing progressive neurodegenerative disease such as mitochondrial disorder, fatty acid oxidation disorder, and other progressive myoclonic epilepsies.

■ PROGNOSIS

Overall mortality with SE is around 20%. Short-term fatality rate for RSE is 16–39%. There is always a risk of neuronal injury with ongoing RSE. Mortality of SRSE is 30–40% with poor functional outcome in 75% of survivors. Various MRI findings have been described in children with RSE. These hypoxic–ischemic changes following RSE have been called as hypoxic–ischemic brain injury (HIBI). Changes are evident in watershed areas (areas between those supplied by anterior cerebral artery/middle cerebral artery (ACA/MCA) and MCA/posterior cerebral artery (PCA)] where there is a paucity of blood supply following a hypoxic event **(Fig. 1)**.

Flowchart 1: Algorithm for management of status epilepticus in children.

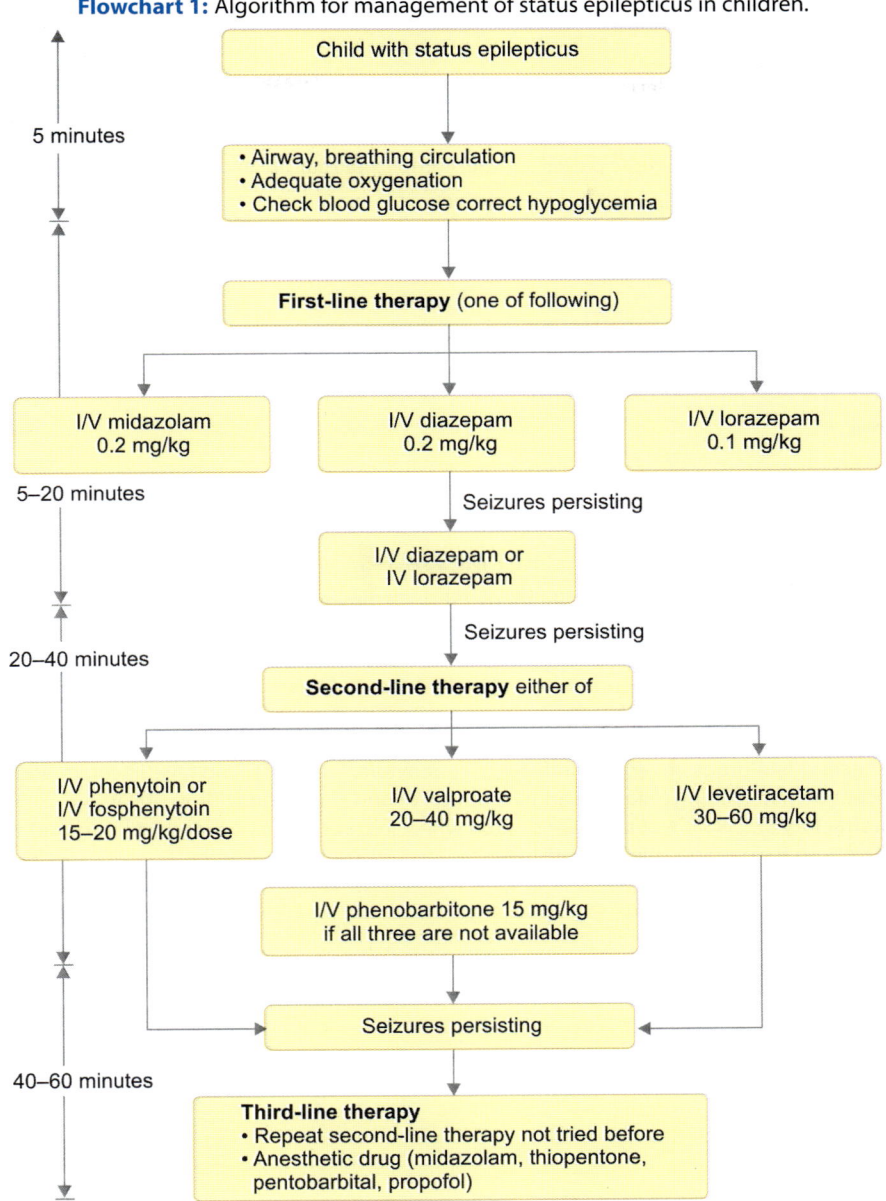

Status epilepticus severity scoring (STESS) scores have been used in adults for prediction of mortality among patients presenting with SE **(Table 6)**. The score is based on four criteria—consciousness, worst seizure type, age, and history of previous seizure. It is an excellent simple tool for predicting mortality and guide aggressive early treatment among those with favorable scores.

The management protocol for SE is summarized in **Flowchart 1**.

TABLE 6: Status epilepticus severity scoring (STESS).

Factor description		Score
Consciousness	Alert/somnolescent/confused	0
	Stuporous/comatose	1
Worst seizure type	Simple partial seizure, complex partial, absence, and myoclonic	0
	Generalized convulsive	1
	Nonconvulsive status in coma	2
Age	<65 years	0
	>65 years	2
History of previous seizure	Yes	0
	No or unknown	1
Total score		**0–6**

Note: Favorable score for survival is 0–2.

KEY MESSAGES

- There are two timelines in status epilepticus (SE)—T1 beyond which seizure should be regarded as continuous seizure activity and T2 is a timeline beyond which there is a clear risk of long-term complication.
- SE is classified under four axis—semiology (Axis 1), etiology (Axis 2), EEG descriptor (Axis 3), and age (Axis 4).
- Benzodiazepines remain the first drug of choice for the initial management of SE.
- All the second-line drugs are equally effective—phenytoin, valproate, and levetiracetam and there is no concept of mini-loading following administration of one antiepileptic drug (AED).
- Super-refractory SE (SRSE) would be considered when seizures persist beyond 24 hours and there are limited options for treating children with SRSE.

CHAPTER 35: Treatment of Infections of Nervous System

■ INTRODUCTION

Infections in the central nervous system (CNS) are broadly divided into bacterial, viral, protozoal, and fungal infections. Risk factors for children to develop CNS infections include daycare attendance, lack of immunization, poor hygiene, and low socioeconomic status. This chapter presents an overview of the management of specific CNS infections.

■ MENINGITIS

The majority of the cases of pyogenic meningitis are clustered below 5 years of age. The three most common organisms that result in pyogenic meningitis are *Haemophilus influenzae* type B, *Streptococcus pneumoniae*, and *Neisseria meningitidis*. Other organisms that cause meningitis include *Staphylococcus aureus, Escherichia coli, Klebsiella* spp., and *Acinetobacter* spp. *Pseudomonas, Salmonella,* and *Citrobacter* are other rare causes of pyogenic meningitis. The causative organism varies with the underlying risk factor **(Box 1)**.

The majority of children present with nonspecific symptoms such as fever, excessive irritability, repeated vomiting, lethargy, or refusal to feed. Meningeal signs, signs of raised intracranial pressure, may be absent in infants and young children. Hence, clinical suspicion with laboratory confirmation is essential for the diagnosis of pyogenic meningitis. In children with papilledema, focal neurological deficit, refractory seizures, and Glasgow Coma Score (GCS) <12, neuroimaging should be performed before performing lumbar puncture. Immediate complications in untreated patients include shock, raised intracranial pressure, seizure, and syndrome of inappropriate antidiuretic hormone secretion (SIADH). Early empirical antibiotic treatment is essential to prevent short- and long-term complications **(Table 1)**.

Penicillin is no longer used as the first-line antibiotic for empirical treatment of pyogenic meningitis. Rather with the emergence of resistance in *Pneumococcus* to penicillin and third-generation cephalosporins, a combination of ceftriaxone and vancomycin is recommended as the first line for empirical

---

BOX 1: Risk factors for acute bacterial meningitis and its implicating organism.

Immunocompromised state:
- Complement deficiency (Meningococcemia)
- T-cell defect (*Listeria monocytogenes*)

Asplenia or following splenectomy:
- Pneumococcal meningitis
- *Haemophilus influenzae* type B meningitis

Skull base fracture, meningomyelocele, CSF shunt, and neurosurgical procedure:
- *Staphylococcus epidermidis* (Coagulase-negative staphylococci)
- *Staphylococcus aureus*
- *Escherichia coli/Klebsiella* spp.

(CSF: cerebrospinal fluid)

TABLE 1: Initial or empirical antibiotic therapy for bacterial meningitis.		
Age	Initial antibiotic	Alternative
Neonate	Cefotaxime plus amikacin	Ampicillin (for listeria)
2 months to 5 years	Ceftriaxone or cefotaxime plus vancomycin	Meropenem plus vancomycin or linezolid

- *Ampicillin:* 300 mg/kg/24 hours, in four divided doses (maximum: 12 g/day)
- *Ceftriaxone:* 100 mg/kg/24 hours, in two divided doses (maximum: 4 g/day)
- *Cefotaxime:* 200 mg/kg/24 hours, in four divided doses (maximum: 12 g/day)
- *Vancomycin:* 60 mg/kg/24 hours, in three to four divided doses (maximum: 4 g/day)
- *Meropenem:* 120 mg/kg/24 hours, in three divided doses (maximum: 6 g/day)
- *Amikacin:* 15 mg/kg/24 hours, in three divided doses (maximum: 1.5 g/day)
- *Linezolid:* 10 mg/kg/dose 8 hourly (maximum: 600 mg/dose)

management of children with pyogenic meningitis. The antibiotic can be revised based on the culture reports of cerebrospinal fluid (CSF) and blood and clinical response to empirical treatment. The duration of treatment would ideally depend on the isolate in the CSF culture: *Haemophilus* (7–10 days), *Meningococcus* (7 days), *Pneumococcus* (14 days), *Staphylococcus* (14–21 days), and *Listeria* (21 days). Empirical treatment should be ideally continued for a minimum of 14 days among children with meningitis when the organism could not be isolated. Children with partial or no response should always be evaluated for complications, including subdural effusion and hydrocephalus, which may require neurosurgical intervention. A meta-analysis has shown that adjunctive corticosteroids (low dose) use is associated with reduced risk of hearing loss and neurological sequelae in children with acute bacterial meningitis.

■ ENCEPHALITIS

A case of acute encephalitis syndrome (AES) is defined as *"A person of any age, at any time of the year, with acute onset of fever and a change in mental status (including symptoms such as confusion, disorientation, coma, or inability to talk) and/or new onset of seizures (excluding simple febrile seizures)".* Encephalitis is a pathological diagnosis signifying inflammation of the brain. The term "encephalopathy" refers to an alteration in consciousness or diffuse cerebral dysfunction that may result from traumatic, infective, inflammatory, and metabolic causes. Hence, all encephalitis result in encephalopathy, but not all encephalopathies have encephalitis.

Most common causes of encephalitis are enterovirus, herpes simplex virus (HSV) type 1 and type 2, varicella Zoster virus (VZV), Epstein–Barr virus (EBV), Japanese encephalitis (JE) virus, cytomegalovirus (CMV), and human herpes virus (HHV) type 6 (HHV-6). Children with acute viral encephalitis often present with fever, seizure, and altered sensorium with or without focal neurological deficit. The presence of dystonia and other extrapyramidal features favor JE. The presence of parotitis raises the possibility of mumps virus as the causative agent. History of preceding diarrheal illness favors enterovirus and the presence of petechiae, and bleeding manifestations would raise the possibility of dengue encephalitis or dengue-associated encephalopathy.

Children with acute viral encephalitis are often treated conservatively. Management of seizures, raised intracranial pressure,

TABLE 2: Specific treatment in children with acute viral encephalitis.

Condition	Treatment
Herpes encephalitis and Varicella-Zoster infection	IV acyclovir (20 mg/kg/dose 8 hourly) for 21 days
CMV encephalitis	Intravenous ganciclovir 5 mg/kg three times a day along with IV foscarnet 60 mg/kg 8 hourly
H1N1 encephalitis	Oseltamivir [>12 months: 30 mg BD (<15 kg), 45 mg BD (16–23 kg), 60 mg BD (24–40 kg); 75 mg BD (>40 kg)] [<3 months: 12 mg BD; 3–5 months: 20 mg BD; 6–11 months: 25 mg BD]

(CMV: cytomegalovirus)

and peripheral circulatory failure takes precedence over specific therapies. There are no specific antiviral therapies except for herpes simplex virus, varicella zoster virus, CMV encephalitis, and H1N1-associated encephalitis **(Table 2)**. Isolation of organisms in CSF is essential for the institution of specific treatment except for empirical treatment with acyclovir. One may consider stopping empirical acyclovir once CSF testing for HSV is negative. The role of intravenous immunoglobulin and minocycline is controversial in the treatment of Japanese encephalitis.

■ TUBERCULAR MENINGITIS

Tubercular meningitis (TBM) is a common cause of subacute to chronic encephalitis in Indian children. TBM is characterized by CSF lymphocytic pleocytosis, raised CSF proteins, and low CSF sugars, with or without isolation of tubercular bacilli. Tubercular bacilli may be detected by Ziehl–Neelsen staining, culture, nucleic acid amplification (NAA) test, or polymerase chain reaction (PCR). Neuroimaging findings of basal exudates, hydrocephalus, vascular stroke involving basal ganglia, or meningeal enhancement are highly suggestive of TBM.

As per the joint statement of the Indian Academy of Pediatrics and Revised National Tuberculosis Control Program (RNTCP) guidelines (2019), any new microbiologically confirmed extrapulmonary tuberculosis should be treated with 2 months of isoniazid, rifampicin, pyrazinamide, and ethambutol (HRZE) followed by 4 months of HRE. As per National Tuberculosis Elimination Program (NTEP), 2 months of HRZE/S followed by 10 months of HRE is recommended. However, many experts consider 6 months of treatment to be inadequate for TBM. The World Health Organization (WHO) recommends 12 months of treatment with 2 months of HRZES (S = streptomycin) followed by 10 months of HRE. Doses of HRZE include 10, 15, 35, and 20 mg/kg, respectively, on a daily basis **(Box 2)**. Drugs with good CNS penetration include isoniazid, pyrazinamide, ethionamide, fluoroquinolones (ofloxacin, levofloxacin), and linezolid. Trials are ongoing for higher doses of rifampicin (30 mg/kg), regimen in which ethambutol is replaced with levofloxacin, and use of aspirin for the first 8 weeks to reduce the risk of new infarction. Tumor necrosis factor (TNF) alpha inhibitors like thalidomide and anti-TNF alpha monoclonal antibodies like infliximab and adalimumab and soluble TNF

BOX 2: Antitubercular drug treatment for tubercular meningitis.

Drug treatment of tubercular meningitis as per IAP and NTEP (2022)
- Two combination drugs are available:
  - Three-drug combination $H_{50}R_{75}Z_{150}$ (pediatric designated as tablet P)
  - Adult $H_{75}R_{150}Z_{400}E_{275}$ (tablet for adults designated as tablet A)
  - 100 mg tablet of ethambutol (tablet E)
- Prescription of combination drugs as per the weight: (2 months of HRZE/S followed by 8–10 months of HRE)
  - 4–7 kg: 1P + 1E
  - 8–11 kg: 2P + 2E
  - 12–15 kg: 3P + 3E
  - 16–24 kg: 4P + 4E
  - 25–29 kg: 3P + 3E + 1A
  - 30–39 kg: 2P + 2E + 2A

(IAP: Indian Academy of Pediatrics; NTEP: National Tuberculosis Elimination Program)

alpha fusion protein (etanercept) are some of the host-directed therapies that act on dysregulated host immune response in TBM. Thalidomide and infliximab have been tried in optochiasmatic arachnoiditis and steroid-resistant paradoxical reactions.

Steroids are recommended for all children with TBM along with antitubercular drugs. Oral prednisolone is given in the dose of 1–2 mg/kg/day for 4 weeks followed by slow tapering over the next 4 weeks. The alternative is oral dexamethasone 0.15 mg/kg/dose every 6 hours. Oral pyridoxine is recommended along with antitubercular drugs considering the high dose of isoniazid and the presence of malnutrition predisposing these children to this micronutrient deficiency.

Management of Complications of Tubercular Meningitis

- *Paradoxical upgrading reaction:* It should be considered among children with new tuberculoma or enlargement of pre-existing tuberculoma once antitubercular therapy (ATT) has been started. This should be managed with high-dose steroids along with the continuation of ATT. Pulse methylprednisolone (30 mg/kg/day) for 5 days followed by oral prednisolone for 3–4 weeks or till clinical improvement is suggested for the management of paradoxical reaction. It needs to be differentiated from drug resistant tuberculosis.
- Other complications including opto-chiasmatic arachnoiditis and spinal arachnoiditis are also managed with high-dose steroids. However, these clinical conditions often require long-term steroids or steroid-sparing immunomodulators such as thalidomide, levamisole, and interferon-gamma therapy.
- *Tubercular vasculitis:* In the light of current evidence, there is no role of aspirin in the prophylaxis of stroke or treatment of tubercular vasculitis. Aspirin use is restricted to only those with moyamoya disease secondary to TBM.
- *Hydrocephalus:* The majority of patients with TBM would often require surgical intervention except in those with normal sensorium and no focal neurological deficit. Two major options for surgical interventions include ventriculoperitoneal (VP) shunt and third ventriculostomy. Many neurosurgeons consider that patients with grade III–IV hydrocephalus with features of raised intracranial pressure would require external ventricular drainage (EVD) prior to definitive surgery. The presence of clinical improvement with EVD would guide the need for shunt surgery. Endoscopic third ventriculostomy (ETV) has a limited role and is technically difficult in TBM as basal exudates and inflammation often obscure the base of the third ventricle for access.

NEUROCYSTICERCOSIS

Neurocysticercosis (NCC) is caused by the larval form of the tapeworm *Taenia solium*. It is the most common cause of the first unprovoked seizure and acquired epilepsy in endemic areas of developing countries. It can present variably depending on the location and stage of cysts in the nervous system and the host immune response. Apart from seizure, headache, cognitive decline, extrapyramidal movement disorder, and behavioral problems are common among children with NCC. NCC evolves through stages of vesicular, colloidal, granulonodular, and calcified lesions. NCC can affect any part of the brain. Parenchymal lesions often present with seizures.

The diagnosis of NCC is often radiological. Presence of a cystic lesion (the center of a NCC lesion looks bright on T2 and dark on T1 image) with eccentric scolex favors vesicular or colloidal stages of NCC. NCC is considered active or viable in vesicular, colloidal, and granulonodular stages. In contrast, tuberculoma has caseous material that looks isointense or hypointense (dark) on a T2-weighted image. The majority of NCC are small, have well-defined margins, may be single or multiple, and few may look matted together with the presence of significant perilesional edema. Parenchymal NCC often involve gray matter and white matter junctions. In contrast, tuberculoma often prefers the base of the brain and their cisterns. Both NCC and tuberculoma have ring-enhancing lesions **(Table 3)**. Calcified lesions can also have perilesional edema. Calcified lesions are best appreciated on susceptibility-weighted images (SWI) where it reveals blooming effect [calcified lesion looks dark on SWI and gradient echo (GRE) images]. The mainstay of treatment for NCC with a viable cyst is antihelminthic therapy. Calcified lesions are by convention not treated with antihelminthic therapy. The drug of choice is albendazole (15 mg/kg/day in two divided doses) for 14 days, although studies have shown that shorter duration (7 days) of albendazole is not inferior to 14 days or 28 days of therapy **(Flowchart 1)**. Repeat imaging (MRI brain) is preferably performed 6–12 months after the antihelminthic treatment. If the lesion is still active, then a combination of albendazole and praziquantel would be administered. If the lesion had calcified, then antiseizure medications would be administered for 2 years. At the end of 2 years of seizure freedom, if the EEG is normal, antiseizure medications are withdrawn.

BRAIN ABSCESS

Brain abscess refers to focal infection of brain parenchyma that evolves into a collection

TABLE 3: Radiological appearance of neurocysticercosis (NCC) and tuberculoma.

Neurocysticercosis	Tuberculoma
Lesion <20 mm	Lesion >20 mm
Commonly affects gray-matter and white-matter junction (supratentorial)	Commonly involves basal cisterns and infratentorial stage
T2 core appears hyperintense with hypointense scolex	T2 hypointense core
Meningeal involvement unlikely	Meningeal involvement more likely
In multiple NCC, we may see different stages of NCC (few in colloidal and few in nodular-calcified stage)	In multiple tuberculoma, they are all in the same stage and may be conglomerate

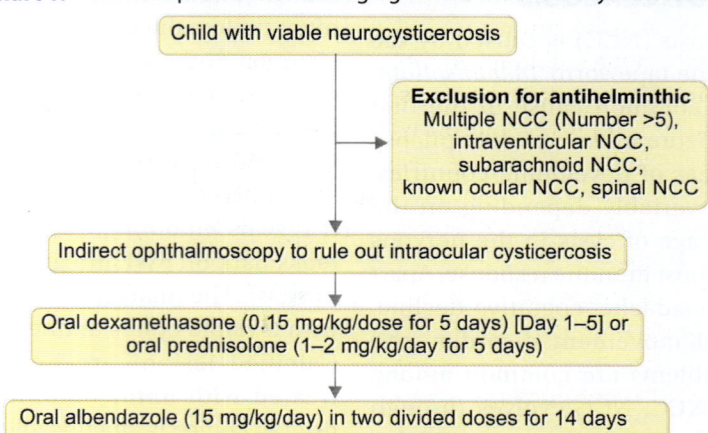

Flowchart 1: Treatment protocol for managing a child with neurocysticercosis (NCC).

of pus. Development of brain abscess leads to pressure symptoms, features of raised intracranial pressure, and evidence of midline shift. The infection reaches the brain either through contagious spread from an infection of ear and sinuses or through hematogenous spread from a distant focus of infection. In rare cases, it may follow an open traumatic skull fracture. Children with cyanotic congenital heart disease, sinus or otogenic infection, immunocompromised state, penetrating skull fractures, and VP shunt are at risk for development of brain abscess. The majority of brain abscess is caused by *Streptococcus*, gram-negative anaerobic bacilli, Enterobacteriaceae, and *Staphylococcus aureus*. In contrast, a spinal epidural abscess is most commonly caused by *Staphylococcus aureus*. The clinical symptoms of brain abscess are often nonspecific such as fever, seizure, focal neurological deficit, altered sensorium, and features of raised intracranial pressure.

Neuroimaging, preferably MRI brain with contrast, is essential for the diagnosis of brain abscess. Three key radiological differentials of brain abscess include tuberculoma, cryptococcoma, and toxoplasmosis. The latter two often involve basal ganglia and are more common in immunocompromised patients. Tuberculoma often affects the base of the brain (infratentorial location), although it may involve supratentorial brain parenchyma also.

A combination of third-generation cephalosporin (cefotaxime or ceftriaxone) with vancomycin (or cloxacillin) and metronidazole is the standard empirical antibiotic therapy **(Table 4)**. In immunocompromised patients, voriconazole and trimethoprim–sulfamethoxazole can be added. In post neurosurgical brain abscess, combination of

TABLE 4: Treatment of brain abscess.

Antibiotic	Doses
Ceftriaxone	100 mg/kg/day in two divided doses
Cefotaxime	200 mg/kg/day in two divided doses
Metronidazole	30 mg/kg/day in three divided doses
Vancomycin	60 mg/kg/day in four divided doses
Cloxacillin	200 mg/kg/day in four divided doses

carbapenem with vancomycin or linezolid is recommended. A total duration of 6-8 weeks is preferred among children with brain abscess. Antibiotics can often be revised based on the culture report. Children who fail to respond clinically, with no decrease in the size despite 3-4 weeks of appropriate antibiotics, may then require surgical intervention. An abscess >2.5 cm that is multiloculated and fungal abscess need surgical drainage (stereotactic aspiration) at the outset of diagnosis. The European Society of Clinical Microbiology guidelines recommend excision of brain abscess where feasible except for toxoplasmosis. The guidelines also recommend the use of adjunctive glucocorticoids in cases with severe perilesional edema or impending herniation. Incision (laminectomy) and drainage are the treatment of choice for spinal epidural abscess along with 6-8 weeks of intravenous antibiotics.

ACUTE INFECTIVE TRANSVERSE MYELITIS

Children with acute flaccid symmetrical motor and sensory weakness with or without bladder involvement and with a definitive sensory dermatome should raise clinical suspicion of acute transverse myelitis (ATM). This group of idiopathic transverse myelitis is treated with pulse methylprednisolone 30 mg/kg/day for 5 days followed by oral prednisolone (1-2 mg/kg/day for the next 4 weeks followed by slow tapering). However, if these symptoms develop along with ongoing fever, rash, or systemic illness, infective causes of myelopathy should also be considered. These children often have meningismus and concurrent systemic infection and may be immunocompromised. Most of these children often have CSF pleocytosis with raised CSF proteins. It is often clinically indistinguishable from idiopathic transverse myelitis. Common viral causes of infective myelopathy include HSV, HHV-6, VZV, CMV, and EBV. Other uncommon infections include measles, mumps, dengue, coxsackievirus, NCC, *Mycoplasma* infection, borreliosis, and tuberculosis. CSF evaluation with the isolation of organisms by PCR or serology and culture is mandatory for the diagnosis of infective myelopathy.

INFECTIVE CAUSES OF PERIPHERAL NEUROPATHY

The most common infections that affect the peripheral nervous system in children include HIV, leprosy, diphtheria, and paralytic forms of rabies. Types of infective neuropathy include polyradiculoneuropathy (Lyme disease), distal symmetrical polyneuropathy (HIV), mononeuritis multiplex (leprosy), and demyelinating polyneuropathy (diphtheria).

Children with bulbar weakness followed by descending motor weakness involving neck muscles and upper limb followed by lower limb muscles should raise the suspicion of postdiphtheritic polyneuropathy. Children with this condition usually have a history of swelling in the neck (bull neck) in the recent past (3-5 weeks) and are partly immunized or unimmunized children. Postdiphtheritic polyneuropathy is often considered pure motor neuropathy that can be demonstrated and confirmed in the nerve conduction study.

HIV-infected children may present with a tingling sensation in feet, sensory loss, pain, and distal muscle weakness. This may also develop following antiretroviral drugs such as stavudine and didanosine. Any child with unexplained skin ulcerations in feet in the endemic area must be always evaluated for leprosy. Children tend to have anesthetic skin patch with thickened nerves along with sensory-motor weakness.

Paralytic rabies can have GBS-like clinical presentation. Rabies must be suspected among children with large animal bite (grade III–IV) in the recent past. These patients, although they receive antirabies vaccination (ARV), often fail to receive rabies-specific immunoglobulin indicated in grade III–IV animal bites. Paralytic rabies must also be suspected when there is a focal paralysis in a part of the body where the animal had bitten in the recent past.

MYOSITIS

Myositis refers to inflammation of the skeletal muscle, manifesting clinically with pain, weakness, muscle tenderness, and swelling. It can result from bacterial, fungal, or viral infections. Generalized involvement of muscles is called *polymyositis*. If pus is formed within the muscles, usually secondary to hematogenous spread, it is called *pyomyositis*. The majority of bacterial organisms result in focal infection of the muscle, and viral and fungal organisms often cause polymyositis.

The most common organism implicated in pyomyositis is *Staphylococcus aureus*. Group A *Streptococcus* infection often results in necrotizing myositis. *Brucella, Salmonella, Mycoplasma, Pseudomonas,* and *Clostridium* species are other uncommon causes of bacterial myositis. *Clostridium* species result in gas gangrene. Among the viral causes, influenza virus A and B are the most common implicated organism for tropical viral myositis. Other uncommon viral causes of myositis include HIV, human T-cell lymphotropic virus (HTLV), and dengue virus. *Candida* is the most common fungal cause for myositis. The most common parasite for muscle involvement is *Trichinella spiralis*. The other parasites include malaria, cysticercosis, and sarcocystis.

OTHER BACTERIAL CNS INFECTIONS

Other bacterial infections that affect the CNS include *Borrelia, Leptospira, Mycoplasma,* and *Treponema* **(Table 5)**. *Bartonella* species is known to result in cat-scratch disease (CSD). Neurological involvement is uncommon in CSD. In the endemic area for CSD, any child with acute encephalopathy with skin papule and regional lymphadenopathy must be considered for the diagnosis of CSD. Rarely, CSD can result in retrobulbar neuritis presenting with acute vision loss. It is a self-limited illness and often does not require antibiotics. Any child with hypopigmented or reddish skin lesions with loss of sensation, thick peripheral nerves, presence of peripheral neuropathy, and/or trigeminal neuralgia must be considered for infection by *Mycobacterium leprae*. A combination of rifampicin, dapsone, and clofazimine or minocycline is used for the treatment of leprosy.

VIRAL INFECTIONS OF CENTRAL NERVOUS SYSTEM

Viral infections can affect the CNS resulting in various clinical syndromes including meningoencephalitis, acute cerebellar ataxia, and acute flaccid paralysis **(Table 6)**. These may also present as intrauterine infection. Most common organisms implicated with meningoencephalitis include herpes simplex virus, Epstein–Barr virus, CMV, and West Nile virus. See **Chapter 11** on approach to a child with altered sensorium and coma to understand the differentiating clinical features and radiological findings of each viral infection.

Herpes simplex virus, varicella-zoster virus, CMV, and nonpolio enterovirus may result in Guillain–Barré syndrome and ATM.

TABLE 5: Clinical features, laboratory diagnosis, and management of children with central nervous system (CNS) bacterial infections.

Disease	Clinical features	Laboratory diagnosis	Management
Lyme disease (*Borrelia burgdorferi*)	Cranial neuropathy especially facial nerve palsy, subacute to chronic meningitis, radiculitis, neuritis in presence of erythema migrans	• CSF lymphocytosis with CSF raised protein • Confirmation by EIA or • IgG/IgM Western blot testing	Doxycycline (1–2 mg/kg BD) or amoxicillin (50 mg/kg/day in three divided doses) or cefuroxime axetil (30 mg/kg/day in two divided doses) for 14–21 days
Leptospirosis (caused by *Leptospira*)	High-grade fever, severe headache and myalgia, and conjunctival congestion starting to recover followed by neurological involvement (aseptic meningitis). Child may have jaundice, renal failure, and hemorrhage	ELISA and latex agglutination testing for antibody for Leptospirosis	Doxycycline (1–2 mg/kg BD) or ceftriaxone (100 mg/kg/day in two divided doses)
Mycoplasma pneumoniae infection	*Mycoplasma* infection is associated with encephalitis, acute disseminated encephalomyelitis, acute cerebellitis, and acute flaccid paralysis	PCR for *Mycoplasma* from respiratory secretion. Antibody testing has high false positivity rate and not used for diagnosis	Azithromycin (10 mg/kg/dose BD) or doxycycline (1–2 mg/kg BD)
Congenital syphilis (neurological)	In context of maternal syphilis, infants may present with features of acute meningitis, stroke, and hydrocephalus	CSF analysis may reveal CSF lymphocytosis, raised proteins, and low sugar. VDRL and RPR antibody testing in CSF and serum is considered for diagnosis. EIA testing for treponema is highly sensitive	Crystalline penicillin (3 lakh IU/kg/day in four to six divided doses)

(CSF: cerebrospinal fluid; EIA: enzyme immunoassay; ELISA: enzyme-linked immunosorbent assay; PCR: polymerase chain reaction; RPR: rapid plasma regain; VDRL: Venereal disease research laboratory)

West Nile virus and enterovirus 71 may result in flaccid paralysis secondary to anterior horn cell involvement. Varicella has been typically associated with acute cerebellar ataxia **(Table 6)**. HIV infection can affect both the central and peripheral nervous systems **(Table 7)**. There is an emerging role of metagenomic next-generation sequencing (NGS) in establishing the infective etiology in acute encephalitis syndrome.

FUNGAL INFECTIONS OF CENTRAL NERVOUS SYSTEM

Yeast including *Candida* and *Cryptococcus*, molds including *Aspergillus* and mucormycosis, and dimorphic fungi including *Histoplasma capsulatum*, *Blastomyces dermatitidis*, and *Coccidioides immitis* can infect the CNS. Immunocompromised children, those on immunomodulators,

TABLE 6: Clinical features, laboratory diagnosis, and management of children with central nervous system (CNS) viral infections.

Viral infection	Neurological features	Diagnosis and treatment (if any)
Zika virus	• Guillain–Barré-like syndrome around 1 week after viral prodrome (fever, malaise, arthralgia, and rash) • Maternal infection, which often remains asymptomatic, results in microcephaly in baby, intracranial infection, and optic nerve hypoplasia	• Zika virus-specific IgM antibody testing by ELISA • RT-PCR testing in serum • Zika virus RNA isolation from CSF
Dengue virus	• *Dengue encephalopathy:* Altered sensorium in severe dengue infection (liver failure, metabolic acidosis, severe hyponatremia, shock, and DIC) with normal CSF analysis • *Dengue encephalitis:* Presence of encephalopathy with CSF pleocytosis and presence of dengue virus RNA or NS1 antigen in CSF • Dengue-associated Guillain–Barré syndrome or rhabdomyolysis syndrome • Dengue-associated neuro-ophthalmic complications such as optic neuropathy and maculopathy	Isolation of dengue virus RNA or NS1 antigen in CSF in cases of dengue encephalitis
Influenza virus including H1N1	• *Influenza encephalopathy:* Development of neurological manifestations (seizures, status epilepticus, and encephalopathy) following respiratory illness with often normal MRI study and normal CSF • *ANEC:* Rapid neurological deterioration with extrapyramidal features, seizures, and encephalopathy in an infant associated with influenza infection raises the possibility of ANEC. MRI brain typically shows bilateral symmetrical thalamic and basal ganglia hemorrhagic T2 hyperintensity • Children with *RANBP2* mutation have propensity to develop recurrent ANEC-like illness	• RT-PCR from nasopharyngeal swabs • ELISA antibody testing against hemagglutinin and neuraminidase antigen in serum
Chikungunya virus	• Acute encephalitis-like illness with coma and seizures • Perinatal chikungunya in newborns who are born to mothers with chikungunya; those who survive can develop cerebral palsy and global developmental delay	• IgM antibody capture ELISA (MAC-ELISA) in serum • RT-PCR testing in serum
Nipah virus	• Acute encephalitis [fever, headache, seizures, altered sensorium, marked hypotonia, areflexia, pinpoint pupil, and autonomic manifestations (tachycardia and hypertension)] • Relapsing Nipah virus encephalitis, which occurs several months to years after symptomatic or asymptomatic infection. This results in vasculitis and multiple white matter signal changes	• RT-PCR from nasal swab and CSF • IgG and IgM ELISA

Contd...

Contd...

Viral infection	Neurological features	Diagnosis and treatment (if any)
Mumps	• Aseptic meningitis (fever, headache, and meningeal signs) occurs within days to week after parotid swelling • Mumps encephalitis (early-onset) presents as febrile encephalopathy in presence of parotid swelling • *Postinfectious encephalitis:* It occurs within weeks of parotid swelling	• Lymphocytic pleocytosis with low sugar levels in CSF is suggestive of aseptic meningitis • Aseptic meningitis and mumps encephalitis need symptomatic treatment • Demyelinating lesions often respond to pulse methylprednisolone
Measles	• *Primary measles encephalitis (PME):* It occurs during active measles infection; presents as acute encephalopathy and seizures • *Acute postinfectious measles encephalitis (APME):* It occurs weeks to months after measles; can involve brain and spinal cord; presents as motor weakness, sensory loss, and altered mental status • *Measles inclusion body encephalitis (MIBE):* Drug-resistant seizures with altered sensorium months to years after measles infection; occurs in immuno-compromised children such as those with leukemia • *Subacute sclerosing panencephalitis (SSPE):* It presents with relentlessly progressive myoclonic epilepsy and retinal scars	• *PME:* MRI may show T2 hyperintensity; CSF may show lymphocytosis with raised proteins; measles-specific antibody will be negative in serum and CSF • *APME:* CSF shows myelin basic protein with lymphocytosis and raised protein; MRI shows multifocal T2 hyperintensity; treatment remains IVIG and steroids considering postinfectious/demyelinating pathology • *MIBE:* MRI is usually normal; CSF shows raised measles-specific antibodies • *SSPE:* MRI shows nonspecific white matter signal changes; EEG shows generalized periodic epileptiform discharges; demonstration of antimeasles antibody in CSF
Rabies	• Furious rabies often presents with classical signs of aerophobia and hydrophobia • Paralytic rabies present with ascending flaccid paralysis. It may also present with focal paralysis at the site of rabid animal bite	Viral antigen detection in CSF or corneal smear and RT-PCR for viral antigen detection
Japanese encephalitis virus (JEV)	Fever, headache, and vomiting followed by seizures, altered sensorium (acute febrile encephalopathy) with features of extrapyramidal system involvement (dystonia and choreoathetoid movement), and features of raised intracranial pressure	MRI brain shows symmetrical thalamic and basal ganglia lesion. JEV-specific IgM antibody detection by ELISA in CSF and serum. Treatment is largely supportive

Contd...

Contd...

Viral infection	Neurological features	Diagnosis and treatment (if any)
Chandipura virus	Rapidly progressive illness with fever, seizure, and encephalopathy with high mortality rate	RT-PCR for *Chandipura* virus
Poliomyelitis	• Paralytic poliomyelitis results in asymmetric patchy, flaccid pure motor weakness with or without cranial neuropathy or bulbar involvement • Residual paralysis following an attack of paralytic poliomyelitis is common. Few patients in the late adulthood may develop fresh paralysis called post-polio syndrome	Viral isolation from stool sample

(ANEC: acute necrotizing encephalopathy of childhood; CSF: cerebrospinal fluid; DIC: disseminated intravascular coagulation; ELISA: enzyme-linked immunosorbent assay; IVIG: intravenous immunoglobulin; NS1: nonstructural protein 1; RANBP2: RAN binding protein 2; RT-PCR: reverse transcription–polymerase chain reaction)

TABLE 7: Key clinical features of neurological infection with HIV.

Syndrome	Clinical feature
HIV encephalopathy	• Perinatally acquired HIV infection may present in late infancy with gradual loss of motor and cognitive abilities (progressive) along with generalized spasticity and acquired microcephaly; MRI showing diffuse cortical atrophy with intraparenchymal calcifications similar to TORCH infection • It may also present as global developmental delay/intellectual disability (static)
Other CNS features	Cognitive disturbance, behavioral and neuropsychiatric problems, epilepsy, and cerebrovascular stroke
Opportunistic infections	Toxoplasmosis* (encephalitis with hepatic involvement, can present as multiple ring-enhancing lesions in basal ganglia and thalamus), CMV† (retinitis, encephalitis affecting periventricular white matter, and axonal polyradiculoneuropathy), HSV (encephalitis), cryptococcal meningitis with typical basal ganglia involvement (pseudogelatinous cyst), and tubercular meningitis
Progressive multifocal leukoencephalopathy	Focal motor weakness including ataxia, cognitive impairment, vision impairment; MRI brain shows multifocal white matter T2 hyperintensities in subcortical white matter, cerebellum, and brainstem; diagnosis by *Polyomavirus* JC isolation by PCR
CNS lymphoma	Presents with seizures and focal neurological deficits; MRI shows single or multiple lesions in periventricular location with perilesional edema
Peripheral nervous system involvement	HIV-associated neuropathy (mononeuritis multiplex, symmetrical polyneuropathy, mononeuropathy, radiculopathy); HIV-associated myopathy; HIV-associated myelopathy

*Toxoplasmosis is managed with pyrimethamine–sulfadiazine combination.
†CMV requires ganciclovir plus foscarnet.
(CMV: cytomegalovirus; CNS: central nervous system; HSV: herpes simplex virus; PCR: polymerase chain reaction)

TABLE 8: Common fungal infections of central nervous system.

Fungal infection	Clinical features	Management
Candida	Cerebral abscess (in preterm), meningoencephalitis, ventriculitis, and vasculitis	Amp-B: 1 mg/kg/day or Liposomal Amp-B 3–5 mg/kg/day plus oral flucytosine* (25 mg/kg) for 28 days
Cryptococcosis	Chronic meningitis (fever, headache, nuchal rigidity, vomiting, and focal neurological signs). Children have associated lymphadenopathy, hepatosplenomegaly, and prolonged respiratory findings	Amp-B (1 mg/kg) plus flucytosine (100 mg/kg in four divided doses) for 2 weeks followed by oral fluconazole (12 mg/kg) for 2 months
Aspergillosis	Presence of prolonged fever with features of raised intracranial pressure with preceding prolonged respiratory symptoms. MRI brain shows ICSOL with massive hemorrhage, venous sinus thrombosis, and hemorrhagic infarct/vasculitis	Voriconazole 8 mg/kg/day (2–12 years) or 4 mg/kg/day (>12 years)
Mucormycosis	Infection starts from the sinuses (bloody nasal discharge), orbit (proptosis), and then extends to central nervous system. It affects blood vessels resulting in thrombosis and infarction in brain	Liposomal Amp-B: 3–5 mg/kg/day
Histoplasmosis	Chronic meningitis, focal parenchymal lesion, and vascular stroke can be presenting features	Liposomal Amp-B: 3–5 mg/kg/day for 4–6 weeks followed

*Avoided in neonates <1 month of age.
(Amp-B: amphotericin B; ICSOL: intracranial space-occupying lesion)

and children who have undergone stem cell transplantation are prone to fungal infections. In addition, preterm babies, low-birth-weight babies, those on prolonged parenteral nutrition, and those on prolonged hospital stay are prone to invasive candidiasis. **Table 8** summarizes the key neurological clinical features and management of common fungal infections that affect CNS.

KEY MESSAGES

- Empirical treatment of suspected pyogenic meningitis includes combination of third-generation cephalosporin with vancomycin; the duration of antibiotic treatment will depend on age at presentation and the type of organism isolated.
- Active lesion of NCC is conventionally treated with albendazole for a duration of 7–28 days under the cover of steroids for the initial 5 days.
- Brain abscess is empirically treated with a combination of third-generation cephalosporin with vancomycin and metronidazole.
- HIV, leprosy, diphtheria, and paralytic forms of rabies are the most common infections that affect peripheral nerves.
- Children who are immunocompromised or those on immunomodulators are prone to CNS fungal infections.

CHAPTER 36: Management of Raised Intracranial Pressure

INTRODUCTION

The intracranial compartment consists of brain (80%), cerebral blood volume (10%), and cerebrospinal fluid (10%). An increase in intracranial pressure (ICP) can result from an increase in the volume of either of these compartments **(Box 1)**. Intracranial volume is governed by the extent of cerebral edema that significantly contributes to increasing ICP. There are three main types of cerebral edema—(1) cytotoxic edema, (2) vasogenic edema, and (3) interstitial edema **(Table 1)**. Cerebral edema could be focal as in brain tumor or neurocysticercosis, which may result in cerebral herniation such as uncal herniation.

Increased ICP tends to decrease cerebral perfusion pressure (CPP) and cerebral blood flow. Normal ICP tends to vary with age—neonate (<2 mm Hg), infant (2-6 mm Hg), children (1-15 years): 3-7 mm Hg and adolescents and adults have ICP <15 mm Hg. ICP >20 mm Hg and CPP <40 mm Hg require urgent management. Management of raised ICP is ideally performed in an intensive

BOX 1: Common causes of raised intracranial pressure (ICP) in children.

Common causes of raised ICP:
- *Increase in brain volume:*
    - *Intracranial space-occupying lesion (ICSOL):* Tumor, abscess, and hematoma
    - *Cerebral edema:* Encephalitis, meningitis, hypoxic–ischemic encephalopathy (HIE), traumatic brain injury (TBI), hepatic encephalopathy, Reye syndrome, and stroke
- *Increase in cerebrospinal fluid (CSF) volume:*
    - Hydrocephalus
    - Choroid plexus papilloma
- *Increase in blood volume:*
    - Vascular malformation
    - Cerebral venous thrombosis
- *Meningitis and encephalitis*

TABLE 1: Types of cerebral edema and its etiopathogenesis.

Types of cerebral edema	Pathogenesis	Cause
Cytotoxic edema	Increased water content is localized intracellularly (gray matter involvement)	Ischemia and profound metabolic derangements
Vasogenic edema	Disruption of BBB leading to increased permeability (white matter involvement)	Tumors, inflammatory lesions, and traumatic tissue damage
Interstitial edema	Increased transependymal flow from the intraventricular compartment to the brain parenchyma	Obstructive hydrocephalus

(BBB: blood–brain barrier)

care unit (ICU) setting. It would be ideal to monitor the ICP while managing children with coma and raised ICP.

PHYSIOLOGICAL BASIS

The main objective of the management of raised ICP would be to reduce the secondary neuronal injury from hypoxia, hypertension, hypotension, and hypercarbia. Secondary neuronal injury may worsen the survival and increase morbidities among the survivors. Hence, apart from measures to reduce ICP, crucial steps include maintaining normal oxygen saturation, normal pCO_2, normal temperature, and control of seizures.

The target PaO_2 is 60–80 mm Hg. Once the PaO_2 falls to <60 mm Hg, there will be cerebral vessel dilatation resulting in increased cerebral blood flow and thus, further increasing the ICP. Similarly, hypercarbia (pCO_2 >40 mm Hg) results in cerebral vasodilation resulting in raised ICP. Hence, pCO_2 is targeted between 35 and 40 mm Hg. Also, cerebral vasodilatation results from hypotension below the level of autoregulation. If hypotension is not appropriately managed, it increases the risk of ischemia. This means hypoxia, hypercarbia, and hypotension result in cerebral vasodilation resulting in increased ICP.

In contrast, hypertension beyond the range of autoregulation and hypocarbia (below 25–30 mm Hg) results in cerebral vasoconstriction that may increase the risk of further ischemia. Hence, the treatment is targeted to prevent hypoxia, hypercarbia, and hypotension **(Fig. 1)**.

CLINICAL SIGNS OF RAISED INTRACRANIAL PRESSURE

Recognizing signs of impending herniation and features of raised ICP are essential. Raised ICP must be suspected in all children

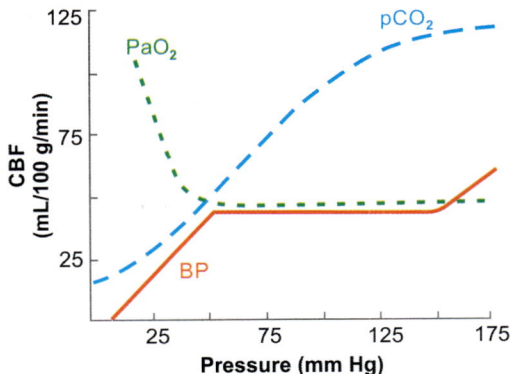

Fig. 1: There is a steep rise in cerebral blood flow (CBF) once partial pressure of oxygen (PaO_2) falls below a threshold, and blood pressure (BP) rises above the range of autoregulation. Note that once BP falls below the threshold, there is a steep decline in CBF. Partial pressure of carbon dioxide (pCO_2) follows a sigmoid curve with the rise in CBF with a rise in pCO_2.

with altered sensorium such as meningitis, head trauma, and encephalitis. Similarly, children with known liver disease or diabetes mellitus presenting with coma must also be considered to have features of raised ICP. The presence of irritability, vomiting, headache, confusion, and decreased alertness are important symptoms of raised ICP. Among the clinical signs, the two most reliable signs are bulging fontanel in infants and the presence of papilledema on fundus evaluation. Few of the other clinical signs that need to be recognized include:

- *Presence of unequal pupil:* Unilateral pupillary dilatation in an unconscious child is indicative of uncal herniation unless proven otherwise.
- *Abnormal respiratory pattern:* The respiratory pattern is abnormal based on the extent of raised ICP with resultant pressure effect on the brainstem and impending herniation—Cheyne-Stokes respiration (diencephalic lesion),

neurogenic hyperventilation (midbrain lesion), and ataxic respiration (medullary lesion).
- *Worsening of sensorium* with fall in Glasgow coma scoring (GCS) and *four* scorings is a reliable indicator of raised ICP.
- Development of unilateral or bilateral *sixth nerve palsy* (false localizing sign).
- *Abnormal posturing:* Decorticate posturing (lesion above midbrain) and decerebrate posturing (lesion below red nucleus at midbrain-pons level) are an indicator of impending herniation.
- Presence of *Cushing triad* (hypertension, bradycardia, and abnormal respiratory pattern)

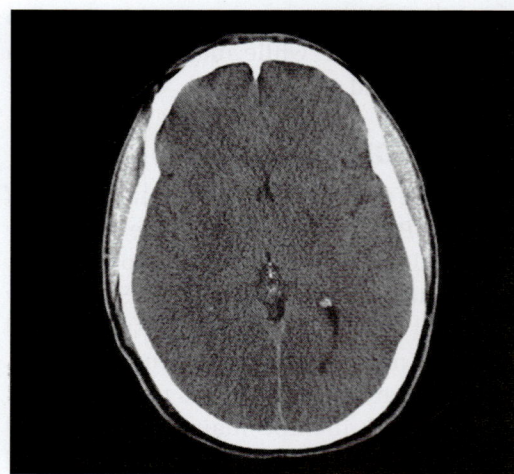

Fig. 2: Computed tomography (CT) brain showing effacement of cortical sulci and loss of gray matter–white matter junction with small chinked ventricles suggestive of diffuse cerebral edema that results in raised intracranial pressure.

■ INVESTIGATIONS

The diagnosis of raised ICP is made on clinical grounds. Neuroimaging provides supportive evidence. Neuroimaging might show effacement of gray matter–white matter junction, loss of differentiation of lenticular nucleus, decreased visualization of sulci and insular ribbon, and lateral ventricles appear small **(Fig. 2)**. A definitive diagnosis of raised ICP is made by measuring ICP.

Monitoring Intracranial Pressure

There are noninvasive and invasive methods to monitor the ICP in children. Noninvasive methods such as transfontanelle pressure transducer are preferred among infants. Point-of-care ultrasonography (POCUS) is gaining popularity in neurocritical care. Transcranial Doppler ultrasonography is a noninvasive investigation that can measure the cerebral blood flow (CBF) from which the ICP can be estimated. Optic nerve sheath diameter (ONSD) can be estimated using POCUS.

Children with GCS <8, those with a rapid decline in GCS scores, those who are ventilated with high-ventilator setting, and those who are on high-sedative drugs or drugs for neuromuscular paralysis such as vecuronium require invasive ICP monitoring. The invasive methods for ICP monitoring include fiberoptic intraparenchymal monitor, subarachnoid bolts, epidural or subdural catheter, and intraventricular catheter. Intraparenchymal and intraventricular catheter placement is technically easy and relatively cheap but has a higher risk of infections. In contrast, subdural or epidural catheters have a lower risk of infections but have poor accuracy of ICP measurement.

■ MANAGEMENT

Goals of Management

The main goal of managing raised ICP is to prevent secondary brain insult. Target is to reduce the ICP to <20–25 mm Hg, while maintain cerebral perfusion pressure (CPP) above 50 mm Hg and systolic BP above the age-appropriate lower limit.

Initial Stabilization

Airway, breathing, and circulation are the critical initial steps in the management of raised ICP. Airway needs to be secured among children with worsening sensorium (fall of GCS by >3), GCS <8, evidence of herniation, inability to maintain airway, pCO_2 >45 mm Hg or <25 mm Hg, and persistent hypoxemia. Rapid-sequence intubation (RSI) is useful among those with raised ICP. Few neuroprotective measures during preinduction include vasopressors (norepinephrine and phenylephrine) and analgesic (fentanyl) that could be used 3 minutes before the induction to avoid rapid elevation of BP during RSI. Ketamine could be used during RSI induction. Sedation may be considered for intubation using either lidocaine (1.5 mg/kg) thiopental or muscle relaxants such as vecuronium. Shock needs to be managed judiciously using appropriate fluids (normal saline 20–40 mL/kg fluid challenge) and inotropes (adrenaline or noradrenaline) to ensure adequate CPP. Uses of hypotonic fluids are discouraged. Maintenance of normothermia and normoglycemia (blood glucose < 120 mg/dL) is known to prevent secondary brain injury.

Sedation for Raised Intracranial Pressure

Following drugs may be used for sedation among intubated patients with raised ICP—morphine (0.1 mg/kg IV), midazolam (0.2–0.3 mg/kg IV), propofol, lidocaine (1–1.5 mg/kg IV), short-acting nondepolarizing neuromuscular blockers (if required) that include vecuronium (0.1 mg/kg IV), atracurium (0.5 mg/kg IV), or rocuronium (0.6–1.2 mg/kg IV).

Prophylactic Antiepileptic Drugs

Short-term prophylactic antiepileptic drugs are recommended among children with raised ICP. Although there is enough evidence to support its use in traumatic patients with raised ICP, its use in nontraumatic patients is limited. Continuous EEG monitoring may be considered, if feasible, to detect subclinical seizure activity among intubated patients. Most centers prefer a short duration of 7 days for prophylactic antiepileptic medication. Phenytoin is commonly used among traumatic raised ICP.

Hyperventilation and Raised Intracranial Pressure

Hyperventilation results in carbon dioxide washout resulting in cerebral vasoconstriction, which in turn decreases the ICP. However, hyperventilation also results in a reduction of global cerebral blood flow. With pCO_2 25–30 mm Hg, there is a reduction in regional blood flow and once pCO_2 <10 mm Hg, it results in a reduction in cerebral oxygen consumption. Most of the effects are transient (>6 hours can result in a rebound increase in ICP with normalization of pCO_2). Owing to these concerns, early, prolonged, and severe hyperventilation are discouraged during the management of raised ICP. Moderate hyperventilation with target pCO_2 30–35 mm Hg may be considered.

Head Position and Raised Intracranial Pressure

With every 10° head elevation, there is a decrease of ICP by 1 mm Hg and CPP by 2–3 mm Hg. CPP is at its best in the horizontal position. Hence, among patients with large ischemic strokes in whom there is still a possibility of salvaging tissue in the ischemic penumbra, it may be preferable to keep the head end of the bed flat, except at times of acute ICP crisis. Moderate head elevation (15–45°) may be beneficial, as it reduces ICP, but elevation >45° may be dangerous because of a critical decrease in CPP.

Hypertonic Saline in Raised Intracranial Pressure

Hypertonic saline (HS) results in osmotic mobilization of water across the intact blood–brain barrier, which reduces the cerebral water content. Hypertonic saline dehydrates endothelial cells and erythrocytes, thus increasing the diameter of the vessels and deformability of erythrocytes. It also acts by plasma volume expansion with improved cerebral blood flow. Among traumatic raised ICP, HS also reduces leukocyte adhesion in the traumatized brain. It may be administered as an infusion or bolus dose that is effective at reducing ICP in traumatic brain injury and subarachnoid hemorrhage. Hypertonic saline reduces the ICP but may not improve the overall neurological outcome of the patient. It remains a drug of choice for managing raised ICP among those with hypovolemic shock. There is no consensus on the most optimal concentration of hypertonic saline because all concentrations appear to have favorable effects on ICP. Hypertonic saline can be used as bolus (1 mL/kg over 10–15 minutes) or as continuous infusion (0.5–2 mL/kg/h) to reach a target serum sodium of 145–150 mEq/L.

Concerns with the use of hypertonic saline include:
- Development of central pontine myelinolysis or osmotic demyelination syndrome (ODS), especially with rapid correction of serum sodium and among malnourished children
- Acute heart failure and pulmonary edema from rapid blood volume expansion.
- Among those with disrupted blood–brain barrier, there is a concern of reverse osmosis.
- A fear of rebound edema with continuous infusion.
- Risk of hyperchloremic acidosis, hyperosmolar renal failure, and deranged coagulation with prolonged use of HS.

Mannitol in Raised Intracranial Pressure

Mannitol is useful for the control of raised ICP at doses of 0.25–1 g/kg. Early rheological effects of mannitol include immediate plasma-expanding effect, reduce the hematocrit, increase the deformability of erythrocytes, reduce blood viscosity thus increases CBF with a resultant increase in cerebral oxygen delivery. The delayed osmotic effect of mannitol occurs after 15–30 minutes and lasts for 4–6 hours. Hence, mannitol has a maximum effect within minutes of administration and it is useful in patients with CPP <70 mm Hg.

A single administration of mannitol can have short-term beneficial effects, during which further diagnostic procedures (e.g., CT scan) and interventions (e.g., evacuation of intracranial mass lesions) can be accomplished. It may be used as an intermittent bolus for prolonged therapy for raised ICP. However, in children with arterial hypotension, those with a renal shutdown, those on nephrotoxic drugs, we should avoid the use of mannitol. It is observed that continuous infusion of mannitol is as effective as a bolus.

Mannitol versus Hypertonic Saline

In a meta-analysis among patients with traumatic brain injury, hypertonic saline was more effective than mannitol in ICP management with the pooled relative risk of successful ICP control being 1.06 (95% CI: 1.00–1.13; p = 0.044). Hypertonic saline in comparison to mannitol results in a greater reduction of ICP with a longer duration of effect and lesser treatment failure.

Other Therapies for Raised Intracranial Pressure

Barbiturates are known to reduce the ICP and have been used in refractory intracranial hypertension. However, the side effect such as hypotension limits its wide utility, as any lowering effect on ICP is offset by its indirect lowering of CPP. In the controlled ICU setting, barbiturates may be tried among those refractory to hypertonic saline, mannitol, and other supportive measures. Among children with vasogenic edema secondary to neurocysticercosis, tumors, and other infections, steroids (dexamethasone 0.15 mg/kg/dose) may be administered to reduce ICP. Steroids are also useful in radiation-induced vasogenic edema. However, there is no role of steroids in cytotoxic edema as in patients with stroke or intracranial bleed. There are reports of a possible role of bradykinin β-2 receptor antagonist (Bradycor™) in reducing ICP, but not to be used outside research settings. Therapeutic hypothermia, where hypothermia is usually maintained for 12–72 hours, followed by a period of controlled rewarming over 12–24 hours, has been used at many centers for raised ICP. However, there are concerns of sepsis, cardiac arrhythmia, hemodynamic instability, and coagulopathy with the use of therapeutic hypothermia. Other drugs that are useful for the reduction of ICP include glycerol (useful in edema caused by vascular stroke), furosemide, and acetazolamide (useful in hydrocephalus and in high-altitude illness).

Surgical Treatment in Raised Intracranial Pressure

Recalcitrant intracranial hypertension after head trauma could be managed with craniectomy with duraplasty. Hemicraniectomy may be preferable in focal lesions such as hemorrhagic contusions. Decompressive craniectomy becomes a treatment of choice for intracranial hypertension resistant to conventional treatment and is known to reduce mortality. It is often recommended early in the course considering the goal of prevention of secondary brain injury.

KEY MESSAGES

- The goal of management of raised ICP is to reduce the ICP to <20 mm Hg and maintain cerebral perfusion pressure to >40 mm Hg.
- Bedhead end elevation to 15°, moderate hyperventilation (target pCO_2 between 30 and 35 mm Hg), and maintenance of normothermia and normoglycemia are useful in reducing ICP.
- Hypertonic saline (3% NaCl) is effective in reducing ICP and is preferred among those with hypotensive states and those with renal failure.
- There is a limited role of steroids, barbiturate coma in management of raised ICP in children.
- Decompressive craniectomy is effective and must be attempted early among those children not responsive to conventional medical measures for the reduction of ICP.

CHAPTER 37: Medical Management of Acute Vascular Stroke

■ INTRODUCTION

Stroke is defined as "rapidly developing signs of focal or global disturbance of cerebral function, lasting >24 hours (unless interrupted by surgery or death), with no apparent causes other than that of vascular origin." The incidence of pediatric stroke is 1-6 per 100,000 children per year. Broadly, there are two types of pediatric stroke—(1) ischemic stroke (arterial ischemic or venous thrombosis) (60%), and (2) hemorrhagic stroke (40%). Arterial ischemic stroke (AIS) refers to ischemia conforming to an arterial vascular distribution. AIS includes neonatal stroke (<28 days) and childhood AIS (>28 days). Hemorrhagic stroke is characterized by spontaneous intraparenchymal hemorrhage, intraventricular hemorrhage, or subarachnoid hemorrhage.

■ CLINICAL PRESENTATION

Infants and toddlers with acute stroke often present with seizures, altered sensorium, and irritability. Older children may present with hemiparesis (may not be obvious in the beginning), sensory symptoms (positive and negative), speech disturbances, visual field defects, oculomotor/facial palsy, headache, and vomiting. History of fever may suggest an underlying infective/inflammatory pathology. History of the recent head or neck trauma, recent upper respiratory tract infection, or varicella infection must be elicited. History of a prior cardiac or hematological condition such as sickle cell anemia might give a clue to underlying etiology for vascular stroke **(Table 1)**.

TABLE 1: Basic evaluation in a child with suspected stroke and its rationale.

History and examination	Rationale
History of head or neck trauma	Arterial dissection and intracranial bleed
History of prior cardiac disease	Possibility of thromboembolic stroke
History suggestive of sickle cell anemia	Possibility of hypercoagulable state and moyamoya vasculopathy
History of prior varicella	Varicella-associated vasculopathy
History of trivial head trauma like fall from bed	Think of mineralizing angiopathy
Family history of migraine and past history of recurrent headaches	Hemiplegic migraine

■ CLINICAL APPROACH TO STROKE

Is it a Stroke?

The first step is to think about whether it is a stroke or a mimicker of stroke. If an adult

TABLE 2: Clinical features of common stroke mimics.

Stroke mimics	When to think of these conditions?
Postictal Todd's palsy	History of preceding focal seizure before onset of focal neurological deficit. Todd's palsy usually lasts for <24 hours although it can last for as long as 72 hours
Hemiplegic migraine	History of associated headache with onset of hemiparesis, family history of migraine, and normal neuroimaging
Acute disseminated encephalomyelitis (ADEM)	Presence of hemiparesis or focal neurological deficit with presence of altered sensorium and features of raised ICP. History of preceding febrile illness or vaccination may be present. MRI brain may reveal focal and asymmetric patchy involvement of white matter and/or basal ganglia
Encephalitis	Presence of febrile encephalopathy with focal neurological deficit often points to encephalitis with focal signs as in herpes encephalitis (temporal lobe). MRI brain may reveal hemorrhagic involvement of medial temporal lobe and inferior frontal lobe
Posterior reversible leukoencephalopathy syndrome (PRES)	Sudden onset of focal neurological deficit with presence of hypertension should raise possibility of PRES especially among those with nephrotic syndrome, or those on chemotherapeutic drugs or immunosuppressants. MRI brain may reveal symmetrical T2 hyperintensities in bilateral parieto-occipital region with diffusion restriction
Mitochondrial leukoencephalopathy (POLG related)	Sudden onset of focal neurological deficit with neuroimaging evidence of vascular stroke, but not in any arterial or venous distribution is highly suggestive of mitochondrial disease

presents in casualty with sudden-onset hemiparesis or any focal neurological deficit, it is often presumed to be a vascular stroke, and immediate thrombolysis is lifesaving. However, when children present with sudden onset of focal neurological deficits such as cranial nerve palsy or hemiparesis, there is an extensive list of differentials that should be considered along with ischemic stroke. Common stroke mimics include a postictal state (immediately after a focal seizure), acute disseminated encephalomyelitis, and hemiplegic migraine. **Table 2** lists common clinical conditions that can mimic an acute vascular stroke.

What is the Type of Stroke?

The second step in evaluation is to categorize the type of stroke into an arterial ischemic, arterial embolic, or venous thrombotic or hemorrhagic stroke.

The majority of *arterial ischemic strokes* (AIS) are insidious in onset, and they present with focal motor weakness, speech disturbances, and ataxia.

- *Embolic strokes* often have a predisposing factor such as underlying cardiac lesions or recent postoperative cardiac surgery. Most of the embolic strokes are "gate crashers," they present with hyperacute onset.
- Hemorrhagic strokes and venous thrombotic strokes have sudden-onset weakness that develops over minutes to hours with the presence of altered sensorium, features of raised intracranial pressure, and focal neurological deficit.

What is the Etiology of Stroke?

The etiology of stroke can be attributed to vascular, cardiac, metabolic, hematological, and prothrombotic disorders **(Box 1)**. The

> **BOX 1:** Causes of acute arterial ischemic and hemorrhagic stroke.
>
> *Arterial ischemic stroke:*
> - *Vasculopathies (50–80%):* Focal cerebral arteriopathy, postvaricella arteriopathy, moyamoya disease, arterial dissection, CNS vasculitis
> - *Cardiac:* Congenital heart disease (right-to-left shunt), rheumatic heart disease, infective endocarditis, cardiomyopathies, and cardiac surgeries
> - *Metabolic:* Homocystinuria, MELAS, Leigh's disease; organic acidemias
> - *Hematological:* Sickle cell disease, polycythemia, and thrombocytosis
> - *Prothrombotic states:* Protein C deficiency, protein S deficiency, antithrombin III deficiency, APCR, FVL, LA, APLA, elevated Lp(a), hyperhomocysteinemia, and MTHFR
> *Hemorrhagic stroke:* AV malformations, cavernous malformation, aneurysms, bleeding disorder, and thrombocytopenia

(APCR: activated protein C resistance; APLA: antiphospholipid antibody; AV: arteriovenous; CNS: central nervous system; FVL: factor V Leiden deficiency; LA: lupus anticoagulant; Lp: lipoprotein; MELAS: mitochondrial encephalopathy with lactic acidosis and stroke; MTHFR: methyl-tetra-hydro-folate reductase)

most common etiology for pediatric stroke is arteriopathy. Focal or transient cerebral arteriopathy is the most prevalent cause of AIS in children. Few of these patients may give a history of rash suggestive of varicella (postvaricella arteriopathy). Other infections that have predilection for cerebral vasculature include *Mycoplasma*, Rickettsial, and tuberculosis. Most common cause of stroke in toddlers and infants is cardiac conditions and systemic illnesses.

Clinical clues to the underlying etiology are often evident from the history. For example, presence of underlying cyanotic congenital heart disease or recent cardiac surgery may predispose a child to embolic stroke. Similarly, sickle cell anemia must be considered an important risk factor in certain population. Metabolic etiology such as homocystinuria, Leigh disease, or organic acidemia may be considered among those with failure to thrive, developmental delay, waxing, and waning course with or without encephalopathy. Underlying procoagulant states such as protein C deficiency and protein S deficiency are extremely uncommon, and they are often associated with some other risk factors. For example, we may detect protein C deficiency in a child with cyanotic congenital heart disease presenting with stroke. Protein C deficiency can also be acquired in many conditions such as nephrotic syndrome and chronic liver disease.

The presence of seizures, focal deficits, behavioral changes, and slowly progressive cognitive decline in an older child must raise clinical suspicion of central nervous system (CNS) vasculitis. In India, one must always consider iron deficiency anemia as an important cause of vascular stroke in children. Underlying malignancy, chemotherapeutic drugs, and history of use of recreational drugs may provide vital clues. Clinical clues to underlying etiology are summarized in **Table 3**.

Vascular stroke can also be classified based on vessel size (small, medium, and large vessel arteriopathy), temporal course (static or progressive), and etiology (inflammatory or noninflammatory; genetic or acquired). It is difficult to predict the involvement of small vessels or large vessels on history and examination; we often need neuroimaging clues. If there are repeated episodes of stroke with or without cognitive decline, it must raise suspicion of a progressive etiology such as CNS vasculitis or moyamoya disease. There is an emerging interest in genetic factors responsible for pediatric vasculopathy.

A hemorrhagic stroke usually has an obvious etiology, which includes underlying

TABLE 3: Etiology of acute arterial ischemic stroke.

Condition	Key features
Focal cerebral arteriopathy	It is an acquired unilateral nonprogressive monophasic intracranial arteriopathy associated with basal ganglia stroke. It commonly involves distal ICA, and proximal ACA/MCA. History of preceding infection may be elicited
Moyamoya disease	Bilateral progressive stenosis or occlusion of terminal portion of ICA and/or proximal portion of ACA/MCA with vascular collaterals (appearing as puff of smoke on conventional angiography) with predisposition to recurrent strokes
Arterial dissection	Vertebral artery dissection commonly occurs at the lateral masses of C1 and C2. Whereas, carotid artery dissection is usually seen 2–3 cm above the carotid bulb. Arterial dissections are better delineated on CT angiography rather than MRI
CNS vasculitis	• Think of CNS vasculitis when there are newly acquired focal and/or diffuse neurological deficits, and/or psychiatric symptoms including regression in a previously healthy child • It can be progressive or nonprogressive. It may involve small vessels or medium–large vessels

(ACA: anterior cerebral artery; CNS: central nervous system; CT: computed tomography; ICA: internal carotid artery; MCA: middle cerebral artery; MRI: magnetic resonance imaging)

coagulopathy or arteriovenous malformation (AVM)/aneurysm. The majority of older children presenting with hemorrhagic stroke often have underlying AVM. Underlying anomalies (AVM) may not be readily apparent on imaging immediately after an acute hemorrhage; it is better to repeat after 2–8 weeks. Risk factors for venous stroke include otitis media, mastoiditis, neonatal sepsis, and dehydration.

Why there is a Delay in the Diagnosis of Pediatric Stroke?

"Time is brain"—this phrase is often used to act swiftly in saving the brain from further vascular damage in adult patients with stroke. However, there is a remarkable delay within hospital diagnosis of acute pediatric stroke, as MRI brain is time consuming as compared to a quick CT brain in adults. Moreover, there is an extensive list of differentials before we consider vascular stroke to be the cause of focal neurological deficit **(Table 2)**. It is essential to get an MRI brain to differentiate these clinical conditions. In addition, children can have a mild deficit or nonspecific clinical presentations such as headache or repeated vomiting that may be overlooked by parents and naïve pediatrician.

■ NEUROIMAGING IN STROKE

Refer to the basics of neuroimaging in **Chapter 5**. CT brain can miss majority of stroke mimics and can often be normal in the early stages of stroke, besides carrying the risk of radiation exposure. Hence, CT brain is usually not considered appropriate for the initial evaluation of a child with pediatric stroke unless there is a clear history of recent head trauma. Hemorrhages and skull (bony) fractures are better delineated on CT scan as compared to MRI brain. However, where facilities for MRI brain are not available, a screening CT scan can give valuable information **(Fig. 1)**.

An MRI brain with dedicated vascular stroke protocol is suggested for the evaluation of all children with stroke **(Box 2)**. MR angiography is an essential part of this protocol **(Fig. 2)**. All vascular strokes, whether

508 | **SECTION 4:** Common Therapeutic Dilemmas

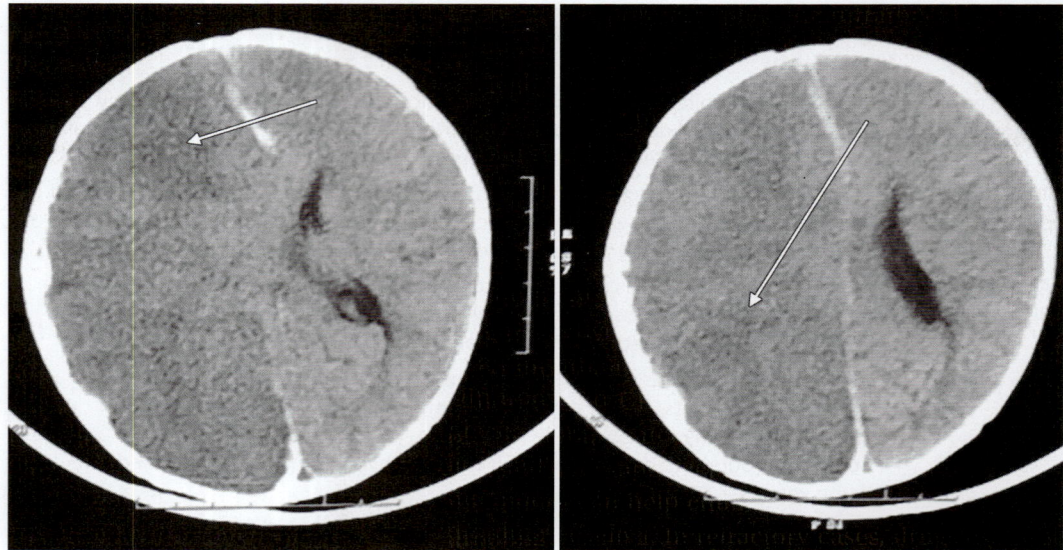

Fig. 1: Noncontrast CT scan head showing hypodensity (arrows) on the right cerebral hemisphere suggestive of vascular stroke.

BOX 2: Suggested magnetic resonance imaging (MRI) brain protocol for stroke.

An MRI brain protocol for acute stroke should include axial T2-weighted fast spin-echo, coronal FLAIR, sagittal T1-weighted spin-echo, DWI in three planes and calculated ADC map, intracerebral 3-D TOF MRA, axial dual-echo STIR and T1-weighted spin-echo through the neck, and extracerebral 2-D TOF MRA of the neck down to the aortic root

(ADC: apparent diffusion coefficient; DWI: diffusion-weighted imaging; FLAIR: fluid-attenuated inversion recovery; MRA: MR angiography; TOF: time of flight)

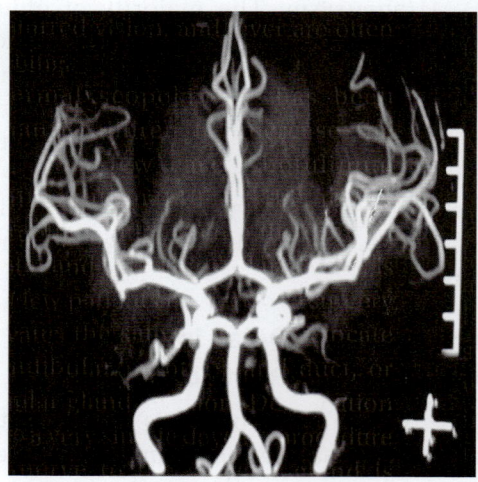

Fig. 2: Normal MR angiography.

it is arterial or venous, look hyperintense on T2-weighted fluid-attenuated inversion recovery **(Figs. 3A and B)** and hypo- or isointense on T1-weighted images. Diffusion restriction on the MRI brain is one of the earliest findings in a child with acute arterial stroke **(Figs. 4 and 5)**. This indicates cytotoxic edema that results from arterial vascular occlusion. Venous strokes are more prone to hemorrhagic transformation when compared to arterial strokes **(Fig. 6)**.

Bilateral symmetrical thalamic and basal ganglia hyperintensity could be seen in deep venous sinus thrombosis. Similarly, the presence of symmetrical parasagittal infarct is suggestive of sagittal sinus thrombosis **(Figs. 7A and B)**. Another clue to differentiate an arterial from venous stroke is contrast enhancement, which is

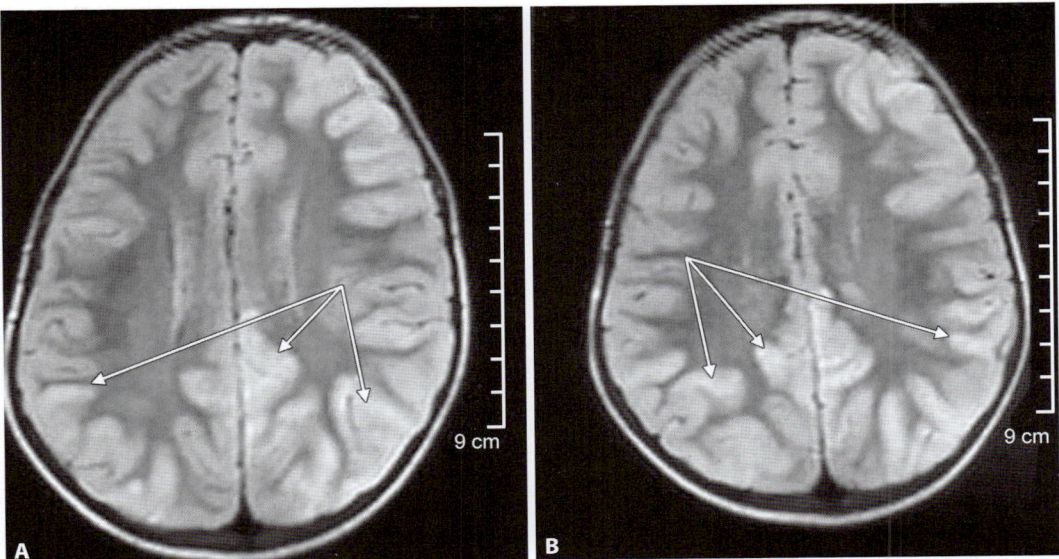

Figs. 3A and B: MRI brain (T2/FLAIR images) showing hyperintensity on bilateral parieto-occipital region. (T2/FLAIR: T2-weighted fluid-attenuated inversion recovery)

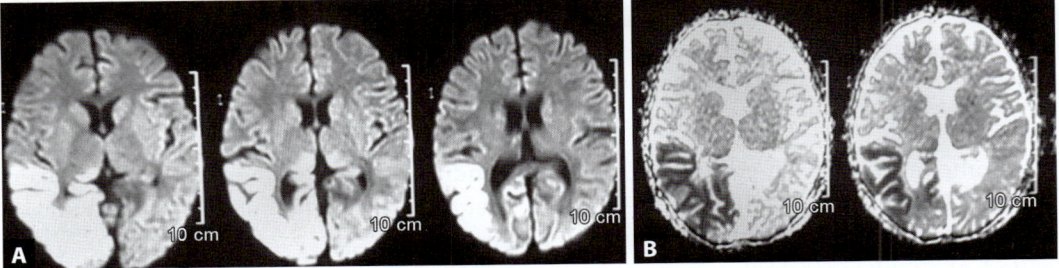

Figs. 4A and B: DWI (A) and ADC map (B) showing diffusion restriction across inferior division of right middle cerebral artery and posterior cerebral artery suggestive of arterial ischemic stroke. (ADC: apparent diffusion coefficient; DWI: diffusion-weighted imaging)

characteristically seen in a garland or ribbon form across arterial ischemic stroke, whereas contrast enhancement is either absent or patchy in a venous stroke. Thrombosed sinuses are often evident as a bright signal in T1-weighted images **(Fig. 6)**. In addition to MR venography, radiologists often look at the venous sinus flow voids among those with suspected venous sinus thrombosis.

Magnetic resonance imaging axial fat-saturated images would be immensely useful to rule out carotid and vertebral artery dissection. MR angiography is an additional tool to look for the architecture of cerebrovascular vessels for diagnosis of moyamoya vasculopathy **(Fig. 8)**. Other scans for MR venography are useful to screen for venous drainage.

Distribution of vascular stroke gives a clue to the underlying diagnosis. Hemispheric strokes (involvement of one entire hemisphere) is unlikely with arterial ischemic stroke, one may consider other possible differentials such as hemiconvulsion–hemiplegia epilepsy

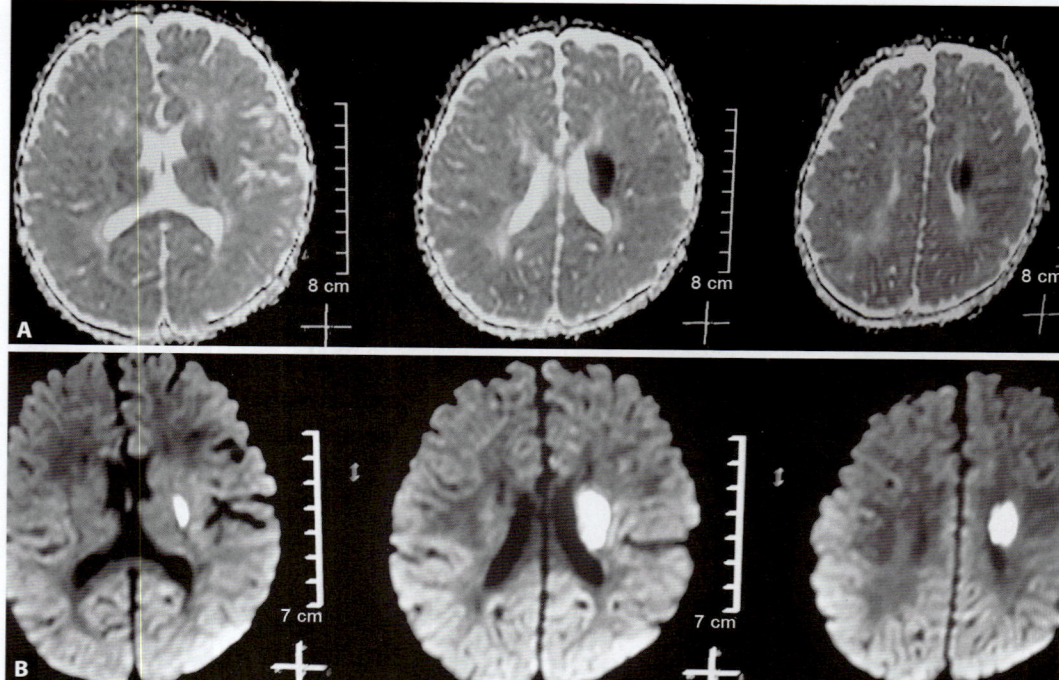

Figs. 5A and B: ADC map (A) and DWI images (B) showing diffusion restriction across the left basal ganglia suggestive of left lenticulostriate arterial ischemic stroke. (ADC: apparent diffusion coefficient; DWI: diffusion-weighted imaging)

syndrome or Rasmussen encephalitis **(Figs. 9A and B)**. The involvement of the entire cerebral cortex with sparing of the cerebellum called as "white cerebellar sign" is seen in hypoxic–ischemic brain injury (HIBI) **(Fig. 10)**. The involvement of watershed zones [areas between anterior cerebral artery (ACA) and middle cerebral artery (MCA), between MCA and posterior cerebral artery (PCA)] suggests HIBI **(Fig. 11)**. Bilateral symmetrical parieto-occipital lesions with rapid clinical improvement and resolution of these lesions on follow-up images performed within 4 weeks are highly suggestive of posterior reversible leukoencephalopathy (PRES) **(Figs. 12A and B)**. Bilateral asymmetric patchy white matter hyperintensities are highly suggestive of acute disseminated encephalomyelitis (ADEM) **(Fig. 13)**. These conditions are common stroke mimickers that need to be differentiated from a vascular stroke.

Digital subtraction angiography is an invasive procedure restricted to clarify suspected aneurysms and arteriovenous (AV) malformation, especially when there is a hemorrhagic stroke and MRA is not contributory. CT angiography is a useful noninvasive alternative to screen for underlying aneurysms and AV malformations. In any child with hemorrhagic stroke, once underlying coagulopathy has been ruled out, one should always keep the possibility of underlying AV malformation.

■ INVESTIGATIONS

All children with acute pediatric stroke must be screened for underlying congenital

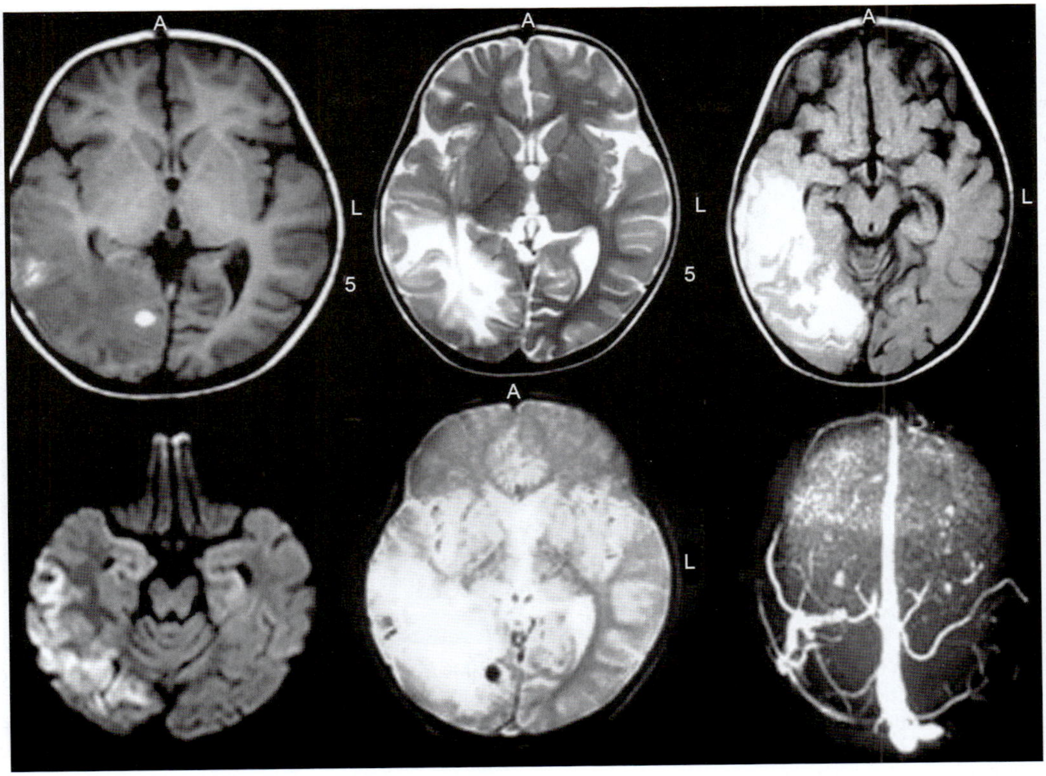

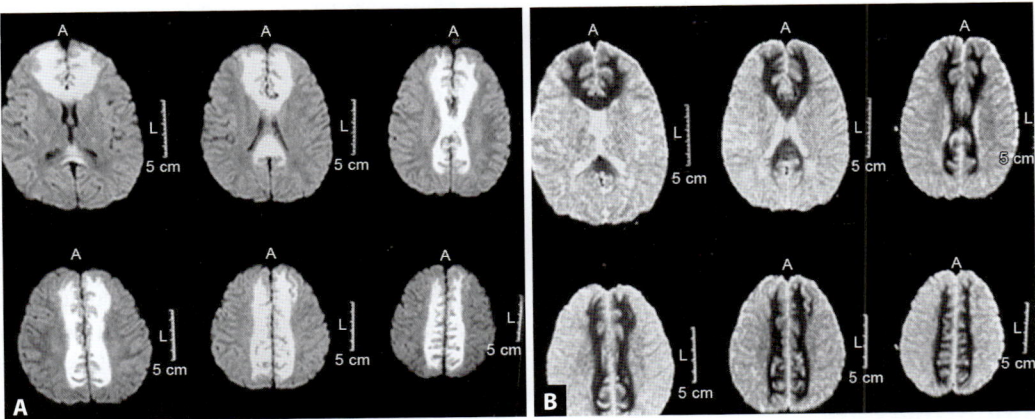

Fig. 6: MRI brain (top panel and left to right) shows T1 patchy hyperintensity, T2 hyperintensity, and FLAIR hyperintensities in right parieto-occipital region with (lower panel and left to right) diffusion restriction evident on DWI images, blooming effect on SWI images with MRV showing attenuation of bilateral transverse sinus suggestive of transverse sinus thrombosis. (DWI: diffusion-weighted imaging; SWI: susceptibility-weighted imaging; MRV: magnetic resonance venography; FLAIR: fluid-attenuated inversion recovery)

Figs. 7A and B: MRI brain shows diffusion restriction—(A) Looks bright on DWI and (B) Dark on ADC map—in bilateral parasagittal area along the distribution of superior sagittal sinus suggestive of sagittal sinus thrombosis. (ADC: apparent diffusion coefficient; DWI: diffusion-weighted imaging)

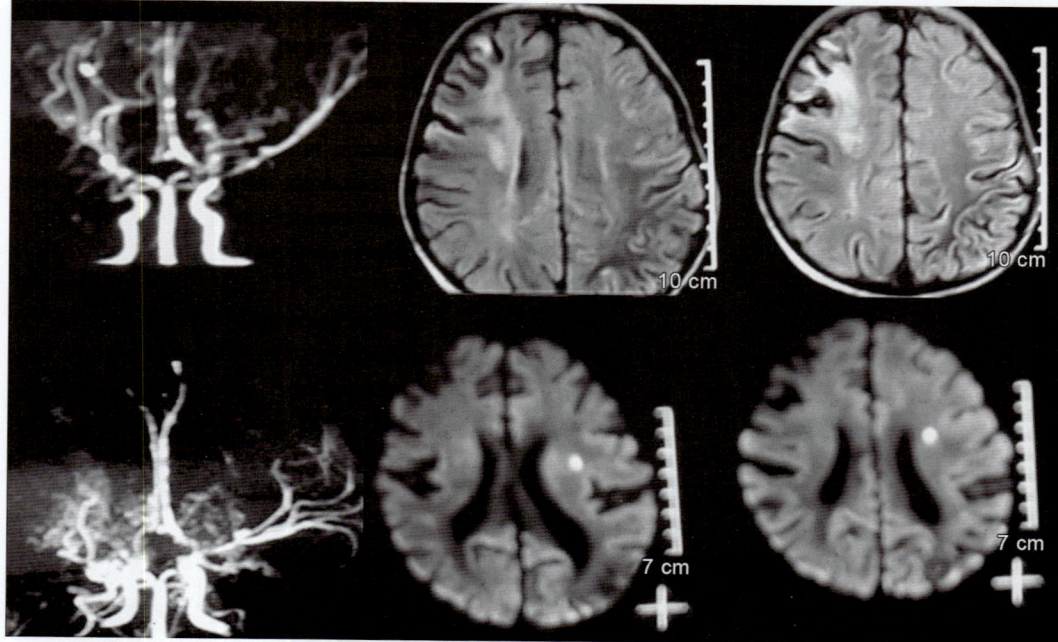

Fig. 8: MRI brain (T2/FLAIR image) showing gliosis in right MCA territory suggestive of an old infarct, with diffusion restriction in the left basal ganglia suggestive of superimposed new infarct. MR angiography reveals obstruction at the level of distal ICA and proximal MCA/ACA with extensive collaterals suggestive of moyamoya disease. (ACA: anterior cerebral artery; MCA: middle cerebral artery; ICA: internal carotid artery; T2/FLAIR: T2-weighted fluid-attenuated inversion recovery)

or acquired heart disease even if any other evident cause is obvious. Bubble-contrast echocardiography might be useful to detect a patent foramen ovale. If the bubble study is positive, four-extremity Doppler study may be considered. Transesophageal echocardiography is useful to detect a patent foramen ovale with a shunt. Preliminary workup in a child with acute stroke is summarized in **Table 4**.

MANAGEMENT OF A CHILD WITH ACUTE STROKE

Supportive Care

The mainstay in the treatment of acute stroke is to maintain normothermia, normal oxygenation and normal glucose, treatment of hypertension, ensuring proper nutrition, early mobilization; treat dehydration (if any); treat anemia (decide for the need of blood transfusion). At present, there is no role of prophylactic antiepileptic drugs. Early recognition of raised ICP is crucial among children with large ischemic stroke. Continuous ICP monitoring would immensely guide the therapeutic decision. It is prudent to involve the neurosurgical team in refractory raised ICP for the need for early surgical decompression. This should be anticipated among children with large ischemic stroke. **Table 5** summarizes the critical supportive measures for managing a child with acute stroke.

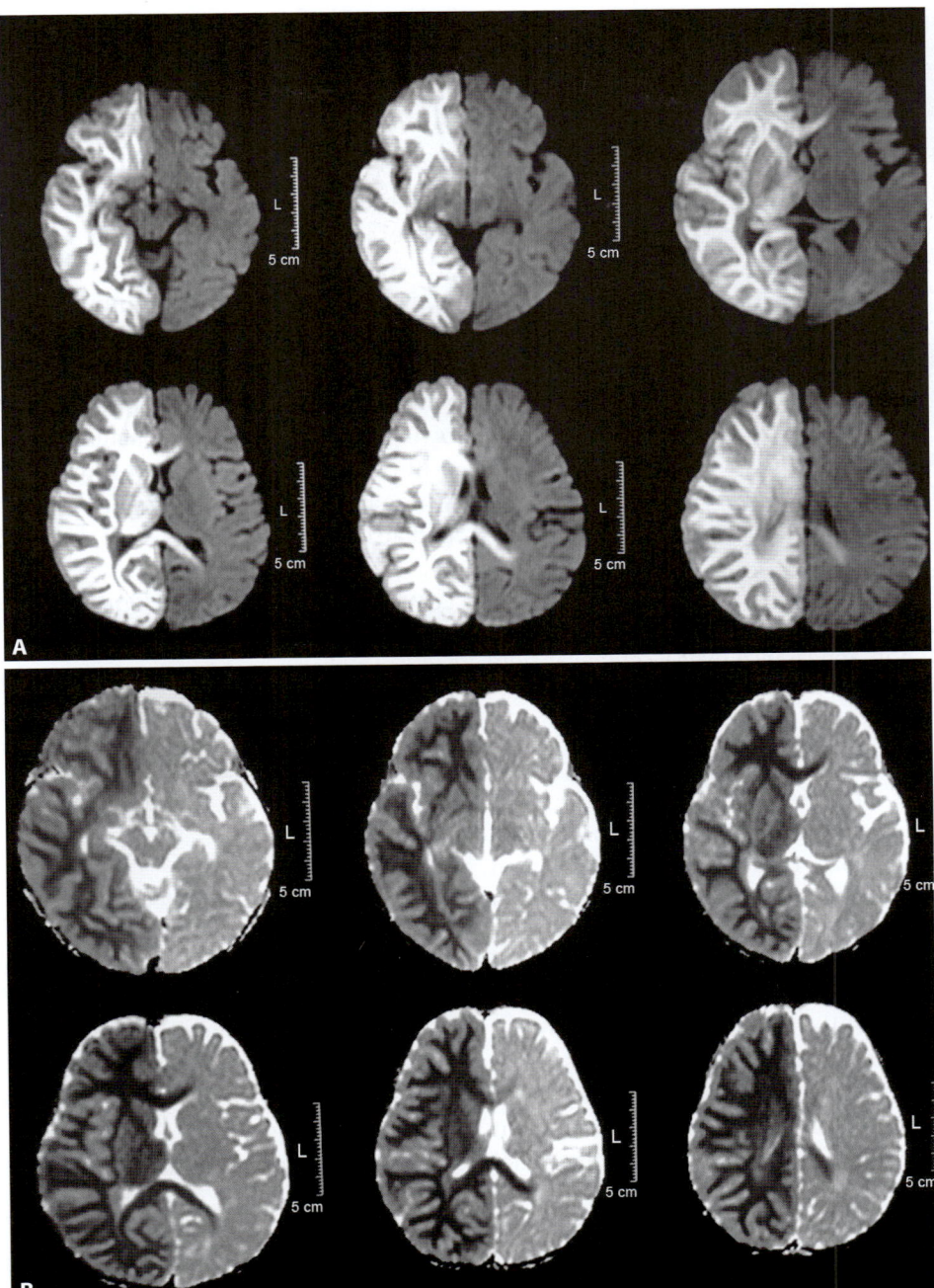

Figs. 9A and B: (A) DWI images and (B) ADC map of the brain showing diffusion restriction across the entire right hemisphere in a child who presented with left focal status epilepticus and left-sided hemiparesis. He subsequently developed focal epilepsy suggesting a clinical diagnosis of hemiconvulsion–hemiplegia epilepsy syndrome. (ADC: apparent diffusion coefficient; DWI: diffusion-weighted imaging)

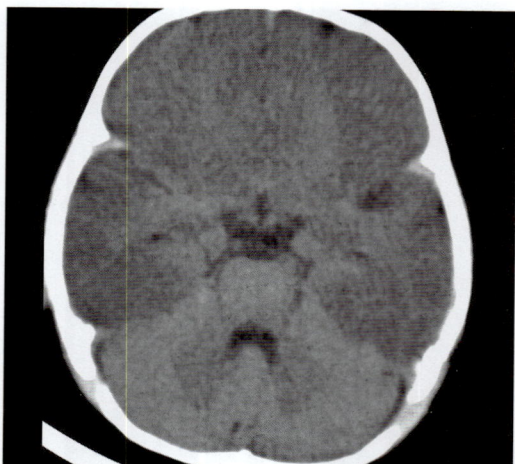

Fig. 10: Computed tomography (CT) brain of a child who was brought to casualty with altered sensorium and features of raised intracranial pressure following refractory status epilepticus. CT brain reveals diffuse hypodensity across the entire cerebrum with sparing of cerebellum giving it a "bright" appearance (white cerebellar sign) suggestive of diffuse hypoxic damage.

Thrombolysis

There is no role of thrombolytic agents (alteplase) for the management of arterial ischemic stroke. Its use has been associated with increased mortality and morbidity at discharge. Its role may be considered in selected patients with cerebral venous sinus thrombosis. Ambiguities exist on the use of tPA (tissue plasminogen activator) owing to lack of data on its safety, and dosage in children (the fibrinolytic system is immature). Moreover, most pediatric AIS often present beyond 6 hours, and there are wide differential for acute onset hemiplegia in children. Hence, outside a research setting, there is *no role of thrombolysis* as of now in management of a child with acute stroke, irrespective of etiology. Children who are diagnosed within 4.5 hours of presentation with convincing evidence of large-vessel occlusion may be considered for tPA (0.9 mg/kg to maximum 90 mg) on case-to-case basis with consensus of stroke specialist.

Antithrombotic: Aspirin vs. Low-molecular-weight Heparin

An antiplatelet drug such as aspirin is preferred in conditions with rapid flow or stenosis where because of platelet activation, platelet-rich thrombus is formed. Anticoagulants such as low-molecular-weight heparin (LMWH) is useful in conditions with slow stasis, prothrombotic states where owing to activation of the coagulation system, a fibrin-rich thrombus is formed. **Table 6** summarizes the management strategies in pediatric stroke.

Low-molecular-weight Heparin

The LMWH is preferred over heparin considering its subcutaneous ease of administration. Only weekly or monthly factor Xa monitoring (target factor Xa activity is 0.5–1.0 IU/mL) is required among children on LMWH.

Indications for LMWH:
- Risk of recurrent cardiac embolism
- Cerebral venous sinus thrombosis
- Selected hypercoagulable state or known prothrombotic condition
- Extracranial arterial dissection
- It may be considered in children after arterial ischemic stroke pending investigations.
- Recurrence of the stroke on aspirin

Dose of LMWH: <2 months: 1.5 mg/kg/dose 12 hourly; >2 months: 1 mg/kg/dose 12 hourly

Warfarin

It has been used for long-term anticoagulant action to prevent recurrent stroke among those with existing cardiac etiology prone

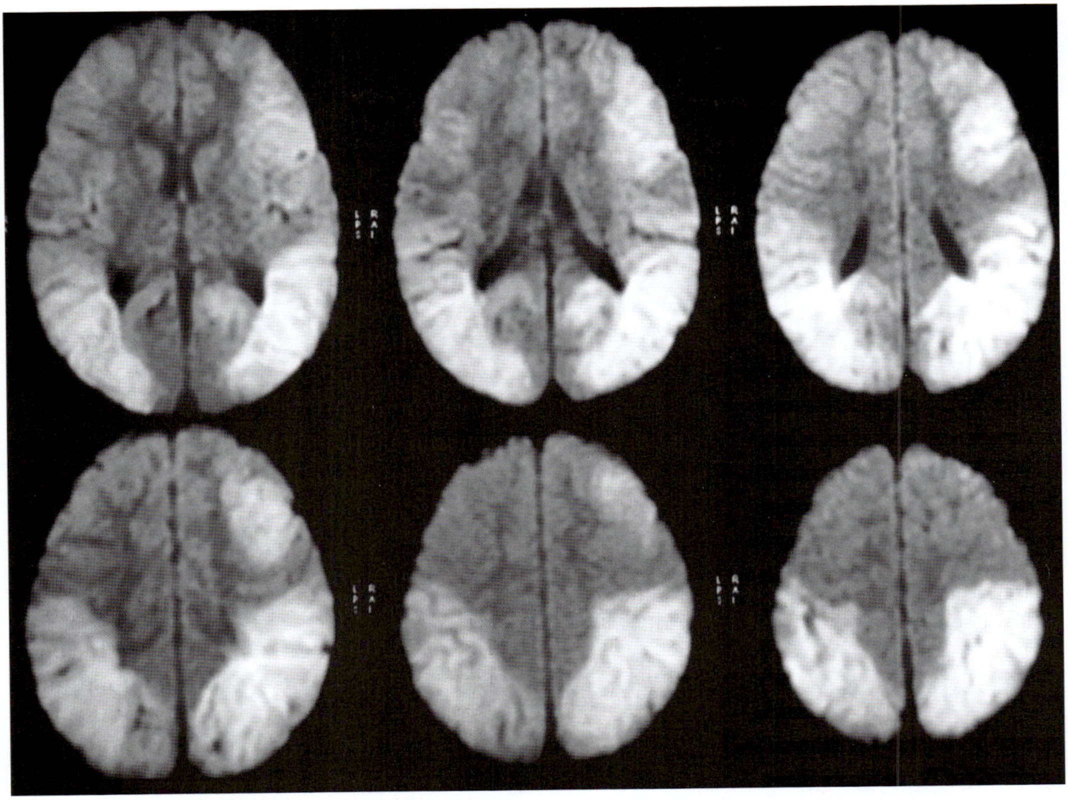

Fig. 11: DWI images of brain showing watershed infarcts following near drowning.
(DWI: diffusion-weighted imaging)

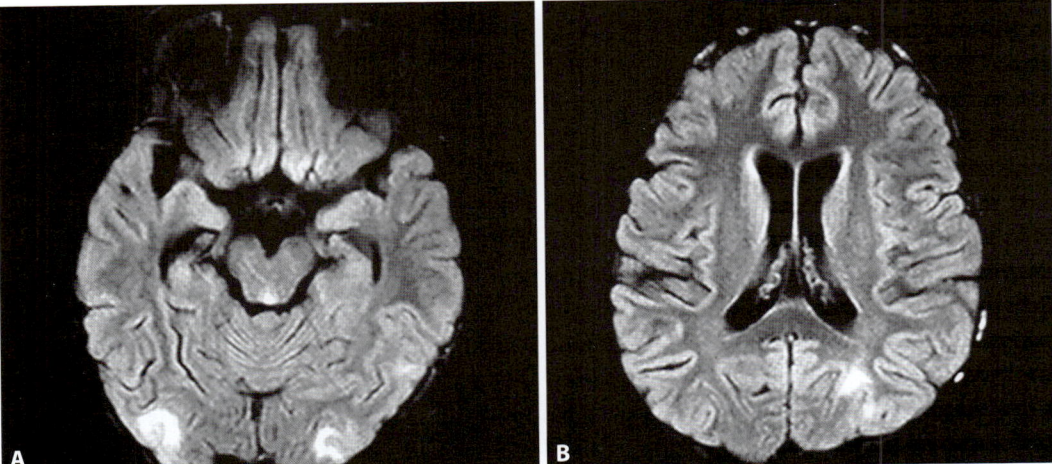

Figs. 12A and B: Fluid-attenuated inversion recovery (FLAIR) images showing hyperintensity in the bilateral occipital region suggestive of posterior reversible leukoencephalopathy syndrome in a child with nephrotic syndrome brought to casualty with focal neurological deficit and hypertension.

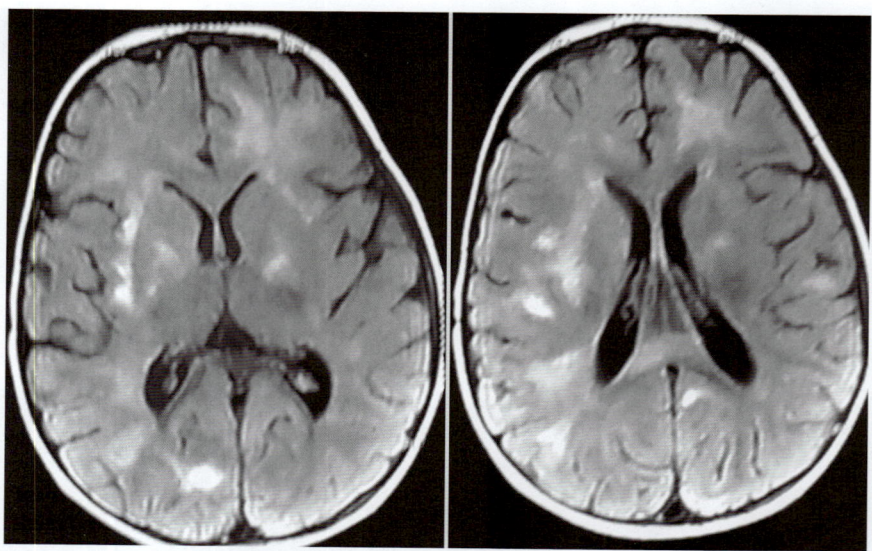

Fig. 13: Fluid-attenuated inversion recovery (FLAIR) images of brain show bilateral discrete patchy asymmetrical hyperintensity in a child with focal neurological deficit and altered sensorium suggestive of acute disseminated encephalomyelitis (ADEM).

TABLE 4: Investigations in a child with acute stroke.

Investigation	Rationale
Protein C, protein S, antithrombin III levels, and fibrinogen level	These may be falsely decreased in acute stage. Hence, better performed after 3 months following the stroke
Thrombophilia screen including MTHFR mutation, mutation in *prothrombin* gene (G20210A polymorphism), factor V Leiden mutation	To look for underlying thrombophilic conditions
Serum homocysteine levels	To look for evidence of hyperhomocysteinemia
Antiphospholipid antibody (APLA)	To look for acquired thrombophilic state
Lipid profile including serum lipoprotein A level	To look for hyperlipidemia
Complete blood count with peripheral smear and serum ferritin and serum iron level	To screen for iron deficiency anemia
Hemoglobin electrophoresis	To screen for sickle cell anemia and other hemoglobinopathies, especially in endemic zones

to recurrent embolism, cerebral venous sinus thrombosis, arterial dissection, and selected hypercoagulable state such as congenital protein C, protein S deficiency, and antithrombin-III deficiency.

Dose: 0.2 mg/kg, dose titration is based on the target INR of 2–3

- *If INR is 2–3:* No dose change
- *If INR 1.5–1.9:* Increase dose by 10%
- *If INR 1.1–1.4:* Increase dose by 20%

TABLE 5: Supportive care for children with acute stroke.

Supportive measure	Management
Normothermia	Children with acute stroke are best nursed between 36.5 and 37°. Hyperthermia is known to be associated with poor neurological outcome. However, therapeutic hypothermia has not shown any proven benefit in management of children with acute stroke
Normal oxygen saturation	Children with acute stroke need to maintain oxygen saturation between 96 and 99%. Hyperoxia (SpO_2 = 100%) is as harmful as hypoxia for acute stroke
Normal blood pressure	Management of hypotension is mandatory with fluids and vasopressors. Appropriate fluid management is essential to maintain adequate cerebral perfusion pressure. Sudden fluctuation in blood pressure may lead to adverse neurological outcomes
Normoglycemia	Hyperglycemia was independently associated with poor neurological outcome
Normal intracranial pressure	Management strategies for reduction of increased intracranial pressure includes bed elevation 15–30°, hyperventilation to a target pCO_2 of 25–30 mm Hg, hyperosmolar therapy (3% NaCl or mannitol), ventriculostomy, external ventricular drainage, and decompressive craniectomy
Management of seizure	It is important to manage the seizures in children with acute stroke
Prevention of deep venous thrombosis	Prophylactic stockings can prevent deep venous thrombosis in paralyzed legs

(pCO_2: partial pressure of carbon dioxide; SpO_2: oxygen saturation)

TABLE 6: Management strategies in pediatric stroke.

Condition	Treatment of choice
AIS with nonmoyamoya vasculopathy	Aspirin or LMWH
AIS with moyamoya vasculopathy	Aspirin and revascularization surgery
AIS with extracranial arterial dissection	LMWH for 6 months
AIS with cardioembolic phenomena	LMWH till corrective surgery
CVST with or without hemorrhagic transformation	LMWH for 3–6 months
Hemorrhagic intraparenchymal bleed	Get CT angiography or digital subtraction angiography to diagnose and manage underlying AV malformation

(AIS: arterial ischemic stroke; CVST: cerebral venous sinus thrombosis; LMWH: low-molecular-weight heparin)

- *If INR 3.1–3.5:* Decrease dose by 10%
- *If INR > 3.5:* Withhold warfarin

Aspirin

Aspirin is commonly used for secondary prevention of arterial ischemic stroke in children in whom infarction is not due to sickle cell disease, not at risk of recurrent cardiac embolism or severe hypercoagulable state.

Dose: 3–5 mg/kg/day in the acute stage and 1–3 mg/kg for secondary prophylaxis (withhold the drug during varicella and influenza).

Children on aspirin should be vaccinated annually with the influenza vaccine, and varicella vaccine. These vaccines preferably must be administered before starting aspirin.

Treatment of the Underlying Cause

- Treat coagulation factor deficiency with coagulation factor/vitamin K.
- Prescribe folic acid/vitamin B_{12} in *MTHFR* mutation (homozygous) or those with hyperhomocysteinemia.
- Low-cholesterol diet and if required, statins for hypercholesterolemia.
- Correction (surgical) of complex congenital heart disease, resection of atrial myxoma.
- Revascularization surgery among those with moyamoya disease, especially among those with recurrent transient ischemic attack (TIA) and those with cognitive decline.
- *Surgical correction of aneurysms or AV malformations:* AV malformations are also amenable to stereotactic radiotherapy and neuroradiology intervention.
- *Surgical or catheterization-mediated closure of patent foramen ovale (PFO):* It is not very clear, if PFO closure leads to a reduction in stroke recurrence.
- *Exchange transfusion:* Among children with sickle cell anemia presenting with acute stroke, exchange transfusion to decrease the percentage of HbS to <30% might be required. Subsequently, regular blood transfusion to keep HbS < 30–50% is desirable with regular monitoring for need of chelation. Moyamoya vasculopathy in children with sickle cell anemia will require surgical revascularization.
- Steroids/cyclophosphamide is often recommended for biopsy-proven CNS vasculitis.

Surgical Management

- Children with acute parenchymal hemorrhage
- Posterior circulation stroke patients might develop obstructive hydrocephalus requiring surgical intervention.
- Decompressive craniotomy and lumbo-peritoneal shunt might be required in children with large MCA stroke with raised intracranial pressure not amenable to medical management.
- Revascularization surgery for moyamoya vasculopathy detected on conventional angiography

Mechanical Thrombectomy (Endovascular Treatment)

Mechanical thrombectomy of large-vessel occlusive (LVO) disease is a standard of care in adults when initiated within 3 hours of the onset of symptoms. There is limited experience with endovascular therapy using mechanical thrombectomy devices in children. It can be used up to 24 hours in children with LVO and among those children where tPA is contraindicated in consultation with stroke specialists.

Perinatal Stroke

Perinatal stroke refers to stroke occurring between 28 weeks of gestation and 28 days of postnatal life. It often presents in neonates with focal seizures or other nonspecific features such as encephalopathy and lethargy. The risk factors for perinatal stroke include maternal chorioamnionitis, premature rupture of membrane, oligohydramnios, neonatal cardiac lesion, neonatal-onset coagulation disorders and genetic disorders including *COL4A1*. The stroke workup will be the same, except that thrombophilia workup is not required as levels of protein C, protein S, and antithrombin will be decreased owing to maternal overlap. Most of the perinatal strokes affect the MCA of the left hemisphere. The majority of perinatal strokes are diagnosed retrospectively when the child or infant presents with hemiplegic cerebral palsy (presumed perinatal stroke).

KEY MESSAGES

- Stroke in children often remains unrecognized considering diverse clinical presentation, a wide list of stroke mimickers, delay in medical attention, and lack of neuroimaging facilities in every medical facility.
- Vasculopathy is the most common cause of pediatric stroke; including moyamoya disease, arterial dissection, and AV malformation.
- Low-molecular-weight heparin is indicated in those with cardioembolic stroke, extracranial arterial dissection, selective hypercoagulable state, and cerebral venous sinus thrombosis.
- Aspirin is indicated among those with vasculopathy-related AIS including moyamoya disease, which requires definitive revascularization surgery.
- Goals of treatment are to optimize recovery, prevent a recurrence, and avoid complications, including those due to unnecessary and potentially harmful interventions.

CHAPTER 38

Management of Developmental Disorders

■ INTRODUCTION

Neurodevelopmental disorders comprise disorders with motor impairment such as cerebral palsy (CP), disorders affecting cognition (intellectual disability), and disorders of impairment of social interaction and communication [autism spectrum disorder (ASD)]. The chapter discusses an overview of the clinical approach and management of children with CP, intellectual disability, and ASD.

MANAGEMENT OF CHILDREN WITH CEREBRAL PALSY

Cerebral palsy is defined as a "group of permanent disorders of the development of *movement and posture*, causing activity limitations that are attributed to *nonprogressive* disturbances that occurred in the developing fetal or infant brain". The two keywords are "disorders of movement and posture" (only those with impairment in movement and posture will qualify for diagnosis of CP) and "nonprogressive disorder" (clinical features will improve with time and will not worsen). The brain injury can occur during the prenatal, perinatal, and postnatal periods up to 2 years of age. The motor disorders of CP are often accompanied by disturbances of sensation, perception, cognition, communication, behavior, epilepsy, and secondary musculoskeletal problems.

TABLE 1: Neurological features and related impairments in children with cerebral palsy.

Neurological features	Associated impairment
• Muscle weakness • Abnormal muscle tone • Balance problems • Loss of selective control • Pathological reflexes • Loss of sensation • Contractures • Deformities	• Intellectual disability • Epilepsy • Vision impairment • Hearing impairment • Speech and communication problem • Swallowing difficulty • Failure to thrive • Respiratory problems • Incontinence

Table 1 enumerates the neurological features and associated impairments in children with CP.

Motor Impairment

The main causes of motor impairment in children with CP include abnormality of muscle tone, weakness of the muscles, loss of selective motor control, and loss of balance **(Fig. 1)**.

- Abnormality of muscle tone manifests as a lack of relaxation of muscles with unnecessary contraction during the movement, resulting in hypertonia.
- Apart from hypertonia, the muscles are weak with a lack of force to generate a particular desired movement.

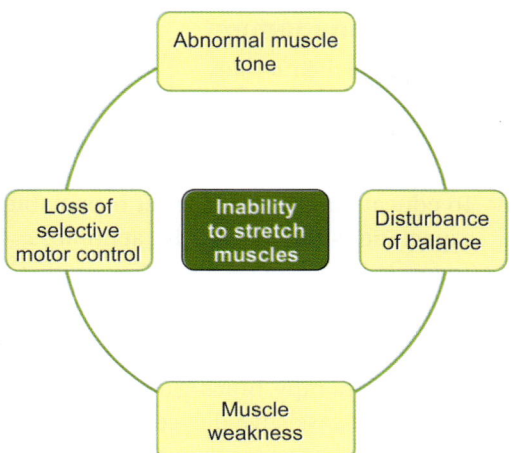

Fig. 1: Key features of motor impairment in children with cerebral palsy.

- When an agonist muscle contracts, the antagonistic muscle has to relax to perform that movement. This phenomenon, called *selective motor control*, may be impaired in children with CP.
- Few children have associated disturbance of balance.

Abnormalities of muscle tone, strength, selectivity, balance, and sensation contribute to primary motor impairment in CP. These *primary impairments* lead to contractures and deformities (*secondary impairment*). This, in turn, results in an adaptive mechanism to counteract these contractures and deformities (*tertiary impairment*). For example, spasticity in gastrocnemius (primary) leads to ankle contractures (secondary) that lead to an adaptive mechanism of hyperextension of the knee (tertiary) to compensate for ankle contractures while walking.

Muscle Involvement

The muscles that are affected in children with CP are biarticular, the ones that cross two joints. In the lower limb, hip adductors, knee flexors, and ankle flexors are commonly affected, and in the upper limb, pronator, wrist flexor, finger flexor, and thumb adductor are affected. These groups of muscles undergo selective contractures. The most common deformities include scoliosis, kyphosis, hip subluxation, hip dislocation, equinus, varus, valgus deformity, femoral internal torsion, and tibial torsion.

Injury to the central nervous system (CNS) can result in loss of inhibitory impulses to lower motor neurons that produce hyperactive stretch reflexes (spasticity, hyperreflexia, clonus, and co-contraction). CNS pathology may also result in loss of connections to lower motor neurons resulting in weakness, loss of selective motor control, poor coordination, and sensory deficits.

Neonatal Reflexes and Advanced Postural Reaction

In a typically developing child, primitive reflexes have to disappear for advanced postural reactions to appear. These reflexes are essential for the development of head control and muscle tone. Most of the primitive reflexes disappear by 4–6 months of age, as the CNS starts maturing. Postural reactions develop during the latter half of the first year and are responsible for the attainment of motor skills. These advanced postural reactions maintain the body in an upright position as a reaction to changes in the body position. They persist lifelong to help maintain balance and movement. These reactions are either poorly developed or absent in children with CP. Hence, they are unable to maintain body posture and gain motor development.

There are three advanced postural reactions: (1) Righting reaction, (2) equilibrium reaction, and (3) protective reaction.

Righting reflex is responsible for maintaining the alignment of the head to the trunk (neck righting reflex) and alignment of head and body to change in position (body righting reflex). Equilibrium reactions provide balance when the center of gravity is disturbed, especially once the child learns to sit and stand to maintain this erect posture. If equilibrium reactions are unable to restore the position, then protective reactions will act to restore the balance. Evaluation of postural reactions **(Box 1 and Table 2)** is essential to plan the therapeutic intervention.

Goals of Management

- To improve the mobility
- To prevent deformity (decrease spasticity, gaining muscle strength, and improve the joint alignment)
- To educate the parents (to set reasonable expectations and do exercise at home)
- To teach daily living skills
- To provide community and social support

Components of rehabilitation: Physiotherapy, occupational therapy, bracing (once the child learns to walk), assistive devices (toddler for mobility), adaptive technology, sports and recreation, and environmental modification are components of rehabilitation. Other treatment options include hyperbaric oxygen therapy, sensory integration, neurodevelopmental therapy, constraint-induced movement therapy (CIMT) for improving hand functions in hemiplegic CP, and Vojta method.

Principles of Physiotherapy

Physiotherapy improves the postural control and also enhances muscle strength, range of motion (decrease spasticity and contractures), joint alignment, and motor balance. It consists of exercise, bracing, and activities toward reaching a specific functional goal.

BOX 1: Clinical evaluation of advanced postural reactions.

Righting reaction (RR):
- RR in prone
- RR in lateral
- RR in flexion
- Neck righting on body
- Labyrinthine righting
- Optical righting

Equilibrium reaction: Slow and fast perturbation at different tilt angles

Protective reaction (PR):
- PR prone
- PR forward
- PR side
- PR backward

TABLE 2: Methods of eliciting common righting reflexes.

Labyrinthine righting reflex	Ability to maintain the head in midline when the infant is held vertically with eyes covered and tilted off the center (infant takes vestibular cue to maintain the balance)
Optical righting reflex	Ability to maintain the head in midline when the infant is held vertically with eyes open and tilted off the center (infant takes the visual cue to maintain the balance)
Body righting reflex	Infants lift his head away from the surface, when the body of the infant touches the surface
Landau righting reflex	When an infant is suspended horizontally in prone position, there is extension of body with head in vertical plane

It should be started from infancy through adolescence. During infancy, the main goal is to stimulate an advanced postural reaction. In toddlers and preschoolers, the main component includes stretching the spastic muscle and strengthening weak muscles. Conventional exercises include active and passive range of motion exercises, stretching exercises to prevent contractures, and strengthening exercises to strengthen the weak spastic and antagonist muscles. Children with CP are prone to osteoporosis. Treatment includes calcium, vitamin D, and oral bisphosphonates.

Management of Contractures

Spastic contractures are initially dynamic, and there is no actual shortening of the muscle. Dynamic contractures are best managed with casting, splinting, and intramuscular use of botulinum toxin type A. Fixed contractures are managed by surgical tendon lengthening. Orthopedic surgeries for contractures are rarely required before 6 years of age. Orthopedic surgery includes tendon lengthening, split transfer, and simple tenotomy. Angular osteotomy and rotational osteotomy are useful for torsional deformities such as femoral anteversion and tibial torsion. A single event, multilevel surgery, can be used to correct all fixed contractures and torsional deformities in a single operative session.

Bracing

Bracing refers to devices that hold extremity in a stable position. It keeps joint in a functional position, increases function, and prevents deformity. Ideally, bracing should be simple, light, but strong. Ankle foot orthosis (AFO) is useful among ambulant children with CP to improve their gait and provide support during the swing and stance phases of the gait. Conventional AFOs are used to correct the equinus deformities. Dorsal shell AFOs or posterior leaf spring AFOs are useful among those with knee hyperextension. Other variants such as floor reaction AFOs are useful among those with excessive knee flexion. Braces often require revision based on the desired response and the child's growth. Other types of AFOs include knee–ankle–foot orthosis, hip abduction orthosis, thoracic–lumbar-sacral orthosis (TLSO), and hand splints. Serial casting is used at few centers to stretch the spastic muscles to improve the range of motion.

Mobility Devices

Mobility devices intend to help children with CP to explore the surrounding, interact with peers, develop balance, and improve their posture. Mobility devices for children with CP include standers, walkers, crutches, and cranes. Standers provide support to maintain an erect posture, enable weight bearing, and decrease muscle tone. Prone frames are useful among few children, but better avoided in children with severe extensor spasticity and poor head control. Other supports to maintain ambulation include walkers, gait poles or sticks, crutches, and wheelchairs. Wheelchairs can be either manual or powered. Wheelchairs can be custom-molded based on individual cases.

Management of Spasticity

Management of spasticity should be in conjunction with physiotherapy. It is reemphasized to the reader that an isolated reduction of hypertonia might not be beneficial as the underlying muscles are weak, and there is a loss of selective control and balance. Oral medications for

TABLE 3: Antispasticity medications for children in cerebral palsy.

Drug	Dose	Practice points
Baclofen (5 mg, 10 mg tablet; 5 mg/5 mL syrups)	10–15 mg/day in three divided doses; increase it by 5 mg biweekly to maximum of 40–60 mg/day	• Sedation is a major side effect • Slow withdrawal should be done to avoid rebound increase in spasticity • Avoid baclofen in children with epilepsy/seizures • Baclofen is a good choice when the child has mixed signs of spasticity and dystonia
Tizanidine (2 mg tablet)	2–4 mg/day in three to four divided doses; titrate it by 2 mg biweekly to a maximum tolerable dose or a cumulative dose of 36 mg/day	• Avoid its use in children with liver disease or deranged liver functions • Major adverse effects include sedation, hypotension, and dry mouth
Diazepam (valium) 5 mg tablet	0.2–0.8 mg/kg/day in three to four divided doses	• Drowsiness, weakness, and ataxia are the main side effects • It can be used for a short term during the crises • It is a good choice when sleep problems are a major issue • Slow withdrawal is recommended • Avoid long-term use for the fear of drug dependence

spasticity include baclofen [binds to gamma-aminobutyric acid (GABA) receptor in the spinal cord], tizanidine (central α-2 agonist), and diazepam **(Table 3)**. Other rarely used drugs for spasticity include dantrolene and clonidine.

Selective dorsal rhizotomy involves cutting selective dorsal rootlets at L2–S2 level among diplegic children aged above 3 years with pure spasticity. This procedure requires intensive physiotherapy after the surgery. The concerns of this procedure include the development of scoliosis, hip instability, and urinary incontinence. These postoperative concerns have discouraged the success of this procedure.

Intrathecal baclofen through pump is useful among children with spastic quadriplegic CP aged above 3 years with Gross Motor Function Classification System (GMFCS) IV and V. Intramuscular onabotulinum toxin (Botox) acts by impairing the neurotransmission at the neuromuscular junction (NMJ) and thus weakens the muscle. It is short acting and its effects last for 3–4 months.

Other treatment modalities for children with spastic CP include electric stimulation therapy including transcutaneous electric nerve stimulation (TENS) and neuromuscular electric stimulation (NMES). Gait rehabilitation includes robot-assisted gait training. Virtual reality is emerging development in neurorehabilitation.

Management of Dystonia

The treatment of children with dyskinetic CP includes trihexyphenidyl, tetrabenazine, baclofen, levodopa, and gabapentin. Other therapeutic options include intrathecal baclofen and deep brain stimulation. Other medications, including botulinum toxin, lacked sufficient evidence on improvement in dystonia among children with CP.

Trihexyphenidyl is a centrally acting anticholinergic drug, which is a competitive inhibitor of acetylcholine with a direct antispasmodic effect on smooth muscle. It is started at a dose of 0.2 mg/kg/day in 1st week, 0.5 mg/kg/day in 2nd week, 1 mg/kg/day in 3rd week, 2 mg/kg/day in 4th week, and the same 2 mg/kg/day will be continued for the next 8 weeks. Tetrabenazine is an antidopaminergic drug useful in children with associated choreoathetoid movement as in children with dyskinetic CP. A trial of levodopa is suggested, especially when a clinical diagnosis of CP is not convincing, or dystonia is unexplained.

Management of Status Dystonicus

Dystonic spasm of more than 72 hours with the presence of fever, dehydration, hyperkalemia, hypocalcemia, acidosis, hyperCKemia (elevated creatine phosphokinase levels), and myoglobinuria with or without end-organ dysfunction suggests status dystonicus. The following measures need to be ensured:
- Intravenous rehydration
- Antipyretics, cooling blankets, and analgesics
- Sedatives (chloral hydrate 30–100 mg/kg every 6 hourly)
- Can start with a trial of oral or parenteral clonidine (0.2–2.0 µg/kg/h)
- Continue trihexyphenidyl and tetrabenazine in maximum tolerable doses. Other treatment options include baclofen, benzodiazepine, and gabapentin.
- Treat triggering factors such as infection (broad-spectrum antibiotic)
- Management of pain is essential; minimize noxious stimuli.
- If there is no response, IV midazolam or propofol or neuromuscular relaxant such as suxamethonium will be required in an intensive care unit (ICU) setting.
- In nonresponders, plan for intrathecal baclofen, deep brain stimulation, or pallidotomy.
- Consider avoiding clonazepam as few cases of worsening of dystonia are reported.

Management of Drooling of Saliva

Drooling of saliva is often secondary to hypersensitive mouth, lack of jaw stability, open mouth, and inadequate lip closure in children with CP. Simple measures of oral physiotherapy such as massaging of face, lips, and gums and keeping ice cubes around the mouth can help children with excessive drooling of saliva. In refractory cases, drugs such as glycopyrrolate (0.5–2 mg/day in two to three divided doses) can be useful. Side effects of dry mouth, constipation, urinary retention, blurred vision, and fever are often quite disturbing.

Transdermal scopolamine has been used in many children to decrease the sialorrhea. In a few cases, botulinum toxin administration (10–40 IU) under ultrasonographic guidance into the salivary gland (parotid and submandibular glands) is useful. Very few patients may require surgery that denervates the salivary gland, relocate the submandibular/parotid gland duct, or submandibular gland excision. Denervation surgeries are a very simple daycare procedure where the nerve to the salivary gland is excised by approaching through the middle ear.

Management of Feeding Difficulties

Common feeding problems include persistent drooling of saliva, inability to open the mouth owing to oromandibular dystonia, difficulty in chewing/swallowing, and gastroesophageal reflux disease. Children with CP are often advised to give frequent small feeds rather than an attempt at feeding meals at specified times. It would be good to give small pieces of solid food or preferably soft mashed food. The child may be placed in a sitting position while feeding. Shallow spoons are preferable to long spoons so the food is placed in the middle of the tongue. The therapist may advise applying pressure on temporomandibular joints to maintain jaw stability while the child is chewing the food.

Gastroesophageal reflux disease must be screened using GERD nuclear scans. Children with severe GERD often require medications, including prokinetic (metoclopramide) drugs along with ranitidine or pantoprazole. Thick feeds are recommended among children with severe GERD. Percutaneous endoscopic gastrostomy (PEG) and jejunostomy are common interventions to improve the nutritional status of children with CP. However, feeding through PEG requires strict asepsis, and there is always an increased risk of infection, severe GERD, and aspiration. Constipation is quite common in children with CP. Measures to address constipation include adequate fluids, plenty of fruits, and fruit juices. Lactulose and polyethylene glycol (PEG) are commonly prescribed for constipation. Children with speech difficulty can be provided with augmentative and alternative communication devices.

Management of Sleep and Behavioral Problems

Sleep problems are often addressed by ensuring good sleep hygiene. Medications, including melatonin (3 mg), clonidine, or diphenhydramine, are useful in sleep induction. Melatonin is the most commonly used medication, which is given half an hour before sleep. Excessive behavioral issues such as disruptive behavior and aggressive behavior that disrupt the activities of daily living often require medications including risperidone (start at 0.25–0.5 mg, with gradual hike).

Occupational Therapy

Occupational therapy focuses on teaching a child age-appropriate self-care activities such as dressing, bathing, and brushing teeth. Hand and upper extremity functions can be improved in the child through play and purposeful activity. Play improves mental capacity and provides psychological satisfaction. Play activities, like other activities, should be picked so that they "fit" a child's level of development and help him/her move one step further. Sports and recreation, including swimming and horseback riding (normalize muscle tone, decrease contractures, improve head control, and trunk balance), are useful. Assistive devices such as feeding aids are available in various shapes, thickness, and angles of spoon and fork according to the child's coordination. Picture symbols or use of high-end electronic technology can be used as an aid to communication.

Special Education

Special education focuses on children with disabilities for the achievement of their educational goals. It includes measures to support their education at the school. Some of the common principles of special education are to go stepwise from teaching simple prenumber concepts to concepts of numbers, applications of concepts in daily living, and problem-solving skills. Few simple prenumber concepts are enumerated in **Table 4**.

TABLE 4: Methods of skill training under simple prenumber concepts for children with cerebral palsy/intellectual disability.

Skill	Method of skill training
Measurement	Difference between big/small, tall/short, wide/narrow, and thick/thin
Quantity	Difference between more/less and few/many
Capacity/volume	Difference between more/less and full/empty with liquids
Weighing	Difference between heavy/light
Shapes	Circle, triangle, square, and rectangle
Colors	Recognition of colors red, yellow, blue, green, black, and white
Matching	Child will match two identical balls
Sorting	Sort out similar balls from a container containing big and small balls
Identifying	The child will point to the big ball when asked
Number skills	Numbers and counting
Application	Money, time, calendar, and capacity
Problem solving	Reading and word-solving problems

MANAGEMENT OF CHILDREN WITH INTELLECTUAL DISABILITY

Individualized educational programs (IEPs) are the mainstay in the management of children with intellectual disability. A detailed assessment of the present level of functioning needs to be determined before planning intervention. Evaluation of vision, hearing, gross motor and fine motor ability, ability to self-care, language ability, cognitive ability, and social and emotional ability need to be determined. There is a limited role of drugs in the management of children with intellectual disability **(Table 5)**. Treatable causes of intellectual disability should never be missed **(Table 6)**.

Assessment

A trained psychologist should perform detailed assessment. Assessment must not be performed during an illness. The environment for evaluation must be conducive, and a note on the cooperation of the child and the ability to understand instructions of the psychologist must be noted. It is essential to perform an assessment of adaptive functioning in terms of the conceptual (academic), social, and practical domains. The most common scales used by clinical psychologists for assessment of intelligence include the Malin Intelligence Scale (MISIC) and the Binet–Kamat Intelligence Scale (BKT). Vineland Social Maturity Scale (VSMS) is the most common tool used for assessment of adaptive functioning. The conceptual domain includes evaluation of memory, language, reading, writing; social domain includes awareness of other's feelings, friendship, and interpersonal communication skills; and practical domain includes personal care and job responsibility. Assessment must be made in the context of associated comorbidities, including seizures, behavioral problems, and motor disabilities including spasticity or dystonia.

Goals of Management

It is essential to set annual goals by setting short-term objectives. For example, one of

TABLE 5: Pharmacological management in children with intellectual disability.

Drug and its target	Dose
Methylphenidate (hyperactivity)	5–10 mg/day for immediate-release and 18 mg for sustained-release tablets; gradually hike every week to achieve the desired effect
Clonidine (hyperactivity)	Start with 0.25–0.5 mg/kg to a maintenance dose of 0.1–0.5 mg/kg
Risperidone (hyperactivity, aggressive behavior, and disruptive behavior)	0.1–0.5 mg/kg in 2–3 divided doses
Fluoxetine (SSRI) (disabling motor stereotypies)	Start at 2.5 mg/day and increase to 10 mg/day

(SSRI: selective serotonin reuptake inhibitor)

TABLE 6: Treatable causes of intellectual disability.

Causes of intellectual disability	Specific treatment
Mucopolysaccharidosis (MPS type 4)	Enzyme replacement therapy
Congenital hypothyroidism	Thyroxine
Phenylketonuria	Low phenylalanine diet
Cerebral creatinine deficiency	Creatine supplement
Menkes disease	Copper histidine

Note: Visit https://www.tidebc.org/ for identifying treatable causes of intellectual disability in children.

your goals could be that you want the child to become independent in indicating for toilet needs in the next 1 year. To achieve the same, short-term objectives such as "number of dry days in a week" may be monitored. Parents can be provided with instructions to maintain a urine log, where a routine timing for passing urine is noted for a week; just a few minutes before that time, the child may be taken to toilet and encouraged to pass urine. If he or she passes, then a reward may be provided.

Task Analysis

Each task shall be broken into individual components before teaching the child. This process of breaking each task into small teaching steps is called task analysis. For example, to eat a biscuit independently, the task may be split into reaching the kitchen, reaching for the biscuit jar, opening the jar, picking up a biscuit and so on. A child with an intellectual disability will often take a long time before accomplishing a task.

A *functional approach* to a child with an intellectual disability focuses on enabling the child to perform day-to-day activities. In contrast, a *lifespan approach* focuses on adaptive needs for that developmental age. For example, in a child of 4 years, the focus would be on school readiness and training of culturally acceptable adaptive behaviors. In a child of 9 years, the focus of training would be academic skills and personal developmental skills to enable him for vocational training.

Comprehensive Management

Speech therapists, audiologists, occupational therapists, physiotherapists, special educators, and clinical psychologists to handle challenging behaviors are a part of a comprehensive team of rehabilitation specialists. It is essential to make a placement decision whether the child can attend a regular school, special school, or a daycare center.

MEDICAL TREATMENT OF AUTISM SPECTRUM DISORDER

Behavioral Intervention

Applied behavior analysis (ABA) is a well-established and effective intervention for ASD. Early intensive behavioral intervention (EIBI) is based on principles of ABA that are delivered early (before 5 years) and intensively (25–40 hours a week). The objective of EIBI is to train and teach children how to learn and to equip them to be able to benefit from school-based services. Improvement in areas of language, play, adaptive skills, and vocational skills has been demonstrated among those on EIBI. Other structured programs for ASD include discrete trial training and pivotal response training. Parent-mediated intervention includes their training in a structured behavioral method, which can be applied at home, thus reducing the time at the therapy center, making the intervention more enjoyable and natural.

Pharmacological Treatment

Existing pharmacological treatments are not effective for the core symptoms of ASD. These drugs often act on comorbid symptoms such as hyperactivity, inattention, aggressive, irritable or self-injurious behavior, or rigid, repetitive behavior. Drugs often work as an adjunct to behavioral intervention: Methylphenidate is useful for hyperactivity, risperidone for aggressive and irritable behavior, and aripiprazole for abnormal motor stereotypies and aggressive behavior. Other medications targeting irritable, aggressive, and impulsive behaviors include selective serotonin reuptake inhibitor (SSRI), a tricyclic antidepressant, gabapentin, clonidine, guanfacine, and memantine [N-methyl-D-aspartate (NMDA) receptor antagonist]. Melatonin may be useful for sleep disturbances.

Therapies of Unproven Efficacy (Complementary and Alternate Medicine)

Lack of effective medication for the treatment of ASD creates parental interest in complementary and alternate medicine. None of these interventions in isolation or combination have shown any definitive evidence. There are various dietary supplements and biological and non-biological treatments that have been tried among individuals with ASD **(Table 7)**.

SUPPORT TO FAMILY

Autism and intellectual disability are a lifelong condition with a wide range of fluctuation in the clinical course. The ability to live an independent adult life depends on the severity of the condition and extent of associated intellectual disability. Access to appropriate medical services, educational materials, and social support is required for families. There is a remarkable delay in diagnosis, especially in autism, owing to delay between symptom recognition by parents and final clinical diagnosis of autism. There is an emerging need for infrastructure, trained therapist, and medical insurance to care for children with special needs in India. The prohibitive cost of intensive behavioral intervention in the private sector is a major limiting factor in the care of Indian children with special needs.

TABLE 7: Complementary and alternative medicines for autism spectrum disorder.

Supplements	Other biological treatment	Nonbiological treatment
Vitamin B_6 (pyridoxine)	Gluten-/casein-free diet	Craniosacral manipulation
Omega-3 fatty acid	Immunoglobulin and pentoxifylline	Facilitated communication
Magnesium	Gastrointestinal medication (secretin triggering factor for digestion)	Yoga and reiki
Vitamin A	Hyperbaric oxygen therapy	Chiropractic therapy
Vitamin C	Chelation (DMSA and DMPS)	Auditory integration training

(DMPS: 2,3-dimercapto-1-propanesulfonic acid; DMSA: dimercaptosuccinic acid)

Right for Person with Disability (RPWD) act bill has been notified by the Government of India in its official gazette on December 28th, 2016, which covers ASD as one of 21 disabilities. The National Trust for welfare of persons with autism, CP, mental retardation, and multiple disabilities is a statutory body of the Ministry of Social Justice and Empowerment to enable and empower persons with disabilities including ASD. There are large numbers of government schemes for the benefit of children with intellectual disability and ASD.

KEY MESSAGES

- CP is a disorder of movement and posture, which results from nonprogressive injury to the brain in the antenatal, natal, or postnatal period.
- The motor impairment in children with CP results from a combination of abnormality of muscle tone, weakness of the muscles, loss of selective motor control, and loss of balance.
- Spasticity responds to medications including baclofen and tizanidine; choreoathetosis responds to tetrabenazine; and dystonia responds to trihexyphenidyl, baclofen, and gabapentin.
- IEPs remain the mainstay in the management of children with intellectual disabilities.
- There is a limited role of medications in the management of children with intellectual disability and ASD except for disturbing aggressive or disruptive behaviors.

CHAPTER 39

Treatment of Neuropathies and Myopathies

■ INTRODUCTION

In this chapter, we deal with the medical treatment of a few selected treatable neuromuscular conditions in children. Supportive treatment remains the mainstay in the majority of children with chronic neuropathies and myopathies. A clinical approach to diagnosis is dealt with in other chapters.

■ SPINAL MUSCULAR ATROPHY

SMN gene is present in the long arm of chromosome 5 (5q). There are two copies of SMN gene—SMN1 and SMN2, which are present in each chromosome 5 (**Fig. 1**). SMN2 gene is identical to SMN1 gene except for few nucleotides. In a healthy individual, SMN1 gene produces a functional protein and SMN2 produces a nonfunctional protein. Spinal muscular atrophy is an autosomal-recessive condition, which will manifest either in a homozygous state or in a compound heterozygous state.

In children with spinal muscular atrophy, there is a homozygous deletion of the entire SMN1 gene, or they have a mutation in the exon 7 that makes SMN1 gene behave like SMN2 gene, thus producing a nonfunctional protein. This latter process is called gene conversion mutation. Nearly 95% of 5qSMA patients will have either deletion of SMN1 or gene conversion mutation. It is only in 5% of 5qSMA patients that you have a

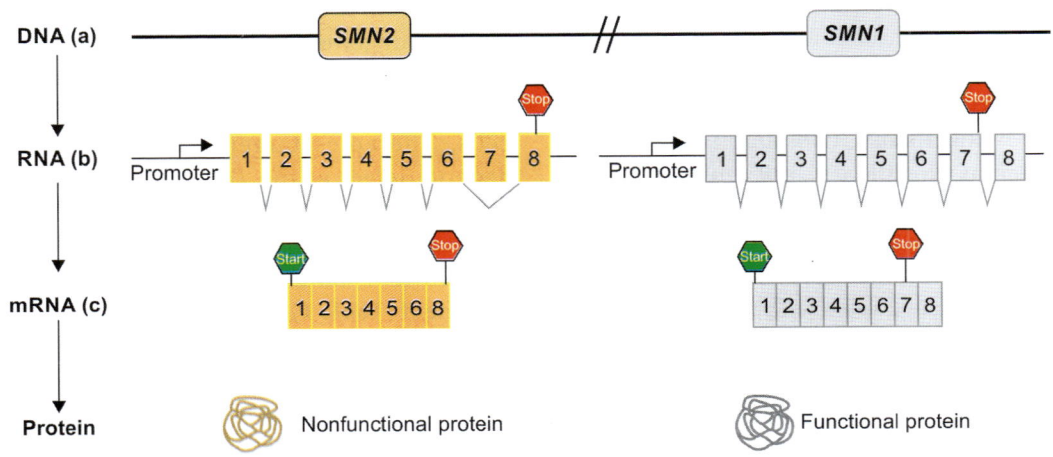

Fig. 1: Normal SMN1 and SMN2 in a healthy child.

point mutation in one chromosome and gene conversion mutation in the other chromosome (compound heterozygous).

Both *SMN1* and *SMN2* are almost the same except for a few nucleotides that are different in *SMN2*. Instead of "T", *SMN2* at exon 7 location has "C" nucleotide. Hence, when *SMN2* gene DNA transcripts into RNA, this site (intron site 7) gets excised and spliced out. This process is called intronic splicing. Hence, the final protein product is a nonfunctional protein in *SMN2*. If we target a process by which this intronic splicing is suppressed, then *SMN2* will produce a good functional protein in spinal cord motor neuron such as *SMN1* even if the entire *SMN1* gene is deleted. This process of blocking the intronic splicing suppressor element is carried out by antisense oligonucleotide (ASO). One such ASO called *Nusinersen* (Spinraza™) is approved for the treatment of children with spinal muscular atrophy.

There are three Food and Drug Administration (FDA) approved treatments for SMA: (1) Nusinersen, (2) Risdiplam, and (3) Onasemnogene abeparvovec-xioi (Zolgenesma). Nusinersen and Risdiplam are SMN2 splice modulators and Zolgensma is a gene therapy. Studies have demonstrated good functional motor improvement with Nusinersen. The drug is now available in India. The other SMN2 splice modulator is Risdiplam. Risdiplam is given orally, whereas Nusinersen is given intrathecally. Both the drugs are useful in all types of SMA. Zolgensma is a gene therapy administered intravenously and is used for children younger than 2 years with SMA with bi-allelic gene mutation in *SMN1* gene.

Apart from Nusinersen, possible targets for the treatment of spinal muscular atrophy include increasing the SMN transcript so that more functional protein can be produced. Drugs known to increase the SMN transcript include sodium valproate and sodium phenylbutyrate (histone deacetylase inhibitor) and hydroxyurea (nonhistone deacetylase inhibitor). Other drugs like aminoglycoside and proteasome inhibitors act on stabilization of SMN protein. Neuroprotective agents, including riluzole, gabapentin, and olesoxime, have been tried with not very encouraging results.

DUCHENNE MUSCULAR DYSTROPHY

Duchenne muscular dystrophy (DMD) is caused by a mutation in the *DMD* gene located on chromosome X (Xp21). It is one of the largest genes with 79 exons. Out of these 79 exons, majority of patients with DMD will have large mutations involving more than one exon. The most common is deletion (85%) followed by duplication of the *DMD* gene. Only very few patients will have a point mutation in the *DMD* gene.

DMD gene produces protein *dystrophin* that links the cytoskeleton of muscle fibers to the extracellular matrix. The absence of dystrophin leads to destabilization of the sarcolemma and thus increased muscle fragility. Three main pathologies in DMD include degeneration of muscle, chronic inflammation in the muscle, and impaired regenerative capacity of muscle precursor cells. Therapies targeted at the level of genetic defect at the *DMD* gene level are called primary treatment strategies, and those targeted at the muscle level to protect from further damage are called secondary treatment **(Table 1)**.

Primary treatment includes exon skipping, stop-codon read-through, gene addition therapy, genome editing, and myoblast transplantation. To understand these complicated terminologies, let us

TABLE 1: Primary and secondary treatment of Duchenne muscular dystrophy.

Primary treatment	Secondary treatment
Exon skipping (eteplirsen)	Anti-inflammatory drugs (corticosteroids)
Stop-codon read-through (ataluren)	Antimyostatin antibodies (domagrozumab and talditercept-α)
Gene addition therapy (microdystrophin through AAV virus)	Drugs that reduce fibrosis (givinostat, coenzyme Q, halofuginone, tamoxifen, and pamrevlumab)
CRISPR-Cas9 genome editing	Drugs that act on calcium metabolism (idebenone and rimeporide)
Myoblast transplantation	Vasodilator drugs [lisinopril (ACE inhibitor), metformin (NO signaling), sildenafil (PDE-5 inhibitor)]

(AAV: adeno-associated virus; ACE: angiotensin-converting enzyme; NO: nitric oxide; PDE: phosphodiesterase)

consider the *DMD* gene to be a bus that needs to reach its destination, that is, the production of dystrophin protein. We know that the bus is not working well, so it is unable to reach its destination. There can be various reasons for the bus not functioning—either there is small puncture in the tyre (deletion of exon), or one entire tyre is missing (large exon deletion), or it is replaced with a tire for a scooter (duplication), or there is premature breakdown of the bus before it reaches its destination (stop codon). Primary treatment targets at reaching the destination, i.e., production of dystrophin protein. If we place a tape (called ASO like eteplirsen) to seal the puncture (missing exon) so that the bus keeps running to reach its destination, it is called exon skipping. However, we know that this is not a solution; it is a temporary measure.

If we break the red signal (stop codon) to reach the destination (functional protein), it is called stop-codon read-through (like ataluren). However, ataluren will be useful only in those buses where there is premature termination (nonsense mutation). It will not work if the tyre is punctured (exons are deleted).

It would be great if we can introduce altogether new buses into the road using a virus [adeno-associated virus (AAV)]. This procedure that looks lucrative is called gene addition therapies or gene therapy. We know how difficult it is to introduce these big new buses (dystrophin is a big gene with 79 exons) into these old roads. So, we choose only the essential components of the bus (microdystrophin) and leave behind rest. Microdystrophin will produce smaller protein and not full dystrophin.

It would be a dream come true if we can repair these existing buses entirely before we start the bus. This complete repair is called *genome editing*. DNA has an inherent capacity to repair itself when injured. We also know that DNA is transcribed to mRNA, which translates into protein. CRISPR-Cas9 technology is used to induce dsDNA break at specific places in genome (where there is a defective gene) so that a defective gene is cut and the rest of the two ends join (repair) before they transcript to mRNA. Hence, although small, it will produce a functional mRNA that will translate into protein. Here, we are correcting the problem even before the bus starts (starts transcription). But we know that it is going to take a long time; it is still in the experimental phase.

Exon Skipping

In a healthy child, the mRNA transcript from the *DMD* gene will produce a functional protein called dystrophin. However, if there is a deletion of one or more exon in the *DMD* gene, it will disrupt the reading frame, thus producing a truncated mRNA that gets degraded. Hence, there is no production of dystrophin. This kind of complete loss of protein owing to change in the reading frame is called "*out-of-frame*" mutation that results in the DMD phenotype.

If there is a deletion of one or more exons whose absence does not stop the reading frame but produces a shorter mRNA, this process is called "*in-frame deletion*" that results in milder phenotype, Becker muscular dystrophy. Hence, if we convert "out-of-frame" deletion to "in-frame deletion", then we will be able to produce a smaller but functional protein that would be better than no protein. This process of "silencing" the reading of deleted exon so that the rest of the exons are read is achieved with an ASO. (This concept was explained above as silencing or sealing the puncture of the tire in the above example.) This process of skipping a nonexisting or default exon so that the reading frame is preserved is called "exon skipping" **(Figs. 2A to C)**. Hence, "exon skipping" would convert a DMD phenotype into the BMD phenotype.

Deletion of exons 45 to 55 in the *DMD* gene is considered as "hotspot" location where the most common deletion/duplications are seen. ASO that targets exon 51 is the most commonly used ASO for exon skipping in DMD. Names of ASOs that have been used in clinical trials of DMD patients include 2′OMePS (trade name is Drisapersen) and PMO (trade name is Eteplirsen). Apart from exon 51, other exon targets such as exon 45 are under clinical trial. Eteplirsen has been approved by the FDA and is used in many patients across the globe in research settings. Other exon-skipping agents include Golodirsen (exon skipping 45) and Casimersen (exon skipping 53).

Read-through Exon

Nearly 10% of DMD patients are a result of nonsense mutation in the *DMD* gene. Nonsense mutation refers to a single nucleotide change in the exon of *DMD* gene resulting in premature termination of translation, resulting in a truncated protein. Typically, the ribosome reads through the mRNA till it reaches a normal stop codon, which terminates the protein production. However, when there is a premature stop codon in the mRNA owing to nonsense mutation, it results in premature termination of translation, thus producing a small and truncated protein. If we can find a drug that can "*read through*" or ignore the premature stop codon and continue to read the rest of the mRNA, this drug would then probably restore the functional protein, as it will stop at a normal stop codon and produce a normal protein. Ataluren (previously called PTC124) selectively induces read-through of premature stop codon and not the normal stop codon. The results of clinical trials on ataluren are not very promising. There are ongoing clinical trials of ataluren in India for selected patients of DMD with a nonsense mutation. Gentamicin and NPC-14 are other drugs that work through the "read-through" principle.

Vector-mediated Gene Therapy (Gene Addition Therapy)

If there is an absent gene, one can try to introduce that gene through a viral vector. However, the *DMD* gene is very big and adenovirus (AAV) has a very small capacity. There are four domains in the *DMD* gene—(1) actin-binding amino-terminal domain, (2) central rod domain, (3) cysteine-rich domain, and (4) carboxy terminus. Of these four, N-terminal and cysteine-rich domains are mandatory; deletion of the other two

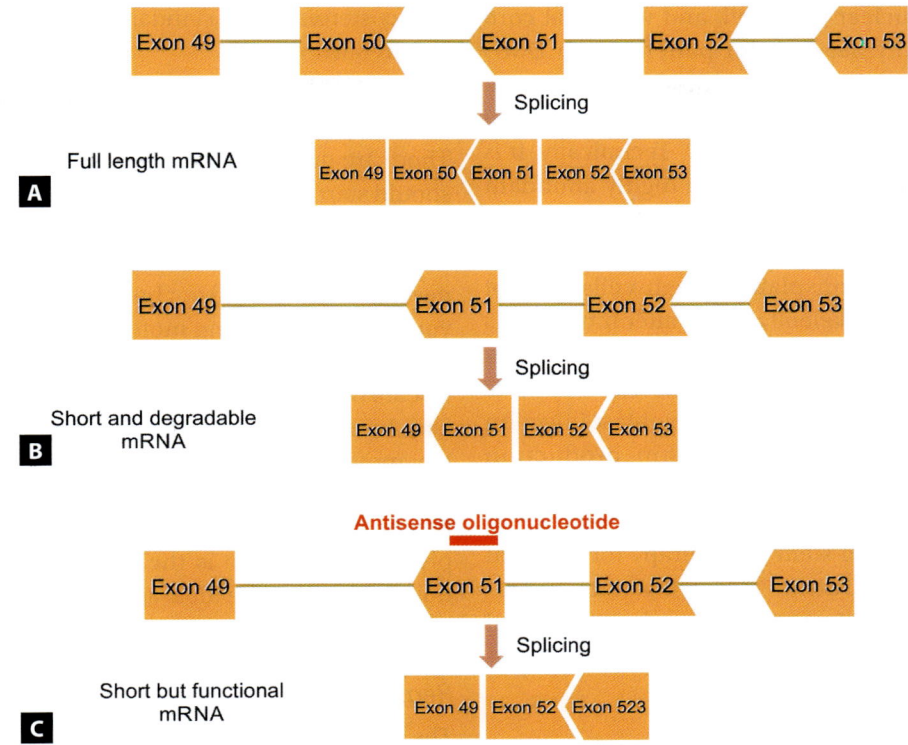

Figs. 2A to C: The concept of exon skipping: (A) Normal DMD gene transcript; (B) Exon 50 deletion; (C) Exon 51 skipping for exon 50 deletion.

domains may not severely affect the function of the protein. Hence, why not pack only small dystrophin gene (micro- or mini-dystrophin) that has these essential domains of *DMD* gene into the AAV vector. When the AAV vector is introduced locally into the muscle, it should ideally produce functional dystrophin protein, thus improving the function of that muscle. This process is called vector-mediated gene transfer therapy. Recently, in June 2023, Elevidys (first gene therapy for DMD) has been approved by the FDA for the treatment of ambulatory boys aged 4 and 5 years.

Stem Cell Transplantation

Instead of introducing a part of the gene through a vector, if we introduce an entirely new cell with a functional dystrophin gene, it might restore the dystrophin protein. So where do we get that new cell: If we get it from a matched donor, it is called "allogeneic stem cell transplantation." If we get it from the same person, modify the cell genetically, and then send it back to him again, it is called "autologous stem cell transplantation." Which cell do I choose to transplant? It could be a satellite cell that is normally found beneath the muscle fiber or a myoblast or a mesoangioblast that, when injected into the vessel, goes through the vessel into the muscle and differentiates into muscle fiber. The other cells include umbilical cord mesenchymal cells and bone marrow-derived mononuclear cells. Clinical trials using mesoangioblast, bone marrow-derived mononuclear stem cell, and umbilical cord mesenchymal cells for patients with DMD have not yielded any significant improvement.

There are major issues with the use of stem cell therapy for DMD. Technically, it is challenging as muscle is a highly abundant tissue, and muscle stem cells have limited proliferative capacity in in vitro conditions. Moreover, transplanted stem cells are not taken up by skeletal muscle after intravenous delivery, thus limiting its acceptance at the donor site. Can we inject it locally? It is demonstrated that direct myoblast injection resulted in local dystrophin production around the site of injection, but how many muscles will we inject? These are inherent limitations of stem cell therapy for children with DMD. Outside research setting, at present such treatments are strongly discouraged for patients with DMD.

Corticosteroids

Complement activation and invasion by macrophages and T-cell activation have been demonstrated in the necrotic muscles of children with DMD. Corticosteroids are known to improve the muscle strength and function in children with DMD, although the precise mechanism of action is not clear. It slows the natural decline in muscle strength. The drug is known to preserve important functions like independent walking, ability to rise from the floor, and ability to climb stairs. It also delays the onset of scoliosis and improves cardiac functions. For a long time, corticosteroids are a standard of care, among children with DMD.

Indications

There are no clear indications as to when we should start steroids in a child diagnosed with DMD. In clinical practice, it is commenced during the plateau phase of motor development. It need not be started when the young child is gaining motor milestones. By convention, steroids are never started before 2 years of age. But once he reaches a plateau (say, by 4 years of age) when he is not gaining any motor milestone, that is the correct time to start the drug. Similarly, once the child has begun declining already as in late clinical presentation, there is the limited utility of this drug. Hence, an ideal age to start steroids would be 3–5 years.

Regimen

The conventional practice is to give 0.75 mg/kg of oral prednisolone or 0.9 mg/kg of deflazacort daily for ambulatory children with DMD. Oral prednisolone is a preferred choice owing to low cost and easy availability **(Table 2)**. There are multiple regimens like daily, weekday drug with weekend off, 10 days on and 10 days off regimen, alternate-day drug administration, and high-dose weekend-only regimen. Although studies have compared various regimens, most of them have looked at short-term gains rather than long-term gains. As of now, the conventional practice is to give daily steroids for children with DMD. Once

TABLE 2: Steroid dose and schedule in children with Duchenne muscular dystrophy (DMD).

Steroid	Indication	Dose
Prednisolone	Ambulatory children aged beyond 2 years in the plateau phase	0.75 mg/kg/day
Deflazacort	Ambulatory children aged beyond 2 years in the plateau phase	0.9 mg/kg/day
Prednisolone	Children with DMD who become nonambulatory	0.25 mg/kg/day

TABLE 3: Monitoring on oral corticosteroids.

Monitoring parameter	Frequency
Weight and height	6 monthly
Pubertal development beyond 9 years	Annually
Calcium and serum vitamin D level	Annually
Pulmonary assessment including sleep studies	Annually in ambulatory phase and 6 monthly once the child becomes nonambulatory
Echocardiography or cardiac MRI (cardiac assessment)	Annually
Scoliosis monitoring	Annually

the patient is nonambulatory or develops side effects to steroids, the dose is reduced to 0.25 mg/kg/day. Steroids are best taken after the breakfast. The most common side effects include weight gain, growth restriction, risk of osteoporosis, behavioral problems, cataracts, and delayed puberty. It would have been so good if we have corticosteroid that functions with an anti-inflammatory mechanism but has no side-effect profile. This led to the discovery of a drug called vamorolone that has demonstrated anti-inflammatory effects without any change in biomarkers such as insulin resistance, adrenal suppression, or weight gain. This looks promising, but we need more research on the same. **Table 3** summarizes the monitoring parameters while the child is on steroids. The need for calcium and vitamin D supplementation may be considered when indicated.

Other Treatment for Duchenne Muscular Dystrophy

Other drugs that target patients with DMD include anti-inflammatory, anti-oxidant, and antifibrotic drugs such as *halofuginone* and *idebenone*. Myostatin pathway inhibitor such as *givinostat* and drugs for utrophin upregulation such as *SMT-C1100* are under clinical trial. Myostatin regulates skeletal muscle mass. Suppression of myostatin will result in an increased size of muscle fibers. This principle is used for drugs such as givinostat, which is a myostatin pathway inhibitor. Utrophin, on other hand, is a dystrophin homolog that is similar to the C-terminal domain of dystrophin. Drugs such as SMT-C1100 that upregulate utrophin will increase this homolog leading to functional improvement. Clinical trials are underway with these drugs. Exercise induces ischemia in patients of DMD. Drugs that target the nitric oxide pathway, such as sildenafil and tadalafil, can alleviate exercise-induced ischemia and improve the functional status of children with DMD.

Supportive Care

In children with cardiac compromise and those children with borderline cardiac dysfunction in terms of low ejection fraction, angiotensin-converting-enzyme (ACE) inhibitors and/or β-blockers are prescribed. Echocardiography must be performed at least once in 2 years for the first 10 years of life and then subsequently, it must be done annually **(Table 3)**. Children with DMD are prone to recurrent chest infections; immunization with the annual influenza vaccine and pneumococcal vaccine is recommended. It is essential to additionally vaccinate the child with varicella vaccine at least 2 months before starting steroids. Children with respiratory muscle weakness are prone to sleep disorders and inability to expectorate the cough. Hence, these children benefit from cough-assistive devices. The need for noninvasive mechanical home ventilation should be assessed. Idebenone (Coenzyme Q analog) is known to improve the respiratory functions. Range of motion and stretching exercises along with low-impact aerobic exercise such as walking and cycling are advised for children with DMD.

JUVENILE MYASTHENIA GRAVIS

Juvenile myasthenia gravis (JMG) has a marked resemblance to adult myasthenia gravis. There are antibodies that are directed against the postsynaptic acetylcholine receptor (AChR) resulting in defective postsynaptic transmission. It manifests clinically with ptosis (unilateral or bilateral), diplopia, and rarely complete ophthalmoplegia. Uncommon neuromuscular weakness includes dysphagia, dysarthria, and respiratory muscle weakness.

In contrast to adults with generalized weakness, children usually present with ocular myasthenia. JMG is considered "seropositive" when there are elevated antibodies to the acetylcholine receptor. Those who are seronegative may demonstrate antibodies to muscle-specific kinase (MuSK).

The mainstay of treatment includes increasing the availability of acetylcholine neurotransmitters and immunomodulatory therapy to combat the autoimmune process **(Fig. 3)**. Pyridostigmine is the commonly prescribed medication for myasthenia gravis. It is an acetylcholinesterase inhibitor that is prescribed in the dose of 0.5–1 mg/kg/dose given three times a day, gradually increased to a maximum of 7 mg/kg/day (maximum 60 mg/day). Apart from acquired myasthenia, children with congenital myasthenic syndrome may respond to pyridostigmine (1–1.5 mg/kg/day). Salbutamol and ephedrine are β2-adrenergic receptor agonists found useful in few types of congenital myasthenia (DOK-7 related and end-plate acetylcholinesterase deficiency).

Among the immunomodulators, plasmapheresis and intravenous immunoglobulin

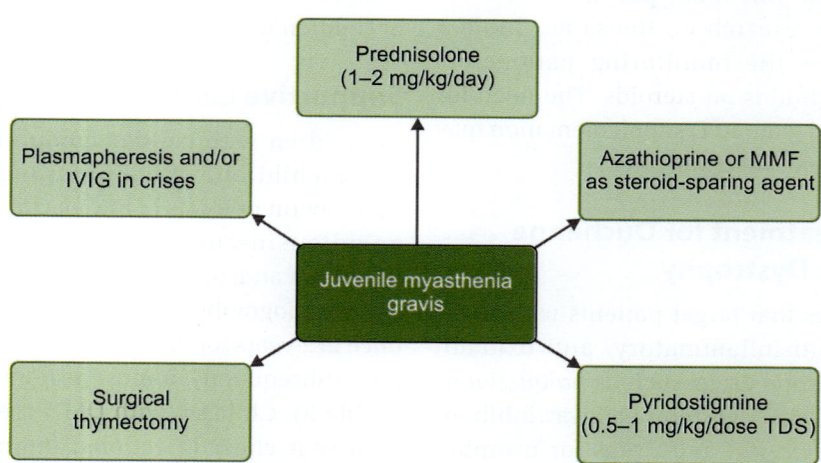

Fig. 3: Therapeutic options for juvenile myasthenia gravis. (IVIG: intravenous immunoglobulin; MMF: mycophenolate mofetil)

(IVIG) are the therapeutic options, especially among those with myasthenic crises. Corticosteroids, including prednisolone, form the mainstay of immunomodulatory therapy. Steroid-sparing agents, including azathioprine and mycophenolate mofetil (MMF), are also used among children with JMG. Thymectomy is indicated among those with thymoma in JMG. There is limited evidence on the role of thymectomy among those without thymoma. Parents should be provided with a list of drugs that are contraindicated in JMG, especially aminoglycosides, tetracycline, and D penicillamine. The anesthetist must be informed in case of surgery to avoid neuromuscular blockers.

JUVENILE DERMATOMYOSITIS

Children with juvenile dermatomyositis often present with chronic, progressive weakness of proximal muscles. Other features include cutaneous manifestations (Gottron papule, heliotrope rash, shawl sign) and elevated creatine kinase levels. Electromyography (EMG) may reveal fibrillations with high-frequency repetitive discharges and short-duration small-amplitude myopathic potentials. Chronic inflammatory changes are observed on muscle biopsy. Daily steroids are considered the mainstay of treatment for children diagnosed with juvenile dermatomyositis. Prednisolone is started at a dose of 2 mg/kg/day with gradual tapering by 2–4 weeks over a period of 10–12 months. In severe presentation, pulse methylprednisolone (30 mg/kg/day for 5 days) and/or IVIG (2 g/kg spread over 4–5 days) can be used to tide over the crises. In such severe presentations, children are started simultaneously on oral methotrexate (1 mg/kg weekly once) along with oral steroids. Other immunomodulators that have been used for refractory cases include rituximab, cyclophosphamide, tacrolimus, and MMF.

GUILLAIN–BARRÉ SYNDROME

Immunomodulatory treatment remains the mainstay of therapy for children with Guillain–Barré syndrome (GBS). Rapidly progressive disease course, inability to walk independently, and the presence of respiratory or bulbar involvement are indications for treatment in children with GBS. Fall in single breath count, presence of neck flexor weakness, difficulty in breathing, and fall in vital capacity are red flag signs to decide for the need of mechanical ventilation.

Intravenous immunoglobulin and *plasma exchange therapy* (PLEX) are the most effective immunomodulatory treatment in children with GBS. They act against the antibodies that result in nerve dysfunction. They are also known to downregulate β-cell-mediated antibody production and complement inhibition. Both the therapies are known to shorten the hospital stay and time to recovery of independent ambulation. They need to be started as soon as possible, preferably within 2 weeks from the onset of illness.

Intravenous immunoglobulin is preferred over plasmapheresis in most of the centers, as it is easily available and is easy to administer. IVIG is given in a dose of 2 g/kg, administered over 2–5 days. Plasma exchange is performed to a volume of 250 mL/kg with 5–6 cycles on alternate days over 10 days. The clinical response begins 3–7 days from the commencement of treatment during which clinical progression may occur. A combination or sequential treatment of IVIG and plasma exchange has not proven any superiority over the individual therapy. There are no clear indications for the second course of IVIG. However, children who achieved plateau phase with no improvement after 4 weeks can be tried on combination of plasma exchange followed by IVIG or a second course of IVIG can be given. There is no role of corticosteroids in the management of GBS.

Gabapentin is often required for pain management in children with GBS. GBS is a polyradiculoneuropathy that often results in excruciating pain in the limbs. Few children require opioid analgesics. Once the pain subsides, physiotherapy must be initiated. One must ensure the care of the back and of eyes and address issues of constipation and urinary retention. Adequate fluids and nutrition must be ensured during the acute phase of the illness.

The majority of children recover within 6 months from the onset of illness with 80% achieving ambulation at the end of 1 year. The demyelinating variant of GBS improves more completely when compared to the axonal variant. Few children might have unexcitable nerves where it becomes difficult to characterize the type of neuropathy. These children might have a poor outcome. Severity at presentation, respiratory or bulbar involvement at presentation, and prolonged need for mechanical ventilation are significant predictors of poor functional recovery.

CHRONIC INFLAMMATORY DEMYELINATING POLYNEUROPATHY

Three therapies are known to improve the functional status of children with chronic inflammatory demyelinating polyneuropathy (CIDP)—(1) IVIG, (2) corticosteroids, and (3) plasmapheresis. Children who are nonambulatory and those with motor or sensory disabilities are candidates for immunomodulatory therapy. Majority of treatment is for long duration; hence, the choice of immunomodulatory treatment needs to be decided based on cost, availability, and possible side effects of each treatment.

Intravenous immunoglobulin is the most commonly used immunomodulatory treatment for children with CIDP. The majority of centers use monthly IVIG at 2 g/kg over 2 days. Once there is a good functional recovery, gradually, the interval between IVIG is increased to once in 6–8 weeks. Most of the patients receive this therapy for a variable duration of 6–12 months. Oral prednisolone at a dose of 1–2 mg/kg/day for a duration of 6–12 months is known to be as effective as IVIG in the treatment of children with CIDP. Few centers use initial pulse methylprednisolone (30 mg/kg/day for 3–5 days) followed by oral steroids. The majority of the centers prefer IVIG over oral steroids for the side effect profile of the latter. With cost as a limiting factor, steroids are recommended as the first line. PLEX has also demonstrated efficacy in CIDP. However, the facility of PLEX is not available in all centers. Moreover, the cost and safety of PLEX need to be weighed. Some of the common adverse effects of chronic PLEX therapy include anemia, hypocalcemia, and recurrent infection owing to hypoimmunoglobulinemia.

MYOTONIC DISORDERS

Myotonic disorders comprise myotonic dystrophy and nondystrophic myotonia including paramyotonia congenita, and congenita myotonia (Becker and Thomsen). The drugs that are known to improve myotonia include phenytoin, quinine, procainamide, and mexiletine.

KEY MESSAGES

- The advances in the management of neuromuscular diseases have slowed down the progression of the disease.
- Nusinersen, Risdiplam, and Zongensma are the three FDA-approved drugs used for the treatment of children with spinal muscular atrophy.
- In DMD, current treatments cannot stop the relentless loss of muscle tissue and function. The FDA has approved Elevidys, the first gene therapy for children with DMD.
- *CASPR-Cas9*-mediated genome editing is a promising emerging therapy for children with DMD.
- Ataluren is useful among children with nonsense mutation and eteplirsen is useful for exon 51 deletion for the management of DMD.

Index

Page numbers followed by *b* refer to box, *f* refer to figure, *fc* refer to flowchart, and *t* refer to table.

A

AAV *See* Adeno-associated virus
ABA *See* Applied behavior analysis
Abdominothoracic respiration 429
Abduction, dorsal interossei for 84
Abductor pollicis brevis 84
Abetalipoproteinemia 258, 323, 324, 326, 329
Abortions, recurrent 227
Abortive medications 342
Abscess 127
ACA *See* Anterior cerebral artery
Acanthamoeba 168
Acanthocytes, peripheral smear for 329
ACE *See* Angiotensin-converting enzyme
Aceruloplasminemia 309, 446
Acetylcholine 188*f*
 receptor resistance 281
Acetylcholinesterase deficiency 281
Achilles tendon contractures 285
Acid-fast bacilli 169*f*
Acinetobacter spp. 485
Acoustic neuroma 153
Actin-binding amino-terminal domain 534
Acute arterial ischemic
 causes of 506*b*
 stroke, etiology of 507*t*
Acute ataxia 112, 317, 320, 320*t*, 321*fc*
 diagnosis of 318*t*
Acute disseminated
 encephalitis 308
 encephalomyelitis 137, 137*f*, 212, 213, 228*f*, 321, 399, 414, 516*f*
Acute encephalitis syndrome 486
Acute flaccid paralysis 414, 423, 423*t*
 causes of 414*t*, 415*t*
Acute inflammatory demyelinating polyneuropathy 414
Acute motor sensory axonal
 neuropathy 414, 422
 polyneuropathy 7

ADC *See* Apparent diffusion coefficient
Adduction, palmar interossei for 84
ADEM *See* Acute disseminated encephalomyelitis
Adeno-associated virus 533
Adenosine deaminase
 deficiency 292
Adenosylsuccinate lyase
 deficiency 292
ADHD *See* Attention deficit hyperactivity disorder
ADI-R *See* Autism diagnostic interview revised
ADOS *See* Autism diagnostic observation schedule
Adrenaline 4
Adrenergic neurons 39
Adrenocorticotropic hormone 39
Adrenoleukodystrophy 258, 261, 323, 329
Advanced postural
 reaction 521, 522*b*
 reflexes 42
AED *See* Antiepileptic drug
Aerobic exercise, low-impact 538
AFP *See* Alpha-fetoprotein
Agnosia 65
Agraphesthesia 65
Agyricpachygyric cortex 138*f*
AICA *See* Anterior inferior cerebellar artery
Airway, establishing 213
AIS *See* Arterial ischemic stroke
Akinetic rigid syndrome 303
Albumin 170
ALD *See* Adrenoleukodystrophy
Alexander disease 258, 261, 263*f*, 266
Alleles 177
Allogeneic stem cell
 transplantation 535
Alpha fusion protein 488
Alpha-amino-3-hydroxyl-5-methyl-4-isoxazole propionate 469
Alpha-fetoprotein 330
Altered sensorium 19*fc*, 212, 222
 history of 214

AMAN *See* Acute motor axonal neuropathy
Amblyopia 68
Aminoacidopathy 226
Amitriptyline 342
AMPA *See* Alpha-amino-3-hydroxyl-5-methyl-4-isoxazole propionate
AMP-B *See* Amphotericin B
Amphetamine 309
Amphotericin B 497
AMSAN *See* Acute motor sensory axonal neuropathy
Amygdala 38
 controls aggression 38
AN *See* Auditory nerve
ANA *See* Antinuclear antibody
ANCA *See* Antineutrophil cytoplasmic antibody
Anderson syndrome 277
ANEC *See* Acute necrotizing encephalopathy of childhood
Anemia 216, 374, 380, 540
 chronic 337
Anencephaly 353, 354
Aneurysms 518
Angelman syndrome 179, 181
Angiography, role of 231
Angiostrongylus 167
Angiotensin-converting
 enzyme 533
Angular gyrus, isolated lesion of 21
Anisotropy 127
Ankle
 clonus 88
 dorsiflexion 378
Ankle joint
 bilateral 380
 movement at 87
Anosognosia 65
Antalgic gait 92
Antenatal history 368, 425, 455
Anterior cerebral artery 28, 29, 507, 510
 branch of 27
Anterior horn cell 273, 278, 414, 424, 428
 pathology 76, 414

Anthropometric parameters 395
Anthropometry 278, 374, 386, 429, 437, 449
Antibiotic 490
  initial 486
Anticardiolipin 308
Anticonvulsant-like phenytoin 318
Antidepressant, tricyclic 529
Antidromic conduction 157
Antiepileptic drug 145, 318, 465, 468, 469t, 470, 471, 471t, 473, 474, 482
  classification of 465b
  discontinuing 474
  first-line 466t
  level monitoring 474
  newer 468t
  prescription, general principles of 471
  second-line 467t
  side effect of 472, 473t
  therapy, duration of 474
  use of 473
Antiganglioside antibody 422
  testing 422
Antigravity movement, lack of 424
Antineutrophil cytoplasmic antibody 231
Antinuclear antibody 231
Antiphospholipid antibody 506
  syndrome 308
Anti-seizure
  drug 465
  medication 349, 465
Antisense oligonucleotide 532
Antistreptolysin 312
Antitubercular drug treatment 488b
Antitubercular treatment 390
Anxiety 38, 231, 290, 299
  disorders, rumination in 299
AOA *See* Ataxia with oculomotor apraxia
APCR *See* Activated protein C resistance
Apgar scores 234
Aphasia
  expressive 20
  receptive 21
  type of 21fc
APLA *See* Antiphospholipid antibody
Aplasia 75
Apparent diffusion coefficient 227f, 508, 509f, 510f, 513f
Apraxia 65
Arachnoid mater 31
Arcuate nucleus 39
Argyll-Robertson pupil 35

Arm recoil 102
Aromatic l-amino acid decarboxylase deficiency 446
Arterial ischemic stroke 136f, 224, 504, 505, 509f, 510f, 517
Arteriovenous 213, 506
  malformation 122, 128
ASA *See* Anterior spinal artery
ASD *See* Autism spectrum disorder
Aseptic meningitis 495
Ash-leaf macule 238f
ASO *See* Antisense oligonucleotide
Asomatognosia 65
Asperger syndrome 289
Aspergillosis 497
Aspergillus 493
Asphyxia
  perinatal 211, 236f, 370, 373
  prolonged 224
Aspirin 514, 517
Astrocytes *See also* Glial fibrillary acidic protein
Astrocytoma 323
Asymmetric tonic neck reflex 41, 42f
Asynergia 318
AT *See* Ataxia telangiectasia
Ataxia 268, 276, 285, 316, 317, 324, 326, 327, 303
  chronic progressive 329, 450
  diagnosis of 316
  drug-induced 319
  etiology of 324
  hereditary 323
  history of 448
  presence of 112, 319
  progression of 319
  telangiectasia 240f, 259, 323, 324, 327, 330
  unilateral 317
  vestibular 107, 316, 316t
Ataxic disorders 316
Ataxic dysarthria 22
Athetoid movements 303
Athetosis 304, 379
ATM *See* Acute transverse myelitis
Atrophy 173
ATT *See* Antitubercular treatment
Attention span 57
  testing 58f
Attention-deficit hyperactivity disorder 289, 296, 300b, 310
Auditory cortex 32
Auditory pathway 32
Auditory radiation 32
Aura 200, 209
Autism 289, 294, 295

diagnostic observation schedule 290
Autism spectrum disorder 281, 289, 290, 290fc, 291b, 291t, 292b, 295, 344, 520, 530t
  diagnosis of 233
  medical treatment of 529
  screening for 294
Autistic regression 295, 296
Autistic trait, early screening for 294
Autoimmune 308
  n-methyl-d-aspartate receptor encephalitis 295
  workup 229
Autologous stem cell transplantation 535
Automatism 200
Autonomic instability 231
Autonomic nervous system 39
Autonomic system 420, 440
Autonomous bladder 190
Autosomal dominant inheritance 323
Autosomal recessive
  disorder 258
  inheritance 323, 361
AV *See* Arteriovenous
AVED *See* Ataxia with vitamin E deficiency
Awareness, lack of 214
Axillary frecklings 345
Axonal neuropathy 422
Axonal polyneuropathy 6
Axons 4
Azathioprine 539

B

Baclofen 349, 524
Bacterial CNS infections 492
Bacterial infections 493t
Bacterial meningitis 170, 486t
  diagnosis of 170
  risk factors for acute 485b
Bacterial myositis, causes of 492
Ballismus 112, 304, 379
Band-like sensation 407f
Barrington's nucleus 189, 190
Bartonella species 492
Basal ganglia 16, 17, 130, 348f
  anatomy of 17f
  blood supply of 29t
  motor circuit 17f, 18f
  pathology 17
  sparing of 262f
Basal thalamus 130
Basic motor nerve conduction 157f
Basilar artery syndrome 13

Index 545

Basilar impression 323
Basilar migraine 318, 319
BBB *See* Blood-brain barrier
BBE *See* Bickerstaff brainstem encephalitis
BEAP *See* Brainstem-evoked auditory potentials
Becker muscular dystrophy 284, 433, 441
Beevor's sign 84
Behavior 444
    abnormal 293
Behavioral arrest 198
Bell's phenomenon 72
Benedict syndrome 15
Benzodiazepine 525
Bickerstaff brainstem encephalitis 319, 321
Bile alcohol 329
Binet-Kamat intelligence scale 527
Binocular eye movement 69
Biogenic amines 172
Biogenic monoamines, disorders of 171
Biopsy sample, processing of 172
Biotinidase deficiency 324
Birth history 350
BKT *See* Binet-Kamat intelligence scale
Bladder emptying voiding reflex 190*f*
Bladder-sphincter dyssynergia 191
Blastomyces dermatitidis 493
Bleeding per vaginum 368
Blood
    glucose levels 168
    pressure 221
    subacute 118
    sugar 212
    vessel 39
Blood-brain barrier 166, 498
Body
    encephalitis 495
    mass index 437
    parts of 445
    righting reflex 43, 522
    sudden jerk of 201
Bone 123
Bony deformities 374
Borrelia 492
    burgdorferi See also Lyme disease
Botulinum toxin 524
Botulism 414-416
Brachioradialis muscle 441
Bradycardia 500
Bradykinesia 303
Brain 19*f*, 23, 120*f*

    advantages computed tomography of 121*b*
    area of 25, 29, 39, 39*t*
    blood supply of 27
    cisterns of 121*f*
    computed tomography of 118, 223
    dead 20, 55, 387
    disadvantages of computed tomography 121*b*
    injured child syndrome 296
    iron accumulation 252*f*
    limbic system in 38
    lobes of 19, 19*t*, 25
    magnetic resonance imaging of 123, 123*t*, 124*f*, 195, 225
    metabolites 127
    myelination in 130*t*
    normal myelination of 129
    parenchyma 118, 122
    tissue 121
    venous drainage of 29, 30*f*
Brain abscess 122, 127, 215, 224, 489
    leads, development of 490
    treatment of 490*t*
Brain injury
    postnatal 372
    preterm 369
    severe hypoxic 170
Brain tumor 323
    causing ataxia 327
Brainstem 4, 13, 27, 112, 130, 422
    blood supply of 14*f*
    dorsal 260
    encephalitis genetic causes 318
    lesion 112
    reflex 55, 57
    syndromes 15*t*
    tumor, extra-axial 153
Brainstem-evoked auditory potential 151, 152
    normal 152*f*
    waveforms 151*f*
    response audiometry 320
Brazelton neonatal behavior 100
BRCA1 gene mutation 186
Breath holding spells 205
Breathing
    cessation of 101
    type of 429
Brivaracetam 465, 468
Broca motor speech area 24
Brody disease 277
Brucella 492
Brucellosis 260
Brudzinski's sign 98, 98*f*, 109
BS *See* Burst suppression

Buccal midazolam 478
Bulbar dysarthria 22
Bulbar muscle 435
    weakness 427
Bulbar weakness 276, 450
Burst suppression 143, 203

C

Café-au-lait macules 208, 241, 345
Calcium 537
    channel 468, 469
        blocker 309
    channelopathy 277
Calf hypertrophy 76*f*, 285
Calpainopathy 284-286, 288, 438
Canavan disease 258, 261, 266
Candida 168, 493
Carbamazepine 319, 465, 466, 470, 471, 473
Carboxy terminus 534
Carboxylase deficiency, multiple 229
Cardiac involvement 279, 281, 283, 285
Cardiac lesion, Neonatal 518
Cardiac rhythm abnormalities 437
Cardiofaciocutaneous syndrome 457
Cardiogenic syncope 206
Cardiomyopathy 329
    dilated 285
Cardiovascular system 440
Carnitine deficiency 278
Carotid artery, internal 27, 507
CARS *See* Childhood autism rating scale
Cataract 278
Cat-scratch disease 492
Cauda equina 8, 8*f*
Caveolin 173
Caveolinopathy 286
CBF *See* Cerebral blood flow
CBZ *See* Carbamazepine
CDG *See* Congenital disorders of glycosylation
CECT *See* Contrast-enhanced computed tomography
Cefotaxime 490
Ceftriaxone 490
Cell body 3
Cenobamate 465, 468
Central cyanosis and clubbing, presence of 216
Central electrodes 139
Central hypotonia 272
Central nervous system 3, 7, 106, 167, 258, 414, 438, 451,

482, 492, 493t, 494t, 496, 497t, 506, 507, 521
  components of 7f
  examination of 54
  fungal infections of 493
  structural malformation of 373
  vasculitis 308
Central retinal artery occlusion 357
Central visual pathway 153
Centronuclear myopathy 280
Centrotemporal spikes 142, 202
Cerebellar aplasia 323
Cerebellar artery
  anterior inferior 13, 14f
  posterior inferior 14f
Cerebellar astrocytoma 323
Cerebellar ataxia 257, 328, 316
  acute 318
  causes of early-onset 324b
  gait 92
  sudden onset of 321
Cerebellar atrophy 314
Cerebellar dysarthria 444
Cerebellar dysfunction 97, 317
Cerebellar examination 54
Cerebellar function, examination of 96
Cerebellar hemangioblastoma 323
Cerebellar hemispheric lesions 15, 317
Cerebellar lesion 91
Cerebellar sign 111, 119f, 379, 420
Cerebellar system
  assessment of 450
  examination 109
Cerebellar vermis results 317
Cerebellitis 321
  acute 322f
  postinfectious 318
Cerebellum 15, 130, 260, 262f, 340f
  anatomy of 16f
  deep nuclei of 15
  intracranial space-occupying lesion of 319
  modifies motor 15
Cerebral artery
  left anterior 119f
  right middle 509f
  posterior 13, 14f, 509f, 510
Cerebral blood
  flow 499f, 500
  volume 498
Cerebral cortex 21f
  blood supply of 28f
  body parts in 23f
Cerebral creatinine deficiency 528
Cerebral edema
  diffuse 500f
  types of 498, 498t

Cerebral folate deficiency 292
Cerebral hemispheres 18, 119f
Cerebral palsy 239, 246, 247f, 249f-252f, 252t, 367, 520, 520t, 521f, 524t, 527t
  comorbidities of 246f
  contractures in 247fc
  deformities in 247fc
  early signs of 370
  etiology of 247b
  management of 520
  types of 247, 248f, 248t, 252, 252t
Cerebral perfusion pressure 501
Cerebral vasculature, assessment of 128
Cerebral vein
  great 30
  superior 29
Cerebral venous sinus thrombosis 222, 224, 414, 517
Cerebrospinal fluid 31, 118, 166, 167, 170f, 223, 244, 311, 314, 390, 421, 485, 493, 496, 498
  analysis 170
  bacteriology 167, 168
  cytology 167
  flow of 31f
  glucose 168
  gram stain of 168f
  immunoglobulin 169
  pleocytosis 167
  protein 167
  sample 169f
  spaces 121
Cerebrotendinous xanthomatosis 258, 268, 324, 327, 330
Cerebrum 18
  white matter tracts of 24
Cervical spine 155
Cervicomedullary junction 155
CFCS See Communication function classification system
Charcot-Marie-Tooth disease 275, 284, 285
Cherry red spot 240
Chiari malformation 323
Chikungunya virus 494
Childhood autism rating scale 290
Childhood-onset huntington disease 309
Chloramphenicol 358
Chloride channelopathy 277
Cholesterol levels 329
Choline 127
  acetyltransferase deficiency 281
Cholinergic neurons 39
Chorea 304, 310t, 327, 379
  pure forms of 302

Choreiform movement, high-amplitude 304
Choreoathetoid movement 308, 371
Choreoathetosis 75, 112, 276, 379, 445
Chorioamnionitis 368
Chorionic villus sampling 287
Chorioretinitis 240, 351
Choroid epithelial cells 167
Choroid plexus 166
  cauterization 349
Chromosomal disorders 177, 178, 235, 292
Chromosomal microarray 178, 179, 183, 185, 348, 351
  high-resolution 184f
  results of 184fc
Chromosome 180, 182, 531, 532
  long arm of 181
  short arm of 181
Chronic ataxia 322, 324fc, 327, 329, 330fc
  differential diagnosis of 327t
  etiology for 327t
  treatable causes of 324t
Cigarette paper scars 437
Cingulated cortex 38fc
Cingulated gyrus 38
Circle of Willis 27, 28f, 128
Circulation stroke, right posterior 226f
Citrobacter 485
Clasp knife spasticity 112
Clinical isolated syndrome 321
Clinical worsening 227
Clobazam 208, 470
Clofazimine 492
Clonazepam 470
Clonidine 528, 529
Clostridium species 492
Cloxacillin 490
Clubfoot deformities 281
Cluster headache 333
CMA *See* Chromosomal microarray
CMD *See* Congenital muscular dystrophy
CMT *See* Charcot-Marie-Tooth disease
CMV *See* Cytomegalovirus
CN *See* Cochlear nucleus
CN *See* Cranial nerve
CNS *See* Central nervous system
Coarse facies 257
Coarse postural tremors 314
Cocaine 309
Coccidioides immitis 493
Cochlear nucleus 32, 151f

Coenzyme Q 244
  analog 538
  deficiency 324
Cognitive decline, history of 448
Cognitive impairment 327
Cognitive milestones 51
Cognitive problems 231
Cognitive status 328
Cold caloric test 73, 74*f*
Colliculus, inferior 32, 151*f*
Color vision 66
Coma 20, 55, 212, 213*t*, 216, 224, 224*t*, 387
  depth of 221, 222
  indicator of depth of 226
Common stroke mimics 505*t*
Communication function classification system 251*f*
Complex febrile seizure 207, 208
Compound heterozygous *See also* Chromosome
Compound muscle action potential 163*f*, 286
Compressive myelopathy 405
  causes of 405*t*
Conduct disorder 290
Congenita myotonia 540
Congenital myasthenia 281
  types of 538
Congenital myasthenic syndrome 114, 277, 278, 280, 282, 431
Congenital myopathy 175, 274, 275, 278, 282, 424, 430
  favors 281
  types of 274
Congenital rubella syndrome 351
Consanguinity 227, 425
Consciousness 18, 19*f*, 54, 396, 484
  assessment of 56
  state of 55*t*, 216, 216*t*, 221-223, 387*t*
  structures for 56*f*
Constipation, management of 462
Continuous electroencephalography monitoring, indications of 480*b*
Contralateral cortical atrophy 135
Conventional angiography 231
Cooling blankets 525
Copying skills develop 48
COQ *See* Coenzyme Q
Cord lesion 190
Cornelia de Lange syndrome 236, 351
Corona radiata 130
Corpus callosum 18
  splenium of 130

Cortex, posterior regions of 29
Cortical blindness 358, 360
Cortical bone 124
Cortical functions 108
Cortical lesion 25*t*, 191, 222
Cortical malformation 124, 209
Cortical micturition center 189
Cortical sensation 95
Cortical sulcus 500*f*
Corticobulbar tract 4, 5, 25
Corticospinal fibers 25
Corticospinal pathway 15
Corticospinal tract 25, 26*f*, 112
Corticosteroids 536, 540
Costello syndrome 457
Cough headache, primary 333
Cover-uncover test 35
COX *See* Cytochrome oxidase
CP *See* Cerebral palsy
CPK *See* Creatine phosphokinase
CR *See* Cherry red
Cranial nerve 6*b*, 14, 15, 68, 71, 74, 75, 75*t*, 112, 220*f*, 376, 388, 419, 420, 438
  examination 54, 64, 101, 109, 111, 376, 396
  fiber 14*t*
    types of 13*t*
  functions 108
  history of 214, 404
  nucleus 13
  palsy
    assessment of 450
    multiple 319
    sparing of 116
Cranial neuropathy 422
Craniorachischisis 353, 354
Craniosynostosis 235*f*
Crawling 45*f*
C-reactive protein 313
Creatine
  phosphokinase 323, 432, 446
  transport, disorder of 292
Creeping 45*f*
Cremasteric reflex 90*f*
Cri-du-chat syndrome 236
Critical illness polyneuropathy 415
Cryptococcosis 497
Cryptococcus 168, 493
CSF *See* Cerebrospinal fluid
CSOM *See* Chronic suppurative otitis media
CSWS *See* Continuous spike and wave during sleep
CTX *See* Cerebrotendinous xanthomatosis
Cushing triad 500
CVST *See* Cerebral venous sinus thrombosis

Cyanotic congenital heart disease 215
Cyclophosphamide 518, 539
Cysteine-rich domain 534
Cystic lesion 489
  benign 127
Cytochrome oxidase 174
Cytogenetic investigations 178
Cytogenetic microarray 182, 183
Cytomegalovirus 169, 351, 351*f*, 360, 363, 414, 486, 487, 496
  infection, congenital 251
Cytoplasmic genes 258
Cytotoxic edema 498

D

Dandy-Walker malformation 323
Dapsone 492
DBDs *See* Degenerative brain disorders
Decorticate posturing refers 221
Deep brain stimulation 524
Deep sleep 100
Deep tendon 88
  reflex 12, 22, 26, 92, 102, 116, 221, 272, 316, 408*f*, 409*f*, 410, 422, 430, 440
  loss of 328
  testing 89*f*
Deep venous
  sinus thrombosis 136*f*
  thrombosis, prevention of 517
Deflazacort 536
Degenerating fibers 175*f*
Degenerative brain disorders 257, 258*t*
Dehydration 137
Dehydrogenase deficiency 229
Delirium 55
Deltoid hypertrophy 285
Deltoid muscle, tested 164*f*
Demyelinating central nervous system 321
Demyelinating neuropathy 422
Demyelinating plaque 123
Demyelinating polyneuropathy 6, 422*t*, 491
  early stage of 160*f*
Dengue
  encephalitis 494
  encephalopathy 494
  virus 494
Dense clot sign 231
Dense white matter 263*f*
Dentate nucleus 15
Dentatorubral-pallidoluysian atrophy 326

Deoxyhemoglobin 125
Deoxyribonucleic acid 177
Depigmented nevi 241
Depression 290
Depressive disorders 299
Dermatomyositis 173*f*, 286
    juvenile 539
Detect pneumococcal antigen 169*f*
Detrusor sphincter dyssynergia 191*f*
Developmental disorders,
    management of 520
Dextromethorphan 319
Diabetes mellitus 327
Dialeptic seizures 200
Diamond sign 439
Diazepam 524
    intravenous 478
DIC *See* Disseminated
    intravascular coagulation
Diencephalon 16
Differential leukocyte count 170
Diffusion restriction 225
Diffusion tensor imaging 127
Diffusion-weighted imaging 126,
    508, 509*f*-511*f*, 513*f*
Digit span test 57*f*
Digital subtraction angiography
    128, 231, 510
Dilated pupil, unilateral fixed
    35, 220
Dimercapto-1-propanesulfonic
    acid 530
Dimercaptosuccinic acid 530
DIP *See* Distal interphalangeal joint
Diphtheria *See also* Demyelinating
    polyneuropathy
Diplegia 371
Diplegic gait 92, 371
Diplopia 417, 538
Direct pathway stimulates muscle
    movement 17
Disability 369
Disabling motor stereotypies 528
Disease phenotype 278
Distal interphalangeal joint 85*f*
Distal limb weakness,
    progressive 275
Distal lower limb 107
    weakness 426
Distal predominant weakness 441
Distal upper limb 107
    weakness 276, 426
Diurnal fluctuation 436
Dive bomber 164
DLC *See* Differential leukocyte
    count
DMD *See* Duchenne muscular
    dystrophy

DMPS *See* Dimercapto-1-
    propanesulfonic acid
DNA *See* Deoxyribonucleic acid
Doll's eye reflex *See also*
    Oculocephalic reflex
Doll's eye response 217
Doose syndrome 143, 144, 203
Dopa-responsive dystonia 172, 267,
    307, 446
Dorsal column signs 268
Dorsal root ganglion 159*f*
Down syndrome 180, 180*f*, 236, 237*f*
Dravet syndrome 143, 203, 204, 470
DRG *See* Dorsal root ganglion
DRPLA *See* Dentato-rubro-pallido-
    luysial atrophy
Drug screening 320
DSM-V *See* Diagnostic and
    statistical manual of
    mental disorders-V
DTR *See* Deep tendon reflex
Duchenne muscular dystrophy 174,
    175*f*, 177, 181, 182, 276,
    284, 317, 433, 440*f*,
    532, 536*t*
    treatment for 533*t*, 537
Dumb rabies 417
Dura mater lies 31
DWI *See* Diffusion-weighted
    imaging
Dynamic hip adductor contracture
    380
Dysarthria 316, 318
    types of 22, 22*t*
Dysautonomia 422
Dyscalculia 301
Dysdiadochokinesia 97, 318, 450
Dyselectrolytemia 212, 213
Dysferlin 173
Dysferlinopathy 285, 286, 288
Dysgraphia 300
Dyskinesia 303
Dyskinetic cerebral palsy 368,
    376, 524
Dyslexia 300
Dysmetria 97, 318
Dysmorphism 351
Dysmyelinating 259, 260
Dystonia 112, 206, 257, 276, 304,
    307, 308, 310*t*, 327, 371,
    378, 378*t*, 379, 380, 443,
    445, 450
    history of 445
    management of 524
    worsens 445
Dystrophin 173
Dystrophinopathy 173, 438

E

Ear
    and sinuses, infection of 490
    heel to 102
Echocardiography 329
Edema 498
Edinger–Westphal nucleus 13, 220
EDMD *See* Emery-Dreifuss
    muscular dystrophy
EEG *See* Electroencephalogram
EIA *See* Enzyme immunoassay
Elbow
    extensor 83, 83*f*
    flexor 83, 83*f*
Electric shock 204
Electrocardiogram 329
Electrocardiography 313
Electroclinical syndrome 201
Electrode 139
    active 156
Electroencephalogram 195, 202,
    203, 208, 210, 265,
    296, 320
    basics of 210
Electroencephalography 139, 141,
    147, 226, 251, 311,
    314, 372
    abuses of 145*t*
    pitfalls of 141
    principle of 139
    report 146*t*
    requisition 140
Electromyography 161, 286, 321,
    423, 539
    role of 432
Electron microscopy 172, 173
Elevated free gamma-aminobutyric
    acid 172
ELISA *See* Enzyme-linked
    immunosorbent assay
Embolic strokes 505
EME *See* Early myoclonic epilepsy
Emery-Dreifuss muscular dystrophy
    275, 278, 433
Emotional memory 38
Emotional state, relation to 305
Emotions, reduced sharing of 292
Empirical antibiotic therapy 486*f*
Empty bladder, mechanism of 190*f*
Encephalitis 212, 486
    causes of 486
Encephalocele 354, 355
Encephalomyelitis,
    disseminated 115
Encephalopathy 137, 212, 232*fc*,
    322, 506
    acute 229
        necrotizing 496

causes of 212, 213t
developmental 204, 205
epileptic 204, 205
presence of 112
progressive 254
Endocrine causes 309
Endocrine myopathy 278
Endoscopic third ventriculostomy 349, 488
Endovascular treatment
  See Mechanical thrombectomy
Energy
  deficiency disorders 254
  failure, disorder of 255
Enterobacteriaceae 490
Enterovirus 486
Enterovirus 71 225, 493
Enzyme immunoassay 493
Enzyme-linked immunosorbent assay 169f, 493, 496
  kits 169
Ependymal cells 5
Ependymoma 323
Epigastric sensation 209
Epilepsy 142, 151, 195, 200, 202, 209, 210, 327
  benign 142, 202
  childhood absence 202
  diagnosis of 141, 201
  etiology of 201, 208
  frontal lobe 199
  genetic generalized 205
  juvenile absence 142, 148f, 196, 202, 205, 470
  management of 470
  migrating partial 203
  pediatric 145t
  reflex 140
  risk of future 207
  self-limited 201, 204
  structural 201
  surgery 210
  syndrome 195, 196, 205, 209
  type of 208, 209
Epileptic encephalopathy 143t, 144, 201, 203t, 205
  drug-resistant early-onset 171
Epileptic seizure 195
  self-limited 142t, 202t
Epileptic spasm 197, 198, 100, 201, 204
Epileptiform
  abnormalities 143, 203
  benign 141
  discharges 141
Episodes, multiple 105
Episodic ataxia 323, 323t

Episodic weakness 276
Epithalamus 16
Epithelial cells, single layer of 166
Epstein–Barr virus 321, 486
Equilibrium reaction 522
Erythrocyte
  deformability of 502
  sedimentation rate 231, 313
ES See External sphincter
Escherichia coli 168, 485
ESES See Electrical status epilepticus of sleep
Eslicarbazepine 465, 468
Esotropia 68, 68f
Essential tremors, diagnosis of benign 314
Etanercept 488
Ethambutol 358
Ethionamide 487
Ethosuximide 466, 468
ETX See Ethosuximide
Eutectic mixture local anesthetics 166
Ex vacuo dilatation leads 123
Exaggerated lumbar lordosis 279
Exercise headache, primary 333
Exome sequencing 185, 348
  cost of 186
  interpretations 186fc
Exon skipping 533
  concept of 535f
Exotropia 68, 68f
Extensor plantar 327
Extensor pollicis longus and brevis 84
External sphincter 190f
External ventricular drainage 488
Extramedullary lesion 409f
Extraneural organ 259
Extraneural signs 259t
Extraocular eye movements, supratentorial control of 219f
Extraocular movements 101
Extraocular muscle 34, 36, 435
  weakness 276
Extraocular weakness 417
Extrapyramidal dysarthria 22, 370, 372, 444
Extrapyramidal lesions 91
Extrapyramidal symptoms 268
Extrapyramidal syndrome 445
Extrapyramidal tracts 25
Eye 278
  alignment of 68, 68f
  blinking, unilateral 200
  contact, lack of social use of 292
  look bright 124

of tiger sign 313
open 56, 57, 100, 217
Eye movement 36, 37, 68
  assessment of 217
  common abnormal 37
  interpretation of 218
  supranuclear control of 36, 36f, 36t
  types of abnormal 37t
Eyelid position 72
Ezogabine 465

F

FA See Friedreich ataxia
Facial angiofibroma 239f
Facial dysmorphism 236f
  assessment of 236
Facial expression
  lack of 450
  paucity of 445
Facial involvement 280
Facial muscle 281
  weakness 427
Facial nerve 6, 14
  anatomy course of 71f
Facial sensation 101
Facial weakness 276, 435, 450
Facioscapulohumeral dystrophy 275, 278, 433, 439f
Factor V Leiden deficiency 506
Failure to thrive 281
Familial neonatal seizure, benign 142, 202
FAOD See Fatty acid oxidation disorder
Fascicular architecture 173
Fasciculus
  gracilis 9
  medial longitudinal 15, 219f, 220f
Fascioscapular muscular dystrophy 433
Fastigial nucleus 15
Fat distribution, abnormal 327
Fatty acid oxidation disorder 269f, 270f
FCR See Flexor carpi radialis
Febrile encephalopathy, acute 225t
Febrile illness 115, 215
Febrile infection-related epilepsy syndrome 205
Febrile seizure 207t, 208b, 468
Febrile status epilepticus 207, 208
Feeding difficulties 234, 248, 281, 449
  management of 525
Femoral internal torsion 521

Fentanyl *See also* Analgesic
Ferritin 168
Fertilization 354
Fetal alcohol syndrome 236
Fetal malformation 368
Fetal movement 274
Fever 212
Fiber 39
    across internal capsule 27*f*
    ascending 9
    descending 9
    splitting 287
    type 13, 14
Fibrillations, reveals evidence of 286
Fibroblast activity of hexosaminidase 330
Field of vision 66
Fight *vs.* break resistance 80*f*
Figure of H 69*f*
Filum terminale 8
Fine motor 52
    grasp cubes 47*f*
    milestone 45, 46, 46*t*
    skills 45, 375, 426
Finger
    movement testing 85*f*
    muscles 84
Finger-to-finger test 96
Finger-to-nose test 96, 97*f*
First gene therapy 535
FISH *See* Fluorescent in situ hybridization
Flaccid myelitis, acute 414, 415
Flaccid paraparesis 12
Flaccid weakness 106
Flaccidity 316
FLAIR *See* Fluid attenuated inversion recovery
Flexor carpi radialis 158
Flexor pollicis
    brevis 84
    longus 84
Flexor spasm 201
Floppy baby 424, 432
    examination of 428
    history in 428
Floppy infant 274, 424, 429
    causes of 424*t*
    differential diagnosis of 278
Fluid-attenuated inversion recovery 135*f*, 348*f*, 508, 516*f*
Flunarizine 342
Fluorescent in situ hybridization 178, 180, 185, 243
Fluoroquinolones 487
Fluoxetine 528
Focal epilepsy 151, 199*b*, 200, 201

    drug-resistant 468
    self-limited 205
    syndromes 205
Focal neurological deficit 136
Focal onset 199
Focal seizure, unprovoked 147
Focused neurological examination 109, 110, 406
Foot weakness, distal 435
Foramen of Monro 31
Forearm muscles 83
Formal medical research council 430
Formal sensory system examination 430
Fosphenytoin 479
Fragile X
    syndrome 179, 234, 236, 237*f*, 292, 298, 345
    testing 185
Frequent seizures, direct consequence of 201
Fresh blood, presence of 167
Friedreich ataxia 179, 268, 323, 325, 327, 330
    differential diagnosis of 325*b*
Frontal lobe 19
    dysfunction, bilateral 317
    function 111
FSHD *See* Facioscapulohumeral dystrophy
Functional movement disorder 315
Fundus
    examination 66
    normal 67*f*
Fungal infection 497, 497*t*
Furious rabies 495
FVL *See* Factor V Leiden deficiency
F-wave 158
    latency 162
    response, basis of 160*f*

G

GA *See* Glutaric aciduria
GABA *See* Gamma-aminobutyric acid
Gabapentin 465, 524, 525, 529, 532, 540
Gadopentetic acid 124
Gag reflex, poor 376
Gait 91, 111, 439
    abnormal 315
    abnormalities of 91
    description of 370
    examination 90
Galactosemia 259, 260
γ-aminobutyric acid 469, 524
    pathway 468, 469

Gangliosidosis 258
Gastaut syndrome *See also* Late-onset childhood occipital epilepsy
Gastrocnemius 441
Gastroesophageal reflux disease 251, 291, 437, 526
Gaucher disease, juvenile 264
G-banding karyotype, high-resolution 243
GBS *See* Guillain–Barré syndrome
GDD *See* Global developmental delay
Gene addition therapy 533, 534
Generalized epilepsy syndromes 205
Generalized interictal epileptiform discharges 196
Genetic analysis 287
    indications for 287
Genetic conditions 267
Genetic diagnostic techniques 186
Genetic disease 310, 310*t*, 311, 311*t*
Genetic disorders, groups of 177
Genetic epilepsy 201
Genetic investigations
    advantages of 185*t*
    disadvantages of 185*t*
Genetic panel sequencing 432
Genetic polymorphism 186
Genetic testing 178*t*, 180, 186, 283, 284
Genome editing 533
Genomic techniques 182
GERD *See* Gastroesophageal reflux disease
Gesell figures 48
Giant axonal neuropathy 273
Gigantism 454
Glabellar blink 64
Glasgow coma
    scale 56, 56*t*, 217*t*
    score 485, 500
Glial fibrillary acidic protein 168
Glioma 145
    high-grade 127
Global developmental delay 233, 255, 289, 291, 379
Global hypoxic injury 119
Globus pallidus 29
    evidence of bilateral 133
    externa 17*f*, 18*f*
    interna 17*f*, 18*f*
Glossopharyngeal nerve 6
Glucose transporter 252*f*
    deficiency 204
Glucose-lactate tolerance 329
GLUT *See* Glucose transporter

Glutamate blockers 469
Glutaric aciduria 270f
Glutaryl-coenzyme 229
Gluten-sensitive enteropathy 320
Glycogen storage disorder 283
Glycosylation, congenital disorders of 239f, 255, 327
GMFCS *See* Gross motor functional classification system
Gnathostomata 167
Gomori trichrome stain, modified 174
Gonadotropin-releasing hormone 39
Gottron papule 437, 539
Gower sign 275, 439, 440f
GPE *See* Globus pallidus externa
GPI *See* Globus pallidus interna
Gradient-recalled echo 125
Gram-negative anaerobic bacilli 490
Gram-negative bacilli 168f
Graphesthesia 95
Grasp reflex 64
Gratification 206
Gravity eliminated 86
Gray-matter 120f, 121, 125, 258
  appearance of 124
  function 445
  junction 489
  white matter junction, loss of 500f
Great malleoli 94
Gross motor 44, 52
  examination 45f
  function classification system 249, 378, 431, 524
  milestones 44, 44t
  skills 375
Group atrophy 175
GTCS *See* Generalized tonic-clonic seizure
GTP *See* Guanosine triphosphate
Guanfacine 529
Guanosine triphosphate 310
Guarded procedure 167
Guillain–Barré syndrome 6, 168, 171, 317, 321, 337, 414, 415, 421b, 492, 494, 539

H

H reflex 160
  basis of 161f
Habituation 100
  lack of 101
Haemophilus influenzae 485
Hallervorden-Spatz disease 267
Halofuginone 537
Hamstring muscle 87
Hand weakness, distal 281
Handwashing movement 303
Hartnup disease 319, 320, 323, 324, 327, 329
Head
  bobbing of 318
  compute tomography of 251
  drops 204
  shape 374
  trophy sign, calf on 438
Headache 106, 107, 214, 339b, 489
  acute 335fc, 340b
  causes of 339t
  childhood 334b
  chronic daily 331
  clinical evaluation of 331
  diagnosis of 331
  diary 333
  disorders 332t
  evaluation 338t
  primary 331, 333, 333t, 337
  secondary 331, 332, 337
  tension-type 331, 332, 335
  types of 331, 332, 338
Hearing 371, 444
  assessment 51
  god's voice 62
Hearing loss 361, 363
  acquired 362
  causes of congenital 361fc
  characteristics of 362
  conductive 361
  congenital 362, 362fc, 363fc
  progressive 363
  sensorineural 72, 268, 327, 361
Heavier hammer 88
Heliotrope rash 539
Helminthic infections 167
Hemangioblastoma 323
Hematoma 318
Hemiconvulsion-hemiplegia-epilepsy syndrome 135f, 205, 513f
  diagnosis of 135
Hemiplegia 247, 371
  acute 392, 399fc, 399t
  causes of 392b
  childhood 400fc
  chronic 76
Hemiplegic gait 92, 371
Hemispatial inattention 65
Hemodynamically stable 211
Hemorrhage 127
  intracranial 128
  subacute 123
Hemorrhagic stroke 171, 504, 505, 506b
Hepatic encephalopathy 213
Hepatomegaly 278
Hepatosplenomegaly 241, 257
Hereditary fructose intolerance 255, 269f
Hereditary motor sensory neuropathy 273
  early-onset 114
  polyneuropathy 278
Hereditary neuropathy 428
Hereditary sensory autonomic neuropathy 273
Herpes encephalitis 225, 487
Herpes simplex virus 169, 360, 486, 492, 496
Heterotopia 68, 124, 138, 138f
HFI *See* Hereditary fructose intolerance
HIAA *See* Hydroxyindole acetic acid
Higher cortical function 65, 65t
Higher mental function 111, 208, 372, 387, 396, 419
  components of 54fc
  examination 54
  history of 404
Hip
  abduction 86, 86f
    sign 440
  abductor, testing 86f
  adduction 86, 86f, 87f
  dislocation 521
    rarely 280
  extensor 86, 87f
  flexion 84
    testing 86f
  girdle weakness 435
    proximal 284, 285, 426
  joint, movement at 84
  subluxation 521
    evidence of 374
  surveillance 251
Hippocampal malrotation 209
Hippocampus 38, 38fc
  and olfactory bulb, parts of 4
Histoplasma capsulatum 493
HIV *See* Human immunodeficiency virus
HMSN *See* Hereditary motor sensory neuropathy
Hodgkin's lymphoma 167
Holmes–Adie pupil 35
Holmgren wool test 66
Homocystinuria 506
Homonymous hemianopia 33
Homovanillic acid 172, 446
  urinary excretion of 320
Homunculus 23

Horn cell
  pathology 273
  rules out anterior 282
Horner syndrome 35, 220
HS *See* Hypertonic saline
HSAN *See* Hereditary sensory autonomic neuropathy
HSV *See* Herpes simplex virus
Human cerebral cortex 24*f*
Human herpes virus 486
Human immunodeficiency virus 235, 381, 482, 496*t*
  encephalopathy 496
  infection 254
Human T-cell lymphotropic virus 492
Huntington chorea 179, 267
HV *See* Hyperventilation
HVA *See* Homovanillic acid
Hydranencephaly 344, 452
Hydrocephalus 123, 345, 452, 453, 488
  clinical signs of 457
  congenital 347*f*, 349, 453*f*, 454
Hydronephrosis, development of 462
Hydroxychloroquine 358
Hydroxyindole acetic acid 172, 446
Hyperactive behavior 444
Hyperactivity *See also* Clonidine
Hyperammonemia 213
Hyperckemia 285
Hyperdense 118
Hyperekplexia 206
Hyperkinetic impulse disorder 296
Hyperkinetic movement disorder 303
Hyperreflexia 112
Hypertension 500
Hypertonic saline 502
Hyperventilation 140, 146, 501
Hypocalcemia 540
Hypocontractile bladder 191
Hypodense 118
Hypodontia 261
Hypoglossal nerve 6, 75
  testing for 75
Hypoglycemia 212
Hypoglycemic insult 369
Hypoglycorrhachia 168
Hypoimmunoglobulinemia 540
Hypokalemia 414
Hypokalemic pseudoparalysis 415
Hypokinetic movement disorder 17, 303
Hypomelanosis of ito 208
Hypomyelinating 260
  leukodystrophy 259, 260
  neuropathy, congenital 286

Hypomyelination 129
Hypothalamic hamartoma 204
Hypothalamus 38, 39
Hypothyroid *See also* Endocrinal myopathy
Hypothyroidism, congenital 237*f*, 528
Hypotonia 316
  evidence of 430
  indicative of 427
  peripheral 272, 272*t*, 278
  testing for 78*fc*
Hypoxic-ischemia
  brain injury 170, 510
  secondary 224
Hypsarrhythmia
  classical 147*f*
  evidence of 204

I

IC *See* Inferior colliculus
ICA *See* Internal carotid artery
Ichthyosis 327
ICP *See* Intracranial pressure
ICSOL *See* Intracranial space-occupying lesion
Ictal speech arrest 200
Idebenone 537, 538
Idiopathic intracranial hypertension 337
  headache of 337
Idiopathic transverse myelitis 491
IEM *See* Inborn errors of metabolism
Illness, duration of 110
Illusion 62
Immunoglobulin, intravenous 496, 538*f*, 539
Incontinentia pigmenti 238
Index finger bent and thumb 48
Individual extraocular muscles, actions of 69*t*
Individualized Educational Programs 527
Infant head leads, flexion of 42
Infantile autism 289
Infantile epileptic spasm syndrome 204
Infantile neuroaxonal dystrophy 176, 258
Infantile onset 203
Infantile spasms 468
Infection 120, 360
  recurrent 540
Infectious causes 381
Infectious etiology 201
Infective neuropathy, types of 491

Infective transverse myelitis, acute 491
Inferior pincer grasp 48
Inflammatory demyelinating polyneuropathy, chronic 540
Inflammatory myopathy 173*f*, 281, 286, 427
  dermatomyositis 278
  polymyositis 278
Influenza virus 494
Infrapontine cisterns 121
Inner ear, aplasia of 362
Intact memory 60
Intellectual disability 233, 233*b*, 236*f*, 238*t*, 239, 240*t*, 241*t*, 243, 243*t*, 248, 281, 289, 346, 436, 527*t*, 528*t*
  causes of 236*t*, 244*fc*, 528
  etiology of 234, 235*t*
  management of 527
  severity of 234*b*
  treatable 244*f*
    causes of 528*t*
  unexplained 186
Intensive care unit 56
Intentional tremor 317
Interictal epileptiform discharges 144
Interictal positron emission tomography 210
Intermittent photic stimulation 140
Intermittent porphyria, acute 415
Intermittent prophylaxis, indications for 208
Intermittent-chronic ataxia, causes of 112
Internal capsule 27, 129*f*
  genu of 27
  posterior limb of 29, 129, 259
Internuclear ophthalmoplegia 37
Interpositus nucleus 15
Interstitial edema 498
Intoxication disorder 254, 255
Intracranial bleed 213
Intracranial pressure 213, 231, 232, 318, 321, 344, 390, 399
  benign raised 337
  causes of 498*b*
  clinical signs of raised 499
  decrease raised 212
  management of raised 498
  monitoring 500
Intracranial space-occupying lesion 318, 497
Intramedullary lesion 409*f*
Intrathecal baclofen 524

Intrauterine
 growth restriction 234
 infection 492
Intravascular coagulation,
 disseminated 496
Intravenous 213
Intraventricular bleed 369
Ipsilateral cerebellar signs 319
Ipsilateral side 199
IS *See* Internal sphincter
Ischemic brain injury 482*f*
Ischemic stroke 504
Ishihara card 66, 67*f*
Isolated syndrome 321
Isoniazid 487
 high dose of 488
Isovaleric acidemia 255, 269*f*
Isovaleric aciduria 229
IV *See* Intravenous
IVA *See* Isovaleric acidemia
IVIG *See* Intravenous
 immunoglobulin

J

Japanese encephalitis 225, 226, 414
 virus 486, 495
Jaundice, presence of 216
Jaw jerk, testing 71*f*
JE *See* Japanese encephalitis
Jeavons syndrome 144
Jerky speech 372
Jitteriness 302
Joint
 fixed contractures in 436
 position sensation, testing 93*f*
Joubert syndrome 323

K

Karyotype 178, 180, 181*t*, 185
 blood samples for 180
 report mentions 180
Kayser-Fleischer
 ring 268, 268*f*, 313
 test 446
Kearns–Sayre syndrome 327
Keloids 437
Keratosis pilaris 437
Kernicterus 112
 sequelae 133*f*
Kernig's sign 98*f*, 109
Ketamine 501
KFT *See* Kayser-Fleischer test
Klebsiella spp. 485
Klinefelter syndrome 180

Knee
 extensor 87, 87*f*
 flexor 87*f*
 joint, movement at 87
Krabbe disease 258–261, 266, 445
KSS *See* Kearns–Sayre syndrome
Kyphosis 521

L

LA *See* Lupus anticoagulant
Labyrinth righting reflex 43
Labyrinthine
 ataxia 317
 righting reflex 522
Labyrinthitis 319
Lacosamide 465, 468
Lactate 321, 329
Lactic acid levels 321
Lactic acidosis 506
Lactulose 526
Lafora body disease 176, 264, 314
Laminectomy 491
Laminin 173
Lamotrigine 465, 467, 470, 471, 473
Landau reflex 42, 42*f*
Landau righting reflex 522
Landau–Kleffner syndrome
 143–145, 203, 205, 296, 296*t*
Language 20, 21*f*, 52
 assessment of 62
 dysfunction of 20
 milestones 49, 49*t*
Latency, distal 156
Latex agglutination test 169*f*
Laughs aloud 50
Learning 208
 difficulties 281
 disorder, specific 299–301
 points 400, 401
Leber's hereditary optic
 neuropathy 360
Leber's optic neuropathy 323
Left eyes, adduction of 37
Left temporal epileptiform
 discharges 149*f*
Leg muscles, atrophy of 284
Leg, twisting of 445
Leigh disease 260, 506
Lemniscus, lateral 32, 151*f*
Lennox–Gastaut syndrome 143, 144, 148*f*, 203, 205, 468, 470
Lens
 dislocated 240
 thickening of 34
Lenticulostriate artery stroke 27
Leprosy *See also* Mononeuritis
 multiplex

Leptomeningeal enhancement 7
Leptospira 492, 493
Leptospirosis 225, 493
Lesch–Nyhan syndrome 258, 430
Lesion 91, 112
 at cortex 37, 192
 extent of 223
 localization of 317
 multiple ring-enhancing 133*f*
 site of 92, 221, 424
 vestibular 91
Lethargy 20, 55
Leukodystrophy 259, 261, 308, 309, 313
 classification of 261*fc*
 encountered 261*t*
 patterns of 260*t*
Leukoencephalopathy 259
 reversible 510
Leukomalacia, periventricular 209
LEV *See* Levetiracetam
Levetiracetam 465, 467, 468, 470, 473, 479
Levodopa 524
Levofloxacin 487
LFT *See* Liver function test
LGMD *See* Limb-girdle
 muscular dystrophy
LGS *See* Lennox–Gastaut syndrome
Light reflex 33
Limb
 ataxia 317
 automatism 200
 dystonia, unilateral 200
 flailness of 274
 posterior 129*f*
Limb-girdle
 muscular dystrophy 276, 278, 284, 285, 433
 myasthenia 284
 weakness 441
Limbic system 38
 anatomy of 38*f*
Linezolid 487
Lingual sounds 22
Lipoprotein 329, 506
 low-density 329
Liquid nitrogen, snap frozen in 172
Liver function test 446
LKS *See* Landau-Kleffner syndrome
LL *See* Lateral lemniscus
LL *See* Lower limb
LMN *See* Lower motor neuron
LMWH *See* Low-molecular-weight
 heparin
Locked-in syndrome 20, 55
Lorazepam
 intranasal 478
 intravenous 478

Low birth-weight 234
Low-cholesterol diet 518
Lower limb 92, 111, 157, 158*t*, 248, 279, 377
    proximal 107
    weakness 275
Lower motor neuron 4, 72, 409, 409*f*, 410, 431
    lesion 26, 26*t*
    pathology 258
    weakness 316
Low-molecular-weight heparin 514, 517
    indications for 514
LP *See* Lipoprotein
LR *See* Lateral rectus
LSD *See* Lysosomal storage disorder
LTG *See* Lamotrigine
Lumbar puncture 166, 320, 341
    indications of 208
Lumbosacral spinal level 191
Lupus anticoagulant 506
Luria graphic test 61*f*
Lying-down posture 416
Lyme disease 225, 491, 493
Lysosomal storage disorder 255, 345

M

Macewen's sign 109
Machado-Joseph disease 323
Macrocephaly 257, 258, 343, 344*fc*, 346*fc*, 347, 452
    gene panel testing 348
MAE *See* Myoclonic astatic epilepsy
Magnesium 530
Magnetic resonance
    angiography 128, 128*f*, 231
    spectroscopy 127
    venography 128, 231
Malin intelligence scale 527
Malnutrition 488
    signs of 374
Mannitol saline 502
Maple syrup urine disease 229, 255, 269*f*, 270*f*, 319, 320, 329
Marcus-Gunn pupil 35
Marinesco–Sjögren syndrome 327
Mass spectrometry 351
Maternal chorioamnionitis 518
Maternal fever 350, 368
Maternal transmission 278
Mathematics expression disorders 300
Mature pincer grasp 48*f*
MCA *See* Middle cerebral artery
McArdle disease 281

MCP *See* Metacarpophalangeal
MCPH mutation 351
Measles 495
    antibody 171
    encephalitis
        acute 225, 495
        primary 495
Mechanical thrombectomy 518
Meckel–Gruber syndrome 457
MECP2 gene 296
Medial geniculate body 32
Median nerve, stimulation of 155*f*
Medulla 7
    adrenal 39
Medulloblastoma 323
Megalencephalic leukoencephalopathy 179, 261, 262*f*
Megalencephaly 452
    causes of 457
    classification of 346*fc*, 453*fc*
MELAS *See* Mitochondrial encephalopathy with lactic acidosis and stroke
Melatonin 140, 526
Membrane, premature rupture of 247, 368, 518
Memory 39, 59, 208
    despite normal 62
    long-term 59
    problems 16
    spatial 38
Meningeal enhancement 209
Meningeal sign 109, 379, 398, 420
    examination of 97
Meninges 31
Meningitis 112, 170*t*, 485
    bacterial 224
    causes of chronic 381*t*
    diagnosis of 170
    neonatal 112, 235
    tubercular 224
Meningocele 354, 355
Meningococcemia 215
Meningococcus 168
Menkes disease 528
Mental disorder, statistical manual of 300*b*
Mental disorders-V, diagnostic and statistical manual of 290
Mental retardation 233
Mental status 109, 111
    assessment of 62
MERRF *See* Myoclonic epilepsy with ragged red fiber
Mesial temporal
    lobe epilepsy 199
    sclerosis 135*f*, 209, 210*f*

Metabolic acidosis 213
Metabolic disorders 229, 292, 323
Metabolic etiology 506
Metabolic myopathy 274, 278, 281-283, 427
    indicator of 427
Metabolic problems 109
Metabolic screen 226, 321
Metabolic testing 351
Metabolism, inborn errors of 171, 226, 244, 372
Metacarpophalangeal joints 84, 85*f*
Metachromatic leukodystrophy 260, 261, 262*f*, 266, 266*f*
Metagenomic next-generation sequencing 493
Metathalamus 16
Methylmalonic acidemia 255, 269*f*, 270*f*
Methylmalonic aciduria 229
Methylphenidate 528
Methylprednisolone 540
Methyl-tetra-hydro-folate reductase 506
Metronidazole 490
Mexiletine 540
MFS *See* Miller-Fisher syndrome
Microcephaly 138, 343, 350, 350*fc*, 351*fc*
    primary 235*f*
    severe 350
Microdeletion disorders 181
Microglia 5, 168
    cells 5
    migrates 5
Micturition, neural control of 188*f*
Midazolam
    intramuscular 478
    intranasal 478
Midbrain 15
    blood supply of 13
    brainstem consists of 7
Middle cerebellar
    artery 29, 119*f*, 507, 510
        lenticulostriate branch of 27
    peduncle 129
Migraine 318, 332, 334, 357
    headache, management of acute 342*b*
    probable 334
    with aura 336*b*
    without aura 337*b*
Migrainous headache 334
Migrating partial epilepsy of infancy 203
Migratory focal seizures 143
Milestones 52
Miller–Dieker syndrome 181, 244

Miller–Fisher syndrome 317-319, 321, 414
Minimal conscious state 216
Minocycline 492
Mitochondria, staining for 174*f*
Mitochondrial disorders 258, 266, 292, 307, 327, 329
Mitochondrial encephalopathy 506
Mitochondrial myopathy 278, 281-283, 287, 428, 431
MLC *See* Megalencephalic leukoencephalopathy
MLD *See* Metachromatic leukodystrophy
MLF *See* Medial longitudinal fasciculus
MLPA *See* Multiplex ligation probe amplification
MMA *See* Methylmalonic acidemia
MMD *See* Moyamoya disease
MMF *See* Mycophenolate mofetil
Mobility devices 523
Molecular diagnosis 432
Molecular genetic testing 330
Mondini defect 362
Monogenic disorders 292
Mononeuritis multiplex 6, 491
Mononeuropathy 6
Monoplegia 247
Moro's reflex 41, 41*f*
Mosaicism 178
Motor
 axonal
  neuropathy 162*f*, 422*b*
 polyneuropathy 7
Motor component 70
Motor deficit 234, 370
 history of 370, 371*t*
Motor examination 101, 111
Motor function 108, 216
 classification 436
 gene, survival of 177
Motor homunculus 23*f*
Motor impairment 246, 520
Motor manifestation, absence of 476
Motor movement 293
Motor nerve conduction 156, 158*f*
Motor neurons 4
Motor onset 198
Motor response 56, 57, 217
 to stimuli, assessment of 221
Motor score 56
Motor system 443
 examination 54, 75, 397, 429, 438
Motor unit 6
 components of 6*f*
 potentials 163, 165*f*
 recruitment 164

Motor weakness 316, 417
 symmetric ascending 417
Mouth, position of angle of 72
Movement 316
 abnormal 88, 106, 108, 443
 awareness of 306
 description of 312, 313
 high amplitude 93
 quality and quality of 101
 therapy, constraint-induced 522
Movement disorder 229, 231, 276, 302-305, 305*t*, 306, 306*t*, 309, 309*t*, 310, 311*b*, 310*t*, 379, 379*t*, 443
 classification of 303*b*
 description of 304*t*
 diagnosis of 302
 hyperkinetic 88
 hypokinetic 88
 mixed 309, 309*t*
 onset of 306
Moyamoya
 disease 231
 vasculopathy 134*f*
MPSI *See* Migrating partial epilepsy of infancy
MR *See* Mental retardation
MS *See* Multiple sclerosis
MSUD *See* Maple syrup urine disease
MTHFR *See* Methyl-tetra-hydro-folate reductase
Mucopolysaccharidosis 236, 345, 528
Mucormycosis 497
Multifocal leukoencephalopathy, progressive 496
Multiple café-au-lait macules 239*f*
Multiple injury marks 239*f*
Multiple sclerosis 318, 319, 410
Multiplex ligation 243
 probe amplification 181
Mumps 495
 encephalitis 495
MUPs *See* Motor unit potentials
Murphy's sequence 52, 72
 of hearing 52*f*
Muscle 69, 158, 172, 414, 424
 abdominal 84
 atrophy of 75
 belly 172
 bulk of 75, 438
 hypertrophy 76*f*
 involvement, group of 288
 longest 79*f*
 parts of 172
 pathology 414
 specific kinase 538
 tone, abnormality of 520, 521

Muscle biopsy 172, 173, 174*t*, 284, 286
 current relevance of 175
 driven diagnosis 432
 dystrophic change in 287
 procedure of 172
 role of 283
 site of 172
Muscle fiber 173*t*
 shape of 173
 viscoelastic tension of 429
Muscle pain 436
 rarely sudden onset of 285
Muscle power
 grading of 80*t*
 lack of 424
 testing 10
Muscle weakness 276, 520
 functional assessment of 279
Muscular dystrophy 91, 274, 274*t*, 275, 433, 433*t*, 434
 classical signs in 438
 congenital 114, 175, 274, 280, 282, 424, 436, 437
Muscular gait 91
Musculoskeletal examination 379, 380*t*
Myasthenia 281
 gravis 12, 417
  juvenile 538, 538*f*
 observed in 281
 rules out 282
Myasthenic crises 414, 415
Mycobacterium 168
 leprae 492
 tuberculosis 169
Mycophenolate mofetil 538*f*, 539
Mycoplasma 492, 506
 infection 321
 pneumoniae infection 493
Myelin basic protein 168, 170
Myelinate
 after 130
 before 130
Myelination
 after birth, progression of 130*f*
 delayed 129, 260
Myelitis, transverse 410
Myelocele 354
Myoblast transplantation 533
Myoclonic astatic
 epilepsy 143
 seizures 144
Myoclonic encephalopathy 318, 327
Myoclonic epilepsy 314, 450
 benign 142, 202
 early 143, 203

juvenile 142, 144, 196, 202, 205, 209, 470
progressive 205, 255, 257, 264, 264t, 311, 311t, 450
with ragged red fiber 311
Myoclonic seizures 239f
Myoclonus 304, 309, 327, 379
benign 205
classification of 311b
history of 447
peripheral 309
Myogenic pattern 175t
Myokymia 286
Myopathic pattern 163
Myopathy 273, 427
distal 275
drug-induced 414
treatment of 531
Myositis 492
Myotilin 173
Myotonia 164, 427
congenital 277, 426
evidence of 279
refers 78
Myotonic disorders 540
Myotonic dystrophy
congenital 274, 278, 281, 282, 424
ruling out 281
Myotonic dystrophy *See also* Cataract
Myotubularin 280

N

N-acetyl aspartate 127
NADH *See* Nicotinamide adenine dinucleotide dehydrogenase
NADH-TR *See* Nicotinamide adenine dinucleotide dehydrogenase-tetrazolium reductase
Nasolabial fold, symmetry of 72
National Tuberculosis Elimination Program 488
NBIA *See* Neurodegeneration with brain iron accumulation
NCC *See* Neurocysticercosis
NCL *See* Neuronal ceroid lipofuscinoses
NCS *See* Nerve conduction study
NCSE *See* Nonconvulsive status epilepticus
NDDs *See* Neurodegenerative disorders
Neck extensor 80
muscle power testing 81f
testing 81f
weakness 426, 435

Neck flexor 80
testing 81f
weakness 276, 279, 426, 435
Neck righting reflex 43
Neck stiffness 98f
history of 214
Necrotic myofibers 287
Necrotic tissue 127
Neisseria meningitidis 485
Nemaline rod 275
myopathy 280
Neocortical temporal lobe epilepsy 199
Neonatal encephalopathy 369
Neonatal intensive care unit 369
Neonatal jaundice 112
exchange transfusion for 369
requiring exchange transfusion 369
Neonatal-onset coagulation disorders 518
Neoplasm 122, 127
Nerve
abducens 6
auditory 101, 151f
biopsy 176
cells 5
cochlear 32, 72
fiber 4
hypertrophy 285
pelvic 190
testing, vestibular 72
Nerve conduction study 7, 155, 161, 162, 162b, 286, 420
parameters of 157f
procedure of 156f
Nervous system
electrophysiological response of 154
functional unit of 4
general organization of 3
organization of 3f
treatment of infections of 485
Neural pathway 32
Neural tube
closure 354f
formation of 353f
Neural tube defect 354-355, 452
classification of 354fc
clinical signs of 457
postnatal management of 461
types of 355f, 355t
Neuralgiform headache attacks, unilateral 337
Neuraxis involvement, specific 427t
Neuritis, traumatic 414, 415
Neuroacanthocytosis 446
Neuroacanthosis 309

Neuroanatomical localization 112, 113, 272
Neuroanatomical site 222, 223
Neuroanatomy 317
clinical 3
Neuroblastoma syndrome 318
Neurocutaneous markers 298, 345, 457
evidence of 374
Neurocutaneous syndromes 238t
Neurocysticercosis 120, 122, 125f, 232, 399, 474, 489, 489t, 490fc
Neurodegeneration 252
Neurodegenerative disease 259, 259t, 450t
Neurodegenerative disorder 254, 255, 257, 257t, 289, 443
classification of 256t
diagnosis of 154
Neurodevelopmental disorders 520
Neurodevelopmental therapy 522
Neurofibromatosis 178, 208, 238, 239f, 292
Neurogenic
bladder 191f
pattern 163, 175t
process 165
Neuroglial cells 5
Neuroimaging 118, 209, 340, 421
indications for 341
Neurological complaints, description of 106
Neurological diagnosis 104, 110
Neurological disease 106
genetic evaluation in 177
Neurological evaluation 1, 279
Neurological examination 104, 109b, 110, 111t, 114, 319, 379, 386, 440, 450
neonatal 99
part of 98
Neurological history 104, 105t
Neurological illness 106f, 113, 387, 387t
Neurological infection 496t
Neurological practice 109
Neurological symptoms 104, 107t, 358
Neurological weakness 107
Neurometabolic disorders 254, 267, 269f, 270f, 309, 309t, 373
classification of 255t
Neuromuscular care 280b
Neuromuscular causes 428
Neuromuscular disease 441
role of 286

Index 557

Neuromuscular disorders 273*b*, 278*t*, 432
Neuromuscular electric stimulation 524
Neuromuscular imaging 287
Neuromuscular junction 39, 414, 424, 524
   disorder 414
Neuromuscular transmission 427, 428
   disorder 273
Neuromuscular weakness 12, 272, 273, 302
   extent of 420
Neuromyelitis optica *See also* Multiple sclerosis
Neuron 3, 4
   structure of 4*f*
Neuronal ceroid lipofuscinosis 154, 261, 264, 308, 314, 360
   juvenile 267
Neuronal death, clear risk of 476
Neuronal injury 476
Neuronal network, alteration of 476
Neuronopathy 272, 426, 427
Neuron-specific enolase 168
Neuropathic gait 91
Neuropathology laboratory 172
Neuropathy 272, 273, 426
   treatment of 531
Neurophysiologic evaluation 139
Neuropsychiatric manifestations, predominance of 223
Neurotransmitter disorder 446
Neutral position 423
Newer drugs 480
Next generation sequencing 175, 178, 179, 185, 186
NGS *See* Next generation sequencing
Nicotinamide adenine dinucleotide dehydrogenase 174
   stain 173
   tetrazolium reductase 173
Niemann–Pick disease 308
Nipah virus 225, 494
Nitrazepam 470
Nitric oxide 533
Nitrofurantoin 337
NMDA *See* N-methyl d-aspartate
NMES *See* Neuromuscular electric stimulation
N-methyl-D-aspartate 231, 482
   receptor 213
   encephalitis 170
NMJ *See* Neuromuscular junction
NMO *See* Neuromyelitis optica
NO *See* Nitric oxide

Nocturnal frontal lobe epilepsy 142, 202
Nocturnal tonic seizures 204
Nonbiological treatment 530
Noncompressive myelopathy 405, 409*f*
   causes of 405*t*
Nonconvulsive status epilepticus 145, 151, 477
Noninfectious causes 381
Nonmotor onset 198
Nonpolio enterovirus 492
Nonprogressive ataxia *See also* Progressive ataxia
Nonstructural protein 1 496
Nonsyndromic hereditary hearing loss 362
Nonsyndromic monogenic disorder 361
Nontraumatic headache, presence of 340
Noonan syndrome 457
Noradrenaline 4, 188*f*
Norepinephrine 501
Normal bladder function 189
Normal sural nerve sensory response 159*f*
NS1 *See* Nonstructural protein 1
NTEP *See* National Tuberculosis Elimination Program
Nucleotide sequence 185
Nusinersen 532
Nystagmus 70, 316, 318, 450
   central 70, 70*t*
   peripheral 70, 70*t*
   rotational 72

O

OA *See* Organic acidemia
Obesity 454
Obstructive hydrocephalus 347
Obtundation 20, 56
Occipital epilepsy
   early-onset childhood 202
   late-onset childhood 142, 202
Occipital lobe 19
   seizure 200
Occipitofrontal circumference 344, 350
Occupational therapy 526
Ocular blindness 358
Ocular bobbing 37
Ocular dysmetria 37
Ocular flutter 37
Ocular motility 34
Ocular movement 70
   disorders 16

Ocular myoclonus 37
Ocular reflexes 33
Ocular sign 240, 328
Ocular symptoms 358
Ocular telangiectasia 240*f*
Oculocephalic reflex 74, 217
   abnormalities of 219
Oculomotor apraxia 327, 328, 330
   ataxia with 325
Oculomotor nerve 6, 14
ODS *See* Osmotic demyelination syndrome
OFC *See* Occipitofrontal circumference
Ofloxacin 487
Ohtahara syndrome 143, 147*f*, 203
Olesoxime 532
Olfactory bulb 38
Olfactory nerve 6, 64, 101
Oligodendrocyte *See also* Myelin basic protein
Oligohydramnios 518
Olivary nucleus, superior 151*f*
Olivopontocerebellar degeneration 323
Omega-3 fatty acid 530
One and half syndrome 37
ONSD *See* Optic nerve sheath diameter
Open neural tube defects, types of 354*t*
Open spina bifida 353
Ophthalmoplegia 36, 281
   external 36
   internal 36
Opportunistic infections 496
Opsoclonus 37
   myoclonus ataxia syndrome 320, 322
Optic atrophy 32, 67*f*, 360
Optic chiasma 33*f*
   lesion at 33
Optic nerve 6, 14, 32, 64
   lesion 32, 33*f*
   sheath diameter 500
Optic neuritis 220
Optic radiations 33*f*
Optic tract lesion 33
Optical righting reflex 522
Oral corticosteroids 537*t*
Organelle disorders 254, 255
Organic acidemia 226, 270*f*, 309, 506
Organomegaly 345
Oromandibular dystonia 376
Oromotor dyskinesia 376
Ortho methyl dopa 172
Orthodromic conduction 157

Orthopedic ailments, management of 462
Osmotic demyelination syndrome 502
Oto-acoustic-emission 362
Overlapping symptoms 299
OXC *See* Oxcarbazepine
Oxcarbazepine 465, 467, 470, 471, 473
Oxidative stains 174

P

PA *See* Propionic acidemia
PAG *See* Periaqueductal gray matter
Pain
   and temperature, testing 94
   perception of 216
Palmaris longus 158
Palpebral fissure, width of 72
Panayiotopoulos syndrome 144, 202
Pantothenate kinase-associated neurodegeneration 446, 450
Papilledema 67f, 349
   fundoscopic examination for 359
Parachute reflex 42, 43, 43f
Parahippocampal gyrus 38
Paralysis starting, descending 416
Paralytic rabies 492, 495
Paramyotonia congenita 540
Paraplegia 402, 410fc
Parasomnias 206
Paraspinal contractures 279
Parasympathetic innervation 192
Parasympathetic nervous system 39
Parasympathetic system 188
Parent-teacher meetings 314
Parietal lobe 19
   lesion 33
   seizure 200
Parkinson disease, juvenile 446
Parkinsonian gait 92
Parkinsonian movement disorder 303
Parkinsonism 304, 379
Paroxysmal disorders 195
Paroxysmal dyskinesia 206
   exercise-induced 307
Paroxysmal hemicranias 333
Paroxysmal kinesigenic dyskinesia 307
Paroxysmal movement disorder 307, 307t
Paroxysmal nonkinesigenic dyskinesia 307

Paroxysmal tonic upward gaze 206
Paroxysmal torticollis, benign 206, 303
PAS *See* Periodic acid–Schiff
Passive movement 378
Passive tone assessment 102t
Patent foramen ovale 518
Pathogenic polymerase gamma 330
PB *See* Phenobarbitone
PCA *See* Posterior cerebral artery
PCR *See* Polymerase chain reaction
PDE *See* Phosphodiesterase
PDH *See* Pyruvate dehydrogenase
PE *See* Phenytoin equivalent
Pediatric stroke 517t
   diagnosis of 507
   types of 504
Pedunculopontine nucleus 18f
PEG *See* Polyethylene glycol
Pelizaeus–Merzbacher disease 261
   diagnosis of 263f
Pellagra-like rash 327
PEM *See* Protein-energy-malnutrition
Pendular jerk 450
Penicillin, pneumococcus to 485
Pentose phosphate pathway 255
Perianal sensation, loss of 12
Periaqueductal gray matter 189
Periodic acid–Schiff 174, 311
   staining 174
Periodic epileptiform discharges 145
Periodic interictal epileptiform discharges 1550f
Peripheral nerve 6, 12, 155, 278, 414
   pathology 414
Peripheral nervous system 3, 5, 258, 496
   lesion in 113
Peripheral neuropathy 327, 328
   drug-induced 414
   evidence of 329
   infective causes of 491
Peripontine cistern 121
Periventricular chunky calcification 351f
Permanent vision loss *See also* Transient vision loss
Persistent vegetative state 55
Personal social development 50
Pervasive developmental disorder 289
PFA *See* Paroxysmal fast activity
Pharyngo-cervico-brachial variant 414
Phenobarbitone 465, 466, 471, 473, 479
   intravenous 478

Phenomena 126
Phenotype, clinical 143, 203, 261
Phenylephrine 501
Phenylketonuria 255, 292, 350, 528
Phenytoin 234, 319, 337, 465, 466, 470, 471, 473, 479, 540
   equivalent 479
Phonophobia 334
Phoria *See also* Latent squint
Phosphodiesterase 533
Photic stimulation 139, 146
Photophobia 334
PHT *See* Phenytoin
Physical examination 405
Physiological basis 499
Physiotherapy, principles of 522
Phytanic acid 330
PICA *See* Posterior inferior cerebellar artery
Pin-hole test 358
Pinpoint pupil 221
PIP *See* Proximal interphalangeal
Pituitary gland, tumors of 33
PKAN *See* Pantothenate kinase-associated neurodegeneration
PKU *See* Phenylketonuria
PL *See* Palmaris longus
Planning test 178
Plantar reflex 10
Plantar response 90f, 102
   methods of 90f
Plasma
   amino acid 321
   exchange therapy 539
PMC *See* Pontine micturition center
PMD *See* Pelizaeus-Merzbacher disease
PME *See* Progressive myoclonic epilepsy
Pneumococcus 168
PNPO *See* Pyridoxine 5'-phosphate oxidase
PNS *See* Peripheral nervous system
Point-of-care ultrasonography 500
POLG *See* Pathogenic polymerase gamma
Poliomyelitis 421, 496
   acute 414, 415
Polyethylene glycol 526
Polyhydramnios 274
Polymerase chain reaction 178, 185, 351, 363, 390, 493, 496
Polymerase gamma 482
Polymyositis 492
Polyneuropathy 6
   distal symmetrical 491

Index 559

Polyradiculoneuropathy 418, 420, 491
Polyradiculopathy 117
Polytherapy, avoid 472
Pompe disease *See also* Metabolic myopathy
Pompe myopathy 431
Pons 7
  communicates signals 13
Pontine micturition center 189
Popliteal angle 102
Port-wine stain 239*f*
Postconcussion 318
Postdiphtheritic paralysis 416
Postdiphtheritic polyneuropathy 415, 491
Posterior column sensation 92, 92*t*, 328
Posterior reversible leukoencephalopathy syndrome 399
Postganglionic lesion 159*f*
Postganglionic parasympathetic 39
Postganglionic sympathetic neurons 39
Postictal aphasia 200
Postictal nose wiping 200
Postinfectious encephalitis 495
Postnatal history 456
Postsynaptic acetylcholine receptor 538
Posture 102*f*, 428
  abnormal 443, 500
  and gait 377, 405
  and tone 101
  fine control of 316
Power examination 78
PPN *See* Pedunculopontine nucleus
PPP *See* Pentose phosphate pathway
Prader-Willi syndrome 179, 181, 244
Prechtl neonatal behavioral scale 100, 100*t*
Prednisolone 536
Predominant extrapyramidal syndrome 267*t*
Predominant sensory symptoms 418
Preganglionic lesion 159*f*
Preimplantation genetic diagnosis 287
Prematurity 234
Preoptic nucleus 39
Presenting illness 416
Preterm infants 345
Primitive reflex 102
  assessment of 41
  persistence of 375

Procainamide 540
Progressive ataxia 323, 323*b*
  metabolic causes of 328
Progressive ataxia *See also* Nonprogressive ataxia
Progressive disorders 240
Progressive dystonia, differential diagnosis of 267*t*
Prolactin, secrete releasing hormone for 39
Prolonged fever, presence of 133
PROM *See* Premature rupture of membranes
Prominent scapular winging 285
Prophylactic antiepileptic drugs 501
Propionic acidemia 269*f*
Propionic aciduria 229
Propranolol 342
Proprioception, testing 92
Prosopognosia 65
Protein 173
  C deficiency 506
  C resistance, activated 506
  energy malnutrition 431
  intrathecal synthesis of 167
  nonfunctional 532
Proximal shoulder 428
  girdle weakness 281
Proximal upper limb 107
  weakness 276, 426
PS *See* Photic stimulation
Pseudoathetosis 93*f*
Pseudomonas 485, 492
Pseudoregression 112
Pseudotumor cerebri 359
Psychiatric manifestation, onset of 229
Psychogenic paroxysmal nonepileptic events 206
Psychomotor activity 62
Pterygoid 70
  muscles, lateral 70, 75
Ptosis 35, 69, 220, 275, 276, 281, 417
  evidence of 282
Pubertal development 537
Puberty, delayed 454
Pudendal nerve stopped firing 189
Pupil 35, 67
  abnormalities of 34, 35*t*
  unequal 499
Pupillary abnormality 35
Pupillary light reflex pathway 34*f*
Pupillary reaction 69
Pupillary reflex, assessment of 220
Pupillary size, assessment of 220
Pure cerebellar signs, clinical phenotype of 328
Pure sensory ataxic variant 414

Purine metabolism, disorder of 292
Pyogenic meningitis
  cases of 485
  treated 168
Pyomyositis 492
Pyramidal lesion 91
Pyramidal tract 116, 129, 445
Pyrazinamide 487
Pyridostigmine 538
Pyridoxine *See also* Vitamin B_6
Pyridoxine 5'-phosphate oxidase deficiency 269*f*
Pyruvate 321
  dehydrogenase 324
    deficiency 258, 270*f*, 323

Q

QT syndrome 206
Quadriparesis 117
Quadriplegia 371
Quadriplegic cerebral palsy 248
Quinine 540

R

Rabies 415, 495
Radicular pain 12
Radiodigital grasp 45
Radiological phenotype 261
Ragged red fiber 327, 450
Raised intracranial pressure 108, 332, 344, 358, 452, 456, 490, 500*f*, 501-503
  sedation for 501
Ramsay–Hunt syndrome 323
Ramus
  anterior 8
  posterior 8
RAN binding protein 2 496
RANBP2 *See* RAN binding protein 2
Range of motion 80
Rapid plasma regain 493
Rapid-sequence intubation 501
Rash, presence of 216
Rassmussen syndrome 205
Reaction, righting 522
Reading skills, testing 63*f*
Recalcitrant intracranial hypertension 503
Recent memory 59
  testing 59
Recording electrodes 156
Rectal diazepam 478
Recurrent artery of Huebner 27
Recurrent ataxia, causes of
  acute 318*b*

Index

Reflex
  abdominal 10, 90*f*
  neonatal 521
  propping 43, 43*f*
  released 63, 64*f*
  suck 64
  superficial 88, 90*f*, 410
Refractory status epilepticus 479, 482*f*
  etiology of 482*t*
Refsum disease 268, 323, 327, 329, 330
Regimen 536
Rehabilitation, components of 522
Rehydration, intravenous 525
Relative afferent pupillary defect 68*f*, 220
Relevant systemic examination 440
Repetitive speech *See also* Stereotyped speech
Respiration
  regular 100
  type of 221, 221*t*
Respiratory depression, risk of 479
Respiratory failure 279, 281
Respiratory function 216
Respiratory muscle weakness 427
Respiratory pattern
  abnormal 499, 500
  assessment of 221
Respiratory rate 221
Restless behavior 444
Resultant injuries 315
Retigabine 465, 468
Retinal degeneration 268
Retinal vascular disorder 357
Retinal vein occlusion 357
Retinitis pigmentosa 327
Retinoblastoma 360
Rett syndrome 289
Reverse transcription-polymerase chain reaction 496
Reversible encephalopathy syndrome 216
Rheumatic heart disease, underlying 313
Rhomberg sign 72, 73*f*, 93*f*, 96*f*
Ribcage abnormality 345
Rifampicin, combination of 492
Right centrotemporal epileptiform discharges 149*f*
Right common peroneal nerve injury 12
Right eye 36
  abduction of 37
Right genioglossus turns tongue 75
Right hemiplegic posture, description of 250*f*
Right hemispheric lesion 150*f*
Righting reflexes, assessment of 43
Rigidity 77, 378, 378*t*
Riluzole 532
Rinne's test 72
Risdiplam 532
Risperidone 528
Rituximab 539
Rizatriptan 342
Rolandic epilepsy 144, 470
Rolandic seizures 151
RoM *See* Range of motion
Romberg sign 316, 317
  positive 12
Rotavirus 225
RPR *See* Rapid plasma regain
RR *See* Righting reaction
RT-PCR *See* Reverse transcription-polymerase chain reaction
Rubinstein–Taybi syndrome 236
Rufinamide 465, 468, 470, 473
Ryanodine receptor 280

S

Saccades, slow 327
Saccadic movements, testing 69*f*
Sagittal sinus
  joins 128
  thrombosis 511*ff*
Saliva
  drooling of 376
  management of drooling of 525
Salmonella 485, 492
Sample headache diary 336*f*
Sandifer syndrome 205, 303
Sanger sequencing 178, 179, 185
Sarcoglycan 173
Sarcoglycanopathy 285, 286, 288, 441
SCA *See* Spinocerebellar ataxia
Scalp 139
Scapular winging 82, 438*f*
  testing 83*f*
Scapuloperoneal dystrophy 275
Scapuloperoneal weakness 275
Scarf sign 102, 378
Schirmer test 72
Schwann cells 5
Schwartz–Jampel syndrome 277
Sclerosing panencephalitis, subacute 150*f*, 168, 171, 254, 306, 495
Scoliosis 521
  monitoring 537
SCQ *See* Social communication questionnaire
SD *See* Standard deviation
SDH *See* Succinate dehydrogenase
SE *See* Status epilepticus
Sea blue histiocytes 330
Seizure 104, 138, 195-197, 204, 206, 213, 214, 222, 231, 248, 444, 469, 489
  activity, continuous 476
  acute 468
  atypical absence 204, 468
  benign neonatal 142, 202
  classification 197*fc*, 209
  clonic 199
  etiology of 208
  first unprovoked 468
  focal 196
  frontal lobe 199
  generalized 196
  investigations for 209
  management of 476, 517
  migrating partial 143
  neonatal 112, 369
  partial 197
  refractory 485
  semiology 199, 200, 200*t*
  simple febrile 207, 208
  simple partial 198
  types of 144, 196, 198, 198*t*, 200, 207, 208, 210
  unprovoked 206
Selective dorsal rhizotomy 524
Selective motor control 521
Selective serotonin reuptake inhibitor 528, 529
Sensation
  loss of 16
  move 157
Sensorium 216, 420
  assessment of 216
  states of altered 100*fc*
  worsening of 500
Sensory 420, 444
  and motor nerve conduction 329
  ataxia 316, 317
  ataxic gait 91
  component 70
  deficit 234
  dermatomal levels 11*f*
  dermatome 10, 10*t*
  disturbances 291
  examination 103, 111
  fibers 190
  function 108
  function disorders 234
  ganglion 6

Index 561

inattention 65
motor weakness 491
pelvic nerve 189
Sensory loss
    areflexia with 285
    patterns of 95*f*
Sensory nerve
    action potential 155, 159*f*, 162, 421
    conduction study 157, 159*f*
Sensory system 398, 440
    examination 54, 92, 109, 379, 420, 430
    involvement 113, 427
Serum
    cholesterol 329
    creatine phosphokinase level 286
    glutamic pyruvic transaminase 223
    phytanic acid 329
    vitamin
        D 537
        E 269
Sex chromosomes 180
Shawl sign 539
Short tau inversion recovery 125
Shoulder
    abduction 81, 82*f*
        across chest 82, 82*f*
        muscle power 81
    adduction 82, 82*f*
        muscle power 80
Shoulder-girdle weakness 435
Shuddering spells 205, 303
Shunt
    failure 349, 455
    infection 349, 349*f*, 455, 455*f*
    malfunction 349*f*, 455*f*
    ventriculoperitoneal 488
Sialidosis 264
Sigmoid sinus 128
Signal intensity 124
Single nucleotide polymorphism 181, 182*f*, 184*f*, 185
Single-gene disorders 177, 178
Sinus, superior sagittal 31
Sjögren-Larsson syndrome 260
Skeletal abnormality 345
Skeletal deformities 281
Skeletal muscle 39
Skill 527
    biopsy 176
    training, method of 527, 527*t*
Skull 109, 121
    examination of 98, 379
    shape 351
    sutures of 100*f*

SLE *See* Systemic lupus erythematosus
Sleep 208
    and behavioral problems, management of 526
    benign epileptiform transients of 141
    considering excessive movement artifacts 140
    disturbances 234, 291
    electrical status epilepticus of 295
    electroencephalography, normal 144*f*
    relation to 305
    slow 140
    spindles 139
    wave during 143, 203
Sleep-wake cycle 55, 214, 216
Slit ventricle syndrome 349, 349*t*, 455, 455*t*
Small reactive pupil, unilateral 220
Small reddish spots 215
Smith-Lemli-Opitz syndrome 292, 351
SMN1 gene 531
SMN2 gene 531
Smoke appearance, puff of 134*f*
Smooth muscle, dystrophin expression in 176
SNAP *See* Sensory nerve action potential
SNC *See* Substantia nigra pars compacta
Snout reflex 64
SNP *See* Single nucleotide polymorphism
SNR *See* Substantia nigra pars reticulata
Social communication
    disorder 295
    questionnaire 290, 294
Social interaction 208
Social milestones 50
Sodium
    channel 469
    channelopathy 277
    valproate 465, 470, 473, 479
Soft palate 22
Soft tissue 121
    image 122*f*
SOL *See* Space-occupying lesion
Somatosensory-evoked potential 154, 155
Somnolence 20
Space-occupying lesion 399
Spastic diplegia 131, 249*f*, 375
    mimics of 252*t*

Spastic diplegic cerebral palsy 368
Spastic dysarthria 22, 444
Spastic paraparesis 12
Spastic quadriplegic cerebral palsy 368
Spastic weakness 106
Spasticity 77, 116, 246, 257, 276, 316, 378, 378*t*
    combination of 308
    management of 523
    presence of 116
Special senses 32
Spectrum disorder 289
Speech 22, 370, 375, 396, 444, 445
    assessment of 62
    description of 22, 370
    difficulty in 449
    disturbance in 63*fc*
    expressive motor component of 20
Sphincter 188, 190*f*
Spina bifida occulta 354, 355
Spinal accessory nerve 6, 14, 74
Spinal artery, anterior 14*f*
Spinal cord 7, 10, 12, 113, 422
    ascending tracts of 9*t*
    cross-section of 8*f*
    descending tracts of 9*t*
    hemisection of 11
    lesion 191, 414
    level 10
    malformations 356*f*
    segments of 6*f*
    structure 8*f*
    tracts of 9*f*
Spinal dermatome 10
Spinal muscular atrophy 114, 114*t*, 177, 181, 183*f*, 424, 431, 441, 531
    type 2 282
    type 3 284
Spinal nerve 8, 9*t*
Spinal segment 9
Spine examination 98, 99, 109, 379
    testing 99*f*
Spinocerebellar ataxia 179, 326, 326*t*, 330, 446
    types of 326
Spinocerebellar atrophy 327
    type of 330
Spinocerebellar tract 9
Spino-olivary tract 9
Spinothalamic tract carrying sensation 8
Squint 35
    concomitant 36
    latent 35
    paralytic 36

SR *See* Superficial reflex
SSPE *See* Subacute sclerosing panencephalitis
SSRI *See* Selective serotonin reuptake inhibitor
Staphylococcus aureus 485, 490, 492
Static illness 113
Static weakness 276
Station, abnormalities of 91*t*
Status dystonicus, management of 525
Status epilepticus 147, 476, 477
   classification of 476
   management of 476, 478, 479*t*, 483*fc*
   mechanisms for super-refractory 481
   severity scoring 483, 484*t*
   super-refractory 481
   taxonomical classification of 477*t*
   therapy of 479*t*
   treatment of 478*t*
Stem cell transplantation 535
Stereognosis 95
Stereotactic aspiration 491
Stereotyped motor movement 293
Stereotyped speech 293
Sternocleidomastoid muscle 74
Steroid 488, 518, 536
   sparing agents 539
STESS *See* Status epilepticus severity scoring
Stiffness 443
Stimulation, distal 158
Stimuli, painful 217
STIR *See* Short tau inversion recovery
Stiripentol 465, 468, 470
STN *See* Subthalamic nucleus
Storage disorders 309
Strabismus 35
Streptococcus 490
   infection 492
   pneumoniae 485
Streptomycin 358
Stroke 21, 504, 504*t*, 506
   acute 512, 516*t*, 517*t*
   brain protocol for 508*b*
   etiology of 505
   mimics 505
   neuroimaging in 507
   perinatal 518
   posterior circulation 319
   treatment of acute 512
Stupor 20, 56
Sturge-Weber syndrome 120, 204, 238, 239*f*

Subarachnoid space 7, 122
   benign enlargement of 344, 452
Subcortical cyst 261, 262*f*
Subcutaneous fat pads 239*f*
Subdural effusion, chronic 453
Subdural window 121
Substantia nigra pars
   compacta 18*f*
   reticulata 17*f*, 18*f*
Subthalamic nucleus 17*f*, 18*f*
Subtle hemiplegia, testing 97*f*
Subtraction 61
Succinate dehydrogenase 173, 174
Succinic semialdehyde dehydrogenase 292
Sudden jerks, multiple episodes of 199
Sulfamethoxazole 490
Sun-setting sign 346, 347*f*
Supportive care 423, 512, 537
Suppurative otitis media, chronic 213, 215
Suprasellar aneurysm 33
Supratentorial tumors 323
Susceptibility-weighted image 125
Sutures, overriding of 235*f*
Sweat gland 39
Sweating, lack of 113
Symmetric tonic neck reflex 42
Sympathetic nervous system, activation of 39
Synapse 4
Synaptic damage, marker of 170
Syncope 206
Syndromic epilepsy diagnosis 208
Syndromic megalencephaly 452
Syndromic microcephaly 351
Syphilis, congenital 493
Systemic lupus erythematosus 308, 381

T

Tachypnea 429
Tacrolimus 539
Tactile sensation, testing 94, 94*f*
Taenia solium 167, 489
Tandem walk 90
Tay-Sachs disease 257, 258
TBM *See* Tubercular meningitis
Tegmentum pontis 129
Telangiectasia 259, 327
Temporal lobe 19
   seizures 200
Tendon 156
TENS *See* Transcutaneous electric nerve stimulation
Tetrabenazine 524, 525

Tetracycline 337
Thalamic syndromes 16
Thalamostriate vein 30
Thalamus 16, 29
   anterior 38*fc*
   ventrolateral nucleus of 18*f*
Therapeutic dilemmas, common 463
Therapeutic drug monitoring 474
Third ventricle, distention of 33
Thomsen and Becker disease 277
Thrombolysis 514
Thrombolytic agents, role of 514
Thrombosed sinus 125
Thumb
   abduction of 84
   extension of 84
   movement at 84
Thyroid stimulating hormone 39
TIA *See* Transient ischemic attack
Tibial nerve 157
   tested 160*f*
Tibial torsion 521
Tibialis anterior 288
Tick paralysis 414, 415
Tics 303, 379
Tissue 118
   diagnosis 166
   plasminogen activator 514
Tizanidine 349, 524
TLC *See* Total leukocyte count
TM *See* Transverse myelitis
Tone
   abnormalities 302, 367
   assessment 302, 377, 429
      interpretation 77*fc*
   modified Ashworth grading of 378*t*
   testing 77*f*
Tongue 22
   fasciculation, presence of 279
   movement of 75
   muscle weakness 276
   thrusting movement 376
Tonic seizures 468
Tonic-clonic seizure
   focal to bilateral 198
   generalized 142, 143, 203
Topiramate 342, 465, 467, 470, 471, 473
TORCH infection *See Toxoplasma gondii*, other agents, rubella, cytomegalovirus, and herpes simplex virus infection
Torticollis
   combination of 303
   paroxysmal episodes of 303

Index

Total creatine phosphokinase 432
Total leukocyte count 170
Toxoplasma gondii 360
  other agents, rubella, cytomegalovirus, and herpes simplex virus infection 234, 361, 370
TPM *See* Topiramate
Trail making test 61*f*
Transcortical motor aphasia 20
Transcortical sensory aphasia 20
Transcutaneous electric nerve stimulation 524
Transient ischemic attack 518
Transient visual obscuration 337
Transudate-like albumin 170
Transverse myelitis, acute 414, 415, 491
Transverse sinus
  bilateral 511*f*
  continues 30
  thrombosis 511*f*
Trapezius muscle 74
Trapezoid body 32
Trauma, signs of 216
Tremors 303, 305, 327, 379
Treponema 492
Trichinella spiralis 492
Triclofos 140
Trigeminal autonomic cephalgia 332
Trigeminal nerve 6, 14, 70
  sensory component of 71*f*
Trigeminal neuralgia 337
Trihexyphenidyl 524, 525
Trimethoprim 490
Triple repeat disorders 179
Triptans 342
Trisomy 13 180
Trivial febrile illness 281
Trochlear nerve 6, 14
Trophy sign, calf heads on 439*f*
Tropia 35
Truncal ataxia 276, 317
Truncal weakness 276, 426, 435
TUBBA4 mutation 176
Tubercular bacilli 487
  isolation of 487
Tubercular meningitis 170, 381, 390*t*, 487, 488*b*
  complications of 488
  diagnosis of 224*f*
  management of 488
Tubercular vasculitis 488
Tuberculoma 122, 209, 489, 489*t*, 490
  brain suggestive of 133*f*
Tuberculosis 506

Tuberous sclerosis 120, 238, 238*f*, 239*f*, 292
Tumbling E chart 66*f*
Tumor necrosis factor 487
Turner syndrome 177, 180
Turning head 43
Twisting 443

U

UCD *See* Urea cycle disorder
UL *See* Upper limb
Ullrich
  muscular dystrophy 427
  variant 437
UMN *See* Upper motor neuron
Unverricht-Lundborg disease 264, 314
Upper arm muscles 83
Upper limb 92, 158*t*, 111, 248, 377, 416
  and trunk: 279
  weakness 276
Upper motor neuron 4*f*, 316, 409, 409*f*, 410
  lesion 26, 26*t*, 62
Upper quadrantanopic hemianopia 33
Urea cycle disorders 226, 254, 270*f*
Uremic encephalopathy 213
Urinary bladder 188, 418, 420
  neural control of 188
Urinary continence, loss of 444
Urinary gas chromatography 351
Urinary tract infection 246*f*, 368
Urine
  amino acid 321, 329
  formation 188
  passage of 190
  retention of 190*f*
  storage 190*f*
  reflex 189

V

Vagus nerve 6, 14
Valgus deformity 521
Valley sign 76*f*, 438, 439*f*
Valparin 234
Valproate 465, 468
  acid 471
Valproic acid 466
Vancomycin 490
Vanillylmandelic acid 320
Varicella-zoster
  infection 487
  virus 486, 492
Vascular etiology 308

Vascular lesion 145
Vascular malformation
  absence of 347
  detection of 125
Vascular origin 504
Vascular stroke 506
  acute 504
  distribution of 509
  etiology for 504
Vasogenic edema 498
Vasopressors 501
VDRL *See* Venereal disease research laboratory
Vector-mediated gene therapy 534
Vein of Galen 30, 128
Venereal disease research laboratory 493
Venography, role of 231
Venous circulation 31
Venous sinus 120*f*
  thrombosis 30, 215
  diagnose 128
Venous system, superficial 29
Venous thrombosis 125, 504
Ventral suspension 102
  face down 42
Ventral tegmentum 16
Ventricles, enlargement of 31
Ventricular hypertrophy 329
Ventrolateral thalamus 129
Verbal pain unresponsiveness 217
Verbal response 56, 217
Verbal stimulation 57, 217
Vermal aplasia 323
Vertebrobasilar artery injury 319
Vertebrobasilar occlusion 318
Vertex 152
Vertigo 316
  benign paroxysmal 318
  tinnitus 70
Very long-chain fatty acid 329
Very low-density lipoprotein 329
Vestibular-ocular reflex 217
Vestibulocochlear nerve 6, 14
VGB *See* Vigabatrin
VGKC *See* Voltage-gated potassium channel
Vibration
  sensation, testing 94
  sense 316
Vigabatrin 465, 467, 471, 473
Vineland social maturity scale 527
Violent flinging movements 315
Viral encephalitis 106
  acute 487*t*
Viral infection 492, 494, 494*t*, 495, 496

Viral meningitis 170
Viral myositis 12, 414, 415
Virus 496
Vision 267t, 444
   assessment 51, 101
   comprehensive assessment of 301
   testing field of 66f
Vision loss 106, 108, 357, 359fc
   acute 357, 359fc
   binocular 358
   causes of chronic 360fc
   chronic 360
   fluctuation in 358
   neurological cause of 358
   onset of 357
   transient 358
   traumatic acute 357fc
Visual acuity 64
   assessment of 358
Visual assessment milestones 51f
Visual cortex, region of 358
Visual field defects 33f
Visual fixation 70
Visual impairment 360
Visual pathway 32
Visual-evoked potential scan 153, 251
Vital sign 215, 373, 386, 395, 405, 428
   description 374
Vitamin
   A 337, 530
   B_{12} deficiency 11, 12
   B_6 530
   C 530
   D deficiency 337
      signs of 278
   deficiency 374

E

   deficiency 268, 324, 326, 327, 330
   level 329
   supplementation 327
Voice, altered 416
Voltage-gated potassium channel 213
Voluntary motor activity, modulators of 26
Voluntary movement, impaired performance of 302
Vomiting 214
von Hippel-Lindau disease *See also* Cerebellar hemangioblastoma
Voriconazole 490
VPA *See* Valproic acid
VSMS *See* Vineland social maturity scale
VWM *See* Vanishing white matter

W

Walker-Warburg syndrome 457
Warfarin 234, 514
Waveform, morphology of 477
Weakness 7, 12, 26, 106, 246, 285, 316
   description of 403
   distal 285
   extent of 393, 426, 435
   onset of 393
   pattern of 274, 275, 408f, 417, 433
   progression of 393, 420
   symmetry of 417
   worsening of 427
Weber syndrome 15
Weber test 72
Weight loss, presence of 109

West syndrome 143, 151, 203, 470
West-Nile virus 225, 493
White cerebellar sign 224, 510, 514f, 519f
White-matter 120f, 125, 258, 456
   abnormality 260
      types of 260t
   degenerative brain disease 308
   degenerative disease 445
   disease, vanishing 261
   junction 489
   periventricular 260
   subcortical 260
Whole-exome sequencing 185
Whole-genome sequencing 185
William syndrome 181, 236, 237f, 298, 351
Wilson disease 267, 268f, 309, 323, 446, 450
Wobbly gait 106, 107
Worst seizure type 484
Wrist
   extension 83, 84f
   flexion 83, 84f

X

X chromosome 177, 180
   structural defects 177
X-inactivation 177
X-linked inheritance 323, 437

Z

Ziehl-Neelsen stain 168, 169f, 487
Zigzag figure 334
Zika virus 494
ZNS *See* Zonisamide
Zolgensma 532
Zonisamide 465, 467, 470, 471, 473
ZSM *See* Zonisamide